Lippincott's Illustrated Reviews: Biochemistry

Lippincott's Illustrated Reviews: Biochemistry

Pamela C. Champe, Ph.D.
Department of Biochemistry
University of Medicine and Dentistry of New Jersey—
Robert Wood Johnson Medical School
Piscataway, New Jersey

Richard A. Harvey, Ph.D.
Department of Biochemistry
University of Medicine and Dentistry of New Jersey—
Robert Wood Johnson Medical School
Piscataway, New Jersey

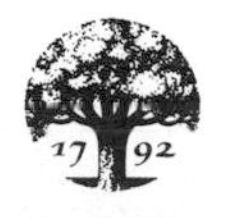

J. B. LIPPINCOTT COMPANY
Philadelphia
London · New York · São Paulo
Mexico City · St. Louis · Sydney

Acquisitions Editor: David Barnes
Sponsoring Editor: Sanford Robinson
Manuscript Editor: Leslie E. Hoeltzel
Art Director: Tracy Baldwin
Production Manager: Kathleen P. Dunn
Production Coordinator: Larry Bryant
Compositor: Ruttle, Shaw & Wetherill, Inc.
Printer/Binder: Malloy Lithographing

 Printed in the United States of America. For information write J. B. Lippincott Company, East Washington Square, Philadelphia, Pennsylvania 19105.

8 9 10 11 12 13 14

Library of Congress Cataloging-in-Publication Data

Champe, Pamela C.
Biochemistry

(Lippincott's illustrated reviews)
Includes index.
1. Biological chemistry—Outlines, syllabi, etc.
2. Biological chemistry—Examinations, questions, etc.
I. Harvey, Richard A. II. Title. III. Series.
[DNLM: 1. Biochemistry—outlines. QU 18 C451b]
QP518.3.C48 574.19'2'0202 87-2919
ISBN 0-397-50801-8

The authors and publisher have exerted every effort to ensure that drug selection and dosage set forth in this text are in accord with current recommendations and practice at the time of publication. However, in view of ongoing research, changes in government regulations, and the constant flow of information relating to drug therapy and drug reactions, the reader is urged to check the package insert for each drug for any change in indications and dosage and for added warnings and precautions. This is particularly important when the recommended agent is a new or infrequently employed drug.

Dedicated to Marilyn and Sewell . . .

for the many reasons
known only to them

Preface

Who will find this book useful

Lippincott's Illustrated Reviews: Biochemistry integrates and summarizes the essentials of medical biochemistry for [1] students in the health-related professions who are preparing for licensure examinations (*e.g.,* National Board Examination Part I, FLEX, ECFMG, FMGEM) and [2] professionals who wish to review or update their knowledge in this rapidly expanding area of biomedical science. Its purpose is to use a high-information-density outline format, summary figures, and practice questions to teach this complex material.

How to use this book

TEXT *Illustrated Reviews* uses a unique expanded outline format that allows you to review and absorb facts and concepts rapidly. The current knowledge in the field of medical biochemistry has been "predigested" and the relevant information recast in a hierarchical organization. Important facts and concepts are shown in bold print, whereas enzymes are featured in a light typeface. This organization permits you to rapidly understand and remember the significant relationships among facts and concepts.

ILLUSTRATIONS *Lippincott's Illustrated Reviews* contains more than 400 original illustrations, each carefully crafted to complement and amplify the text. Abstract concepts have been visualized and inscrutable tables replaced with understandable figures. For example, the concept of Recommended Dietary Allowances takes on new life as a graphic (p. 298) in which you can instantly see the 10-million-fold difference in the body's need for protein (a macronutrient) compared to the requirement for vitamin B_{12} (a micronutrient).

TEXT AND ILLUSTRATIONS *Illustrated Reviews* features a new kind of diagram in which biochemical processes are illustrated with a blend of graphics and summary comments. This marriage of text and art allows you to integrate a body of knowledge without the distraction of constantly shifting from text to illustrations. For example, to sort out the intricacies of amino acid metabolism in an ordinary textbook would require repeated skipping from text to figures. By contrast, *Illustrated Reviews* reveals the major pathways and their connections at a glance. This illustration (p. 250) highlights the important enzyme-deficiency diseases and shows the significant nitrogen-containing products derived from amino acids—all on one integrative figure.

QUESTIONS AND ANSWERS Practice questions of the type used by the National Boards of Medical Examiners are liberally interspersed throughout the text so that you can check your progress in mastering the material. Answers with explanations are provided so that you know both the correct answer and why the distractors are incorrect. Further, these explained answers are contained in a special section at the end of the book, next to the original questions. Thus you can confirm the correct answer to a study question without the disorientation of turning from page to page.

FINDING INFORMATION *Lippincott's Illustrated Reviews* provides an extensive network of more than 300 cross-references. Thus, when you encounter a new block of information, you are immediately directed by page citations to related sections, which reinforces and expands the original material. This elaborate matrix of references provides a cross-fertilization that increases learning and retention, allowing you to end up with the "big picture." Further, an extensive index of more than 2000 citations lets you instantly pinpoint the answer to specific questions.

Acknowledgments

We wish to thank the following artists for their patience and skill in preparing the art for this book: Jo Gershman, art director; Robert Glessman, senior artist; Charles Venancio, Thomas Churac, and Andrea Martin, contributing artists. We gratefully acknowledge the many helpful comments of our colleagues in the Department of Biochemistry at the Rutgers Medical School. The editors and production staff of the J. B. Lippincott Company were a constant source of encouragement and discipline.

Brief Contents

Expanded Table of Contents

UNIT I: Protein Structure and Function

UNIT II: Carbohydrate Metabolism

UNIT IV: Lipid Metabolism

UNIT V: Nitrogen Metabolism

UNIT I: Protein Structure and Function

Structure of Amino Acids

1

I. OVERVIEW

Proteins are the most abundant and functionally diverse molecules in living systems. Virtually every life process depends on this class of molecules. For example, enzymes and polypeptide hormones direct and regulate metabolism in the body, whereas contractile proteins in muscle permit movement. In bone, the protein collagen forms a framework for the deposition of calcium phosphate crystals, acting like the steel cables in reinforced concrete. In the bloodstream, proteins such as hemoglobin and serum albumin shuttle molecules essential to life, whereas immunoglobulins destroy infectious bacteria and viruses. In short, proteins display an incredible diversity of functions, yet all share the common structural feature of being linear polymers of amino acids. This chapter describes the properties of amino acids; Chapter 2 explores how these simple building blocks are joined to form proteins that have unique three-dimensional structures, making them capable of performing specific biological functions.

II. STRUCTURE OF AMINO ACIDS

Although more than 100 different amino acids have been described in nature, only 20 of these species are commonly found as constituents of mammalian proteins. Each amino acid (except for proline) has a carboxyl group, an amino group, and a distinctive side chain ("R-group") bonded to the α-carbon (Figure 1.1). At physiologic pH (approximately 7.4) the carboxyl group is dissociated to form the negatively charged carboxylate ion ($—COO^-$), and the amino group is protonated ($—NH_3^+$). In proteins these carboxyl and amino groups are combined in peptide linkage and are not available for chemical reaction (except for hydrogen bonds as described on p. 17). Thus, it is the nature of the side chains that ultimately dictates the role an amino acid will play in a protein. It is therefore useful to classify the amino acids according to the polarity of their side chains, that is, whether they are nonpolar, uncharged polar, acidic, or basic (Figure 1.2).

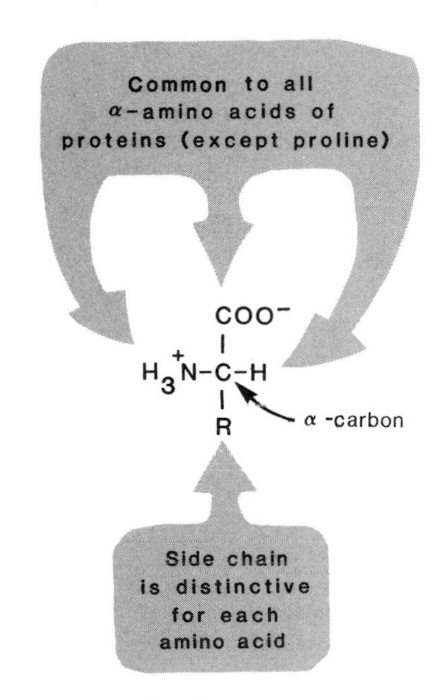

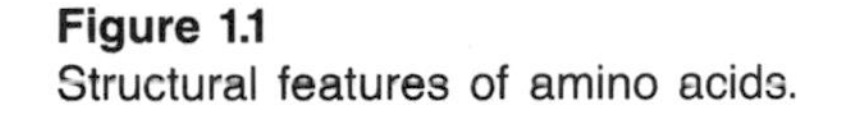

Figure 1.1
Structural features of amino acids.

A. Amino acids with nonpolar side chains

Glycine	=	Gly	Alanine	=	Ala
Valine	=	Val	Leucine	=	Leu

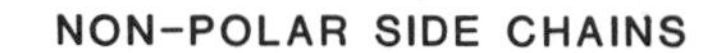

NON-POLAR SIDE CHAINS

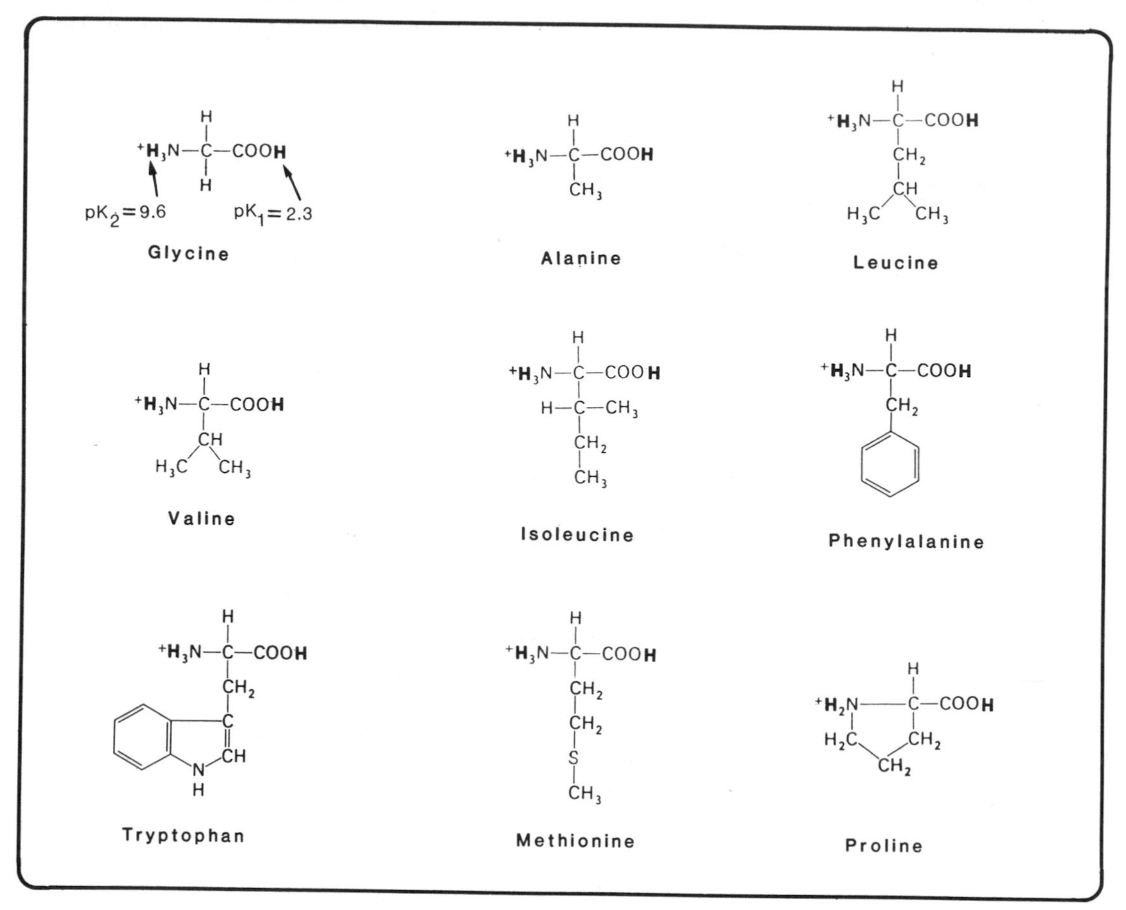

UNCHARGED POLAR SIDE CHAINS

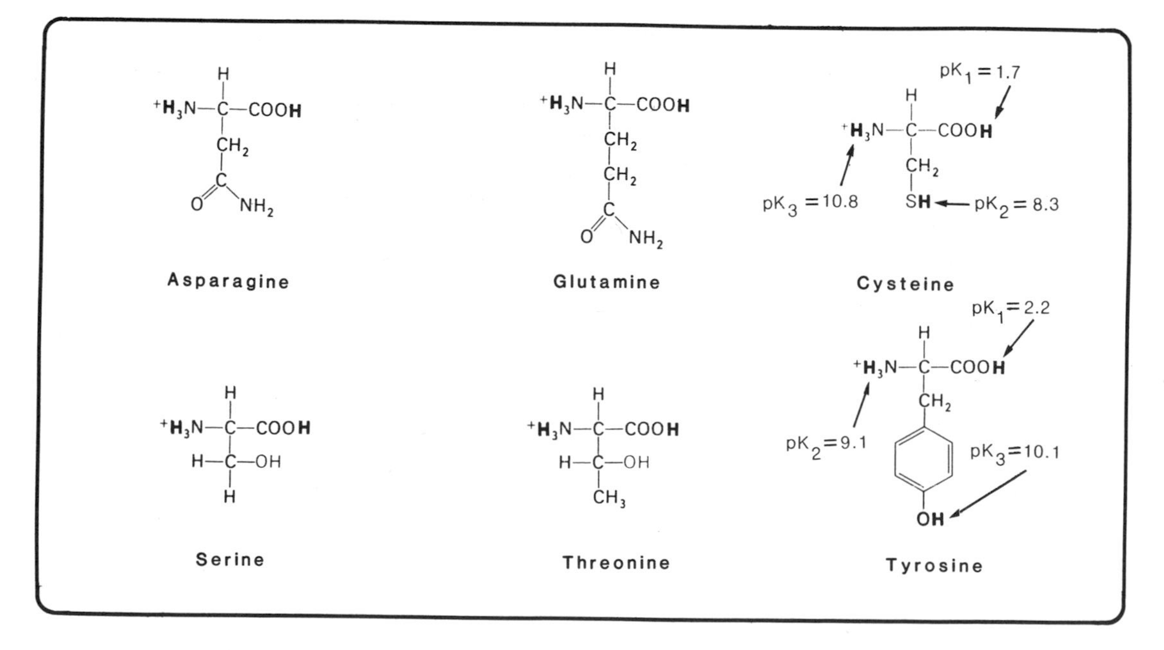

ACIDIC SIDE CHAINS

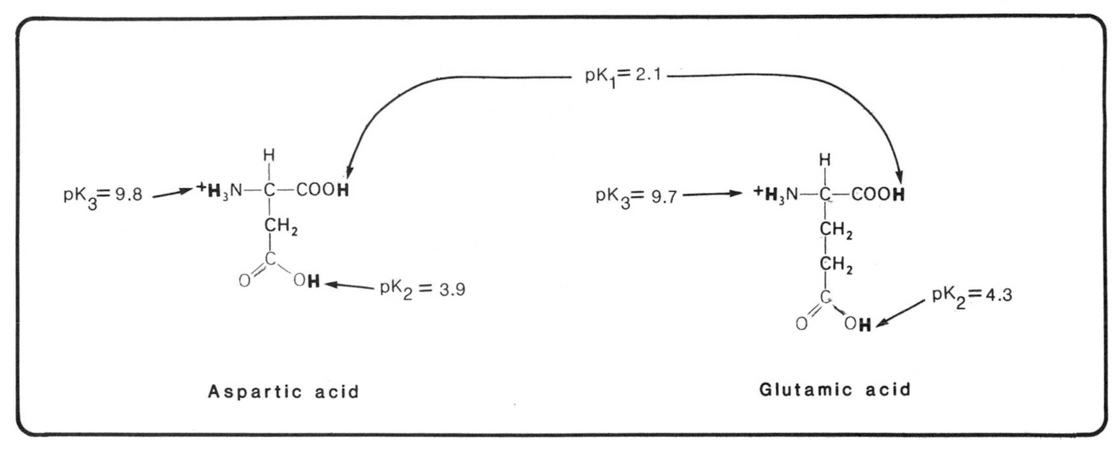

BASIC SIDE CHAINS

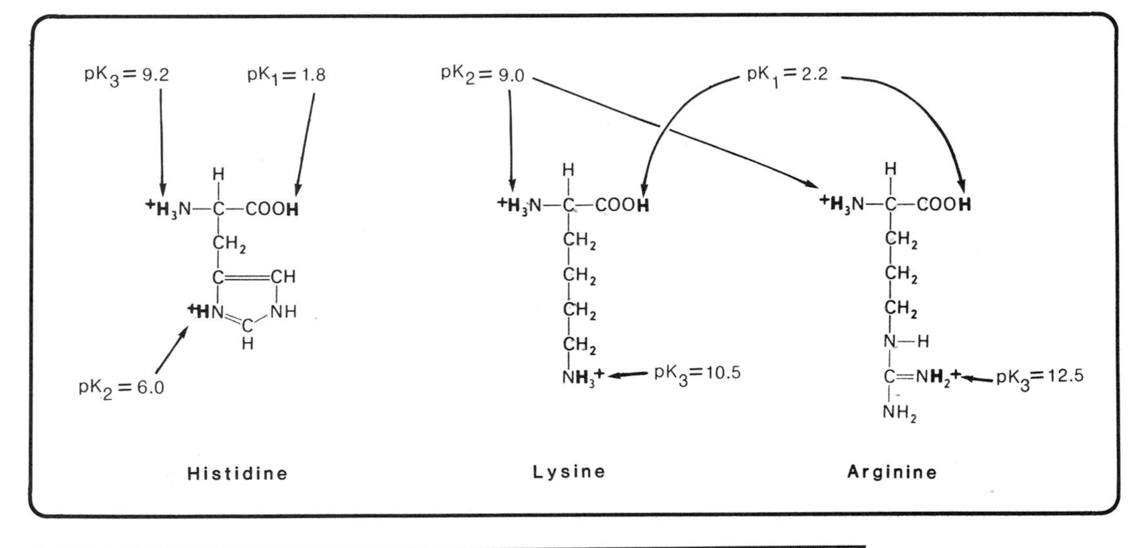

Figure 1.2
Classification of the 20 amino acids found in proteins according to the charge and polarity of their side chains. Each amino acid is shown in its fully protonated form with dissociable hydrogen ions represented in bold print. (For convenience the protonated amino group is shown as $—NH_3^+$ with the understanding that only one hydrogen of the amino group can dissociate.) The pK values for the α-carboxyl and α-amino groups of the nonpolar amino acids are similar to those shown for glycine.

Isoleucine	=	Ile	Phenylalanine	=	Phe
Tryptophan	=	Trp	Methionine	=	Met
Proline	=	Pro			

1. Each of these amino acids has a nonpolar side chain that does not bind or give off protons, or participate in hydrogen or ionic bonds (Figure 1.2).
2. In proteins, the side chains of these amino acids can cluster together because of their hydrophobicity, much like droplets of oil coalesce in aqueous solutions. The importance of these ***hydrophobic interactions*** in stabilizing protein structure will be discussed on p. 17.
3. Proline differs from other amino acids in that it contains an ***imino group,*** rather than an α-amino group.

HN–

Imino group

B. Amino acids with uncharged polar side chains

Asparagine	=	Asn	Glutamine	=	Gln
Cysteine	=	Cys	Serine	=	Ser
Threonine	=	Thr	Tyrosine	=	Tyr

H_2N–

Amino group

1. These amino acids have zero net charge at neutral pH, although the side chains of cysteine and tyrosine can lose a proton at alkaline pH (Figure 1.2).
2. The side chain of cysteine contains a ***sulfhydryl group*** (—SH), which is an important component of the active site of many enzymes. In proteins the —SH groups of two cysteines can condense to form the amino acid cystine, which contains a covalent cross-link called a ***disulfide bond*** (—S—S—). (See p. 18 for a discussion of disulfide bond formation.)
3. Serine, threonine, and tyrosine all contain a polar ***hydroxyl group*** that, in proteins, can participate in hydrogen bond formation (Figure 1.3) or serve as the site of attachment for a phosphate group or a carbohydrate. The side chains of asparagine and glutamine each contain a carbonyl group and an amide group, both of which can also participate in hydrogen bonds or serve as a site of attachment for carbohydrates. (See p. 17 for a discussion of hydrogen bonds.)

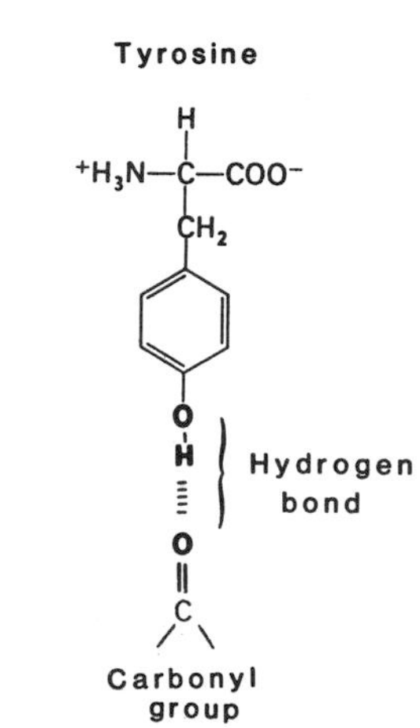

Figure 1.3
Hydrogen bond between the phenolic hydroxyl group of tyrosine and another compound containing a carbonyl oxygen.

C. Amino acids with acidic side chains

Aspartic acid	=	Asp	Glutamic acid	=	Glu

1. The amino acids aspartic and glutamic acid are proton donors: At neutral pH the side chains of these amino acids are fully ionized and contain a ***negatively charged*** carboxylate group ($—COO^-$). They are therefore called aspartate or glutamate to emphasize that at physiologic pH these amino acids are negatively charged (Figure 1.2).

D. Amino acids with basic side chains

Lysine	=	Lys	Arginine	=	Arg
Histidine	=	His			

1. The side chains of the basic amino acids bind protons (Figure 1.2): At physiologic pH the side chains of lysine and arginine are fully ionized and ***positively charged.***
2. In contrast, histidine is weakly basic and the free amino acid largely uncharged at physiologic pH. In proteins, however, the side chain of histidine can be either positively charged or neutral depending on the ionic environment provided by the polypeptide chains of the protein.

Study Questions

Answer A if 1, 2, and 3 are correct
B if 1 and 3 are correct
C if 2 and 4 are correct
D if only 4 is correct
E if all are correct

1.1 Which of the following statements describe(s) the side chain of the amino acid serine?

1. Contains a hydroxyl group
2. Can form disulfide bonds
3. Can participate in hydrogen bonds
4. Is charged at physiologic pH

1.2 Which of the following amino acids has/have a charged side chain at physiologic pH?

1. Aspartic acid
2. Lysine
3. Glutamic acid
4. Asparagine

1.3 Glutamine

1. contains three titratable groups.
2. contains an amide group.
3. is classified as an acidic amino acid.
4. contains a side chain that can form hydrogen bonds in proteins.

1.4 Which of the following statements about amino acids is(are) true?

1. Glycine contains two dissociable hydrogens.
2. Tyrosine is a site of attachment of phosphate groups in proteins.
3. Cysteine is a sulfur-containing amino acid.
4. Glutamine is classified as a basic amino acid.

III. AMINO ACIDS AS BUFFERS

Amino acids contain weakly acidic α-carboxyl groups and weakly basic α-amino groups. In addition, each of the acid and basic amino acids contains an ionizable group in its side chain. Thus, both free amino acids and amino acids combined in peptide linkage can potentially act as buffers. The quantitative relation between $[H^+]$ and weak acids is described by the Henderson-Hasselbalch equation.

A. The Henderson-Hasselbalch equation

1. Consider the release of a proton by a weak acid represented by HA:

$$\underset{\text{weak acid}}{HA} \rightleftarrows \underset{\text{proton}}{H^+} + \underset{\text{salt form or conjugate base}}{A^-}$$

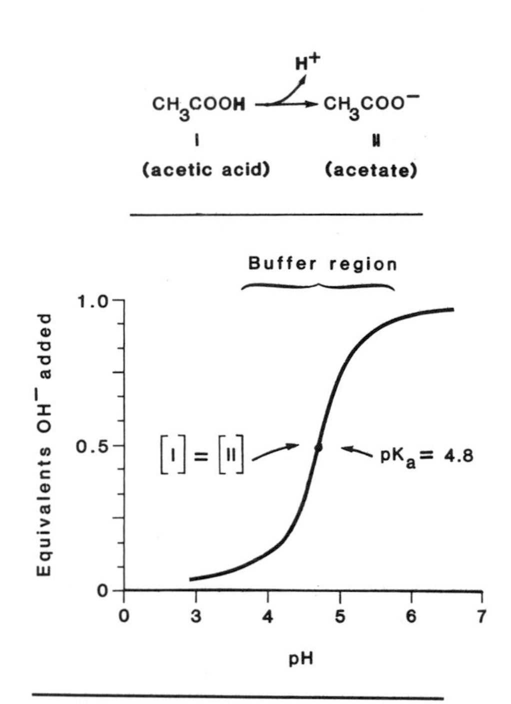

Figure 1.4
Titration curve of acetic acid.

The "salt" or conjugate base, A^-, is the ionized form of a weak acid. By definition, the dissociation constant of the acid, K_a, is

$$K_a = \frac{[H^+]\,[A^-]}{[HA]}$$

By solving for the $[H^+]$ in the above equation, taking the logarithm of both sides of the equation, multiplying both sides of the equation by -1, and substituting $pH = -\log[H^+]$ and $pK_a = -\log K_a$, we obtain the Henderson-Hasselbalch equation:

$$pH = pK_a + \log\frac{[A^-]}{[HA]}$$

which can also be written as

$$pH = pK_a + \log\frac{[\text{conjugate base}]}{[\text{acid form}]}$$

2. The Henderson-Hasselbalch equation can be used to calculate the pH of a solution containing a weak acid after the addition of strong acid or base. For example, Figure 1.4 illustrates the change in pH that occurs when NaOH is added to a solution of acetic acid. This titration curve demonstrates several important concepts:
   a. A ***buffer*** is a solution that resists changes in pH following the addition of strong acid or base. A weak acid and its conjugate base, for example, acetic acid (CH_3—COOH) and acetate (CH_3—COO^-), can serve as a buffer when the pH of a solution is within ±1 pH unit of the pK_a of the weak acid. Maximum buffering capacity occurs at the pK_a. Therefore, a solution containing the acetic acid/acetate buffer pair will resist a change in pH from pH 3.8 to 5.8, with maximum buffering at pH 4.8.
   b. When the pH of a solution is equal to the pK_a, the amount of the salt form is equal to the acid form. As noted above, at this pH the solution will have its maximum buffering capacity.
   c. At pH values less than the pK_a, the protonated acid form (e.g., CH_3—COOH) is the predominant species.
   d. At pH values greater than the pK_a, the deprotonated salt (e.g., CH_3—COO^-) is the predominant species in solution.

Alanine

^+H_3N—C(H)(CH$_3$)—COOH
I
(Fully protonated form)

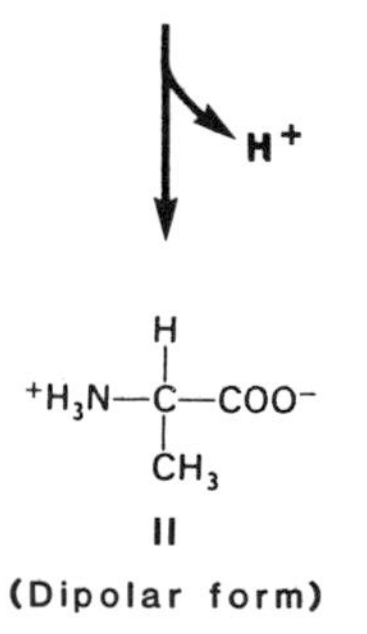

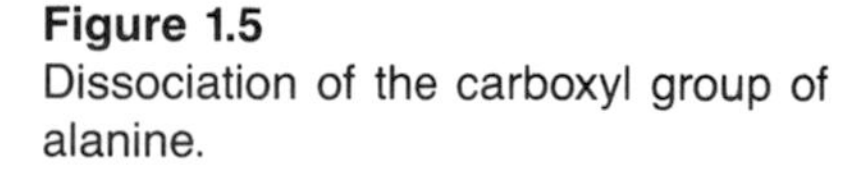

Figure 1.5
Dissociation of the carboxyl group of alanine.

B. The titration of alanine

1. The titration curve of an amino acid can be analyzed in the same way as that described above for acetic acid. For example, consider the amino acid alanine, which contains both a carboxyl and an amino group. At an acidic pH, both of these groups of alanine are protonated (shown in Figure 1.5). The —COOH group of form I can dissociate by donating a proton to the medium, where it binds to a water molecule, producing H_3O^+. This release of a proton results in the formation of the carboxylate group, —COO^-. The structure is shown as form II, which is the dipolar form of the molecule (Figure 1.5). (Note: This form is also called a ***zwitterion,*** and is the ***isoelectric form*** of alanine.

2. The dissociation constant of the carboxyl group is defined as K_1, rather than K_a, since the molecule contains a second titratable group. The Henderson-Hasselbalch equation can be used to analyze the dissociation of the carboxyl group of alanine, as described for acetic acid.

$$K_1 = \frac{[H^+]\ [II]}{[I]}$$

This equation can be rearranged to yield

$$pH = pK_a + \log\frac{[II]}{[I]}$$

or

$$pH = pK_a + \log\frac{[\text{conjugate base}]}{[\text{acid form}]}$$

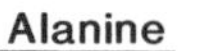

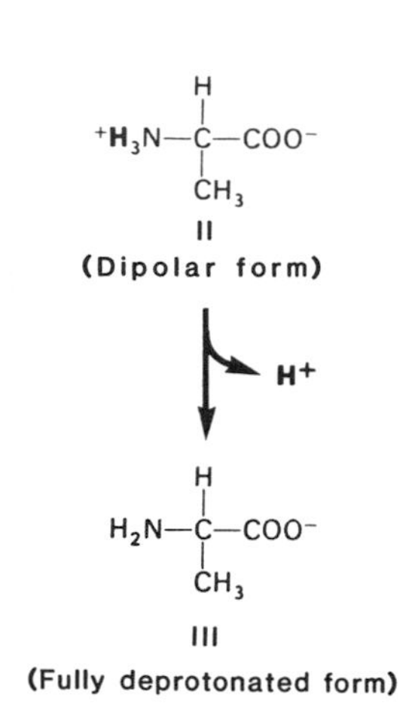

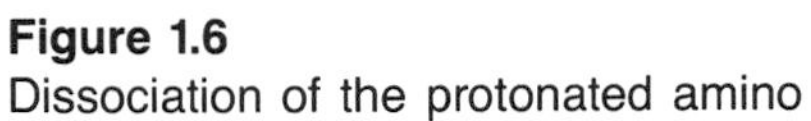

Figure 1.6
Dissociation of the protonated amino group of alanine.

3. The second titratable group of alanine is the amino ($-NH_3^+$) group shown in Figure 1.6. This is a much weaker acid than the —COOH group and therefore has a much smaller dissociation constant, K_2. Release of a proton from the protonated amino group of form II results in the fully deprotonated form of alanine, structure III (Figure 1.6).
4. The sequential dissociation of protons from the carboxyl and amino groups of alanine is summarized below (Figure 1.7). Each of the titratable groups has a pK that is numerically equal to the pH at which exactly half of the protons have been removed from that group. The pK for the most acidic group is pK_1 (—COOH); the pK for the next most acidic group ($-NH_3^+$) is pK_2.

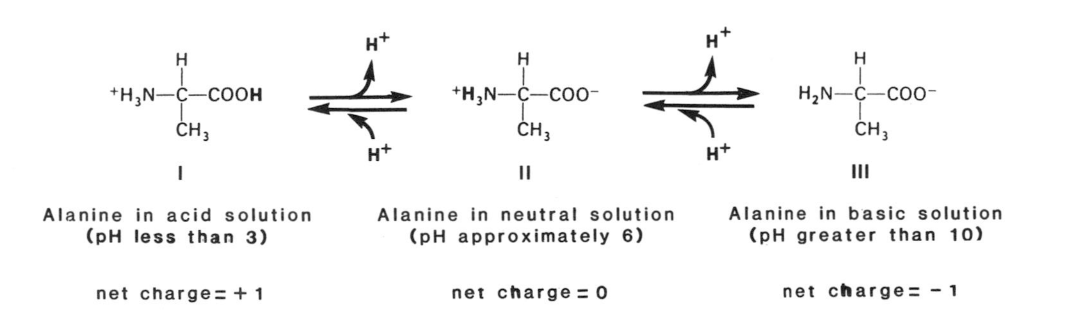

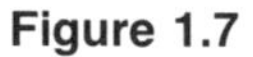

Figure 1.7
Ionic forms of alanine in acidic, neutral, and basic solutions.

5. By applying the Henderson-Hasselbalch equation to each dissociable acidic group, it is possible to calculate the complete titration curve. Figure 1.8 shows the change in pH that occurs during the addition of base to the fully protonated form of alanine (I) to produce the completely deprotonated form (III). Note the following:

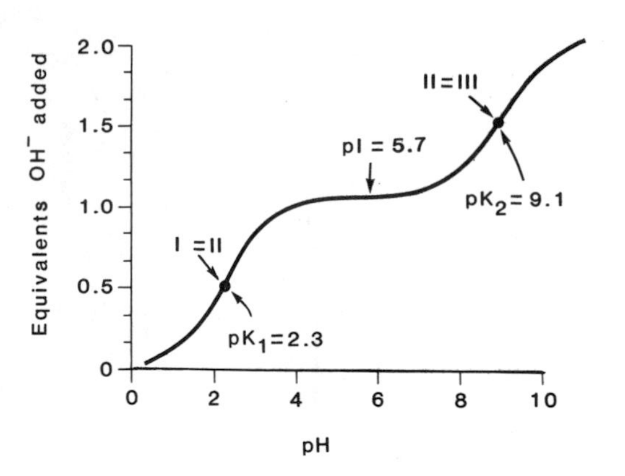

Figure 1.8
The titration curve of alanine.

a. The —COOH/—COO$^-$ pair can serve as a buffer in the region around pK_1, and the —NH_3^+/—NH_2 pair buffers in the region around pK_2.

b. When the pH is equal to pK_1 (2.3), equal amounts of forms I and II of alanine exist in solution. When the pH is equal to pK_2 (9.1), equal amounts of forms II and III are present in solution.

c. At neutral pH, alanine exists predominantly as the dipolar form II in which the amino and carboxyl groups are ionized, but the net charge is zero.

6. The ***isoelectric point*** (pI) is the pH at which a molecule is electrically neutral, that is, where the sum of the positive charges equals the sum of the negative charges.

   a. For an amino acid such as alanine, which has only two dissociable hydrogens (one from the α-carboxyl and one from the α-amino group), the pI is the average of pK_1 and pK_2, pI = (2.3 + 9.1)/2 = 5.7 (Figure 1.8). The pI is thus midway between pK_1 (2.3) and pK_2 (9.1). It corresponds to the pH at which structure II (net charge of zero) predominates, and at which there are also equal amounts of forms I (net charge of +1) and III (net charge of −1).

C. The titration of histidine

1. Histidine is an example of an amino acid that contains three chemical groups, each of which can reversibly gain or lose a proton: the α-carboxyl group, the imidazole group of the side chain, and the α-amino group (Figure 1.9).

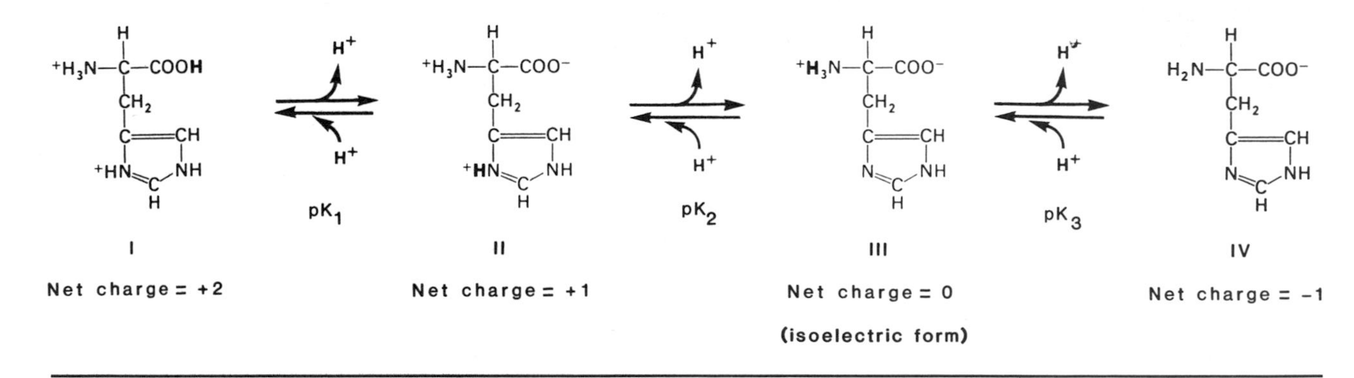

Figure 1.9
Ionic forms of histidine.

2. The R-group of histidine has a pK of 6.0 and can serve as a buffer at physiologic pH.

3. The incremental addition of base to fully protonated histidine results in the sequential removal of protons from the α-carboxyl group (pK_1 = 1.8), the imidazole group (pK_2 = 6.0), and the α-amino group (pK_3 = 9.2). The titration curve is shown in Figure 1.10.

4. The isoelectric point (pI) for histidine is calculated by first identifying the isoelectric form (which has a net charge of zero) of

the amino acid (III in Figure 1.9), then averaging the values of the nearest pK's $(pK_2 + pK_3)/2 = (6.0 + 9.2)/2 = 7.6$) (Figure 1.10). This calculation requires that the isoelectric species be identified. This in turn depends on knowing the order in which the protons are lost from a particular amino acid, since this determines the charges of the intermediate species. The pK values for some of the 20 commonly encountered amino acids are shown in Figure 1.2.

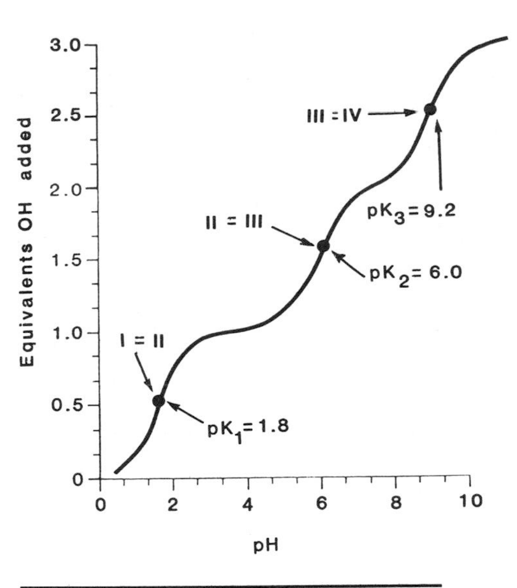

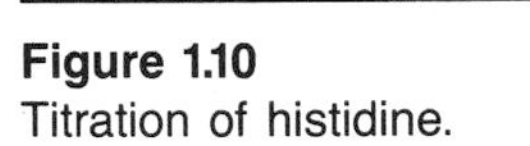

Figure 1.10
Titration of histidine.

Study Questions

Choose the ONE best answer:

1.5 Lysine ($pK_1 = 2.2$, $pK_2 = 9.0$, $pK_3 = 10.5$)

A. contains an amide group.
B. has a charge of +1 when the carboxyl group is protonated.
C. has a pI of 5.6
D. will migrate toward the cathode (negative electrode) during electrophoresis at pH 7.0.
E. has a nonpolar side chain.

1.6 Histidine has a side chain that has a pK_2 of 6.0. Which one of the following amino acids also has a side chain that titrates within about 1.5 pH units of neutrality?

A. Lysine
B. Arginine
C. Threonine
D. Cysteine
E. Hydroxyproline

1.7 The letters A, B, C, D, and E designate regions on the titration curve of glycine ($pK_1 = 2.3$, $pK_2 = 9.6$) shown to the right. Which one of the following descriptions is correct?

A. A is a region of maximal buffering.
B. B is a region of minimal buffering.
C. C is at the isoelectric point (pI).
D. The concentration of $^{+}NH_3—CH_2—COOH$ is maximal in region D.
E. The concentration of $^{+}NH_3—CH_2—COO^{-}$ is maximal in region E.

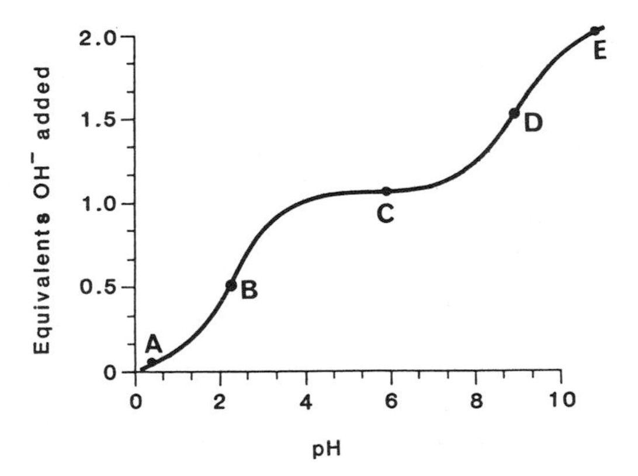

IV. OPTICAL PROPERTIES OF AMINO ACIDS

A. The α-carbon of each amino acid is attached to four different chemical groups and is therefore a ***chiral*** or ***optically active*** carbon atom. Glycine is the single exception since the α-carbon of glycine has two hydrogen substituents and therefore is optically inactive (see p. 46 for a discussion of optical activity).

B. All the amino acids found in proteins are of the L-configuration. However, D-amino acids are found in some antibiotics and in bacterial cell walls.

V. PEPTIDE BOND

A. In proteins, amino acids are joined covalently by peptide bonds that are amide linkages between the α-carboxyl group of one amino acid and the α-amino group of another. For example, glycine and

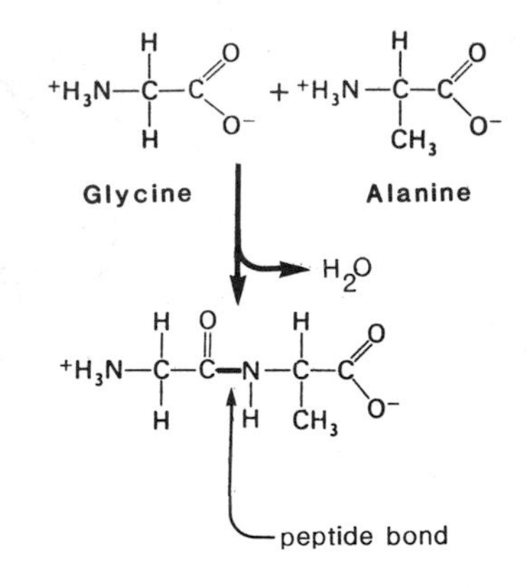

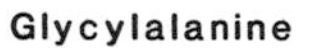

Figure 1.11
Formation of a peptide bond.

alanine can form the dipeptide glycylalanine through the formation of a peptide bond (Figure 1.11). By convention the free amino-end (N-terminal) is written to the left and the free carboxyl-end (C-terminal) to the right. Therefore, all amino sequences are read from the N- to the C-terminal end of the peptide. For example, in Figure 1.11, the order of the amino acids is "glycine, alanine" ***not*** "alanine, glycine".

B. Linkage of many amino acids through peptide bonds results in an unbranched chain called a ***polypeptide***. Each component amino acid in a polypeptide is called a ***residue***. When the compounds are named, all amino acid residues have the end of their names changed from -ine to -yl, except the C-terminal amino acid. For example, a tripeptide composed of N-terminal valine, a central glycine, and C-terminal leucine is called valylglycylleucine.

C. The peptide bond has a ***partial double-bond character*** and therefore is rigid and planar (Figure 1.12); this prevents free rotation around the bond between the carbonyl carbon and the nitrogen of the peptide bond.

D. Like all amide linkages, the peptide bond neither accepts nor gives off protons over the pH range of 2 to 12. Thus, the charged groups present in polypeptides consist solely of the N-terminal amino group, the C-terminal carboxyl group, and any ionized groups present in the side chains of the constituent amino acids.

E. Peptide bonds are not broken by normal handling or by conditions (such as heating alone or high concentrations of urea) that denature proteins. Strong acid or base at elevated temperatures is required to hydrolyze these bonds.

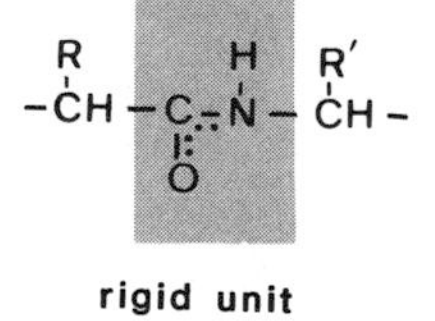

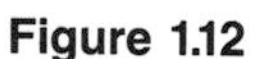
Figure 1.12
Partial double bond character of the peptide bond.

Study Questions

Answer A if 1, 2, and 3 are correct
B if 1 and 3 are correct
C if 2 and 4 are correct
D if only 4 is correct
E if all are correct

1.8 The peptide bond

1. is a special type of amide linkage.
2. has a partial double bond character.
3. is not ionized at physiologic pH.
4. is cleaved by agents that denature proteins, such as organic solvents and high concentrations of urea.

1.9 The peptide alanylglycylserine

1. contains alanine with a free α-amino group.
2. contains three peptide bonds.
3. is optically active.
4. is a dipeptide.

Structure of Proteins

2

I. OVERVIEW

The preceding chapter described the structure of the 20 amino acids found in proteins and the fundamental ways of linking these building blocks by means of the peptide bond. This chapter examines how a linear sequence of amino acids generates a protein molecule with a unique three-dimensional shape. The complexity of protein structure is best analyzed by considering the molecule in terms of four organizational hierarchies, namely, primary, secondary, tertiary, and quaternary structure.

II. PRIMARY STRUCTURE OF PROTEINS

The sequence of amino acids in a protein is called the primary structure. Determining the order of amino acids in a polypeptide chain requires the application of several experimental techniques. First, the amino acid composition is analyzed, that is, the kinds and amounts of amino acids present in the protein are tabulated. Then the identity of the amino acids at the ends of the polypeptide chain is determined. Finally, the original polypeptide is specifically cleaved into smaller fragments, the sequences of which can be determined. These fragments can then be ordered to reconstruct the sequence of the original polypeptide. These techniques are described below:

A. Amino acid composition of polypeptides

1. ***Acid hydrolysis:*** The first step in determining the primary structure of a protein is to identify and quantitate its constituent amino acids. The protein or polypeptide to be analyzed is first hydrolyzed by strong acid at 110° for 24 hours. This treatment cleaves the peptide bonds and releases the individual amino acids. In addition, glutamine and asparagine are hydrolyzed to glutamate and aspartate, respectively, and tryptophan is largely destroyed.
2. ***Chromatography:*** The individual amino acids obtained by acid hydrolysis of the protein are separated by ion exchange chromatography (Figure 2.1). In this method a mixture of amino acids is applied to a column that contains an insoluble ion exchanger. Under the acidic conditions employed all the amino acids have a net positive charge and are bound to the negatively charged ion exchange column. Each amino acid is sequentially released

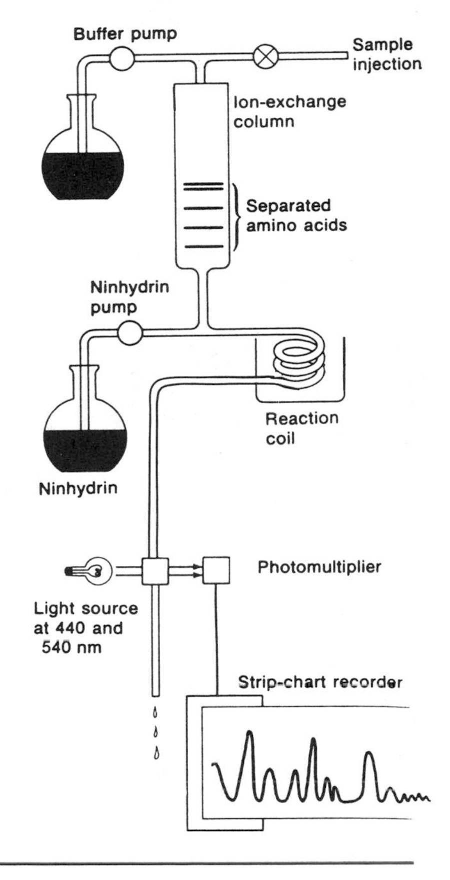

Figure 2.1
Determination of the amino acid composition of a polypeptide using an amino acid analyzer.

from the chromatography column by eluting with solutions of increasing ionic strength and pH (Figure 2.1). As the pH increases, the amino acids lose hydrogen ions, first from the α-carboxyl groups and then from the side chains and α-amino groups. As the amino acids lose hydrogen ions (H^+) they become negatively charged and are released from the resin. Each amino acid emerges from the column at a specific pH and ionic strength.

3. ***Quantitative analysis:*** The separated amino acids contained in the eluant from the column are analyzed quantitatively by heating them with ninhydrin, a reagent that forms a blue compound with most amino acids, ammonia, and amines (but forms a yellow derivative with the imino nitrogen of proline). The amount of each amino acid is determined spectrophotometrically by measuring the amount of light absorbed by the ninhydrin derivative. The absorbance of the amino acid derivatives is recorded continuously on a chart recorder. Each peak on the recorder corresponds to an individual amino acid; the area under each peak is proportional to the amount of that particular amino acid present in the original polypeptide. The amino acid composition is reported as residues of each amino acid per protein molecule. The analysis described above is usually performed by an amino acid analyzer, an automated machine whose components are depicted in Figure 2.1.

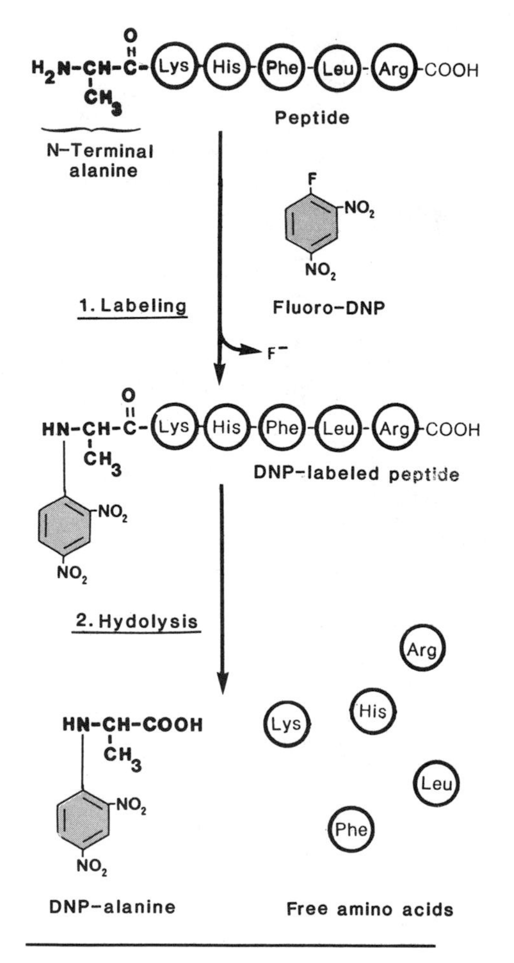

Figure 2.2
Determination of the amino-terminal residue of a polypeptide with fluorodinitrobenzene (Sanger's reagent).

B. Determination of N-terminal amino acid

1. ***Sanger's method:*** Several methods are available to identify the amino acid located at the amino-terminal end of the polypeptide chain. In Sanger's method, fluorodinitrobenzene reacts with α-amino groups of the N-terminal amino acids to form a yellow dinitrophenyl (DNP) derivative of the amino acid (Figure 2.2). The bond linking the DNP group and the amino acid is not cleaved by mild acid hydrolysis. Thus the amino acid that has become the DNP-derivative can be isolated after hydrolysis of the polypeptide. The DNP-amino acid derivative, which corresponds to the N-terminal residue, can be identified by ion exchange chromatography.

2. ***Edman's reagent:*** Phenylisothiocyanate, known as Edmans's reagent, is also used to label the amino-terminal residue (Figure 2.3). The phenylthiohydantoin (PTH) derivative formed can be selectively cleaved from the polypeptide without breaking the peptide bonds between the remaining amino acid residues. Edman's reagent has an advantage over Sanger's reagent in that it can be applied repeatedly on the shortened peptide obtained in the previous cycle. Using automated techniques, the repetition of the method can be used to determine the sequence of more than 100 amino acid residues starting at the amino terminal.

C. Determination of the C-terminal amino acid

1. ***Hydrazine:*** All carbonyl carbons bound in peptide linkage react with hydrazine, forming amino acid hydrazones. However, the C-terminal amino acid does not react with hydrazine, and therefore is liberated as an unmodified amino acid that can be separated from the modified residues and identified.

2. ***Carboxypeptidase:*** This exopeptidase (see p. 225 for a description of this enzyme) sequentially cleaves peptide bonds, starting at

the C-terminal end. The carboxyl-terminal amino acid is thus the first amino acid to be liberated by *carboxypeptidase*.

D. Cleavage of polypeptide into smaller fragments

1. ***Enzymic cleavage:*** *Trypsin* and *chymotrypsin* are pancreatic enzymes commonly used to cleave a protein or polypeptide into fragments that are shortened and therefore more amenable to sequence analysis. *Trypsin* cleaves peptide bonds on the carboxyl side of either lysine or arginine. The fragments produced are called ***tryptic peptides***. *Chymotrypsin* is less specific, favoring cleavage on the carboxyl side of phenylalanine, tyrosine, tryptophan, and other bulky residues (see p. 225 for a description of these enzymes in the digestion of proteins).
2. ***Cyanogen bromide:*** Treatment with cyanogen bromide is also a commonly used method for cleaving a polypeptide. Cyanogen bromide splits the polypeptide chain on the carboxyl side of methionine residues, forming homoserine lactone from methionine (Figure 2.4). The action of this reagent, like that of *trypsin*, is highly specific and usually leads to the production of a limited number of fragments.
3. ***Overlapping peptides:*** The peptides produced by cleavage of a protein with proteolytic enzymes or cyanogen bromide are usually small enough to be sequenced by the Edman degradation. However, even after the sequences of the peptides have been successfully determined, it is not known how the peptides fit together to form the original protein. To determine the position these fragments occupy in the protein, it is necessary to prepare overlapping peptides. These are formed by treating the original protein with reagents that cleave the polypeptide chain at sites different from that used to prepare the original peptides. Overlapping peptides act as bridges in ordering the peptide fragments, since a peptide produced by one reagent will overlap sequences that correspond to the N-terminal and C-terminal sequence of a second fragment produced by a different reagent. For example, Figure 2.5 shows that cleavage of a polypeptide by cyanogen bromide provides an overlap peptide that allows the ordering of the two peptides produced by the action of *trypsin*.
4. ***Polymeric proteins:*** If a protein is composed of more than one type of polypeptide chain, the chains must first be separated before sequence analysis can be performed. Denaturing agents, such as ***urea*** or ***guanidine hydrochloride,*** disrupt noncovalent bonds and serve to dissociate the protein into single chain components. The individual polypeptide chains can be isolated and the amino acid sequence of each determined.

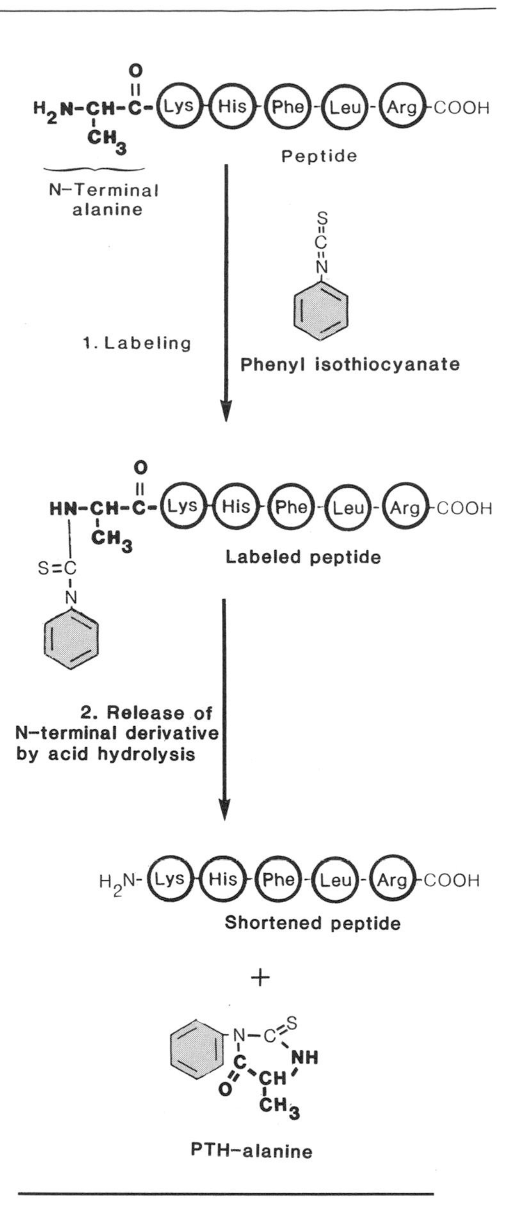

Figure 2.3
Determination of the amino-terminal residue of a polypeptide by the Edman degradation.

Study Questions

Answer A if 1, 2, and 3 are correct
B if 1 and 3 are correct
C if 2 and 4 are correct
D if only 4 is correct
E if all are correct

2.1 Which of the following reagents would be useful in determining the N-terminal amino acid of a polypeptide?

1. Fluorodinitrobenzene
2. Carboxypeptidase
3. Phenylisothiocyanate
4. Cyanogen bromide

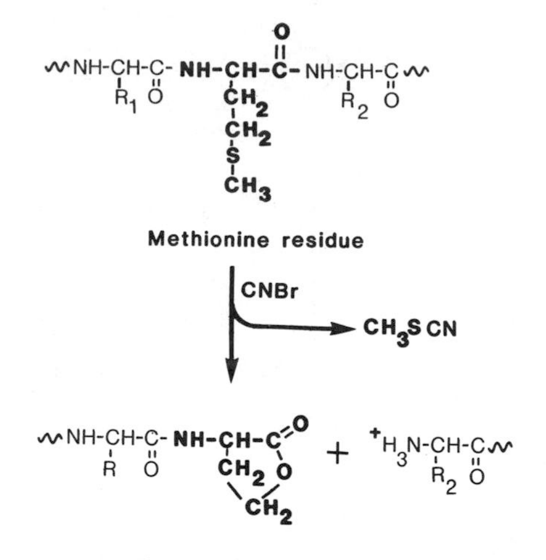

Figure 2.4
Cleavage of peptide bond by cyanogen bromide on the carboxyl side of methionine residues.

2.2 Which of the following correctly describes the expected products obtained when the polypeptide arg-gly-phe-leu-met-lys is treated as indicated below?.

1. Treatment with cyanogen bromide yields two fragments.
2. Treatment with trypsin gives three fragments.
3. Treatment with 6N HCl at 100° gives six products.
4. Treatment with hydrazine yields two fragments.

Choose the ONE best answer:

2.3 You are presented with the following information about a peptide composed of five amino acids:

(a) Amino acid analysis gives equimolar amounts of Ala, Glu, Gly, Lys, and Met.
(b) Digestion of the original peptide with trypsin gives rise to a free amino acid.
(c) Digestion of the original peptide with cyanogen bromide generates two fragments, one of which moves toward the anode and the other toward the cathode when electrophoresed at pH 7.

Which one of the following best describes the structure of the peptide?

A. Lys-Gly-Met-Glu-Ala
B. Gly-Lys-Met-Glu-Ala
C. Lys-Glu-Met-Ala-Gly
D. Gly-Glu-Met-Ala-Lys
E. Glu-Gly-Met-Ala-Lys

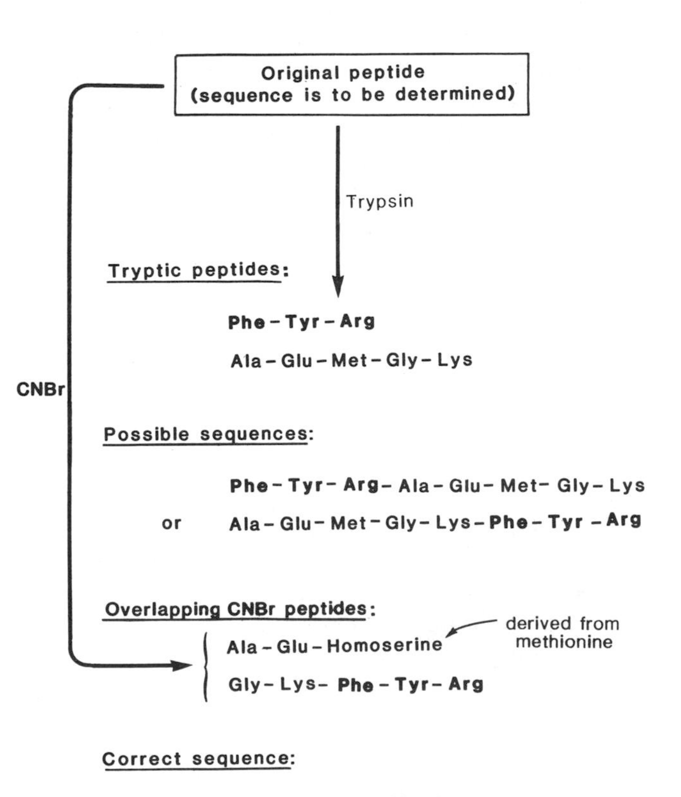

Figure 2.5
Overlapping of peptides produced by the action of *trypsin* and by cyanogen bromide.

2.4 Which one of the following best describes the products obtained when the tripeptide alanylglycylleucine is treated with phenylisothiocyanate followed by mild acid hydrolysis?

A. PTH-alanine, glycylleucine
B. PTH-leucine, alanylglycine
C. PTH-alanine, glycine, leucine
D. PTH-alanylglycylleucine
E. Alanine, glycine, leucine

III. SECONDARY STRUCTURE OF PROTEINS

If proteins contained only primary structure, they would form long, spaghetti-like molecules. However, the polypeptide backbone of proteins does not assume such a random structure, but instead forms regularly repeating structures termed the ***secondary structure***. The α-helix and the β-pleated sheet are examples of secondary structure frequently encountered in proteins. (The triple helix, another example of secondary structure, is unique to collagen and is discussed on p. 32).

A. The α-helix

1. The α-helix is a rod-like structure with the side chains of the amino acids extending outward from the central axis of the coiled polypeptide backbone (Figure 2.6).
2. Hydrogen bonds extend down the spiral from the carbonyl oxygen of one peptide linkage to the —NH— group of a peptide bond four residues ahead in the primary sequence (Figure 2.6). All the carbonyl oxygens and peptide-bonded nitrogens along the polypeptide backbone are hydrogen bonded in the α-helix. These hydrogen bonds are individually weak but collectively are the major force stabilizing the helical structure.
3. Each turn of the helix contains 3.6 amino acids; thus amino acid residues spaced three or four apart in the primary sequence are spatially close together when folded in the α-helix.

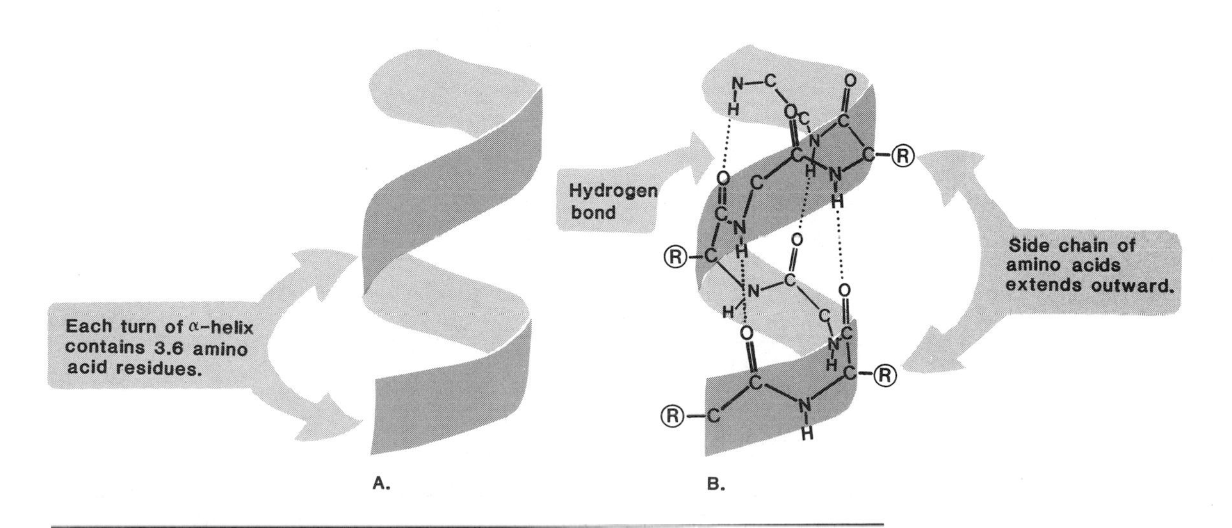

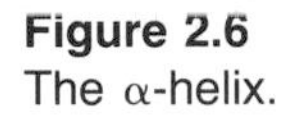
Figure 2.6
The α-helix.

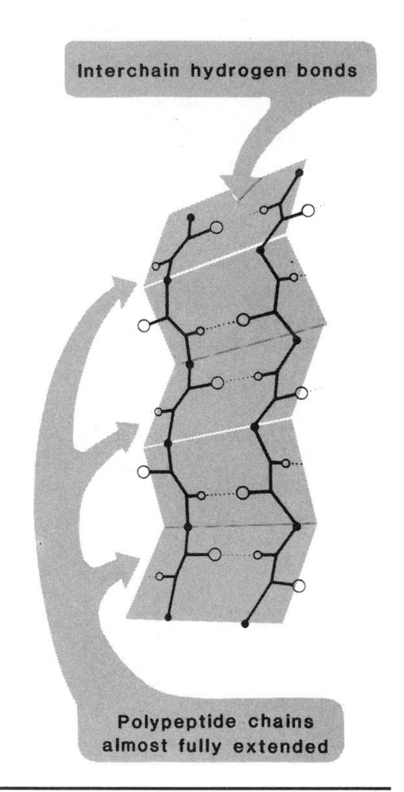

Figure 2.7
Structure of β-sheet.

4. Proline disrupts the α-helix because its imino group is not geometrically compatible with the right-handed spiral of the α-helix. Large numbers of charged amino acids (e.g., glutamate, aspartate, histidine, lysine, and arginine) or amino acids with bulky side chains (e.g., valine, isoleucine, and tryptophan) are also incompatible with the α-helix.
5. The α-helical content of proteins can vary widely, ranging from about 75% for myoglobin and hemoglobin to a virtual absence of helix in *chymotrypsin,* a digestive enzyme secreted by the pancreas.

B. The β-pleated sheet

1. In some proteins, the polypeptide chains line up side by side to form sheets of molecules, called the β-pleated sheet (Figure 2.7).
2. The polypeptide chain is almost fully extended in the β-pleated sheet, rather than being coiled. The structure is stabilized by hydrogen bonds between different polypeptide chains (interchain bonds), in contrast to the intrachain hydrogen bonds of the α-helix.
3. Adjacent strands most commonly run in the opposite direction, that is an antiparallel β-sheet. Silk fibroin is composed almost entirely of this structure. Many globular proteins contain short stretches of β-pleated sheet in which the polypeptide chain changes direction by folding back on its α-helix form in an ***intrachain β bend*** (Figure 2.8).

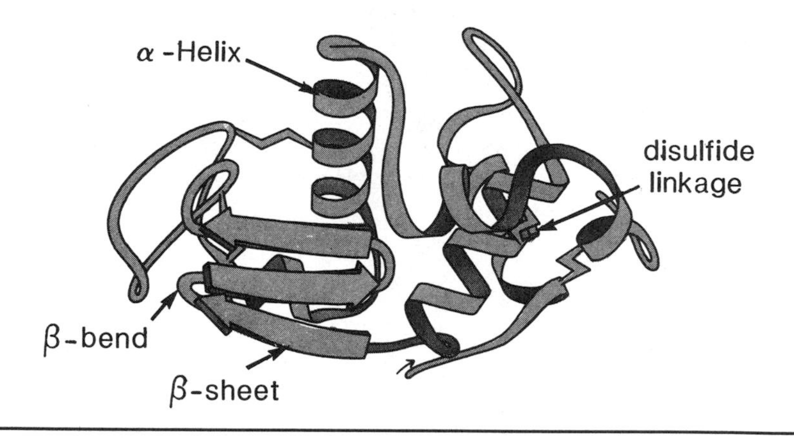

Figure 2.8
Structure of enzyme *lysozyme*. Polypeptide backbone is shown as a ribbon.

IV. TERTIARY STRUCTURE OF PROTEINS

A. Shapes of protein molecules

1. The overall shape or conformation of the protein molecule is called ***tertiary structure***. Most proteins are globular, as opposed to fibrous proteins such as collagen, which is discussed on p. 31. Globular proteins are roughly spherical in overall shape, consisting

of variable amounts of coils with no regular structure, as well as polypeptide chains folded in the α-helix, and β-pleated sheet.

2. For example, *lysozyme* is a relatively small enzyme composed of 129 amino acid in a single polypeptide chain. The protein contains regions of α-helix and β-pleated sheet secondary structures as well as sections in which the polypeptide chain has no regular structure (Figure 2.8).

B. Interactions stabilizing tertiary structure

The unique three-dimensional structure of each protein is determined by its amino acid sequence. Interactions of the amino acid side chains guide the folding of the polypeptide chain to form a compact structure. Four types of interactions cooperate in stabilizing the tertiary structures of globular proteins:

1. ***Hydrophobic interactions:*** Amino acids with nonpolar side chains tend to fold into the interior of the protein molecule where they associate with other hydrophobic amino acids. In contrast, amino acids with polar or charged side chains tend to be located on the surface of the molecule in contact with water molecules of the solvent (Figure 2.9).

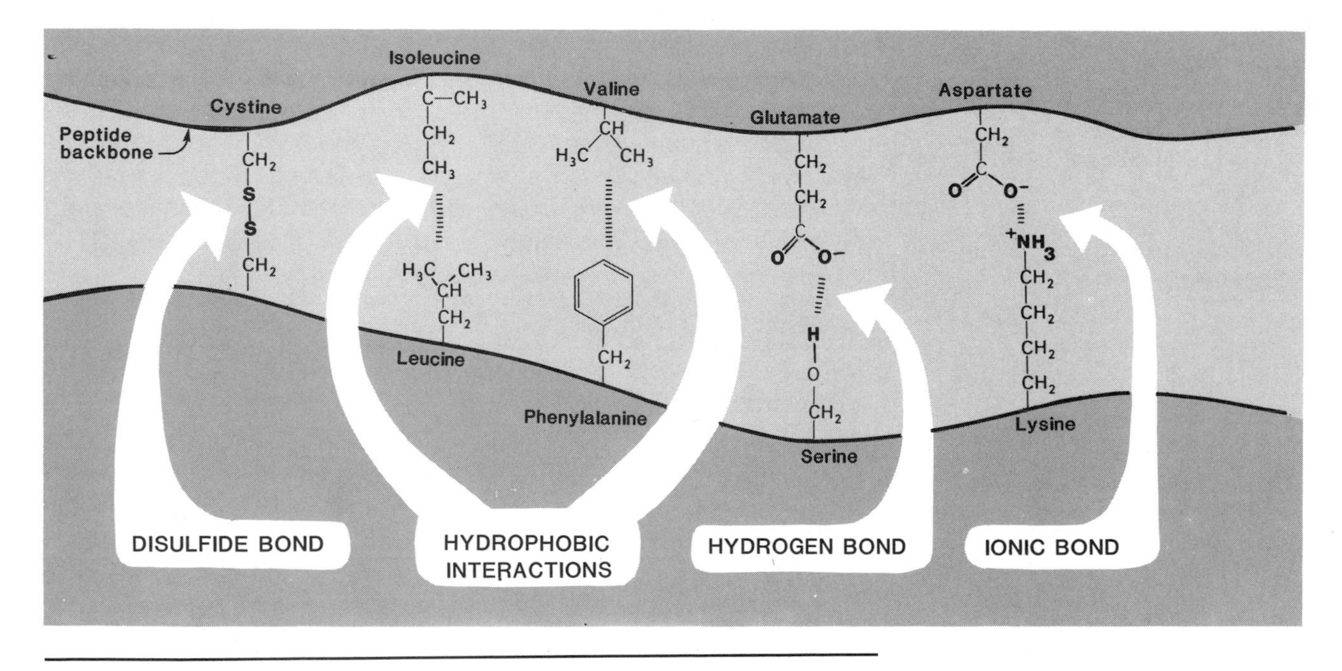

Figure 2.9
Interaction of R-groups of polypeptide chains.

2. ***Hydrogen bonds:*** Amino acid side chains containing loosely bound hydrogens, such as in the alcohol groups of serine and threonine, can form hydrogen bonds with electron-rich atoms such as nitrogen atoms of histidine or the carbonyl oxygen of carboxyl groups, amide groups, and peptide bonds (Figure 2.9).

3. ***Ionic interactions:*** Negatively charged carboxyl groups ($—COO^-$) can interact with positively charged groups, such as the ε-amino ($—NH_3^+$) of lysine (Figure 2.9).

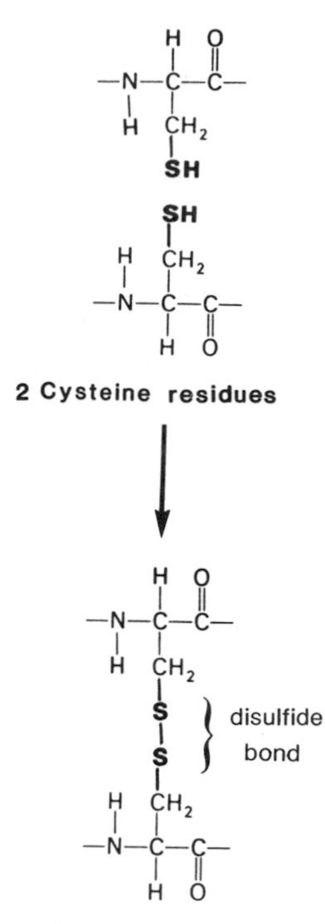

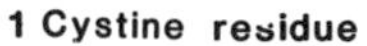

Figure 2.10
Formation of a disulfide bond by the oxidation of two cysteine residues.

4. ***Covalent cross-linkages:*** A disulfide bond is a covalent bond between the thiol group (—SH) of each of two cysteine residues, resulting in the formation of ***cystine*** (Figure 2.10). The two cysteines that participate in the disulfide bond may be separated by many amino acids in the primary sequence of a protein. However, the folding of the polypeptide chain can bring the cysteine residues in proximity and allow covalent bonding of their side chains. The disulfide linkage contributes to the stability of the three-dimensional shape of the protein molecule. Many disulfide bonds are found in proteins that are excreted from the cell. It is thought that these strong, covalent bonds aid in stabilizing the structure of proteins, preventing them from becoming denatured in the various extracellular environments.

C. Domains

1. Frequently the packing of the α-helices and β-sheets forms independent three-dimensional units called domains. These folded structures within the protein tend to be highly organized and often have a specific functional role, such as binding of a substrate or cofactor.

V. QUATERNARY STRUCTURE OF PROTEINS

In proteins containing more than one polypeptide chain, the number as well as the arrangement of the subunits is called the quaternary structure. The subunits are usually held together by noncovalent bonds (hydrophobic interactions, hydrogen and ionic bonds). For example, the enzyme *lactate dehydrogenase* (see p. 117) contains four separate polypeptide chains assembled into a tetrameric protein (Figure 2.11).

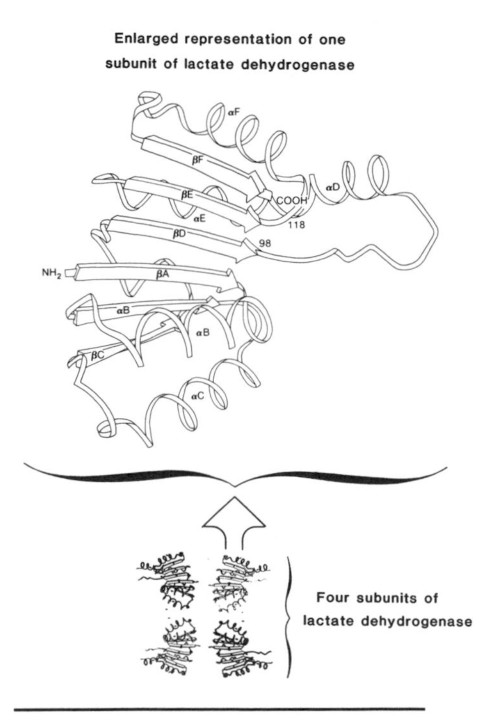

Figure 2.11
Quaternary structure of the enzyme *lactate dehydrogenase.*

VI. DENATURATION OF PROTEINS

A. Reversible denaturation

1. A wide variety of reagents and conditions can lead to protein denaturation—an unfolding and disorganization of the protein structure that is not accompanied by hydrolysis of peptide bonds. Denaturation may be reversible, in which case the protein refolds into its original native structure when the denaturing agent is removed. The refolding process is called ***renaturation***. For example,
   a. *Ribonuclease,* an enzyme that hydrolyzes RNA, comprises a single polypeptide chain that contains four disulfide bonds. In the presence of denaturing agents, such as urea or guanidine hydrochloride, these cystine (—S—S—) residues can be reduced with β-mercaptoethanol to cysteine (—SH) residues (Figure 2.12). The polypeptide of the denatured *ribonuclease* assumes a random structure that has no enzymic activity.
   b. Removal of urea and β-mercaptoethanol in the presence of air leads to oxidation of the sulfhydryls of the denatured enzyme and spontaneous refolding into the native structure. This shows that the information necessary to specify the unique tertiary structure of *ribonuclease* is contained in the amino acid sequence of the enzyme.

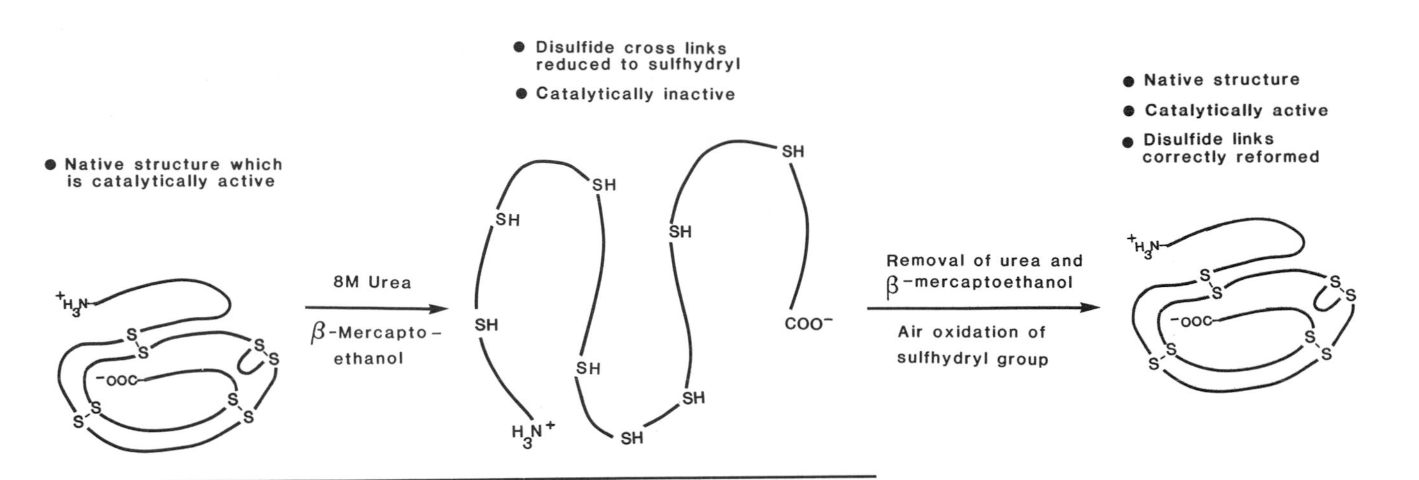

Figure 2.12
Reduction and subsequent renaturation of *ribonuclease*.

B. Irreversible denaturation

1. Denaturing agents can disrupt the hydrogen, ionic, or hydrophobic bonds that stabilize the structure of protein molecules. Therefore, denaturation often leads to an irreversible destruction of all quaternary, tertiary, and secondary structures, producing disordered polypeptide chains.
2. Denaturing agents or conditions that often lead to irreversible denaturation include heat, organic solvents, strong acids or bases, detergents, and ions of heavy metals, such as lead and mercury.

Study Questions

Choose the ONE best answer

2.5 A mutation is most likely to alter the three-dimensional conformation of a protein if

A. it produces a substitution of a hydrophobic amino acid for a hydrophilic amino acid.
B. valine is substituted for leucine.
C. it changes the amino acid at the amino-terminus.
D. it changes the amino acid at the carboxy-terminus.
E. it places proline in the middle of an α-helix.

2.6 Which one of the following types of bonds or interactions is ***least*** important in determining the three-dimensional folding of most proteins?

A. Hydrogen bonds
B. Electrostatic bonds
C. Hydrophobic interactions
D. Disulfide bonds
E. Ester bonds

2.7 Which one of the following amino acids is most likely to be found in the interior of a typical globular protein?

A. Leucine
B. Glutamate
C. Threonine
D. Lysine
E. Arginine

2.8 Which one of the following statements about protein structure is correct?

A. The α-helix is stabilized primarily by ionic interactions between the side chains of amino acids.

B. The formation of a disulfide bond in a protein requires that the two participating cysteine residues be adjacent to each other in the primary sequence of the protein.

C. The stability of quaternary structure in proteins is mainly due to covalent bonds among the subunits.

D. The denaturation of proteins always leads to irreversible loss of secondary and tertiary structure.

E. The information for the correct folding of a protein is contained in the specific sequence of amino acids along the polypeptide chain.

Function of Proteins

3

I. OVERVIEW

The previous chapter described the bonds that stabilize the α-helix and the β-pleated sheet. These structures are the "bricks and mortar" of protein architecture. In combination with other less regular polypeptide conformations, these fundamental structural elements provide a wide diversity of protein structures that have a variety of specialized functions. This chapter examines the relation of structure to function for two families of proteins: the globular hemeproteins and the fibrous collagens.

II. HEMEPROTEINS

Hemeproteins are a group of specialized proteins that contain heme as a tightly bound prosthetic group. The role of the heme group in each protein is dictated by the environment created by the three-dimensional structure of the protein. For example, the heme group of the cytochromes (see p. 105) functions as an electron carrier that is alternately oxidized and reduced. In contrast, the heme group of the enzyme *catalase* is part of the active site of the enzyme that catalyzes the breakdown of hydrogen peroxide. In hemoglobin and myoglobin, the two most abundant hemeproteins in humans, the heme group serves to reversibly bind oxygen.

A. Structure of heme

1. Heme is a complex of protoporphyrin IX and ferrous iron (Fe^{+2}) (see Figure 3.1 and p. 255). The iron is held in the center of the heme molecule by bonds to the four nitrogens of the porphyrin ring.
2. The Fe^{+2} of heme can form two additional bonds, one on each side of the planar porphyrin ring. For example, in cytochrome c these fifth and sixth coordination positions are occupied by a histidine and methionine group of the protein. In myoglobin and hemoglobin, one position is coordinated to a histidine of the protein, whereas the other position is available to bind oxygen (Figure 3.2).
3. Oxidation of the heme component of myoglobin and hemoglobin to the ferric (Fe^{+3}) state forms ***met***myoglobin and ***met***hemoglobin. Neither of these oxidized proteins can bind oxygen, but instead they contain water at the sixth coordinate position of Fe^{+3}.

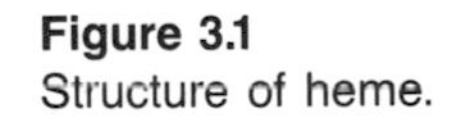

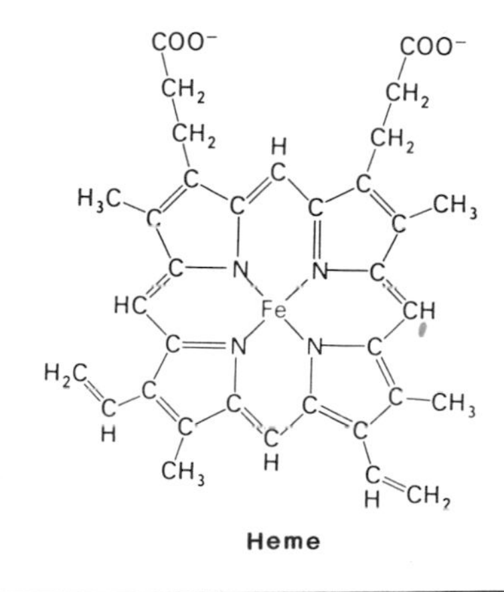

Figure 3.1
Structure of heme.

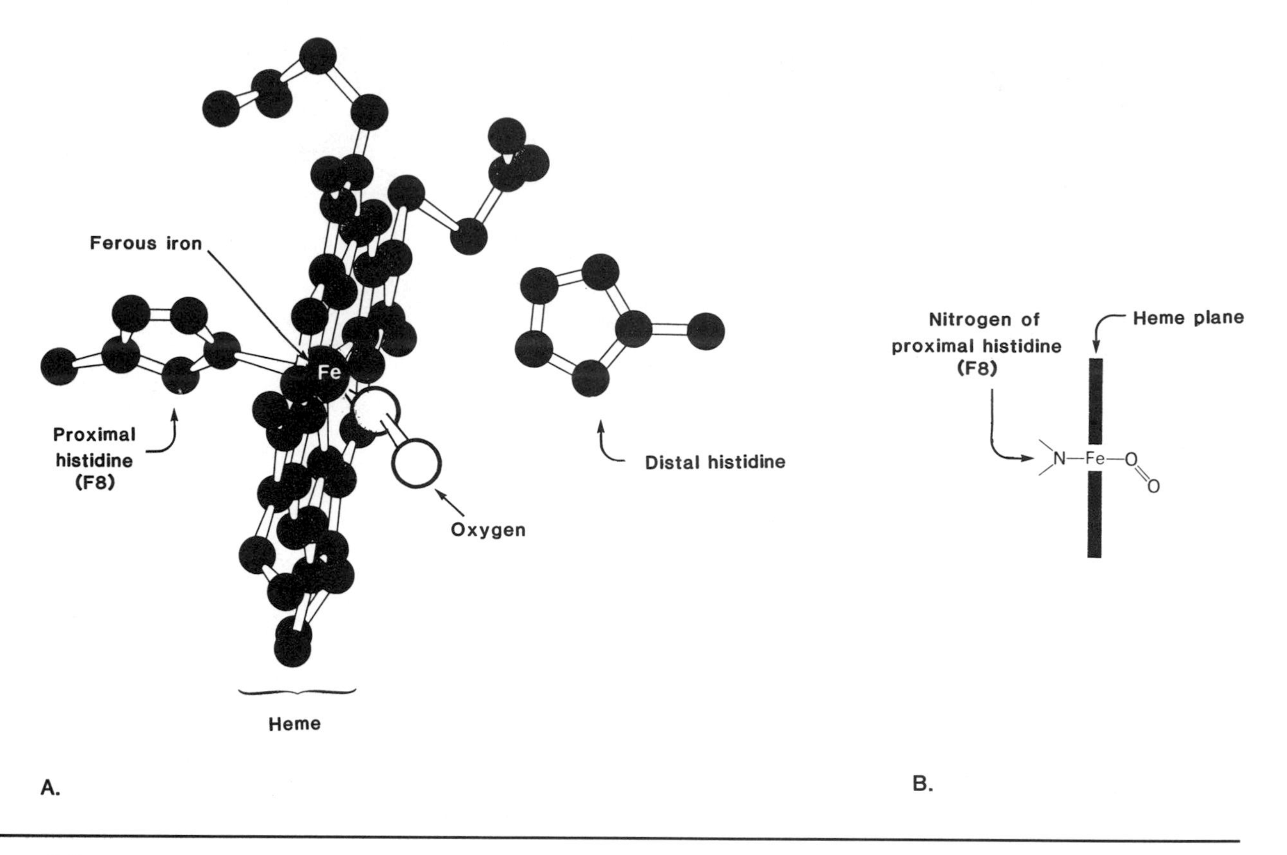

Figure 3.2
A. Model of heme group of myoglobin. **B.** Schematic diagram of the oxygen-binding site in myoglobin.

B. Structure and function of myoglobin

1. Myoglobin, a hemeprotein located primarily in heart and skeletal muscle, functions both as a reservoir for oxygen and as an oxygen carrier that increases the rate of transport of oxygen within the muscle cell.
2. Myoglobin comprises a single polypeptide chain that is structurally similar to the individual polypeptide chains of the hemoglobin molecule. This homology allows myoglobin to serve as a simple model for interpreting some of the more complex properties of hemoglobin.
3. Myoglobin is a compact molecule with approximately 75% of its polypeptide chain folded into eight stretches of α-helix. These α-helical regions are labeled A to G in Figure 3.3. Four of these segments are terminated by the presence of proline, whose five-membered ring cannot be accommodated in an α-helix (see p. 15). The other regions of α-helix are interrupted by bends and loops stabilized by hydrogen and ionic bonds.
4. The interior portion of the myoglobin molecule is composed almost entirely of nonpolar amino acids. For example, the side-chains of alanine, valine, leucine, isoleucine, methionine, and phenylalanine are packed closely together in the center of the molecule, forming a structure stabilized by hydrophobic interactions among these clustered residues (see p. 17). In contrast,

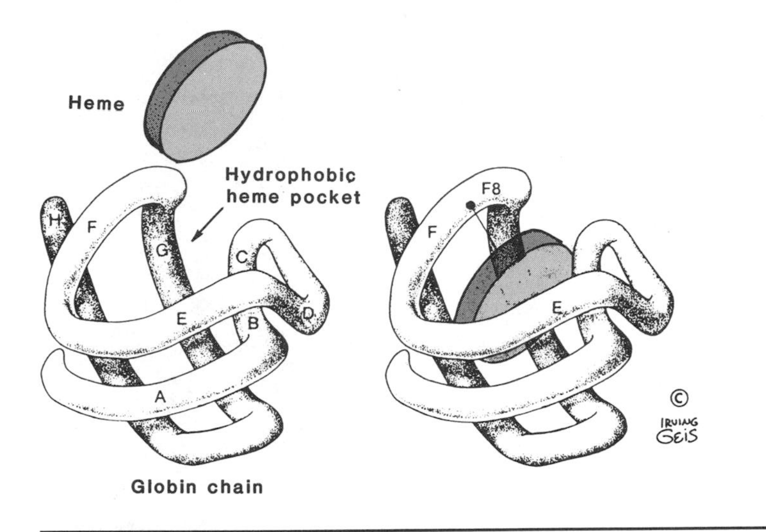

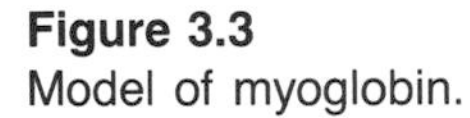
Figure 3.3
Model of myoglobin.

charged amino acids are located almost exclusively on the surface of the myoglobin, where they can form hydrogen bonds with water.

5. The heme group of myoglobin sits in a crevice in the protein. This cavity is lined with nonpolar amino acids, except for two histidine residues (Figure 3.2). One of the histidines, termed the ***proximal*** histidine, binds directly to the iron of heme. The second, or ***distal*** histidine, does not directly interact with the heme groups but helps to stabilize the ferrous form of the iron porphyrin. The protein, or globin, portion of myoglobin thus creates a special microenvironment for the heme that allows the reversible binding of oxygen without the simultaneous oxidation of the ferrous iron.

C. Structure and function of hemoglobin

1. Hemoglobin is found exclusively in the red blood cells, where its main function is to transport oxygen from the lungs to the capillaries of the tissues.
2. Hemoglobin A, the major hemoglobin in adults, comprises four polypeptide chains (two α-chains and two β-chains, $\alpha_2\beta_2$) held together by noncovalent interactions. Each subunit has a helical structure and heme binding pocket similar to that described for myoglobin. However, the tetrameric hemoglobin molecule is structurally and functionally more complex than myoglobin. For example, hemoglobin can transport CO_2 from the tissues to the lung and carry O_2 from the lungs to the cells of the body. Further, the oxygen binding properties of hemoglobin are regulated by the binding of allosteric effectors (see p. 25).
3. The hemoglobin tetramer can be envisioned as comprising two identical dimers, $\alpha_1\beta_1$ and $\alpha_2\beta_2$ (where the numbers refer to dimer 1 and dimer 2). The two polypeptide chains within each dimer are held tightly together. In contrast, the two dimers are able to move with respect to each other. The interactions between these mobile dimers is different in deoxyhemoglobin compared

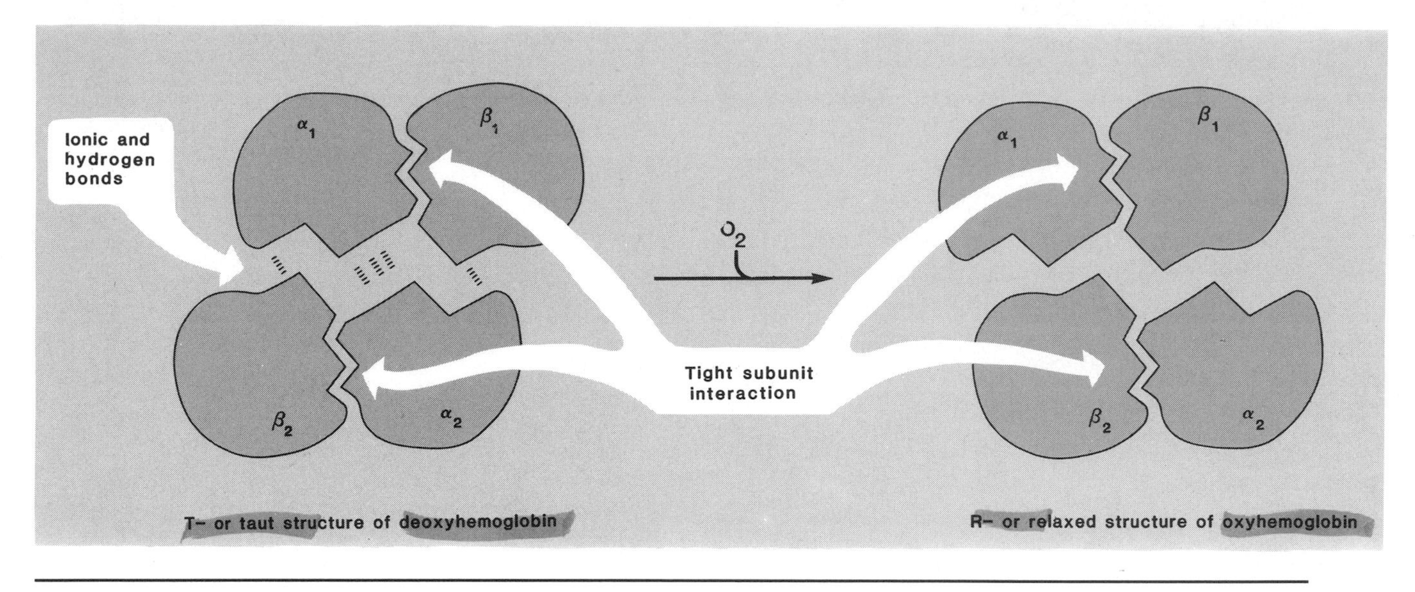

Figure 3.4
Schematic diagram comparing the structure of oxyhemoglobin and deoxyhemoglobin.

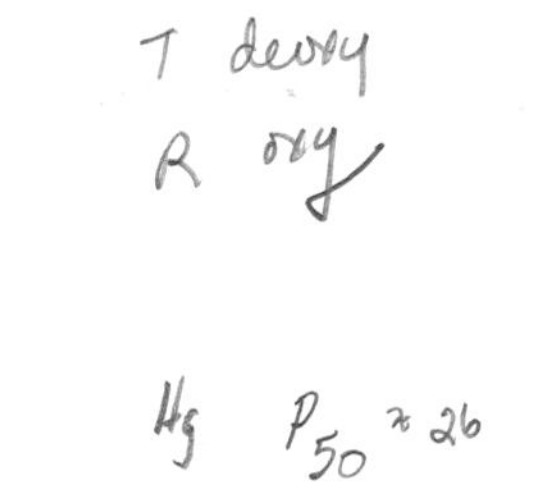

to oxyhemoglobin, and the two dimers occupy different relative positions in deoxyhemoglobin and oxyhemoglobin (Figure 3.4):

a. The deoxy-form of hemoglobin is called the T- or ***taut*** form. The $\alpha_1\beta_1$ and $\alpha_2\beta_2$ dimers interact through a network of ionic bonds and hydrogen bonds that constrain the movement of the polypeptide chains.

b. The binding of oxygen to hemoglobin causes rupture of some of the ionic bonds and hydrogen bonds between the $\alpha_1\beta_1$ and $\alpha_2\beta_2$ dimers. This leads to a structure called the R or ***relaxed*** form in which the polypeptide chains have more freedom of movement.

D. Binding of oxygen to hemoglobin

1. Hemoglobin can bind one oxygen molecule (O_2) at each of its four heme-containing subunits. The saturation of these oxygen binding sites (Y) is defined as the fractional occupancy of the total binding sites. The value of Y can vary between zero (all sites empty) and 100% (all four sites full) (Figure 3.5).

2. A plot of Y measured at different partial pressures of oxygen is called the ***oxygen saturation curve***. The curves for myoglobin and hemoglobin show important differences (Figure 3.5):

   a. Myoglobin has a higher oxygen affinity than hemoglobin. The partial pressure of oxygen needed to achieve half-saturation of the binding sites (P_{50}) is approximately 1 mm Hg for myoglobin and 26 mm Hg for hemoglobin (Figure 3.5). The more tightly oxygen binds, the lower is the P_{50}.

   b. The oxygen dissociation curve for myoglobin has a ***hyperbolic shape*** (see Figure 3.5). This reflects the fact that myoglobin reversibly binds a single molecule of oxygen. Thus oxygenated

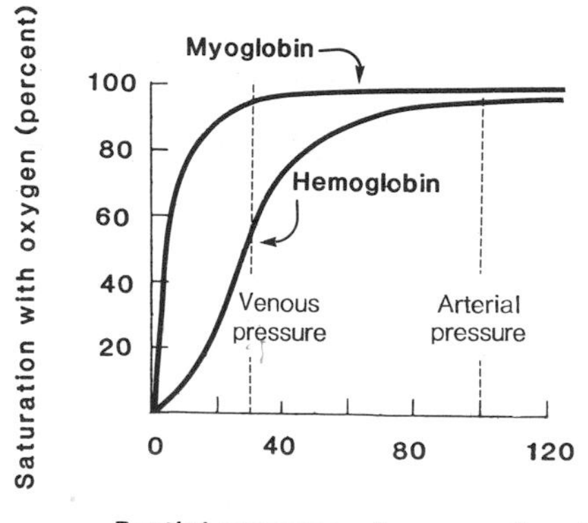

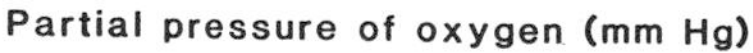

Figure 3.5
Oxygen saturation curve for myoglobin and hemoglobin.

(MbO_2) and deoxygenated (Mb) myoglobin exist in a simple equilibrium:

$$Mb + O_2 \leftrightarrows MbO_2$$

The equilibrium is shifted to the right or the left as oxygen is added to or removed from the system.

c. The oxygen dissociation curve for hemoglobin is ***sigmoidal*** in shape (see Figure 3.5), indicating that the subunits cooperate in binding oxygen. This ***cooperative binding*** results from the fact that the binding of an oxygen molecule at one heme increases the oxygen affinity of the remaining heme groups in the same hemoglobin molecule. Although it is difficult for the first oxygen molecule to bind to hemoglobin, subsequent binding of oxygen occurs with a high affinity as shown by the steep upward curve in the region near 20 to 30 mm Hg (see Figure 3.5).

3. The sigmoidal oxygen binding curve reflects specific structural changes that are initiated at one heme group and transmitted to other heme groups in the hemoglobin tetramer. The net effect is that the affinity of hemoglobin for the last oxygen bound is approximately 300-fold greater than the affinity of the first oxygen bound.

4. The cooperative binding of oxygen allows hemoglobin to deliver more oxygen to the tissues in response to relatively small changes in the partial pressure of oxygen. This can be seen from Figure 3.5, which depicts estimates of the partial pressure of oxygen (PO_2) in the alveoli of the lung and the capillaries of the tissues.

a. In the lung, the concentration of oxygen is high, and hemoglobin becomes virtually saturated (or "loaded") with oxygen (Y = 97%).

b. In peripheral tissues oxyhemoglobin releases (or "unloads") much of its oxygen (Y = 50%) for use in the oxidative metabolism of the tissues.

c. This release of oxygen explains the steep slope of the oxygen dissociation curve over the range of oxygen concentrations that occur in the tissues. A molecule with a hyperbolic oxygen saturation curve, such as myoglobin, could not achieve the same degree of oxygen release over such a limited difference in the range of partial pressures of oxygen present in the peripheral tissues.

E. Allosteric effects

1. ***The Bohr effect:*** The release of oxygen by the hemoglobin is enhanced when the pH is lowered or in the presence of increased partial pressure of CO_2 (see p. 27). Both result in a decreased oxygen affinity of hemoglobin, and therefore a shift to the right in the oxygen saturation curve (Figure 3.6). This change in oxygen binding is called the Bohr effect. Conversely, raising the pH or lowering the concentration of CO_2 results in greater affinity for oxygen and a shift to the left in the oxygen saturation curve.

a. The concentration of both CO_2 and H^+ in the capillaries of metabolically active tissues is higher than that observed in

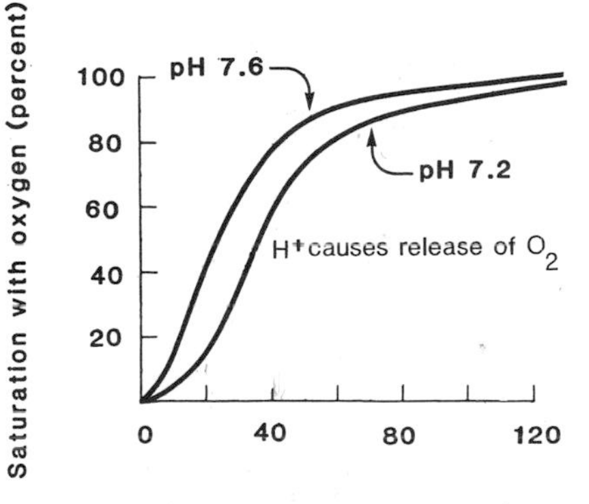

Figure 3.6
Effect of pH on the oxygen affinity of hemoglobin.

alveolar capillaries of the lungs, where CO_2 is released into the expired air. This differential concentration favors the unloading of oxygen in the peripheral tissues and the loading of oxygen in the lung. Thus the oxygen affinity of the hemoglobin molecule responds to small shifts in pH between the lung and oxygen-consuming tissues, thus making hemoglobin a more efficient transporter of oxygen.

b. The Bohr effect reflects the fact that the deoxy-form of hemoglobin has a greater affinity for protons than does oxyhemoglobin. This can be represented schematically as

$$\underset{\text{oxyhemoglobin}}{HbO_2} + H^+ \rightleftarrows \underset{\text{deoxyhemoglobin}}{Hb \cdot H^+} + O_2$$

Specifically, three ionizable groups (a terminal amino group and two histidine side chains) in the β-chains have higher pK_a's (see p. 6) in deoxyhemoglobin than in oxyhemoglobin. Thus, an increase in the concentration of protons (decrease in pH) preferentially stabilizes the deoxy-form of hemoglobin, producing a decrease in oxygen affinity.

2. ***Effect of 2,3-diphosphoglycerate on oxygen affinity:*** 2,3-Diphosphoglycerate (2,3-DPG) is an important regulator of the binding of oxygen to hemoglobin. It is the most abundant organic phosphate in the red blood cell, where it is found in concentrations roughly equivalent to that of hemoglobin. 2,3-DPG is synthesized from intermediates of glycolysis (see p. 115).

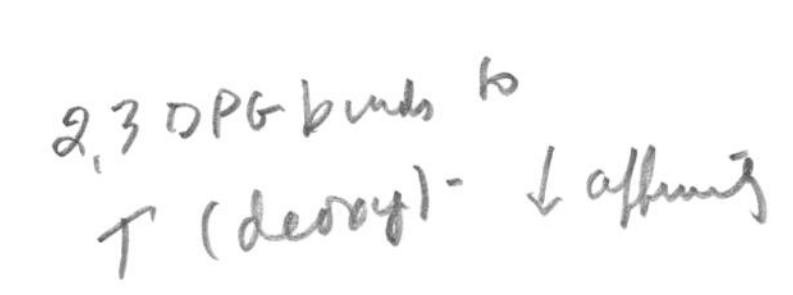

a. Hemoglobin stripped of 2,3-DPG shows a high affinity for oxygen. However, in the red blood cell, the presence of 2,3-DPG significantly reduces the affinity of hemoglobin for oxygen, shifting the oxygen dissociation curve to the right (Figure 3.7). This reduced affinity enables hemoglobin to release oxygen at the partial pressures needed by the tissues for oxidative metabolism.

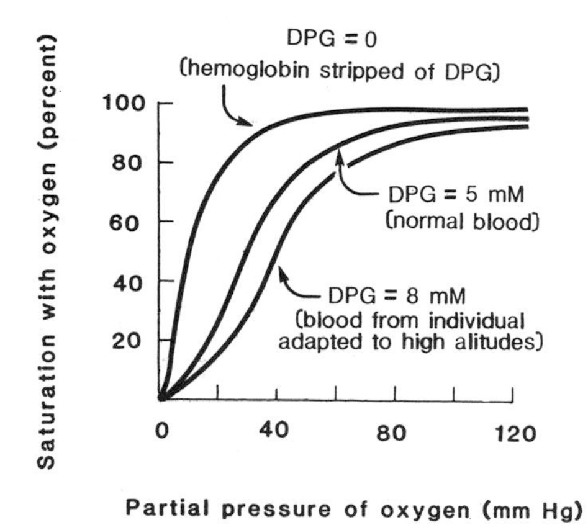

Figure 3.7
Effect of 2,3-diphosphogycerate on the oxygen affinity of hemoglobin.

b. 2,3-DPG decreases the oxygen affinity of hemoglobin by binding to deoxyhemoglobin but ***not*** to oxyhemoglobin. This preferential binding stabilizes the taut configuration of deoxyhemoglobin. The effect of binding 2,3-DPG can be represented schematically as

$$\underset{\text{oxyhemoglobin}}{HbO_2} + \text{2,3-DPG} \rightleftarrows \underset{\text{deoxyhemoglobin}}{Hb \cdot \text{2,3-DPG}} + O_2$$

c. One molecule of 2,3-DPG binds to a pocket in the center of the deoxyhemoglobin tetramer, formed by the two β-chains. This pocket is lined with positively charged amino acids that form ionic bonds with the negatively charged phosphate groups of 2,3-DPG. 2,3-DPG is expelled upon oxygenation of the hemoglobin.

d. The concentration of 2,3-DPG in the red blood cell increases in response to chronic hypoxia, such as that observed in obstructive pulmonary emphysema, high altitudes, or chronic anemia (Figure 3.7). Elevated 2,3-DPG levels lower the oxygen affinity of hemoglobin, allowing greater unloading of oxygen in the capillaries of the tissues.

e. 2,3-DPG is essential for the normal transport function of hemoglobin. For example, storing blood in acid-citrate-dextrose, a formerly widely used medium, leads to a decrease of 2,3-DPG in the red cells. Such blood displays an abnormally high oxygen affinity and fails to unload properly its bound oxygen in the tissues. Hemoglobin, deficient in 2,3-DPG, thus acts as an oxygen "trap," rather than as an oxygen transport system. Although transfused red blood cells are able to restore their depleted supplies of 2,3-DPG in 24 to 48 hours, severely ill patients may be seriously compromised by transfusing large quantities of such "stripped" blood. The decrease in 2,3-DPG can be prevented by adding inosine to the storage medium. Inosine, an uncharged molecule, can enter the red blood cell, where it is converted to 2,3-DPG.

3. ***Binding of CO_2:*** Most of the carbon dioxide produced in metabolism is hydrated and transported as bicarbonate ion. However, some CO_2 is carried as carbamate bound to the uncharged α-amino groups of hemoglobin, which can be shown schematically as follows:

$$\text{Hb—NH}_2 + CO_2 \rightleftarrows \text{Hb—NH—}\underset{\underset{\text{O}}{\|}}{\text{C}}\text{—O}^- + H^+$$

The binding of CO_2 stabilizes the T (taut) or deoxy-form of hemoglobin, resulting in a decrease in its affinity for oxygen, as described on p. 25.

F. Minor hemoglobins

1. ***Hemoglobin A_{1C}:*** Under physiologic conditions, glucose reacts non-enzymically with the N-terminal amino groups of the β-chain of HbA to form hemoglobin A_{1C} (HbA_{1C}, Figure 3.8). Hemoglobin A_{1C} constitutes an average of about 5% of the total hemoglobin of the erythrocyte. However, in individuals with diabetes mellitus (see p. 290 for a description of this disease) the amount is elevated twofold to threefold. The rate of formation of HbA_{1C} is proportional to the concentration of glucose in the blood. The glycosylation of Hb is not reversible. Therefore, once formed, HbA_{1C} persists for the life span of the erythrocyte. Thus, the total HbA_{1C} in a population of red blood cells reflects the average glucose concentration during the previous 6 to 10 weeks. The levels of HbA_{1C} can be used as an index of long-term control of hyperglycemia during the treatment of diabetes (see p. 294).

2. ***Hemoglobin A_2 (HbA_2):*** HbA_2 is a minor component of normal adult hemoglobin, first appearing about 12 weeks after birth and constituting about 2.5% of the total hemoglobin. It comprises two α-chains and two δ-chains.

3. ***Fetal hemoglobin (HbF):*** HbF is a tetramer with two α-chains identical to those in HbA, plus two γ-chains. The γ-chains are similar in amino acid sequence to β-chains of HbA but differ in 37 amino acids.

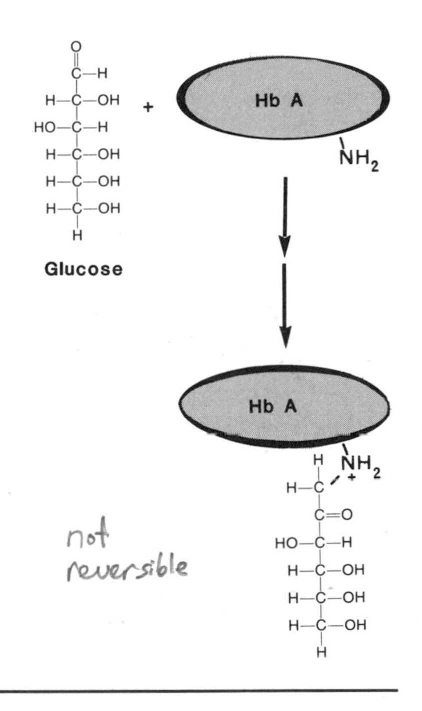

Figure 3.8
Nonenzymic addition of glucose to hemoglobin.

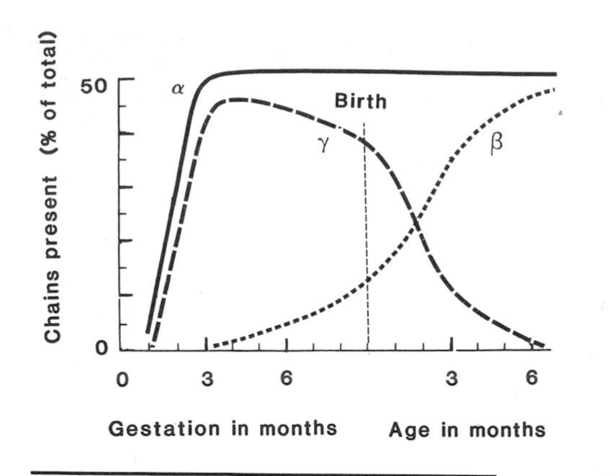

Figure 3.9
Percentage of total polypeptides present in the erythrocyte at various stages of development.

a. HbF is the major hemoglobin found in the fetus and newborn. During the last months of fetal life, HbF accounts for about 60% of the total hemoglobin in the erythrocyte (Figure 3.9). Hemoglobin A synthesis starts at about the eighth month of pregnancy and gradually replaces hemoglobin F.

b. Under physiologic conditions fetal hemoglobin (HbF) has a higher affinity for oxygen than does HbA owing to HbF's binding only weakly to 2,3-DPG. Since 2,3-DPG serves to reduce the affinity of hemoglobin for oxygen, this weak interaction between 2,3-DPG and HbF results in a higher oxygen affinity for HbF relative to HbA. In contrast, if both hemoglobins are stripped of their 2,3-DPG, HbA and HbF have a similar affinity for oxygen.

c. The high oxygen affinity facilitates the transfer of oxygen from the maternal circulation across the placenta to the red blood cells of the fetus. Figure 3.9 shows the relative production of each type of hemoglobin chain during fetal and postnatal life.

III. HEMOGLOBINOPATHIES

Hemoglobinopathies have traditionally been defined as a family of disorders caused either by production of a structurally abnormal hemoglobin molecule or by synthesis of insufficient quantities of normal hemoglobin. Sickle cell anemia and the thalassemia syndromes are two representative hemoglobinopathies that can have severe clinical consequences. Sickle cell anemia results from production of a hemoglobin with an altered amino acid sequence, whereas the thalassemias are caused by decreased production of normal hemoglobin. It is now known that some mutations lead both to alteration of globin structure and to decreased synthesis. These latter mutations are relatively rare and will not be discussed.

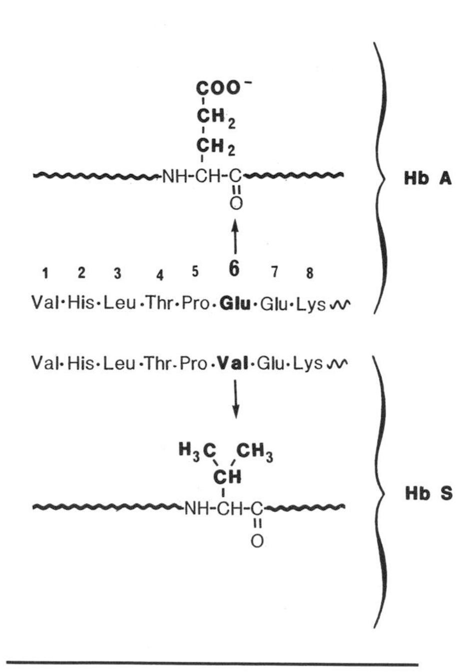

Figure 3.10
Substitution of valine for glutamate in hemoglobin S.

A. Sickle cell anemia

1. Sickle cell anemia, also called ***sickle cell disease,*** is the most common disorder resulting from the production of a variant hemoglobin. It primarily occurs in the black population, affecting 1 in 500 newborn infants in the United States. Sickle cell anemia is a ***homozygous recessive disorder*** occurring in individuals who have inherited two mutant genes (one from each parent) that code for synthesis of the β-chains of the globin molecules (see p. 377 for a discussion of protein synthesis).

2. ***Heterozygotes,*** representing one of ten American blacks, have one normal and one sickle cell gene. The blood cells of such heterozygotes contain both HbS and HbA. These individuals have ***sickle cell trait;*** they usually do not show clinical symptoms.

3. A molecule of HbS contains two normal α-chains and two mutant β-chains in which ***glutamate*** at position six has been ***replaced with valine*** (Figure 3.10).

4. During electrophoresis at alkaline pH, HbS migrates more slowly toward the anode (positive electrode) than does HbA (Figure 3.11). This altered mobility of HbS is due to the absence of two negatively charged glutamate residues in the β-chains, thus rendering HbS

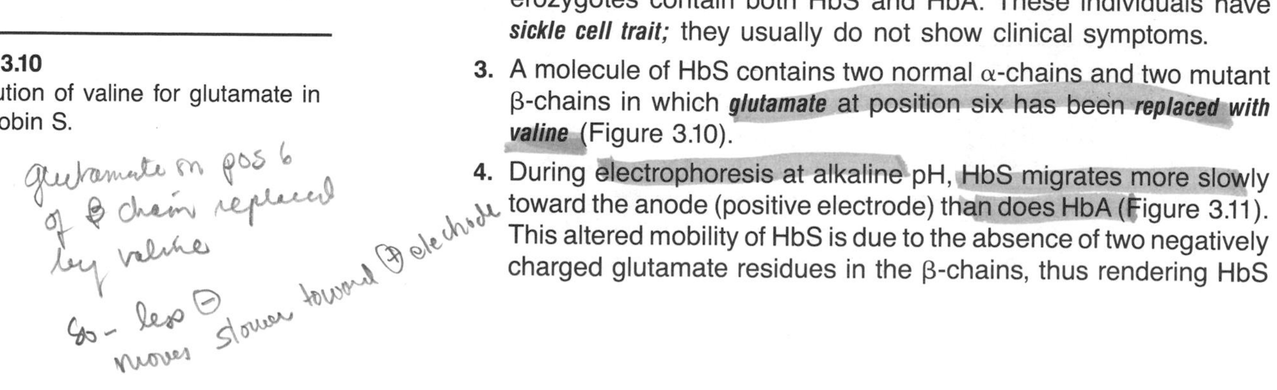

less negative than HbA. Electrophoresis of hemoglobin obtained from lysed red blood cells is routinely used in the diagnosis of sickle cell trait and sickle cell disease.

5. The substitution of the nonpolar side chain of valine for a charged glutamate residue results in a pronounced decrease in the solubility of HbS in its ***deoxygenated*** form. The molecules aggregate to form fibers that deform the red cells into a crescent or sickle shape. Such sickled cells frequently block the flow of blood in the small diameter capillaries. This interruption in the supply of oxygen leads to localized anoxia (oxygen deprivation), which causes pain and eventually death of cells in the vicinity.

6. The extent of sickling and, hence, the severity of disease are increased by any variable that increases the proportion of HbS in the deoxy state, such as
   - decreased oxygen tension caused by high altitude or flying in a nonpressurized plane.
   - increased CO_2 concentration.
   - decreased pH.
   - increased concentration of 2,3-DPG in erythrocytes.

7. The high frequency of the hemoglobin S gene among black Africans, despite its damaging effects in the homozygous state, suggests that a selective advantage exists for those heterozygotes with only one mutant gene. For example, heterozygotes for the sickle cell gene are less susceptible to some forms of malaria. This disease is caused by a parasite, the most dangerous being ***Plasmodium falciparum***. This organism spends an obligatory part of its life cycle in the red blood cell. Since the red blood cells of the heterozygote, as well as the homozygote, have a shorter life span than normal red blood cells, the parasite cannot complete this stage of its development. This may provide a selective advantage to heterozygous individuals living in those regions where malaria is a major cause of death.

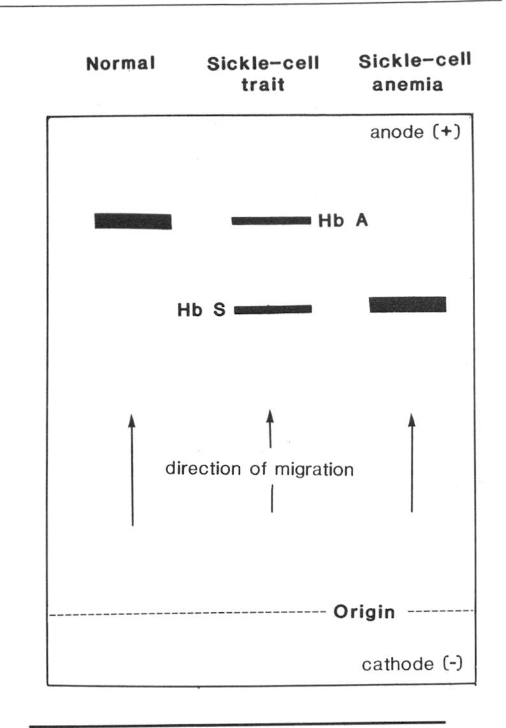

Figure 3.11
Electrophoresis of hemoglobins obtained from individuals who have sickle cell trait or sickle cell disease. Blood from normal individuals contains HbA and is shown for reference.

B. Thalassemias

1. The thalassemias are a group of hereditary hemolytic diseases in which there is an imbalance in the synthesis of globin chains. Normally, synthesis of the α- and β-chains is coordinated so that each α-chain has a β-chain partner. This leads to the formation of $\alpha_2\beta_2$ globin tetramers of hemoglobin A. In the thalassemias, the synthesis of either the α- or β-chain is defective. For example, α-thalassemia syndromes are a group of defects in which the synthesis of α-chains is decreased or absent. The synthesis of the unaffected β-chain continues, however, resulting in the accumulation of β_4 tetramers (hemoglobin H) that tend to precipitate.

2. In the more severe β-thalassemia disorders, synthesis of β-chains is decreased, whereas α-chain synthesis is normal. This leads to the precipitation of aggregates of α-chains, which causes the premature death of cells destined to become mature red blood cells.

3. The decreased synthesis of globin chains seen in various α- and β-thalassemias is not the result of a single type of gene mutation. Rather, each of these syndromes may be caused by a variety

of mutations that have the common feature of interrupting the normal process of protein synthesis described on p. 381. α-Thalassemias are most often due to gene deletions, whereas β-thalassemias are frequently caused by nucleotide substitutions or deletion of one or several nucleotides.

4. Individuals who are homozygous for gene mutations that produce β-thalassemia are designated β° or ***thalassemia major.*** These patients are severely anemic and require regular transfusions of blood. Although this treatment is lifesaving, the cumulative effect of the transfusions is iron overload (a syndrome known as ***hemosiderosis***), which typically causes death between the ages of 15 and 25 years.

5. Individuals who are heterozygous for β-thalassemia are termed β^+ or ***thalassemia minor.*** These individuals make some β-chains and usually do not require specific treatment.

Study Questions

Answer A if 1, 2 and 3 are correct
B if 1 and 3 are correct
C if 2 and 4 are correct
D if only 4 is correct
E if all are correct

3.1 Which of the following statements about the binding of oxygen by hemoglobin is(are) correct?

1. The oxygen affinity of any one heme group depends on the quaternary structure of the molecule.
2. Carbon dioxide lowers the oxygen affinity of hemoglobin by binding to the amino terminal groups of the polypeptide chains.
3. The Bohr effect results in a greater affinity for oxygen at higher pHs.
4. The hemoglobin tetramer binds four molecules of 2,3-DPG.

3.2 Which of the following statements about hemoglobin is(are) correct?

1. The heme groups of hemoglobin are surrounded only by nonpolar side chains of the protein globin.
2. There are no proline residues in hemoglobin because their presence would disrupt the large number of α-helices present in the molecule.
3. Oxyhemoglobin and deoxyhemoglobin have the same affinity for protons (H^+).
4. The polypeptide conformation of hemoglobin allows it to form a stable complex with oxygen without any oxidation of the iron in the heme.

3.3 Which of the following statements is(are) correct about 2,3-diphosphoglycerate:

1. It is formed from an intermediate of the glycolytic pathway.
2. By binding to hemoglobin, it stabilizes the deoxy form of hemoglobin and makes it more difficult for oxygen to bind.
3. It is believed to form ionic bonds with positively charged amino acid R-groups in the center of the hemoglobin molecule.
4. It markedly affects the sigmoidal shape of the oxygen saturation curve for hemoglobin.

3.4 Which of the following hemeproteins would be expected to show a lower (weaker) affinity for oxygen, compared to hemoglobin A at pH 7.4. (Assume that the concentration of 2,3-DPG is 5mM, which is similar to that which occurs in the red blood cell.)

1. Hemoglobin F
2. Methemoglobin A
3. Myoglobin
4. Hemoglobin A at pH 7.2

3.5 You are presented with a patient who has mild anemia and whose hemoglobin has the same electrophoretic mobility (at pH 9.3) as sickle cell hemoglobin (HbS). However, the patient's cells do not sickle on deoxygenation. Which of the following genetic changes can explain the electrophoretic mobility?

1. A mutation that deletes a serine residue from the β-chain.
2. A substitution mutation that replaces a lysine residue in the β-chain with a phenylalanine.
3. A deletion mutation that deletes an arginine residue from the β-chain.
4. A substitution mutation that replaces an alanine residue in the β-chain with an arginine.

3.6 Hemoglobin A and hemoglobin S are the same with respect to which of the following?

1. Amino acid sequence of β-chain
2. Electrophoretic mobility at pH 8.6
3. Solubility in the deoxygenated form
4. Structure of the heme group

IV. COLLAGEN

Collagen is the most abundant protein in the human body. Collagen is not a single protein, but rather refers to a closely related family of rigid, insoluble proteins found in all multicellular organisms. Although these molecules are found throughout the body, their type and organization are dictated by the structural role collagen plays in a particular organ. In some tissues, collagen may be dispersed as a gel that serves to stiffen the structure, as in the extracellular matrix or the vitreous humor of the eye. In other tissues, collagen may be bundled in tight parallel fibers that provide great strength (as in tendons). In the cornea of the eye collagen is stacked so as to transmit light with a minimum of scattering. Collagen of bone occurs as fibers arranged at angles to each other so as to resist mechanical shear from any direction. The polypeptide precursors of the collagen molecule are formed in fibroblasts (or in the related osteoblasts of bone and chondroblasts of cartilage) and are secreted into the extracellular matrix. After enzymic modification the finished collagen monomers aggregate and are cross-linked to form collagen fibrils.

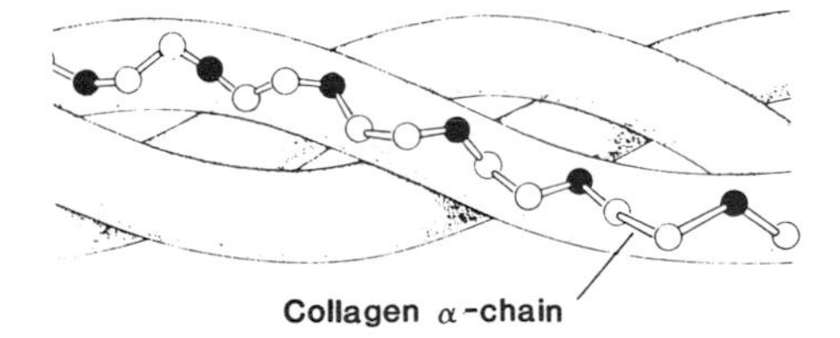

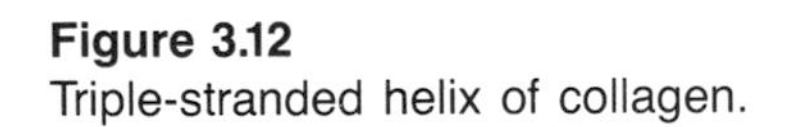

Figure 3.12
Triple-stranded helix of collagen.

A. Structure of collagen

1. ***Types of collagen:*** Collagen molecules each comprise three polypeptides, called ***α-chains,*** which wrap around each other in a triple helix, forming a ropelike structure (Figure 3.12). Variations occur in the amino acid sequence of the α-chains, resulting in structural components that are the same size (approximately 1000 amino acids in length) but with slightly different properties. These α-chains are combined to form the various types of collagen found in the tissues. For example, the most common collagen, type I, contains two chains called α_1, and one chain called α_2.

2. ***Amino acid sequence:*** The primary structure of collagen is unusual in that glycine, the smallest amino acid, is found in every third position of the polypeptide chain. The glycine residues are part of a repeating sequence, —Gly—X—Y—, where X is frequently proline and Y is usually hydroxyproline or hydroxylysine (Figure 3.13). Thus, most of the molecule can be regarded as a polytripeptide whose sequence can be represented as

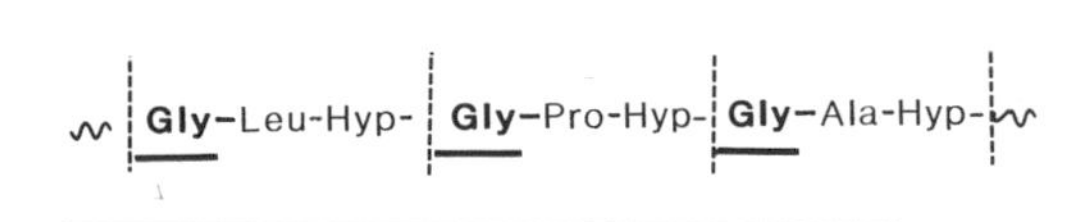

Figure 3.13
Amino acid sequence of a portion of the α_1 chain of collagen.

(—Gly—X—Y—)$_{333}$. Glycine fits into the restricted space where the three chains of the helix come together. The three polypeptide chains are held together by hydrogen bonds between the peptide nitrogen of glycine residues in one chain and the carbonyl oxygen of another.

3. ***Triple helical structure:*** Unlike most globular proteins that are folded into a compact structure, collagen has an elongated triple helical structure that places many of its amino acid side chains on the outside of the molecule. This allows interaction between triple helical molecules that leads to aggregation of collagen into fibers.

4. ***Collagen contains hydroxyproline and hydroxylysine, which are not present in most other proteins:*** Hydroxyproline and hydroxylysine of collagen result from the hydroxylation of certain proline and lysine residues after their incorporation into polypeptide chains. The hydroxylation is thus an example of ***post-translational modification*** (see p. 383). Hydroxyproline is important in stabilizing the triple helical structure.

5. ***The hydroxyl group of the hydroxylysine residues of collagen may be glycosylated.*** Most commonly, a disaccharide of glucose and galactose is attached to the polypeptide chain before helix formation.

B. Biosynthesis of collagen

1. ***Formation of pro-α-chains:*** Collagen is one of many proteins that normally function ***outside*** the cell. Like most proteins synthesized for export, the nascent polypeptide chains of collagen contain a special amino acid sequence at the N-terminal ends of the molecules. This sequence of 50 to 100 amino acids acts as a "signal" that the protein being synthesized is destined to leave the cell. The ***signal sequence*** facilitates the binding of ribosomes to the rough endoplasmic reticulum (RER) and directs the passage of the polypeptide chain into the cisternae of the RER. As with other secretory proteins, the signal sequence is rapidly cleaved in the endoplasmic reticulum to yield a precursor of collagen called a ***pro-α-chain*** (see p. 383 for further discussion of secretory proteins).

2. ***Hydroxylation and glycosylation:*** The pro-α-polypeptide chains are processed by a number of enzymatic steps while the polypeptides are still being synthesized on the ribosome (see p. 381). Proline and lysine residues found in the Y-position of the —Gly—X—Y— sequence can be hydroxylated to form ***hydroxyproline*** and ***hydroxylysine*** residues. These hydroxylation reactions require molecular oxygen and a reducing agent such as ***vitamin C*** (ascorbic acid, see p. 321). Hydroxyproline accounts for about 10% of the total amino acids of collagen, whereas hydroxylysine varies between 0.5% and 5%. Some of the hydroxylysine residues are further modified by glycosylation with glucose or galactose sugars (Figure 3.14).

3. ***Assembly and secretion:*** After hydroxylation and glycosylation, pro-α-chains form ***procollagen,*** a precursor of collagen that has a central region of triple helix surrounded by the nonhelical amino- and carboxyl-terminal extensions called ***propeptides*** (Figure 3.14). The formation of procollagen begins with interchain disulfide

Figure 3.14
Formation of collagen fibers. ►

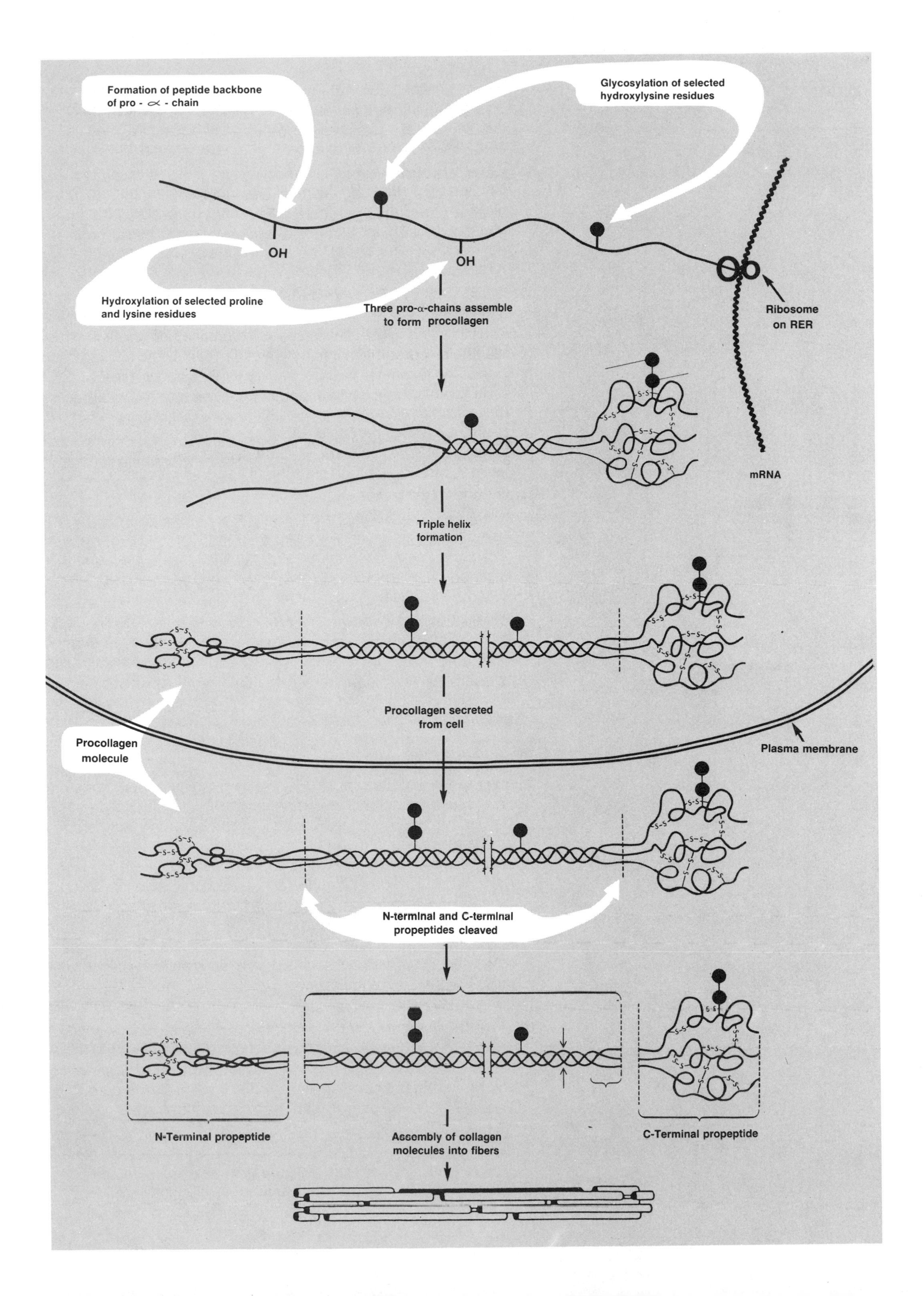

Formation of peptide backbone of pro - α - chain
Glycosylation of selected hydroxylysine residues
OH
OH
Hydroxylation of selected proline and lysine residues
Three pro-α-chains assemble to form procollagen
Ribosome on RER
mRNA
Triple helix formation
Procollagen molecule
Procollagen secreted from cell
Plasma membrane
N-terminal and C-terminal propeptides cleaved
N-Terminal propeptide
Assembly of collagen molecules into fibers
C-Terminal propeptide

bonds between the C-terminal extensions of the pro-α-chains. This brings the three chains into an alignment favorable for helix formation. The procollagen molecules are packaged into vesicles and released into the extracellular space (Figure 3.14).

4. ***Extracellular processing:*** The procollagen molecule, secreted from the fibroblast into the extracellular matrix, is modified by two types of reactions in preparation for fiber formation. First, the N- and C-terminal propeptides are cleaved by extracellular proteases (Figure 3.14). This allows the polypeptide chains to form the triple helical collagen molecule that spontaneously associates into fibrils. Second, the collagen fibrils are strengthened by inter-molecular cross-links. Specific lysyl and hydroxylysyl residues are oxidatively deaminated to aldehydes, which form covalent bridges between different procollagen molecules.

C. Collagen diseases

1. ***Ehlers-Danlos syndrome*** is one of three major groups of disorders that result from inheritable defects in the collagen molecule. This family of related diseases is characterized by stretchy skin and loose joints. Many of the contortionists seen in circus side shows suffer from this syndrome, which may be due to any of several enzyme deficiencies.
2. ***Marfan's syndrome*** is characterized by long spidery fingers and toes. The aorta and pulmonary arteries are structurally weak and have a tendency to rupture. The disease is due to deficient type I collagen formation.
3. ***Osteogenesis imperfecta***, or brittle bone syndrome, is distinguished by bones that easily bend and fracture. Retarded wound healing and a rotated and twisted spine leading to a humpbacked appearance are also common features of the disease.

Study Questions

Answer A if 1, 2 and 3 are correct
B if 1 and 3 are correct
C if 2 and 4 are correct
D if only 4 is correct
E if all are correct

3.7 Which of the following statements about the major collagen type from skin or bone is(are) correct?

1. One third of the amino acid composition of collagen is glycine.
2. Ascorbate is required for the synthesis of triple-helical collagen.
3. Collagen molecules are trimers composed of three monomers each containing approximately 1000 amino acids.
4. Collagen fibrils contain covalent cross-links.

3.8 Complete the numbered statements below with the correct lettered terms.

A if item is associated with (A) only
B if item is associated with (B) only
C if item is associated with both (A) and (B)
D if item is associated with neither (A) nor (B)

(A) Mature collagen fibril
(B) Procollagen

1. contain(s) the amino acid glycine.
2. contain(s) C- and N-terminal extensions (propeptides).
3. contain(s) covalent cross-links.
4. is(are) globular proteins.
5. is(are) intracellular proteins.

Enzymes

4

I. OVERVIEW

Virtually all chemical reactions that occur in biological systems have an energy barrier separating the reactants and the products. This barrier prevents reactions from proceeding in an uncontrolled and spontaneous manner. In cells these reactions are catalyzed by enzymes—specialized proteins that allow reactions to occur at a rate appropriate to the needs of the cell. This chapter examines the nature and mechanism of these catalytic molecules.

II. NOMENCLATURE

A. Some enzymes retain their early trivial names, which give no hint of the associated enzymatic reaction, for example, *trypsin* and *pepsin*.

B. Most commonly-used enzyme names have the suffix "-ase" attached to some intermediate in the reaction, for example, *glucosidase*, or to a description of the action performed, for example, *ribonuclease* and *adenyl cyclase*.

C. The International Union of Biochemists (IUB) has developed a system of nomenclature in which the suffix "-ase" is attached to a fairly complete description of the chemical reaction catalyzed, for example, *D-glyceraldehyde 3-phosphate:NAD oxidoreductase*. The IUB names are unambiguous but are sometimes too cumbersome to be of general use.

III. PROPERTIES OF ENZYMES

A. ***Enzymes are protein catalysts.*** They increase the velocity of a chemical reaction and are not consumed during the reaction they catalyze.

B. ***Enzymes show a high catalytic efficiency.*** Most enzyme-catalyzed reactions proceed from 10^3 to 10^6 times faster than uncatalyzed reactions. Typically each enzyme molecule is capable of transforming 100 to 1000 substrate molecules into product each second.

C. ***Enzymes are highly specific***, catalyzing only one type of chemical reaction. For example, enzymes may act on a particular optical isomer or an isolated chemical group on the substrate.

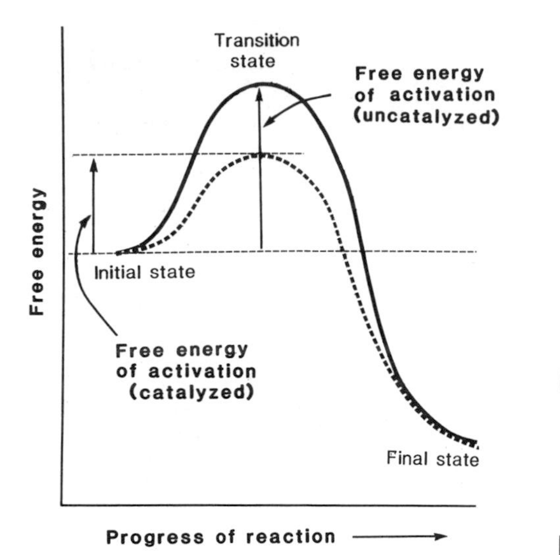

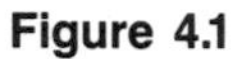

Figure 4.1
Effect of an enzyme on the activation energy of a reaction.

D. ***Some enzymes contain a nonprotein cofactor that is needed for enzymic activity.*** Commonly encountered cofactors include metal ions (e.g., Zn^{++}, Fe^{++}) and derivatives of vitamins (e.g., NAD^{+}, FAD, coenzyme A).

1. ***Holoenzyme*** refers to the enzyme with its cofactor.
2. ***Apoenzyme*** refers to the protein portion of the holoenzyme. In the absence of the appropriate cofactor, the apoenzyme typically does not show biological activity.
3. A ***prosthetic group*** is a tightly bound cofactor that does not dissociate from the enzyme (such as the biotin of *carboxylases,* see p. 127).

E. ***Enzyme activity can be regulated.*** Some enzymes are activated or inhibited by binding allosteric modifiers (see p. 40) or by ***covalent modification*** of the enzyme itself (see p. 41).

IV. THEORY OF ENZYME CATALYSIS

A. ***Activation energy:*** All chemical reactions are impeded by an energy barrier called the ***energy of activation*** (Figure 4.1). The peak of energy represents the transition state during which a high-energy intermediate occurs in the conversion of reactant to product. Because of the activation energy, uncatalyzed chemical reactions generally do not occur spontaneously.

B. ***Energy distribution among molecules:*** For molecules to react they must contain sufficient energy to overcome the energy barrier. Without an enzyme, only a small proportion of a population of molecules possesses enough energy to achieve the transition state between reactant and product. The rate of reaction is determined by the number of such energized molecules. In general, the lower the energy of activation, the faster is the rate of reaction.

C. ***Alternate reaction pathway:*** An enzyme allows a reaction to proceed rapidly under conditions prevailing in the cell by providing an alternate reaction pathway with a lower energy of activation (Figure 4.1). The enzyme does not change the energies of the reactants or products, and therefore does not change the equilibrium of the reaction (see p. 98).

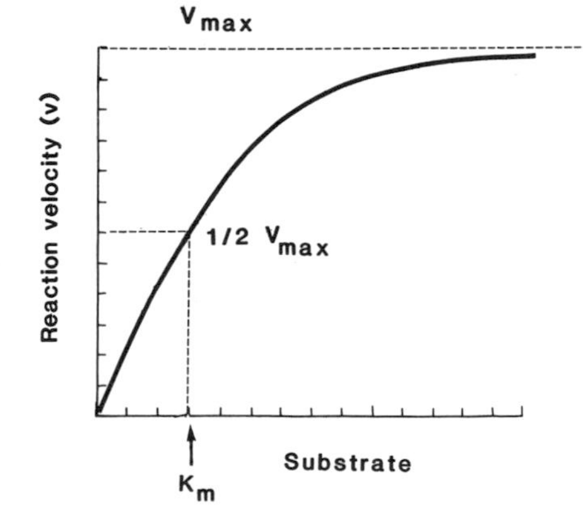

Figure 4.2
Effect of substrate concentration on reaction velocity for an enzyme catalyzed reaction.

V. FACTORS AFFECTING THE VELOCITY OF ENZYME-CATALYZED REACTIONS

A. Substrate concentration

1. The rate of an enzyme-catalyzed reaction increases with substrate concentration until a ***maximal velocity*** (V_m) is reached (Figure 4.2).The leveling off of the reaction rate at high substrate concentrations reflects the saturation of all available binding sites on the enzyme.
2. For enzymes showing Michaelis-Menten kinetics (see p. 37), a plot of reaction velocity against substrate concentration has a shape similar to the hyperbolic oxygen saturation curve of myoglobin (see p. 24). In contrast, allosteric enzymes (see p. 40)

frequently show a sigmoidal curve (see Figure 4.9), similar in shape to the oxygen saturation curve of hemoglobin (see p. 24).

B. Temperature

1. The reaction velocity increases with temperature until a maximum velocity is reached. This increase in reaction velocity is due to the increased number of molecules having sufficient energy to pass over the energy barrier and form the products of the reaction.
2. Further elevation of the temperature results in a decrease in reaction velocity owing to temperature-induced denaturation of the enzyme (Figure 4.3).

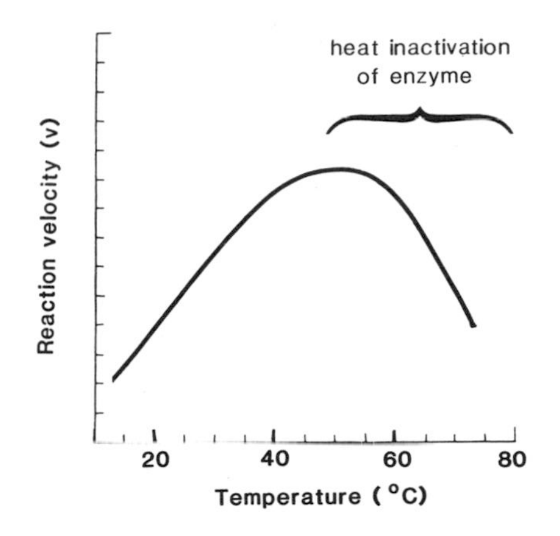

Figure 4.3
Effect of temperature on an enzyme-catalyzed reaction.

C. pH

1. The concentration of H^+ affects reaction velocity in several ways. First, the catalytic process usually requires that the enzyme and substrate have specific chemical groups either in an ionized or un-ionized state in order to interact. For example, catalytic activity may require that an amino group of the enzyme be in the protonated form ($—NH_3^+$). At alkaline pH this group will be deprotonated, and the rate of reaction will therefore decline.
2. Extremes of pH can also lead to denaturation of the enzyme, since the structure of the catalytically active enzyme molecule depends on the ionic character of the amino acid side chains (Figure 4.4).

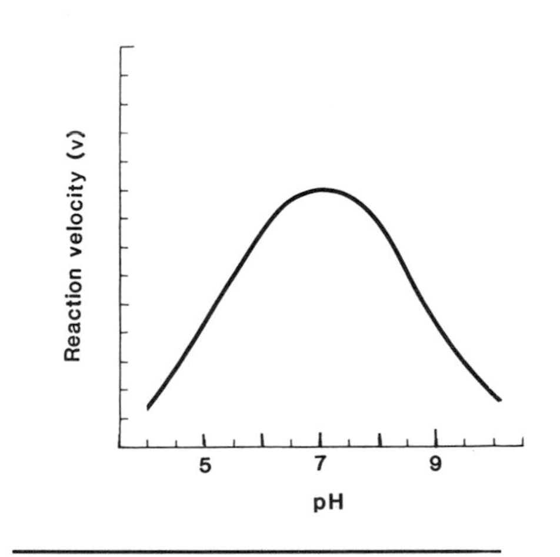

Figure 4.4
Effect of pH on an enzyme-catalyzed reaction.

VI. MICHAELIS-MENTEN EQUATION

A. ***Reaction model:*** The simplest model for an enzyme-catalyzed reaction involving one substrate molecule is represented below:

$$E + S \underset{k_{-1}}{\overset{k_1}{\rightleftarrows}} ES \overset{k_2}{\rightarrow} E + P$$

where S is the substrate
E is the enzyme
ES is the enzyme-substrate complex
k_1, k_{-1}, and k_2 are rate constants

B. ***Michaelis-Menten equation:*** Making certain assumptions, Michaelis and Menten derived the rate expression for this model of enzyme action:

$$v_o = \frac{[V_m][S]}{K_m + [S]}$$

where v_o = initial reaction velocity

V_m = maximal velocity

K_m = Michaelis constant = $\frac{k_{-1} + k_2}{k_1}$

$[S]$ = substrate concentration

C. *The following assumptions are involved in deriving the Michaelis-Menten rate equation:*

1. [S] is much greater than [E], so that the percentage of substrate bound by the enzyme at any one time is small.
2. [ES] does not change with time (the steady-state assumption):
   a. In general, an intermediate in a series of reactions is said to be in steady-state when its rate of synthesis is equal to its rate of degradation. For example, if the reaction velocities of enzyme 1 and enzyme 2 (E_1 and E_2, below) are equal, the concentration of intermediate B will not change with time, that is, it will be in a steady-state.

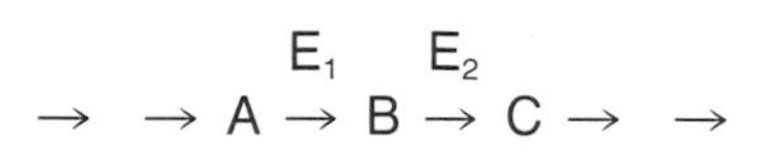

$$\rightarrow \; \rightarrow A \xrightarrow{E_1} B \xrightarrow{E_2} C \rightarrow \; \rightarrow$$

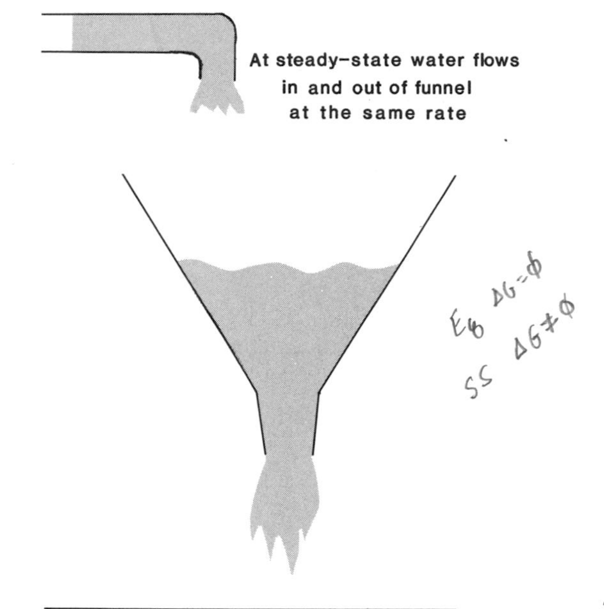

Figure 4.5
Water analogy of the steady-state.

   b. Water flowing into a funnel provides a simple hydraulic analogy of the steady-state (Figure 4.5).The level of water in the funnel (which corresponds to the concentration of an intermediate) will be constant (reach a steady-state) when the influx from above is balanced by the loss of water from the spout of the funnel.
   c. A chemical system in a steady-state differs from a reaction at equilibrium in several important ways:
      1) At equilibrium the concentrations of reactants and products are independent of the amount of enzyme that catalyzes the reaction. In contrast, the steady-state concentration of a substance is determined by the activity of enzymes involved in the formation and degradation of the compound.
      2) There is only one equilibrium ratio of products to reactants that is determined by the free energy of the reaction; however, the steady-state concentration of a compound can vary depending on its rate of formation and degradation.
3. Only ***initial*** reaction velocities are involved, that is, the rate of the reaction is measured as soon as enzyme and substrate are mixed. At that time the concentration of product will be very small, and therefore the rate of the back reaction from P to S can be ignored.

D. Important conclusions about Michaelis-Menten kinetics

1. For an enzyme following Michaelis-Menten kinetics a plot of v_o versus [S] gives a ***hyperbolic curve*** (see Figure 4.2).
2. K_m is a constant, characteristic of an enzyme and a particular substrate, and reflects the affinity of the enzyme for that substrate. K_m is numerically equal to the substrate concentration at which the reaction velocity is equal to ½ V_m. K_m does not vary with the concentration of enzyme.
   a. A numerically small (low) K_m reflects a ***high*** affinity of the enzyme for substrate since a low concentration of substrate is needed to half-saturate the enzyme.
   b. A numerically large (high) K_m reflects a ***low*** affinity of enzyme for substrate, since a high concentration of substrate is needed to half-saturate the enzyme.

c. An enzyme may have different K_m values for different substrates, indicating it has a different affinity for each substrate.

3. When [S] is much less than K_m, the velocity of the reaction is roughly proportional to the substrate concentration. The rate of reaction is then said to be ***first order*** with respect to substrate.

4. When [S] is much greater than K_m, the velocity is constant and equal to V_m. The rate of reaction is then said to be ***pseudo-zero-order*** with respect to substrate concentration.

   a. A substrate concentration that is much greater than K_m is used to assay quantitatively the total activity of a specific enzyme in, for example, plasma samples. Using a high substrate concentration increases the sensitivity of the assay to changes in the amount of enzyme present, since all enzyme molecules will be producing product under these conditions.

5. When $[S] = K_m$ the observed velocity is $\frac{1}{2}\ V_m$.

6. The rate of the reaction is directly proportional to the enzyme concentration.

VII. LINEWEAVER-BURKE PLOT

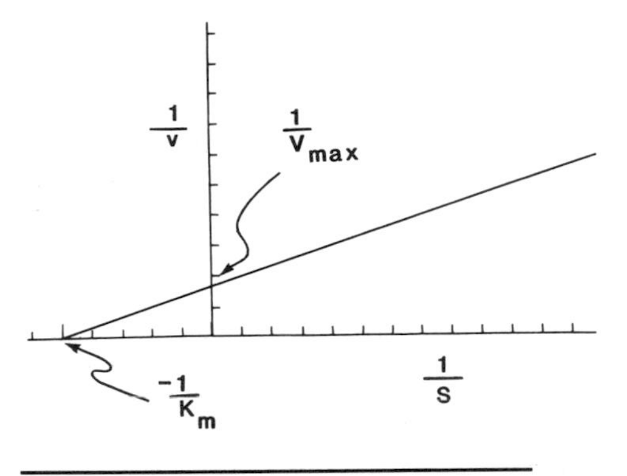

Figure 4.6
Lineweaver-Burke plot.

A. When v_o is plotted against [S], it is not always possible to determine when V_m has been achieved owing to the gradual upward slope of the hyperbolic curve at high substrate concentration. If, however, $1/v_o$ is plotted versus $1/[S]$, a straight line is obtained. This plot is called the ***Lineweaver-Burke plot*** (also called a double reciprocal plot) and can be used to calculate K_m and V_m as well as to determine the mechanism of action of enzyme inhibitors (Figure 4.6).

1. The equation describing this line is

$$\frac{1}{v_o} = \frac{K_m}{V_m[S]} + \frac{1}{V_m}$$

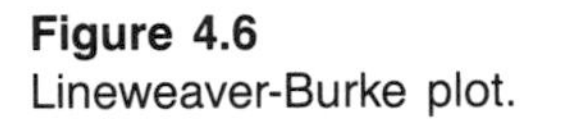

2. The intercept on the x-axis is equal to $-1/K_m$.

3. The intercept on the y-axis is equal to $1/V_m$.

VIII. INHIBITION OF ENZYME ACTIVITY

A. Any substance that can diminish the velocity of an enzyme-catalyzed reaction is called an ***inhibitor.*** The inhibition of enzymes can be classified either as reversible or irreversible:

1. ***Reversible inhibitors:*** These inhibitors bind to enzymes through noncovalent bonds. Dilution of the enzyme-inhibitor complex results in dissociation of the reversibly bound inhibitor and recovery of enzyme activity. Competitive and noncompetitive inhibitors are two commonly encountered sources of reversible inhibition.

2. ***Irreversible inhibition:*** This type of inhibition occurs when an inhibited enzyme does not regain activity upon dilution of the enzyme-inhibitor complex. Some irreversible inhibitors act by forming covalent bonds with specific groups of enzymes; for example,

the neurotoxic effects of certain insecticides are due to their irreversible binding at the catalytic site of the enzyme *acetylcholinesterase*.

B. ***Competitive inhibition:*** This type of inhibition occurs when the inhibitor binds reversibly to the same site that the substrate normally would occupy, and therefore competes with the substrate for that site.

1. ***Effect on V_m:*** The effect of a competitive inhibitor is reversed by increasing [S]. At a sufficiently high substrate concentration the reaction velocity reaches the V_m observed in the absence of inhibitor.
2. ***Effect on K_m:*** A competitive inhibitor increases the apparent K_m for a given substrate, which means that in the presence of a competitive inhibitor more substrate is needed to achieve ½ V_m.
3. ***Effect on Lineweaver-Burke plot:*** Competitive inhibition shows a characteristic Lineweaver-Burke plot in which the reciprocal plot of the inhibited and uninhibited reactions intersects on the Y axis at $1/V_m$ (V_m is unchanged). The inhibited and uninhibited reactions show different X axis intercepts, indicating that the apparent K_m is increased in the presence of the competitive inhibitor (see Figure 4.8).

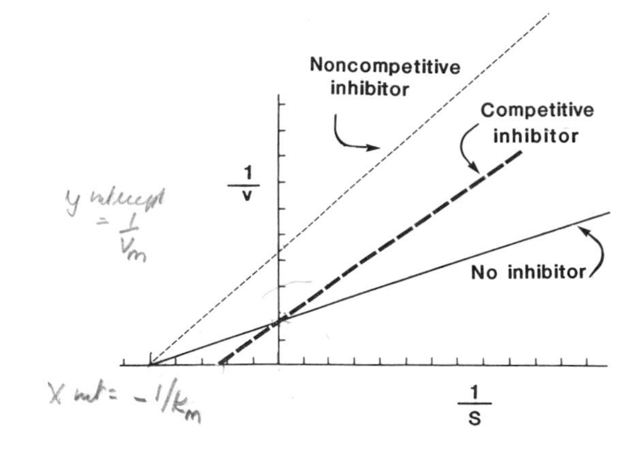

Figure 4.7
Lineweaver-Burke plot of competitive and noncompetitive inhibition of an enzyme.

C. ***Noncompetitive inhibition:*** This type of inhibition occurs when the inhibitor and substrate bind at different sites on the enzyme. The inhibitor can bind either free enzyme or the enzyme-substrate complex, thereby preventing the reactions from occurring.

1. ***Effect on V_m:*** Noncompetitive inhibition cannot be overcome by increasing the concentration of substrate. Thus, noncompetitive inhibitors decrease the V_m of the reaction.
2. ***Effect on K_m:*** Noncompetitive inhibitors do not interfere with the binding of substrate to enzyme. Thus, the enzyme shows the same K_m in the presence and absence of the noncompetitive inhibitor.
3. ***Effect on Lineweaver-Burke plot:*** Noncompetitive inhibition is readily differentiated from competitive inhibition by plotting $1/v_o$ versus 1/[S] and noting that V_m decreases in the presence of a noncompetitive inhibitor, whereas K_m is unchanged (Figure 4.7).

IX. ALLOSTERIC CONTROL OF ENZYME ACTIVITY

A. ***Allosteric binding sites:*** Allosteric enzymes are regulated by molecules called ***effectors*** (also called modifiers or modulators) that noncovalently bind at a site other than the active site. The presence of an allosteric effector can alter the affinity of the enzyme for its substrate or modify the maximal catalytic activity of the enzyme, or both. Effectors that inhibit enzyme activity are termed negative effectors, whereas those that result in an increased enzyme activity are called positive effectors.

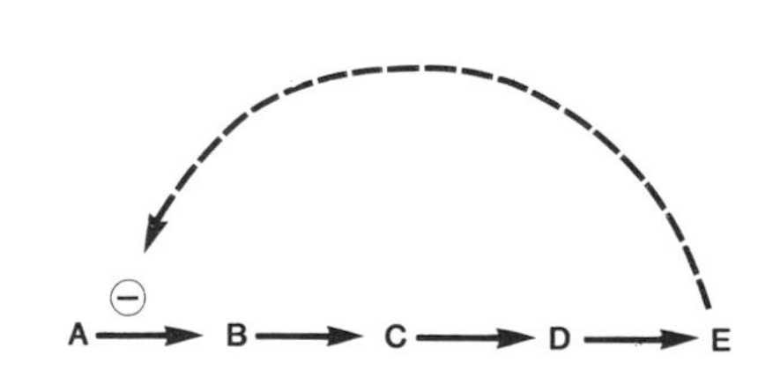

Figure 4.8
Feedback inhibition of a metabolic pathway.

1. The effector may be different from the substrate, in which case the effect is said to be ***heterotropic***. For example, consider the ***feedback inhibition*** shown in Figure 4.8. The enzyme that converts A to B has an allosteric site that binds the end-product E. If the

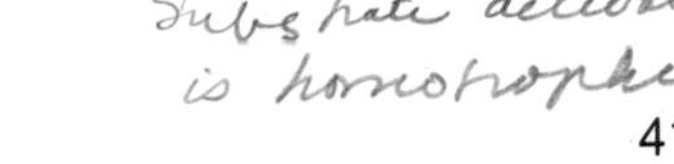

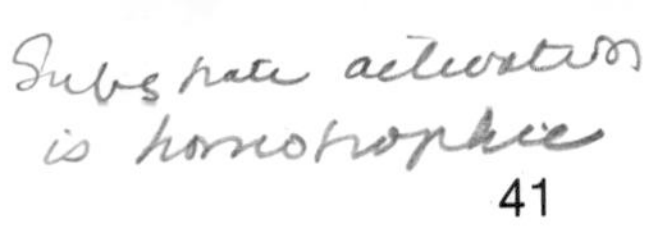

concentration of E increases (because it is not used as rapidly as it is synthesized), the initial enzyme in the pathway is inhibited. Feedback inhibition serves to coordinate the flow of substrate molecules through a series of reactions with the needs of the cell for the product of that particular pathway.

2. When the substrate itself serves as an effector, the effect is said to be ***homotropic***. Most often an allosteric substrate functions as a positive effector. In such a case the presence of a substrate molecule at one site on the enzyme enhances the catalytic properties of the other substrate binding sites. These enzymes show a sigmoidal curve when reaction velocity (v_o) is plotted against substrate concentration, [S] (Figure 4.9). This contrasts with the hyperbolic curve characteristic of enzymes following Michaelis-Menten kinetics.

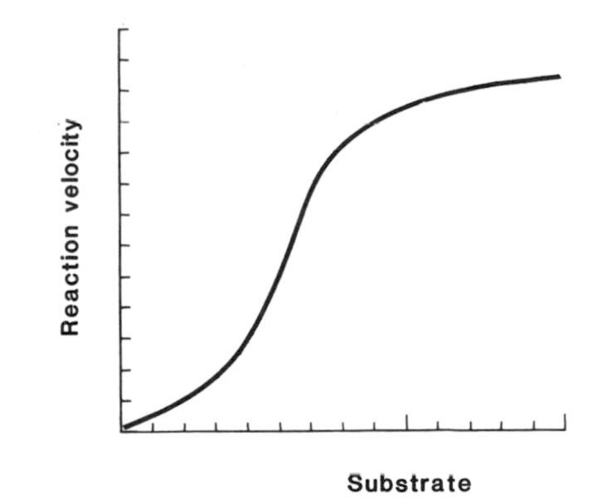

Figure 4.9
Effect of substrate concentration on reaction velocity for an allosteric enzyme.

B. Allosteric enzymes usually contain multiple subunits and frequently catalyze the first committed step in a pathway.

X. REGULATION OF ENZYMES BY COVALENT MODIFICATION

A. Some enzymes may be regulated by covalent modification, most frequently by the addition or removal of phosphate groups from specific serine, threonine, or tyrosine residues of the enzyme (Figure 4.10).

B. Phosphorylation reactions are catalyzed by a family of enzymes, called *protein kinases,* that utilize ATP as a phosphate donor. Phosphate groups are cleaved from phosphorylated enzymes by the action of *phosphoprotein phosphatases.*

C. Depending on the specific enzyme, the phosphorylated form may be more or less active than the unphosphorylated enzyme. For example, phosphorylation of *glycogen phosphorylase* increases activity, whereas the addition of phosphate to *glycogen synthase* results in a less active enzyme (see p. 74).

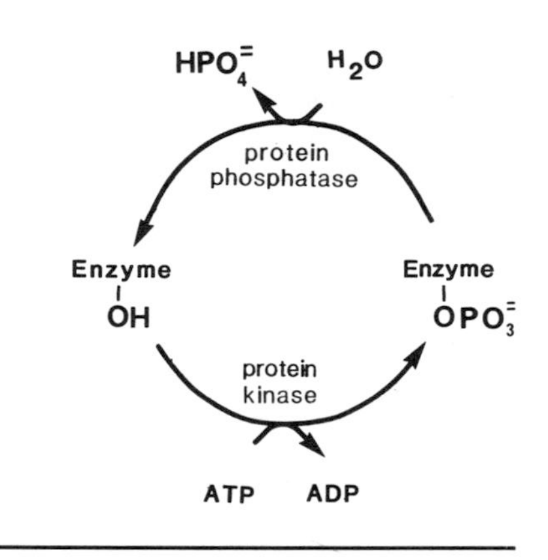

Figure 4.10
Covalent modification by the addition and removal of phosphate groups.

XI. ENZYMES IN CLINICAL DIAGNOSIS

A. Enzymes of normal serum can be classified into two major groups

1. A relatively small group of enzymes are actively secreted into the serum by certain organs. For example, the liver secretes the enzymes involved in blood coagulation.
2. A large group of enzymes are released from cells as a result of normal cell turnover. These enzymes are normally intracellular and have no physiologic function in the plasma.

B. Alteration of serum enzymes levels in disease states

1. A number of diseases that cause tissue damage also result in an increased release of intracellular enzyme into the serum. The activities of many of these enzymes are routinely determined for

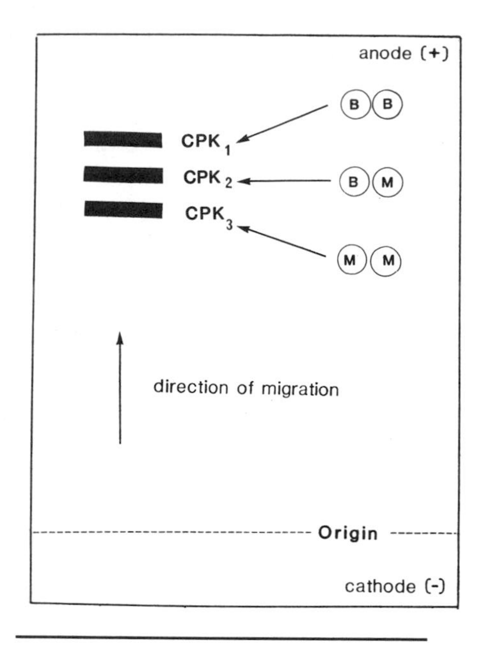

Figure 4.11
Subunit structure and electrophoretic mobility of *creatine phosphokinase* isoenzymes.

diagnostic purposes in diseases of the heart, liver, skeletal muscle, and other tissues.

2. The level of enzymes in the serum frequently correlates with the extent of tissue damage. Thus the degree of elevation of a particular enzyme activity in serum is often useful in evaluating the prognosis of the patient.

C. Serum enzymes as diagnostic tools.

1. ***Organ-specific enzymes:*** Some enzymes are organ-specific in that they show relatively high activity in only one tissue. The presence of increased levels of these enzymes in serum thus reflects damage to the corresponding tissue. For example, the enzymes *fructose 1-phosphate aldolase,* and *sorbitol dehydrogenase* are liver-specific enzymes.
2. ***Organ-specific isoenzymes: Isoenzymes*** (also called ***isozymes***) are enzymes that catalyze the same reaction but differ in their physical properties owing to differences in amino acid sequence. Isoenzymes may contain different numbers of charged amino acids and be separated from each other by electrophoresis. Different organs frequently contain characteristic proportions of different isoenzymes. The pattern of isoenzymes found in the serum may therefore serve as a means of identifying the site of tissue damage.
3. ***Quaternary structure of isozymes:*** Many isoenzymes comprise different subunits in various combinations. For example, *creatine phosphokinase* (see p. 260) occurs as three isoenzymes. Each isoenzyme is a dimer composed of two polypeptides (called B and M subunits) associated in one of three combinations: CPK_1 = BB, CPK_2 = MB and CPK_3 = MM. Each of the CPK isoenzyme shows a characteristic electrophoretic mobility (Figure 4.11).

D. Isoenzymes and diseases of the heart

1. The serum levels of *creatine phosphokinase* (CPK), *lactate dehydrogenase* (LDH), and *glutamate-oxaloacetate transaminase* (GOT) are commonly determined in the diagnosis of myocardial infarction. These enzymes are particularly useful when the electrocardiogram (EKG) is difficult to interpret, such as when there have been previous episodes of heart disease.
2. The hybrid isoenzyme CPK_2 is virtually specific for myocardium. After an acute myocardial infarction, this isoenzyme appears about 4 to 8 hours after chest pain and reaches a peak in activity at about 24 hours (Figure 4.12).
3. *Lactate dehydrogenase* and *glutamate-oxaloacetatetransaminase* are also elevated in the serum after a myocardial infarction. The presence of abnormally high levels of these enzymes can be used to confirm the diagnosis but by themselves are less specific for myocardial infarction than is CPK_2

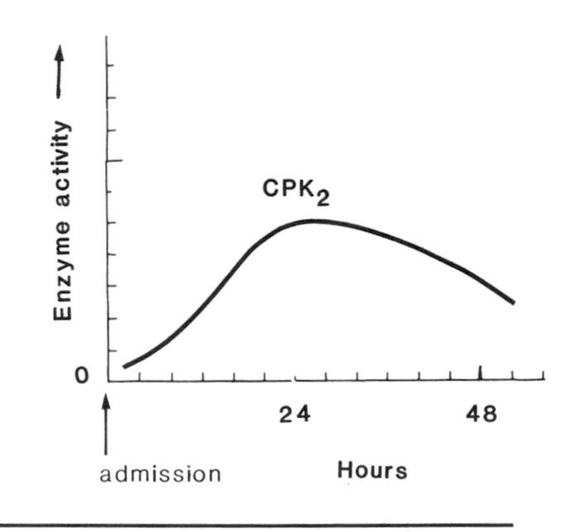

Figure 4.12
Appearance of *creatine phosphokinase* in serum after a myocardial infarction.

Study Questions

Choose the ONE best answer:

4.1 A competitive inhibitor of an enzyme

A. increases K_m without affecting V_m
B. decreases K_m without affecting V_m
C. increases V_m without affecting K_m
D. decreases V_m without affecting K_m
E. decreases both V_m and K_m

4.2 The Michaelis constant, K_m, is

A. numerically equal to ½ V_m.
B. dependent on the enzyme concentration.
C. independent of pH.
D. numerically equal to the substrate concentration that gives half-maximal velocity.
E. increased in the presence of a noncompetitive inhibitor.

4.3 The rate of an enzyme-catalyzed reaction was measured using several substrate concentrations that were much lower than K_m. The dependence of reaction velocity on substrate concentration can best described as

A. independent of enzyme concentration.
B. a constant fraction of V_m.
C. equal to K_m.
D. proportional to the substrate concentration.
E. zero order with respect to substrate.

4.4 Which one of the following statements is NOT characteristic of allosteric enzymes?

A. They frequently catalyze a committed step early in a metabolic pathway.
B. They are often composed of subunits.
C. They frequently show cooperativity for substrate binding.
D. They follow Michaelis-Menten kinetics.
E. The binding of a positive allosteric effector results in an increase in enzymic activity.

4.5 The presence of a noncompetitive inhibitor

A. leads to both an increase in the V_m of a reaction and an increase in the K_m.
B. leads to a decrease in the observed V_m.
C. leads to a decrease in K_m and V_m.
D. leads to an increase in K_m without affecting V_m.
E. increases the steady-state concentration of ES.

4.6 The velocity, v_o, for an enzyme-catalyzed reaction was measured at several substrate concentrations:

[substrate] (moles per liter)	v_o (in millimoles product/min/mg protein)
0.25×10^{-4}	1.0
0.5×10^{-4}	1.7
1×10^{-4}	2.5
20×10^{-4}	5
50×10^{-4}	5

The K_m is approximately

A. 0.25×10^{-4} M.
B. 0.5×10^{-4} M.
C. 1×10^{-4} M.
D. 2×10^{-4} M.
E. 5×10^{-4} M.

UNIT II: Carbohydrate Metabolism

Structure of Carbohydrates

5

I. OVERVIEW

Carbohydrates are the most abundant organic molecules in nature. They have a wide range of functions (Figure 5.1): providing a significant fraction of the energy in the diet of most organisms; mediating much of the intercellular communication; and serving as a structural component of many organisms, including the cell walls of bacteria, the exoskeleton of many insects, and the fibrous cellulose of plants. The generic formula for many of the simpler carbohydrates is $(CH_2O)_n$, hence the name "hydrate of carbon."

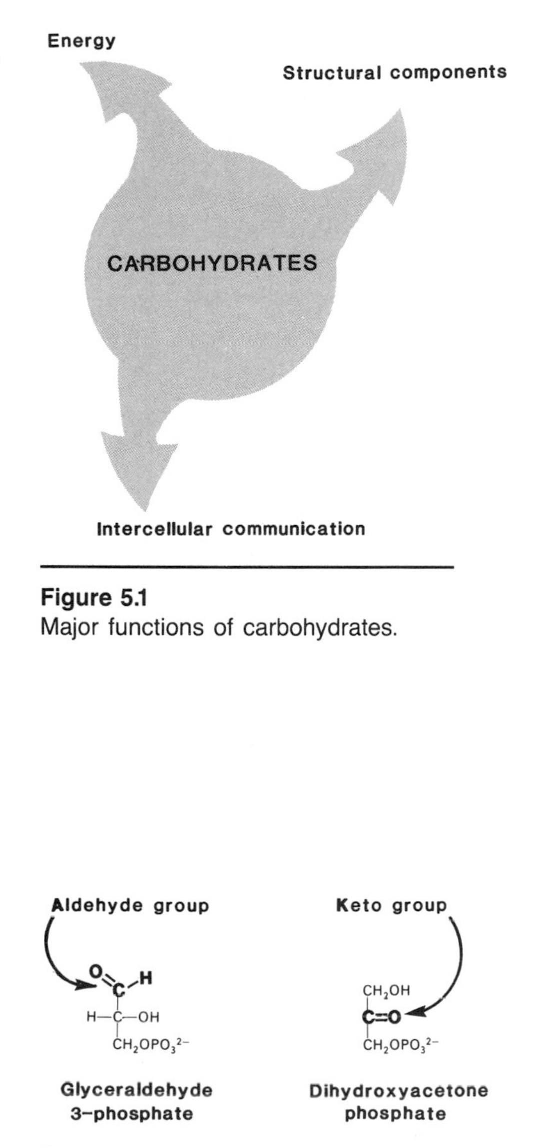

Figure 5.1
Major functions of carbohydrates.

II. CLASSIFICATION AND NOMENCLATURE OF CARBOHYDRATES

A. Monosaccharides

1. Monosaccharides (simple sugar molecules) can be classified according to the number of carbon atoms in the chain. Those found most commonly in humans include the following:

   3 carbons: trioses (e.g,. glyceraldehyde)
   4 carbons: tetroses (e.g., erythrose)
   5 carbons: pentoses (e.g., ribose, ribulose, xylose, xylulose)
   6 carbons: hexoses (e.g., glucose, galactose, mannose, fructose)
   7 carbons: heptoses (e.g., sedoheptulose)
   9 carbons: nonoses (e.g., neuraminic acid)

B. Aldoses and ketoses

1. Carbohydrates with an aldehyde as their most oxidized functional group are called aldoses; those with a keto group as their most oxidized functional group are called ketoses. For example, glyceraldehyde 3-phosphate is an aldose, whereas dihydroxyacetone phosphate is a ketose.
2. Note: The names of aldoses that have a free carbonyl group generally have the suffix ***-ose***. With the exception of fructose, ketoses usually have the suffix ***-ulose*** (Figure 5.2).

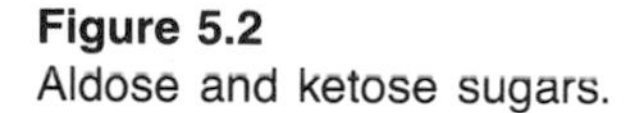

Figure 5.2
Aldose and ketose sugars.

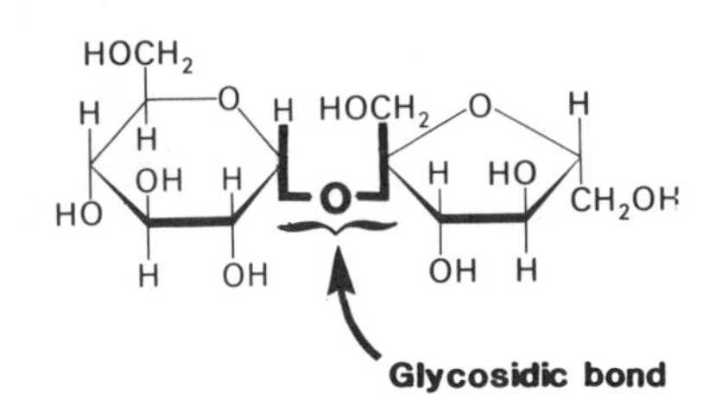

Figure 5.3
A glycosidic bond.

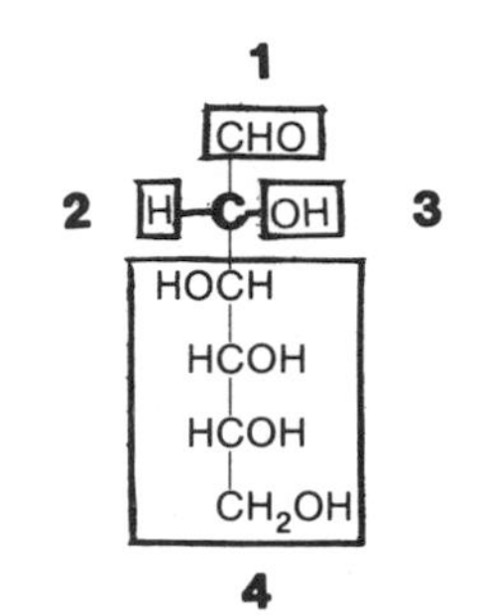

Figure 5.4
Representation of four different chemical groups attached to carbon #2 of glucose.

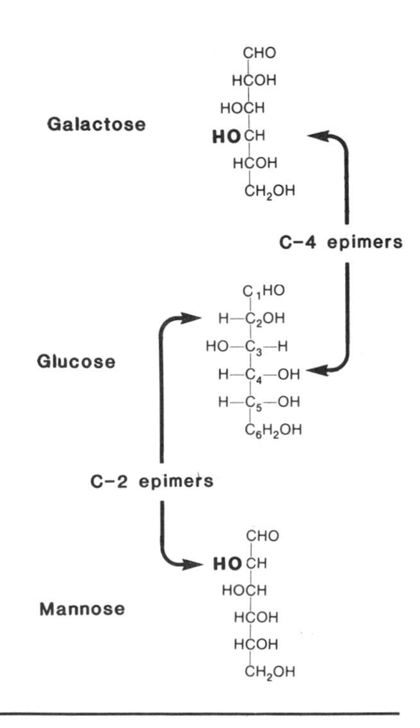

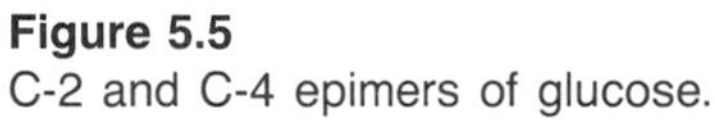

Figure 5.5
C-2 and C-4 epimers of glucose.

C. Glycosides

1. Monosaccharides can be linked by ***glycosidic bonds*** to create larger structures (Figure 5.3). (See p. 49 for a discussion of glycosidic bonds.)
2. ***Disaccharides*** contain two monosaccharides. Examples of these are ***lactose*** (galactose + glucose), ***maltose*** (glucose + glucose), and ***sucrose*** (fructose + glucose).
3. ***Oligosaccharides*** contain from 3 to about 12 monosaccharide units. Examples of these are found in glycoproteins (p. 91).
4. ***Polysaccharides*** contain more than 12 monosaccharide units. They can be hundreds of sugar units in size, and include ***glycogen***—called a ***homopolysaccharide*** because it contains only a single monosaccharide species, glucose (p. 68), and the ***glycosaminoglycans***— termed ***heteropolysaccharides*** because they contain a number of different monosaccharide species (p. 81).

III. STRUCTURE OF MONOSACCHARIDES

A. Asymmetric carbons

1. All monosaccharides have at least one asymmetric (chiral) carbon. An asymmetric carbon has four ***different*** chemical groups attached to it. For example, glucose has four asymmetric carbon atoms: carbons 2, 3, 4, and 5. (Note: The carbons in sugars are numbered beginning at the end with the carbonyl carbon, i.e. the aldehyde or ketone group.) See Figure 5.4 for an example of four different groups surrounding glucose carbon #2.

B. Isomers and epimers

1. Compounds that have the same chemical formula are called ***isomers***. For example, fructose, glucose, mannose, and galactose are all isomers of each other, having the same chemical formula, $C_6H_{12}O_6$.
2. If two monosaccharides differ in conformation around only one particular carbon atom, they are defined as ***epimers*** of each other. (Of course, they are also isomers!)
3. For example, glucose and galactose are ***C-4 epimers***—their structures differ only in the position of the —OH group at carbon #4. Glucose and mannose are ***C-2 epimers***; however, galactose and mannose are NOT epimers—they differ in the position of —OH groups at two carbons (#2 and #4) and therefore are only isomers (Figure 5.5).

C. Enantiomers

1. A special type of isomer is found in the pairs of structures that are mirror images of each other. These "mirror images" are called ***enantiomers*** (Figure 5.6), and the two members of each pair can rotate a plane of polarized light to the same extent but in opposite directions. (Note: Only compounds containing at least one asymmetric carbon are optically active.)
2. If the plane of polarized light is rotated clockwise, the substance causing the rotation is said to be ***dextrorotatory***. If the plane of light

is rotated counterclockwise, the substance is ***levorotatory***. These states are indicated by the notation "d" or "l."

3. The optical properties of sugars (d versus l) are sometimes confused with the standard designation of sugars as "D" or "L," for example, D-glucose. In this case, the letters (which are capitalized) refer to the arrangement of atoms around the asymmetric carbon atom farthest removed from the carbonyl carbon.
4. The vast majority of the sugars in humans are D-sugars. Two notable exceptions are L-fucose (found in glycoproteins, see p. 92), and L-iduronic acid (found in glycosaminoglycans (see p. 81).

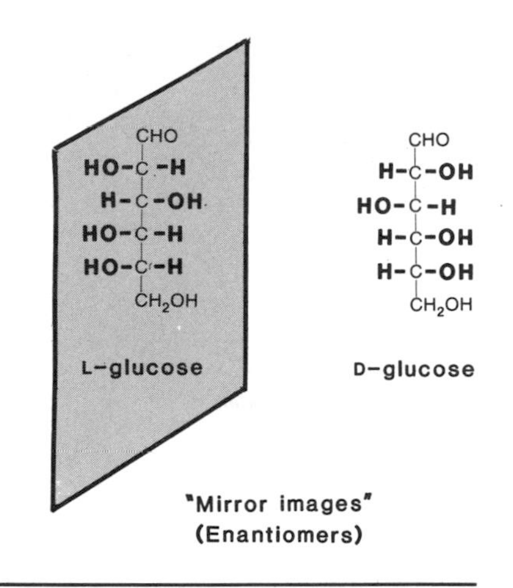

Figure 5.6
Enantiomers of glucose.

D. Hemiacetal and hemiketal rings

1. Less than 1% of each of the sugars with five or more carbons are found in the open chain form. Rather, they are predominantly found in a ring form, where the aldehyde (or ketone) group has reacted with an alcohol group on the same sugar to form a ***hemiacetal*** or ***hemiketal*** ring. If the resulting ring has six members (five carbons and one oxygen), it is a ***pyranose ring***. If it is five-membered (four carbons and one oxygen), it is called a ***furanose ring***.
2. Formation of a hemiacetal results in the creation of a new asymmetric carbon at carbon #1 of an aldose, or carbon #2 of a ketose. This carbon is called the ***anomeric carbon*** and can have two forms: α or β.
   a. For example, two molecules of D-glucose can differ from each other, one having the —OH group on the right in the α-configuration (α-D-glucose) and the other with the —OH on the left in the β-configuration (β-D-glucose). These two sugars are both glucose, but they are ***anomers*** of each other (Figure 5.7).
   b. Enzymes are able to distinguish between these two structures and will use one or the other preferentially.
   c. If the hemiacetal ring is six membered in the above structures, the full name of each sugar would be either α- (or β-) D-glucopyranose. If the ring is five membered, the sugar would be called either α- (or β-) D-glucofuranose.

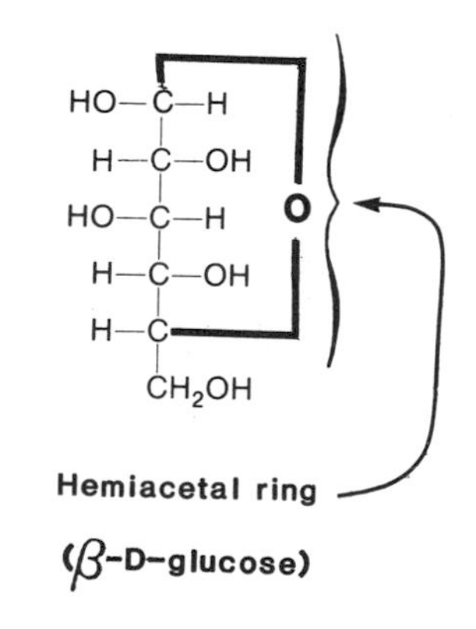

3. The α- and β-forms of a sugar in solution are in equilibrium with each other and can readily be interconverted. For example, if a solution is made of pure D-glucose in water, it will spontaneously equilibrate to produce an equilibrium mixture of about 64% β-pyranose and 36% α-pyranose. This process requires that the ring structure open to the linear form during the interconversion and is called ***mutarotation*** (Figure 5.7).
4. The structure of a sugar can be represented in several ways:
   a. The hemiacetal ring shown in the top structure of Figure 5.8 is called a ***Fischer projection***. The carbon chain is written vertically, with carbon #1 at the top and the hydroxyl and hydrogen substituents written to the left or the right.
   b. A second way of representing this hemiacetal ring is as a ***Haworth projection***, where carbon #1 is drawn farthest to the right. If you consider the plane of the ring to be "flat" on the paper, the —H, —OH, and —CH_2OH groups are located either

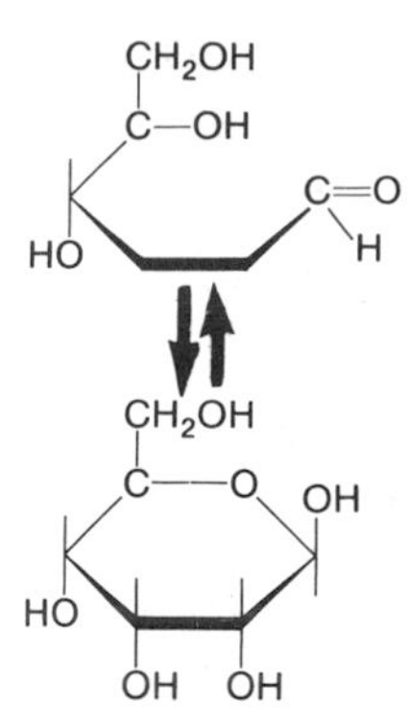

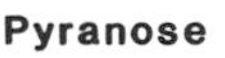
Pyranose

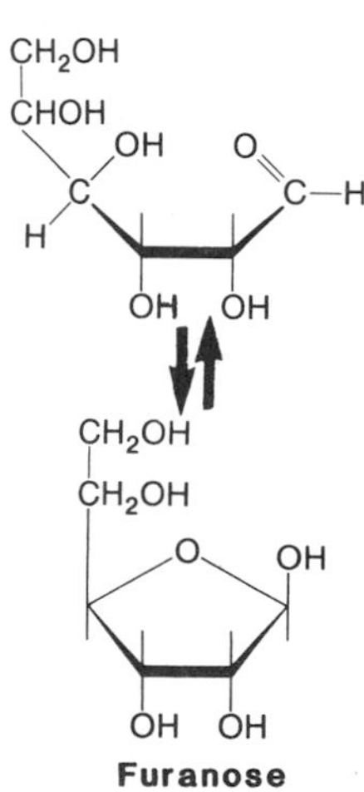
Furanose

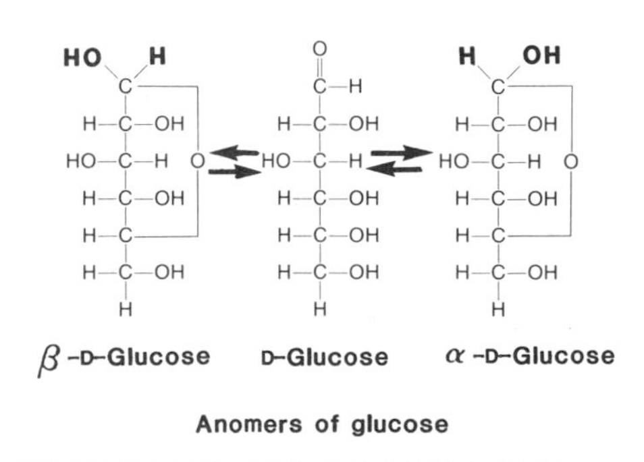

Figure 5.7
The α and β forms of glucose: mutarotation.

"above" or "below" the paper as drawn. (Note: Analysis of this ring structure has shown that it is not a rigid circle, but rather is bent into a conformation resembling either a "chair" or a "boat" (Figure 5.9).)

IV. COMMON CHEMICAL REACTIONS INVOLVING MONOSACCHARIDES

A. Reducing sugars

1. If the oxygen on the anomeric carbon of a sugar is not attached to any other structure, that sugar is called a ***reducing sugar.***
2. A reducing sugar can react with one of several chemical reagents (for example, Tollens, Benedict's, and Fehling's solutions) and reduce the active substance. The ***anomeric carbon*** itself becomes oxidized. Only the state of the oxygen on the anomeric carbon determines whether the sugar is reducing or nonreducing—the other hydroxyl groups on the molecule are not involved.
3. One of the earliest tests for the presence of sugar in the urine of diabetics was a test for reducing sugar (i.e., free glucose). This test, however, could also be positive for reducing sugar in the presence of several other hexoses and pentoses and therefore, while simple, was not diagnostic for diabetes.

B. Oxidation-reduction reactions

1. Oxidation of an aldehyde group at carbon #1 to a carboxyl group produces an ***aldonic acid***. For example, glucose becomes gluconic acid, and galactose becomes galactonic acid.
2. Oxidation of the hydroxymethyl group at carbon #6 produces a ***uronic acid***. For example, glucose becomes glucuronic acid, and galactose becomes galacturonic acid.
3. Reduction of the carbonyl carbon (aldehyde or keto group) produces a new alcohol group. Such compounds are called ***polyols***, for example, glucose is reduced to sorbitol (glucitol) and fructose is reduced to sorbitol and mannitol (see p. 62). Galactose is reduced to galactitol (dulcitol).
4. Reduction of hydroxyl groups produces ***deoxysugars***. For example, ribose is converted to 2-deoxyribose.

COOH
HCOH
HOCH
HCOH
HCOH
CH_2OH

Gluconic acid

CHO
HCOH
HOCH
HOCH
HCOH
COOH

Galacturonic acid

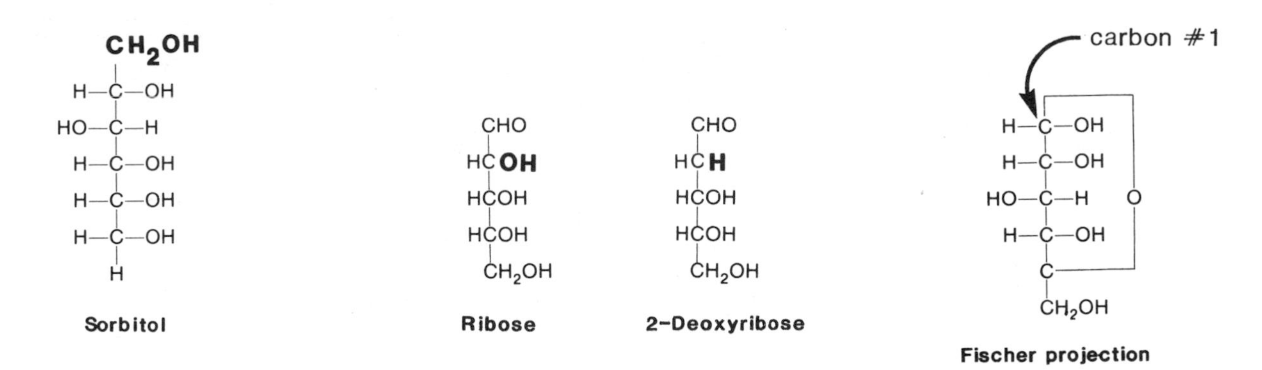

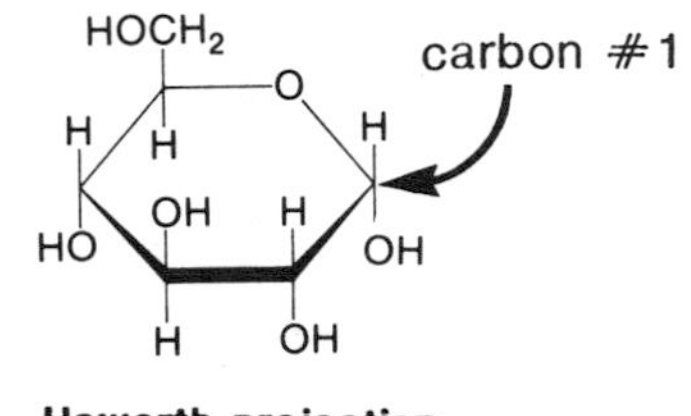

Figure 5.8
Fischer and Haworth projections of a hemiacetal ring.

C. Complex carbohydrates

1. Carbohydrates can also be attached by glycosidic bonds to noncarbohydrate structures to form "complex carbohydrates."
2. The noncarbohydrate portion of the molecule is called the ***aglycone,*** and the entire molecule can be called by the generic name ***glycoside***. The aldose, the carbon #1 of which (or ketose, the carbon #2 of which) participates in the glycosidic link, is called a ***glycosyl***. For example, if the anomeric carbon of glucose participates in such a bond, that sugar is called glucosyl. If the identity of the attached sugar is known, its name can be used, that is, ***gluc***oside or ***galact***oside.
3. If the group on the aglycone to which the sugar is attached is an —OH group, the structure is an ***O-glycoside***. If the group on the aglycone is an $—NH_2$, the structure is an ***N-glycoside***. All sugar-sugar glycosidic bonds are O-type linkages (Figure 5.10). Typical aglycones include purines and pyrimidines (sugar-nucleotides), aromatic rings (such as are found in steroids and bilirubin), proteins (glycoproteins and glycosaminoglycans), and lipids (glycolipids).
4. A sugar, the anomeric carbon of which is in a glycosidic linkage, is no longer a reducing sugar.
5. Glycosidic bonds between sugars are named according to the numbers of the connected carbons and also with regard to the position of the hydroxyl group of the sugar, the anomeric carbon of which is participating in the bond. If that anomeric hydroxyl group is in the α configuration, the linkage is an ***α-bond***. If it is in the β-position, the linkage is a ***β-bond*** (Figure 5.11).
   a. For example, ***lactose*** is synthesized by carbon #1 of a β-galactose forming a glycosidic bond with carbon #4 of glucose. The linkage is therefore a $\beta(1 \rightarrow 4)$ glycosidic bond. Because the anomeric (or reducing) end of the glucose residue is not involved in the glycosidic linkage it (and therefore lactose) remains a ***reducing sugar.***
   b. ***Sucrose,*** on the other hand, is synthesized by carbon #1 of α-glucose, forming a glycosidic bond with carbon #2 of a fructose molecule. The linkage therefore is an $\alpha(1 \rightarrow 2)$ glycosidic bond, and sucrose is ***not a reducing sugar.***

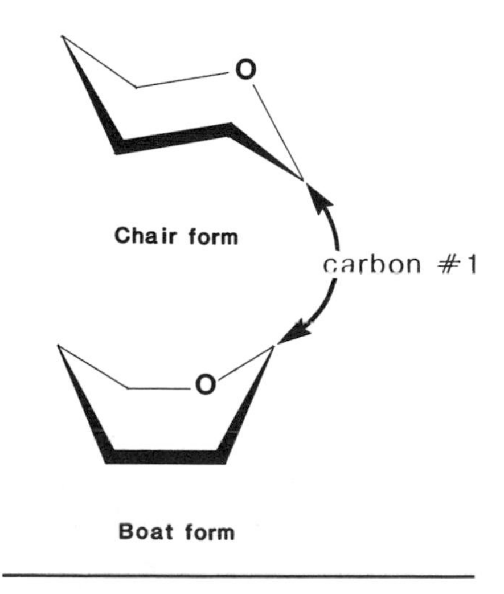

Figure 5.9
"Chair" and "boat" forms of the pyranose ring.

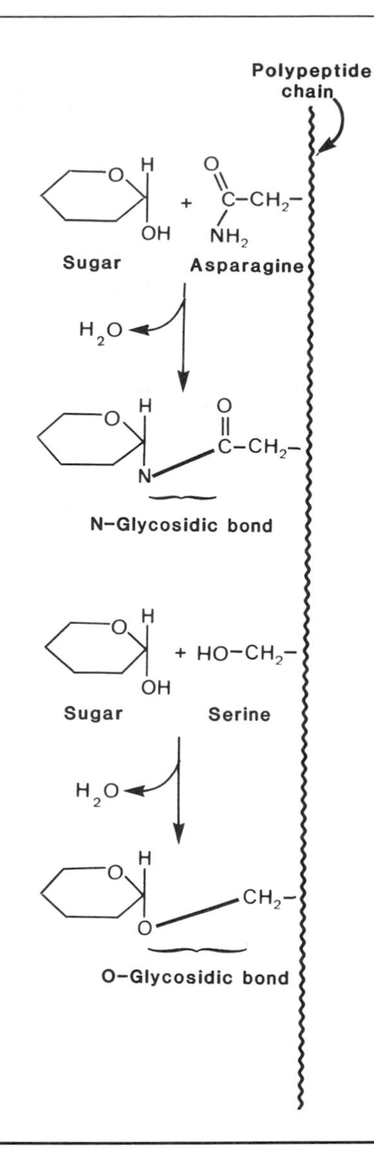

Figure 5.10
Glycosides: N- and O-glycosidic bonds.

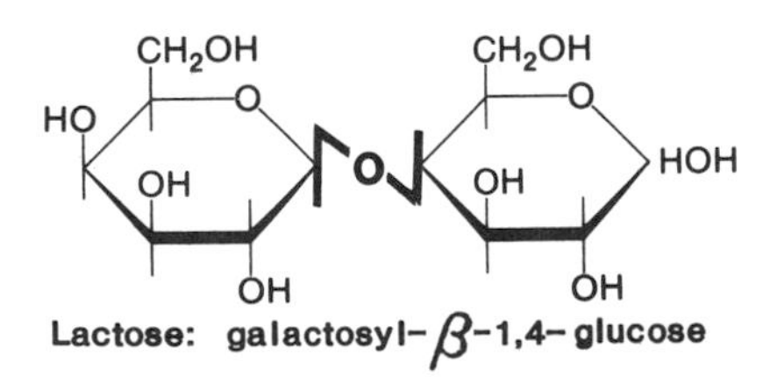

Study Questions

Choose the ONE best answer:

5.1 Which one of the following statements is ***INCORRECT*** regarding the predominant form of α-D-glucose?

A. It is a hemiacetal.
B. It contains five asymmetric carbon atoms.
C. It is a C-4 epimer of galactose.
D. It will rotate a plane of polarized light.
E. In combination with fructose it forms sucrose, which is a nonreducing sugar.

5.2 Which one of the following oxidation-reduction reactions is ***not*** undergone by glucose?

A. Oxidation of the aldehyde group (—CHO) at carbon #1 to a carboxyl group (—COOH) produces gluconic acid.
B. Oxidation of the hydroxymethyl group (—CH_2OH) at carbon #6 to a carboxyl (—COOH) group produces glucuronic acid.
C. Reduction of the aldehyde group at carbon #1 produces sorbitol.
D. Reduction of the hydroxyl group at carbon #3 produces 3-deoxyglucose.
E. Reduction of the hydroxyl group at carbon #2 produces fructose.

5.3 The structure shown below is

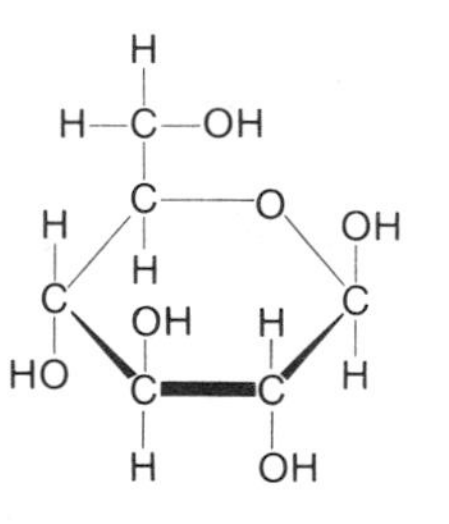

A. α-D-glucopyranose.
B. β-D-glucopyranose.
C. α-D-glucofuranose.
D. β-L-glucopyranose.
E. α-D-fructofuranose.

Answer A if 1, 2 and 3 are correct
B if 1 and 3 are correct
C if 2 and 4 are correct

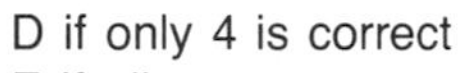
D if only 4 is correct
E if all are correct

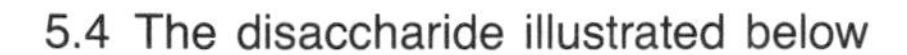
5.4 The disaccharide illustrated below

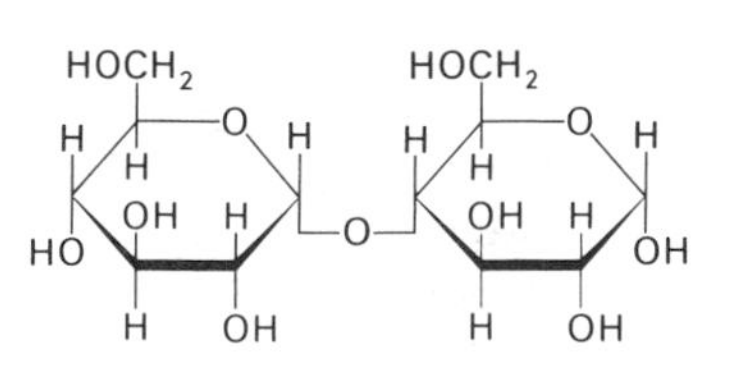

1. contains a β(1→4) glycosidic bond.
2. is a reducing sugar.
3. contains a furanose ring.
4. may undergo mutarotation.

5.5 D-Galactose and D-glucose are

1. enantiomers of each other.
2. isomers of each other.
3. anomers of each other.
4. epimers of each other.

5.6 Which of the following sugars is(are) a ketose sugar(s)?

1. Galactose
2. Fructose
3. Glucose
4. Ribulose

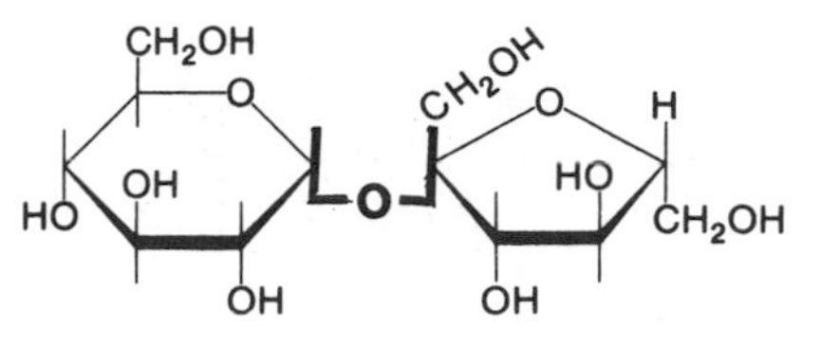

Sucrose: α-D-glucopyranosyl (1,2)-β-D-fructofuranoside

V. DIGESTION OF CARBOHYDRATES

The principal sites of carbohydrate digestion are the mouth and epithelial cells of the intestinal mucosa. There is very little monosaccharide present in diets of mixed animal and plant origin; thus the enzymes needed for degradation of most dietary carbohydrates are primarily *disaccharidases* and *endoglycosidases* (for breaking down oligosaccharides and polysaccharides). A summary of carbohydrate digestion is presented in Figure 5.12. Hydrolysis of glycosidic bonds is catalyzed by a family of *glycosidases* that degrade carbohydrates into their reducing sugar components (Figure 5.13). These enzymes are usually specific for the structure of the glycosyl to be removed and the type of bond to be broken.

A. Digestion of carbohydrates begins in the mouth

1. Dietary starch can be of animal (glycogen) or plant origin (amylose and amylopectin). During mastication, salivary *α-amylase (ptyalin)* acts on dietary starch in a random manner, breaking α-(1→4) bonds.
2. There are both α- and *β-(1→4)-glucosidases* in nature, but humans have little of the latter and are therefore unable to hydrolyze cellulose—a carbohydrate of plant origin containing β-(1→4) bonds between glucose residues.
3. Because both amylopectin and glycogen also contain α-(1→6) bonds, the resulting digest contains a mixture of ***maltose*** (a disaccharide containing two glucose molecules attached by an α-(1→4) linkage that is not attacked by *α-amylase*), ***isomaltose*** (a disaccharide in which two glucose molecules are attacked by an α-(1→6) linkage), some D-glucose, and smaller units of the starch molecule called ***starch dextrins,*** which are partial digestion products.
4. Carbohydrate digestion halts temporarily in the stomach. When the mixture of carbohydrates reaches the stomach, the high acidity inactivates the salivary *α-amylase* and digestion stops temporarily.

B. Further digestion of carbohydrate by pancreatic enzymes in the small intestine

1. When the carbohydrates reach the small intestine, the acidic pH is neutralized by pancreatic juice, and pancreatic *α-amylase* continues the digestion process. This enzyme degrades the

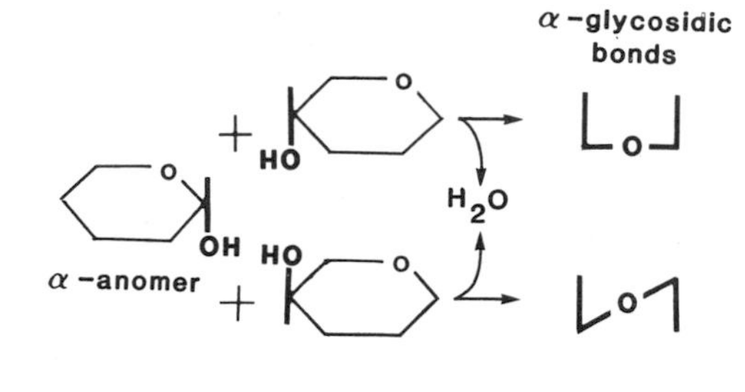

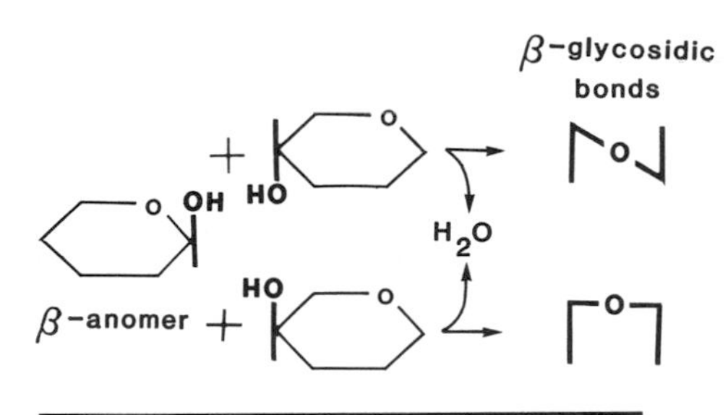

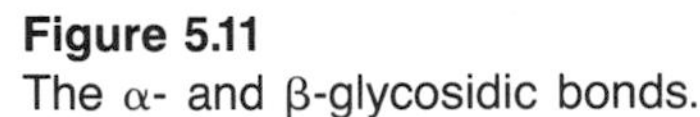

Figure 5.11
The α- and β-glycosidic bonds.

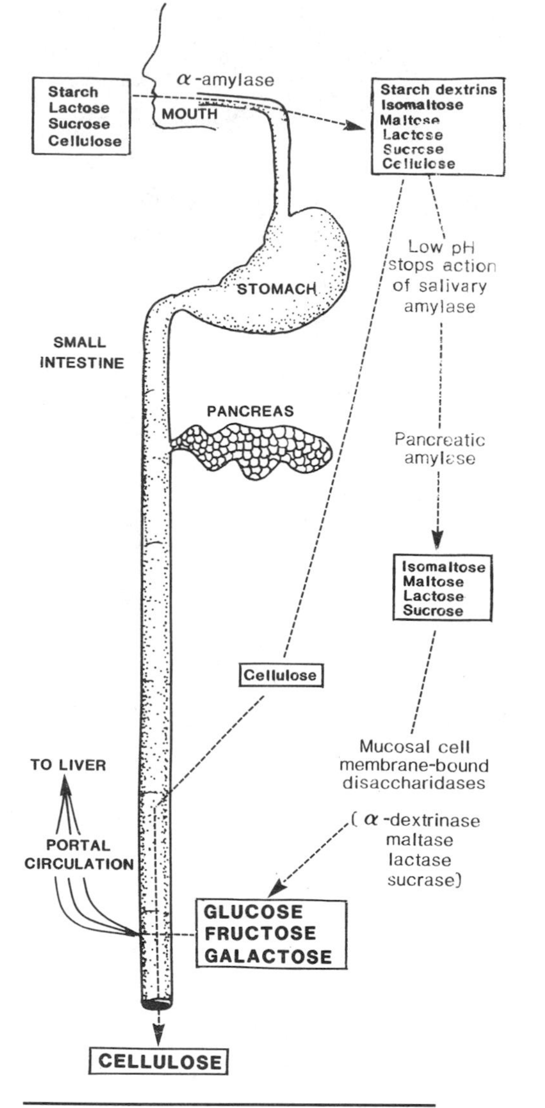

Figure 5.12
Digestion of carbohydrates.

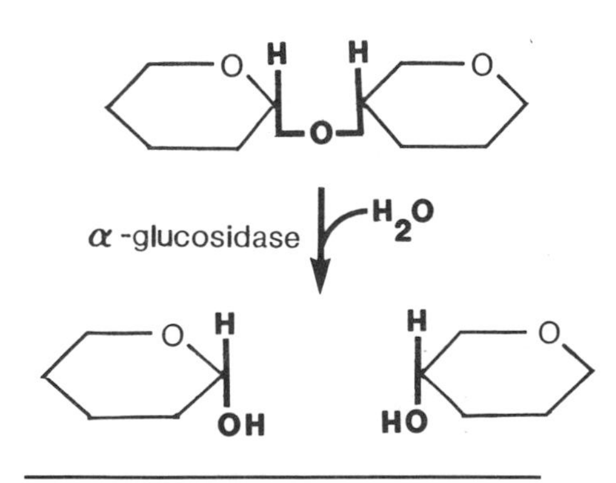

Figure 5.13
Hydrolysis of a glycosidic bond.

remaining starch fragments to disaccharides of maltose and isomaltose.

2. This digestion is rapid and is generally completed by the time the intestinal contents reach the junction of the duodenum and jejunum.

C. Final carbohydrate digestion by enzymes synthesized by the intestinal mucosal cells

1. The final digestive processes occur at the mucosal lining and include the action of several *disaccharidases*. These enzymes are secreted through, and remain associated with, the luminal side of the brush border membranes of the intestinal mucosal cells.
2. The *disaccharidases* include *lactase (β-galactosidase), maltase (α-glucosidase), sucrase (α-fructofuranosidase),* and *α-dextrinase* [*oligo-1,6-glucosidase* that cleaves the α-(1→6) linkages].

D. Absorption of monosaccharides by intestinal mucosal cells

1. Insulin is not required for the uptake of glucose by intestinal cells; however, different sugars have different mechanisms of absorption. For example, galactose and glucose are transported into the mucosal cells by an active, energy-requiring process that involves a specific transport protein and requires sodium ions.

E. Abnormal disaccharide degradation

1. The overall process of carbohydrate digestion and absorption is so efficient in healthy individuals that ordinarily all digestible dietary carbohydrate is absorbed by the time the remaining ingested material reaches the lower jejunum. However, since predominantly monosaccharides are absorbed, any defect in *oligosaccharidase* or *disaccharidase* activity of the intestinal mucosa will cause a passage of undigested carbohydrate into the bowel.
2. As a consequence of the presence of this osmotically active material, water will be drawn from the tissues into the large intestine, causing osmotic diarrhea. This is reinforced by the bacterial metabolism of the remaining carbohydrate to two- and three-carbon compounds plus large volumes of CO_2 and H_2 gas.
3. Hereditary defects of the enzymes *lactase*, *sucrase*, and *α-dextrinase* have been reported in infants and children with disaccharide intolerance or cholesterol malabsorption. (See Figure 5.14 for a summary of normal and abnormal lactose metabolism.)
4. A generalized defect in disaccharide degradation can also be caused by a variety of intestinal diseases, malnutrition, or drugs that injure the mucosa of the small intestine.
5. ***Lactose intolerance*** is also manifested in certain races: adult blacks and Orientals, for example, are less able to metabolize lactose than are individuals of Northern European origin—in fact, up to 90% of Asians and Africans may be *lactase*-deficient as adults. The mechanism by which the enzyme is lost is unknown, but it seems to be determined genetically and is due to a reduction in

the amount of enzyme protein rather than to a modified inactive enzyme. Thus, lactose intolerance may be the single most frequent enzyme deficiency, with as many as 50% of the human race affected. Treatment for this disorder is simply to remove lactose from the diet.

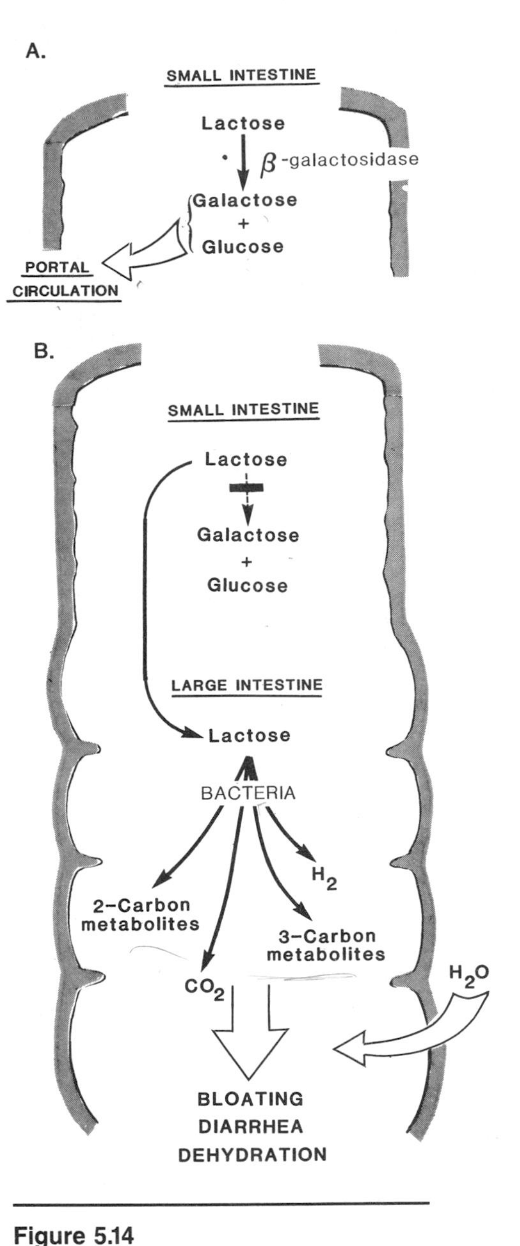

Figure 5.14
Normal **(A)** and abnormal **(B)** lactose metabolism.

Study Questions

Answer A if 1, 2, and 3 are correct
B if 1 and 3 are correct
C if 2 and 4 are correct
D if only 4 is correct
E if all are correct

5.7 Which of the following conditions result in the passage of undigested carbohydrate into the bowel?

1. Deficiency of intestinal lactase
2. Deficiency of salivary α-amylase
3. Malnutrition
4. Deficiency of intestinal glycogen phosphorylase

5.8 Which of the following compounds can be produced from dietary starch by salivary α-amylase?

1. Maltose
2. Starch dextrins
3. Isomaltose
4. Fructose

5.9 Which of the following statements about human disaccharidases is(are) correct?

1. The disaccharidases are produced and secreted by the intestinal mucosal cells.
2. A specific intestinal disaccharidase cleaves $\beta(1 \rightarrow 4)$ glycosidic bonds.
3. The monosaccharides produced by the disaccharidases pass into the portal circulation.
4. Deficiency of a specific disaccharidase has little effect on an individual's ability to digest dietary carbohydrates.

Metabolism of Monosaccharides and Disaccharides

6

I. OVERVIEW

Although many monosaccharides have been identified in nature, only a few sugars appear as metabolic intermediates or as structural components in mammals. Most sugars are rapidly phosphorylated after they enter a cell (Figure 6.1). This "traps" the sugar inside the cell because organic phosphates cannot cross membranes unless there is a specific carrier for that purpose, such as the carrier that transports ADP and ATP across the inner mitochondrial membrane. The exception to this rule of intracellular phosphorylation is the metabolism of polyols (see p. 62).

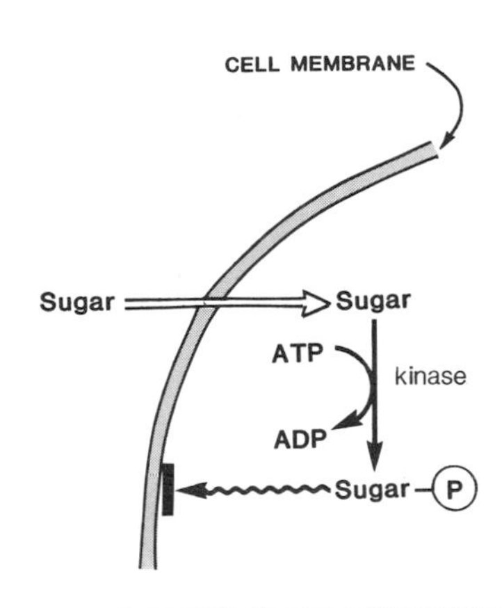

Figure 6.1
Intracellular phosphorylation "traps" sugar inside cells.

II. FRUCTOSE METABOLISM

A. Dietary sources of fructose

1. About 15% to 20% of the calories contained in the American diet is supplied by fructose. The major source of fructose is the disaccharide sucrose (a discussion of its degradation is presented on p. 65).

B. Phosphorylation of fructose

1. For fructose to enter the pathways of intermediary metabolism, it must first be phosphorylated. This can be accomplished by either of two enzymes:
   a. *Hexokinase,* the enzyme that phosphorylates glucose in all cells of the body (see p. 111 for discussion of the phosphorylation of glucose), has a low affinity (i.e., high K_m) for fructose. (See p. 38 for a discussion of the Michaelis constant, K_m.) Therefore, unless the fructose levels of the body become unusually high, little fructose is converted to fructose 6-phosphate by this enzyme (Figure 6.2).
   b. The liver (which processes most of the dietary fructose) and the kidney have an alternate enzyme, *fructokinase,* that converts fructose to fructose 1-phosphate using ATP as the phosphate donor (Figure 6.2).

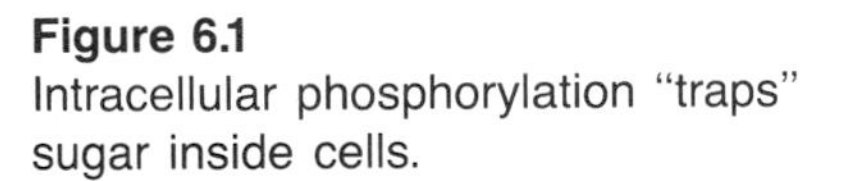

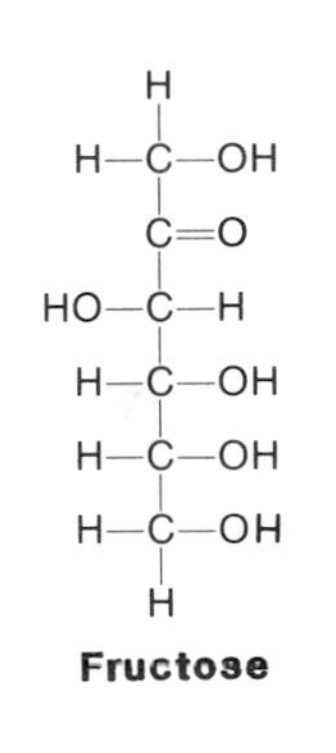

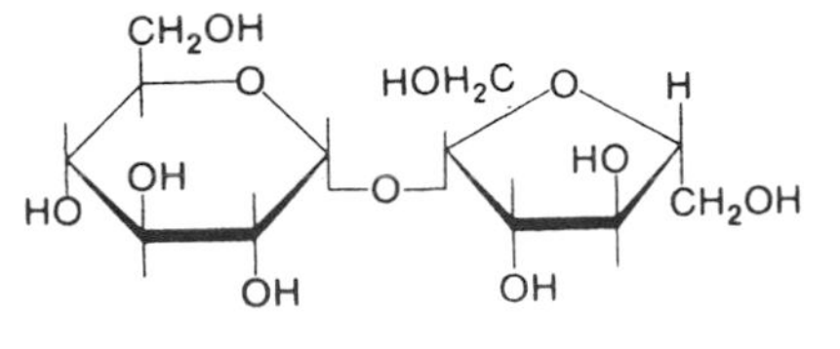

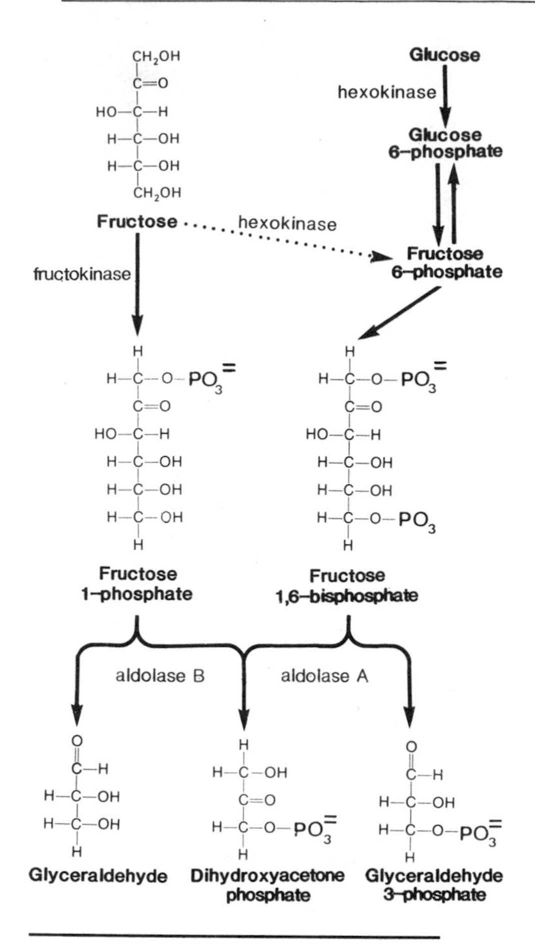

Figure 6.2
Phosphorylation products of fructose and their cleavage.

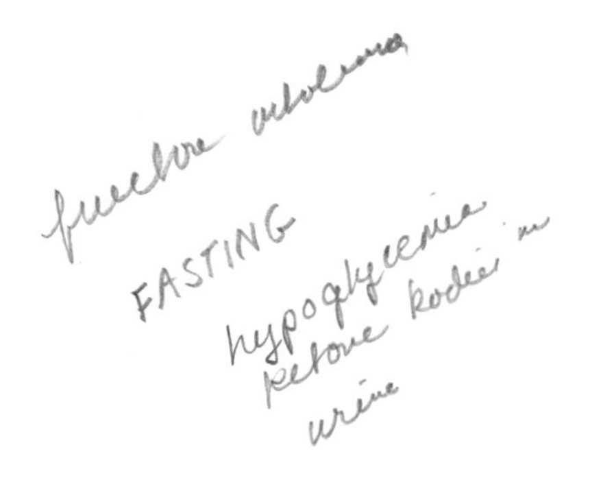

C. Cleavage of fructose 1-phosphate

1. Fructose 1-phosphate is not converted to fructose 1,6-bisphosphate, unlike fructose 6-phosphate, but rather is cleaved directly by *aldolase B* into ***dihydroxyacetone phosphate*** (DHAP) and ***D-glyceraldehyde*** (Figure 6.2).
2. The D-glyceraldehyde produced in this reaction can be metabolized by a number of pathways, including
   a. phosphorylation to glyceraldehyde 3-phosphate, which can enter either glycolysis (see p. 114) or gluconeogenesis (see p. 129)
   b. reduction to glycerol, which can be phosphorylated and serve as a building block for phospholipids (p. 183) or triacylglycerol (see p. 167). A summary of these pathways is included in Figure 6.3.
3. *Aldolase A,* which cleaves fructose 1,6-bisphosphate in glycolysis (see p. 114), is unable to cleave fructose 1-phosphate.

D. Kinetics of fructose metabolism

1. Because the trioses formed from fructose 1-phosphate by-pass the two rate-limiting kinase steps in glycolysis (*hexokinase* and *phosphofructokinase*), the rate of fructose metabolism is more rapid than that of glucose.
2. Elevated levels of dietary fructose significantly elevate the rate of lipogenesis in the liver, owing to the rapid production of acetyl CoA from fructose.
3. Excessive fructose consumption can also adversely affect liver metabolism. For example, the phosphorylation of fructose to fructose 1-phosphate is rapid, whereas the *aldolase B* reaction is relatively slow. This results in a decrease in intracellular inorganic phosphate levels, since much of this phosphate is sequestered in the form of fructose 1-phosphate. The lowered availability of P_i, therefore, limits the rate of production of ATP from ADP + P_i. (Figure 6.4 summarizes this phenomenon.)

E. Disorders of fructose metabolism

A summary of fructose metabolism and genetic diseases associated with this pathway are presented in Figure 6.3.

Study Questions

Choose the ONE best answer:

6.1 In liver, the initial step in the utilization of fructose is its phosphorylation to fructose 1-phosphate. This is followed by

A. phosphorylation to fructose 1,6-biphosphate.
B. cleavage of fructose 1-phosphate to form glyceraldehyde and dihydroxyacetone phosphate.
C. conversion to fructose 6-phosphate by action of a phosphofructomutase.
D. isomerization to glucose 1-phosphate.
E. hydrolysis to fructose followed by isomerization to glucose.

6.2 An individual with fructose intolerance

A. cannot use fructose effectively in glycolysis because of a deficiency in liver fructose 1-phosphate aldolase.
B. cannot produce glucose from fructose 6-phosphate.

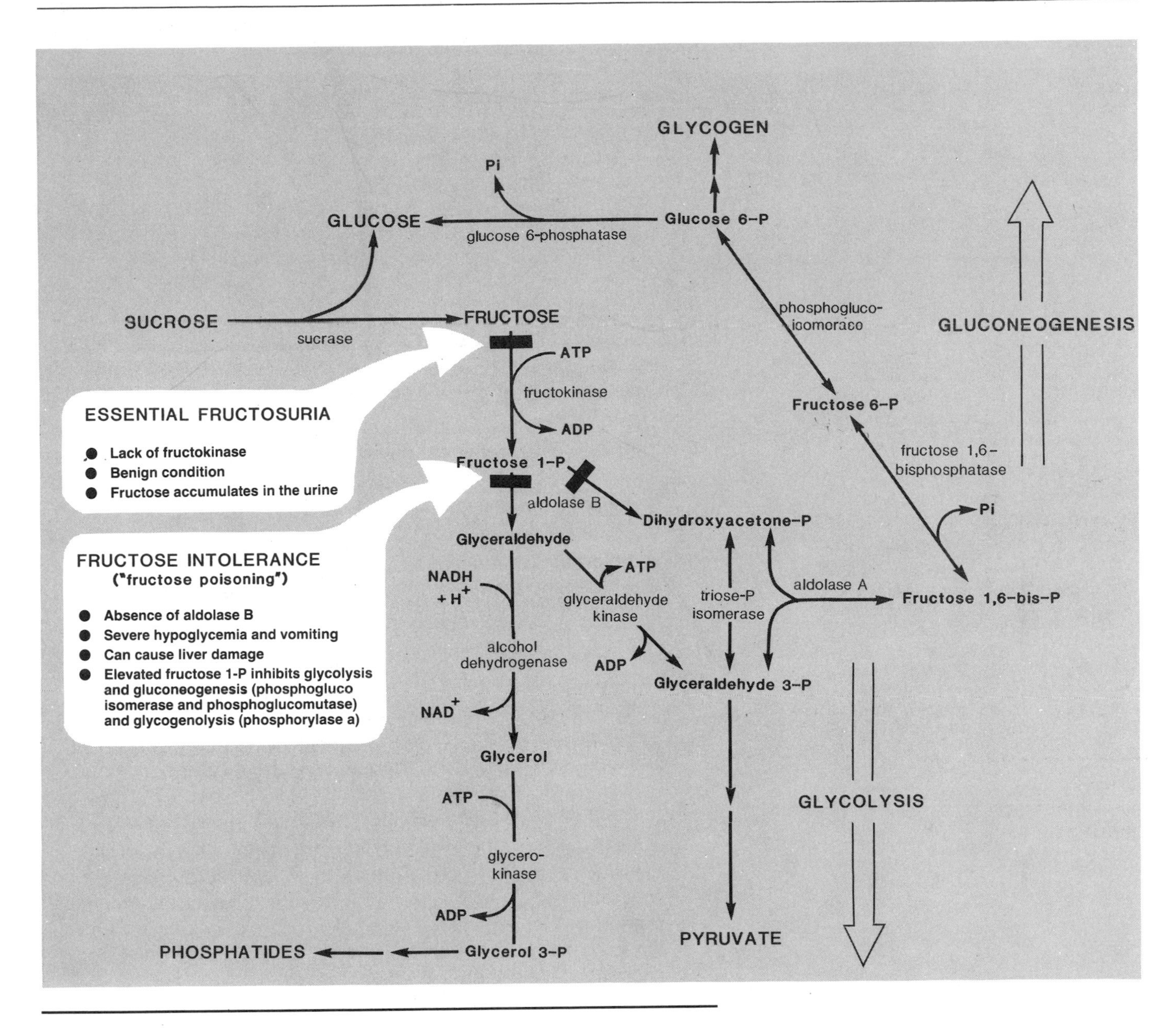

Figure 6.3
Summary of fructose metabolism.

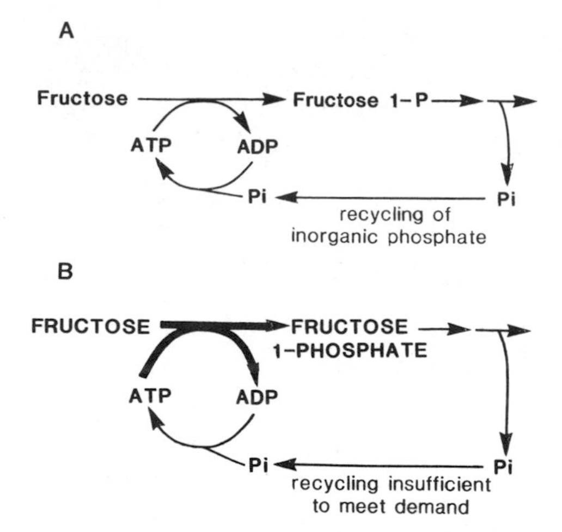

Figure 6.4
A. Moderate consumption of fructose results in an adequate supply of inorganic phosphate for regeneration of ATP. B. Excessive fructose consumption leads to sequestering of inorganic phosphate and, therefore, inadequate regeneration of ATP.

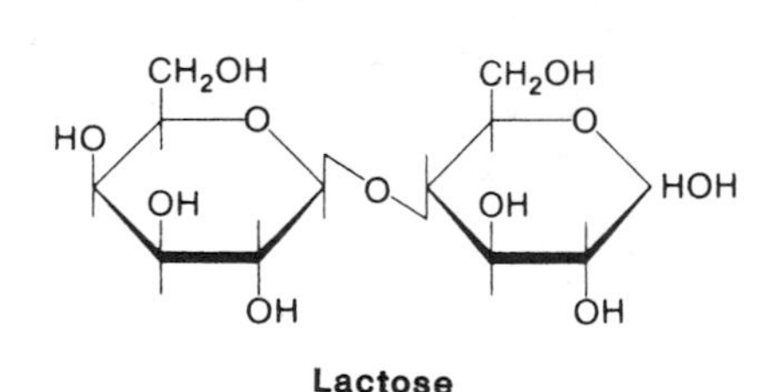

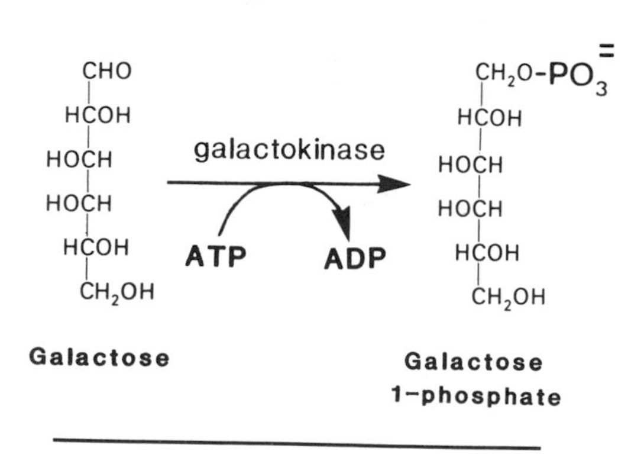

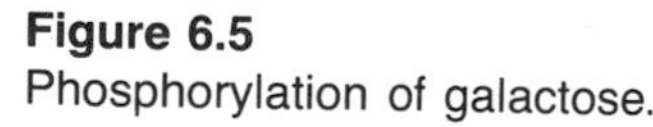

Figure 6.5
Phosphorylation of galactose.

C. cannot convert fructose to fructose 1-phosphate.
D. cannot convert fructose 6-phosphate into fructose 1,6-bisphosphate.
E. cannot produce lactic acid from fructose 6-phosphate.

6.3 Fructosuria is the result of

A. a deficiency of phosphofructokinase.
B. a deficiency of liver fructokinase.
C. elevated levels of liver aldolase B.
D. a deficiency of liver hexokinase.
E. elevated levels of liver fructose 1,6-bisphosphatase.

III. GALACTOSE METABOLISM

A. Dietary sources of galactose

1. The major dietary source of galactose is lactose (β-galactosyl-1 → 4-glucose), obtained from milk and milk products. The digestion of lactose by *β-galactosidase* of the intestinal mucosal cell membrane was discussed on p. 52.
2. Some galactose can also be obtained from the digestion of complex carbohydrates such as glycoproteins and glycolipids, which are important membrane components, as well as from the turnover of the body's own cells.

B. Phosphorylation of galactose

1. Like fructose, D-galactose must be phosphorylated before it can be further metabolized. Most tissues have a specific enzyme for this purpose: *galactokinase,* which produces galactose 1-phosphate (see Figure 6.5). ATP is the phosphate donor.

C. Formation of UDP-galactose

1. Unlike fructose, galactose 1-phosphate cannot enter the glycolytic pathway by a simple cleavage reaction, but rather must first be converted to UDP-galactose (Figure 6.6). This is an exchange reaction in which UMP is removed from UDP-glucose (leaving behind glucose 1-phosphate) and transferred to the galactose 1-phosphate, producing UDP-galactose.
2. The enzyme that catalyzes this reaction, *galactose 1-phosphate uridyl transferase,* is missing in individuals with **galactosemia** (see Figure 6.6).
3. If this enzyme is missing, galactose 1-phosphate, and therefore galactose, will accumulate in the cell. The accumulated galactose will be shunted into side pathways such as that of **galactitol** production. This reaction is catalyzed by the same enzyme, *aldose reductase,* that converts glucose to sorbitol (see p. 62).

D. Use of UDP-galactose as a carbon source for glycolysis or glucogenesis

1. In order for UDP-galactose to enter the mainstream of glucose metabolism, it must first be converted to its C-4 epimer, UDP-glucose, by the enzyme *UDP-hexose 4-epimerase.* (NAD^+ is required for this reaction, becoming alternately reduced then reoxidized, thereby permitting the synthesis of a transient intermediate, 4-keto-hexose).

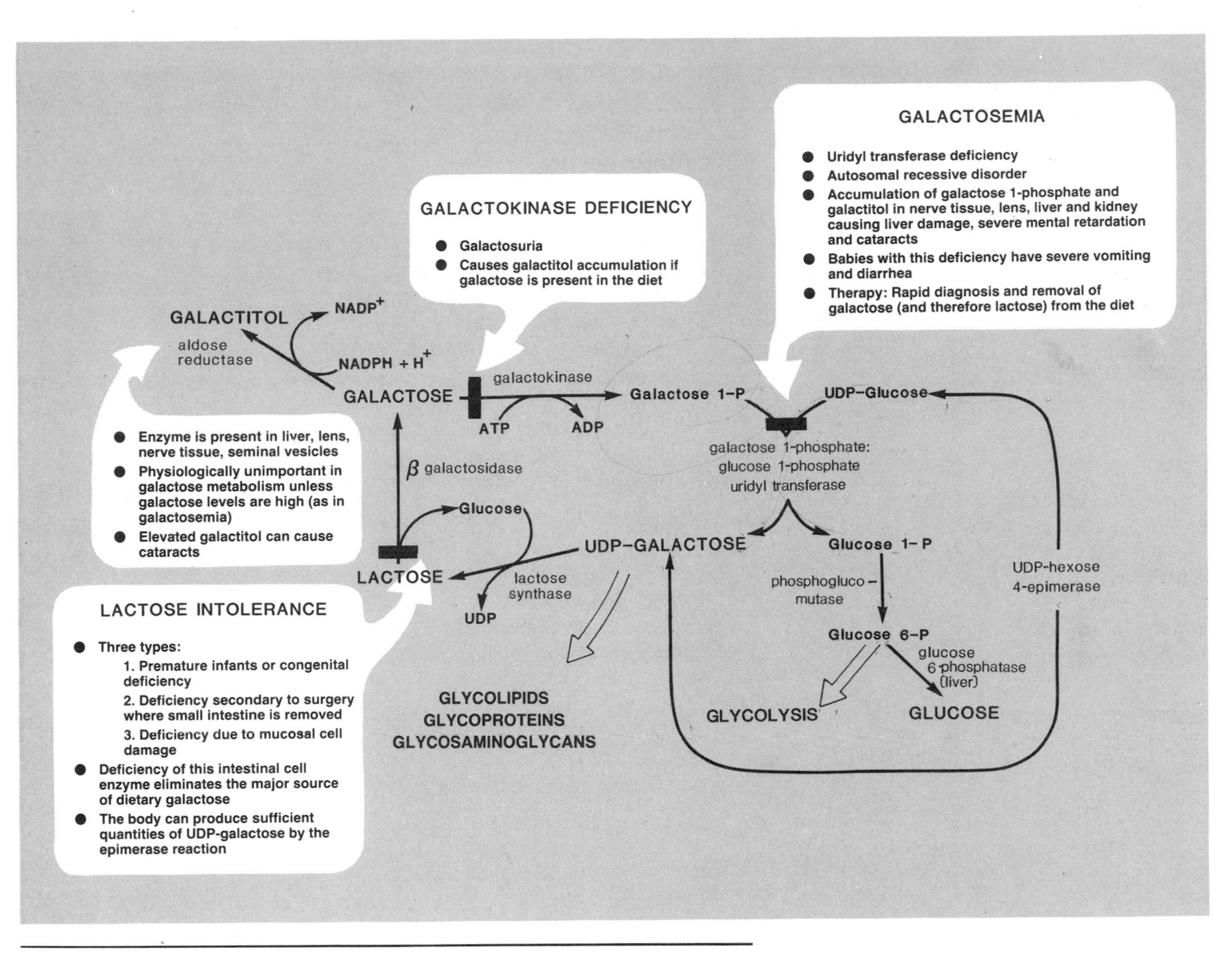

Figure 6.6
Metabolism of galactose.

2. This "new" UDP-glucose can then participate in the *uridyl transferase* reaction described above, converting another galactose 1-phosphate into UDP-galactose and releasing glucose 1-phosphate. The carbons of the original galactose are thus transformed into glucose. (See Figure 6.6 for a summary of this interconversion.)

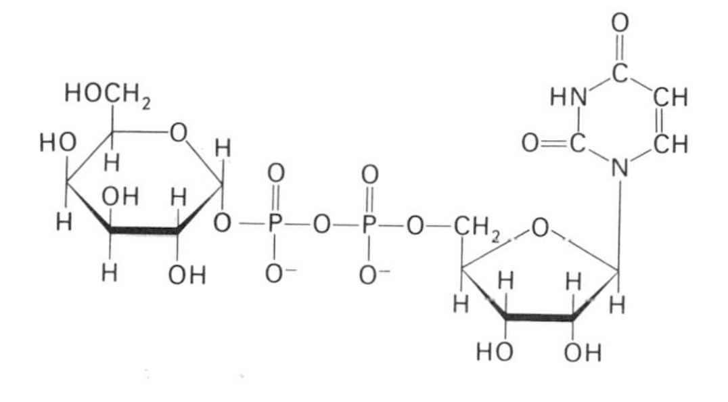

E. Role of UDP-galactose in biosynthetic reactions

1. UDP-galactose can alternatively serve as the donor of galactose units in a number of synthetic pathways, including the synthesis of lactose (see p. 64), glycoproteins (see p. 92), glycolipids (see p. 195), and proteoglycans (see p. 82).

2. Note: If galactose is absent from the diet or cannot be released from lactose owing to a lack of β-*galactosidase,* all tissue requirements for UDP-galactose can be met by the *UDP-hexose 4-epimerase*. (See Figure 6.6 for a summary of galactose metabolism.

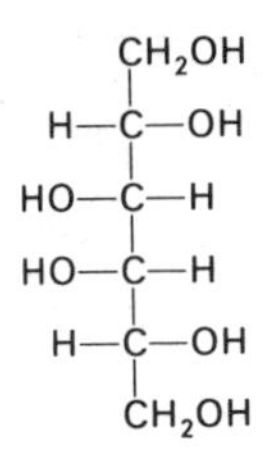

Galactitol

F. Disorders of galactose metabolism

A summary of galactose metabolism and the genetic diseases associated with these pathways is presented in Figure 6.6.

Study Questions

Choose the ONE best answer:

6.4 A galactosemic female can produce lactose because

A. free (nonphosphorylated) galactose is the acceptor of glucose transferred by lactose synthase in the synthesis of lactose.
B. she is able to produce galactose from a glucose metabolite by epimerization.
C. hexokinase can efficiently phosphorylate dietary galactose to galactose 1-phosphate.
D. the enzyme deficient in galactosemia is activated by a hormone produced in the mammary gland.
E. she is able to produce galactose from fructose by isomerization.

6.5 Which one of the following compounds is NOT involved as an intermediate in the metabolic conversion of dietary galactose into blood glucose?

A. UDP-glucose
B. UDP-galactose
C. Glucose 6-phosphate
D. Galactose 6-phosphate
E. Glycogen

6.6 Which of the following statements is true for a mature woman with galactosemia?

A. She can use both hexoses arising from dietary lactose as energy sources.
B. She cannot produce lactose in her mammary glands.
C. She will show a marked decrease in ability to synthesize galactosyl-containing carbohydrates when on a galactose-free diet.
D. When consuming a diet that contains galactose, she will accumulate both galactose 1-phosphate and galactitol in various tissues.
E. She will not be able to convert glucose into UDP-galactose.

6.7 A hereditary childhood disease, galactosemia, is characterized by a

A. high level of liver UDP-galactose.
B. lack of glucose 1-phosphate.
C. very low galactose 1-phosphate uridyltransferase activity in liver.
D. lack of galactokinase.
E. lack of UDP-hexose 4-epimerase.

IV. METABOLISM OF AMINO SUGARS

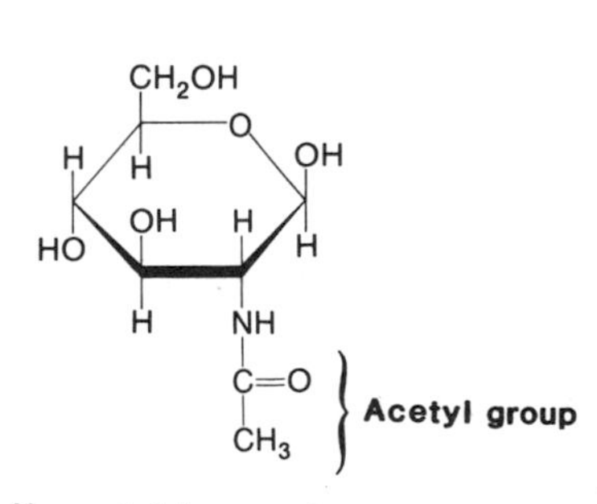

N-acetylglucosamine

The monosaccharide fructose 6-phosphate is the precursor of N-acetylglucosamine, N-acetylgalactosamine, and the sialic acids. In each of these sugars, a hydroxyl group of the precursor has been replaced by an amino group. The amino groups are almost always acetylated.

A. Synthesis of N-acetylglucosamine

1. As shown in Figure 6.7, the nitrogen for the amino group is provided by the amino acid ***glutamine***. The amide nitrogen of glutamine is transferred to fructose 6-phosphate, producing glucosamine 6-phosphate and glutamate. (Note: This reaction is irreversible and is the committed step in amino sugar synthesis.

It is regulated through feedback inhibition by UDP-N-acetylglucosamine.)

2. Glucosamine 6-phosphate is acetylated by acetyl CoA to give N-acetylglucosamine 6-phosphate, which is then converted to N-acetylglucosamine 1-phosphate.
3. For N-acetylglucosamine to be in a form that can be transferred to a growing oligosaccharide chain, it must be converted to a nucleotide derivative—***UDP-N-acetylglucosamine***. The reaction is analogous to that producing UDP-glucose (see p. 68).

B. Synthesis of UDP-N-acetylgalactosamine

1. N-acetylgalactosamine is synthesized by the epimerization of UDP-N-acetylglucosamine, producing UDP-N-acetylgalactosamine (Figure 6.8). This activated amino sugar can then be transferred to a growing oligosaccharide.

C. Synthesis of N-acetylneuraminic acid (NANA)

1. Neuraminic acid is the parent compound of the family of ***sialic acids***, each of which is acetylated at a different site. N-Acetylneuraminic acid is an example of a sialic acid. These compounds are usually found as the terminal carbohydrate residues of oligosaccharide side-chains of glycoproteins.
2. The reactions producing NANA are shown in Figure 6.7. UDP-N-acetylglucosamine is converted in three steps to ***N-acetylmannosamine 6-phosphate***. This compound condenses with ***phosphoenoylpyruvate*** (an intermediate in the glycolytic pathway) to form N-acetylneuraminic acid 9-phosphate. The 9-phosphate is removed hydrolytically, leaving NANA, which can be further acetylated to produce other sialic acids.
3. Before NANA can be added to a growing oligosaccharide, it must be converted into its active form by reacting with CTP. The enzyme *N-acetylneuraminate-CMP-pyrophosphorylase* removes pyrophosphate from the CTP and attaches the remaining CMP to the NANA. This is the only nucleotide sugar in human metabolism in which the carrier nucleotide is a ***monophosphate***.

V. GLUCURONIC ACID METABOLISM

Glucuronic acid, whose structure is that of glucose with an oxidized carbon #6 (—$CH_2OH \rightarrow$—COOH), is an essential component of glycosaminoglycans (see p. 82) and is also required in detoxification reactions of a number of insoluble compounds such as bilirubin and some steroids. In plants and in many mammals other than primates (including man) and guinea pigs, glucuronic acid serves as a precursor of ascorbic acid (vitamin C) (Figure 6.9).

A. Sources of glucuronic acid

1. Glucuronic acid can be obtained from the ***diet***. However, dietary ***inositol*** serving as a precursor for the intracellular synthesis of glucuronic acid provides a quantitatively more significant source of carbons for glucuronic acid in the body.
2. Glucuronic acid can also be obtained from the intracellular lysosomal degradation of ***glycosaminoglycans*** or by the ***uronic acid***

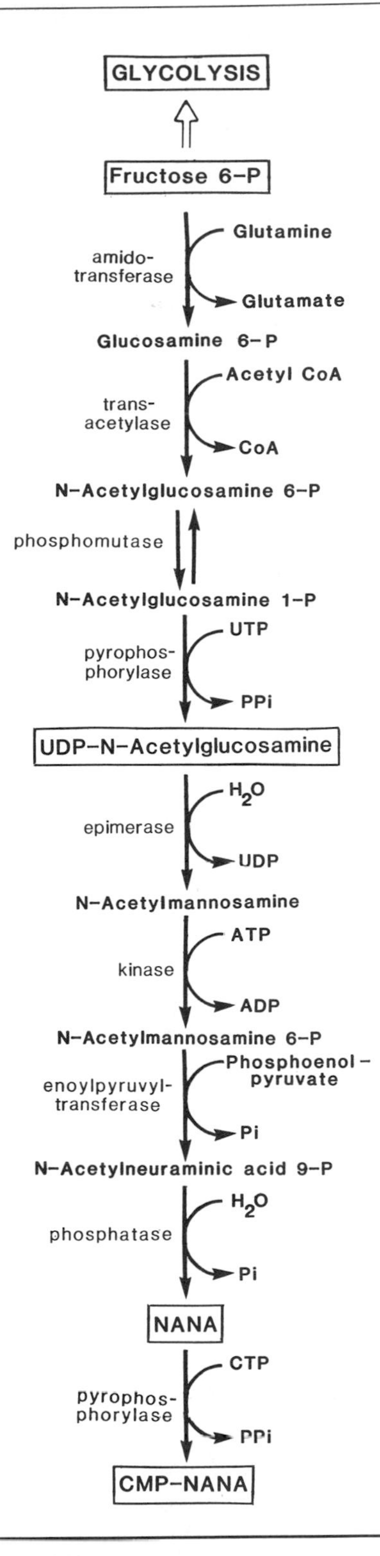

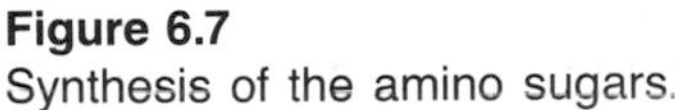

Figure 6.7
Synthesis of the amino sugars.

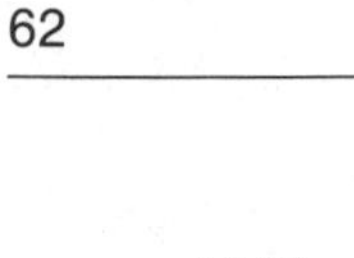

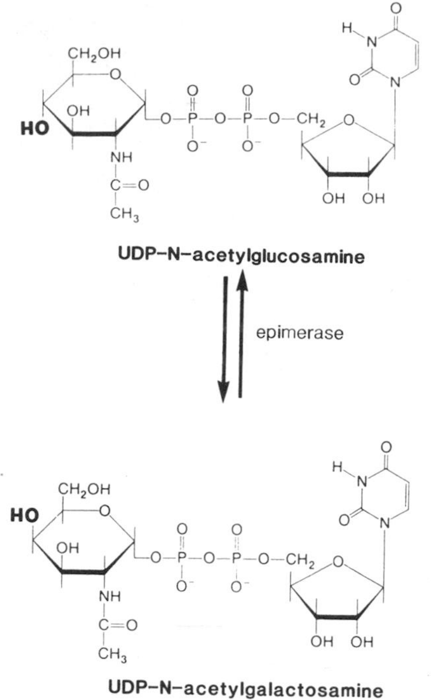

Figure 6.8
Synthesis of UDP-N-acetylgalactosamine.

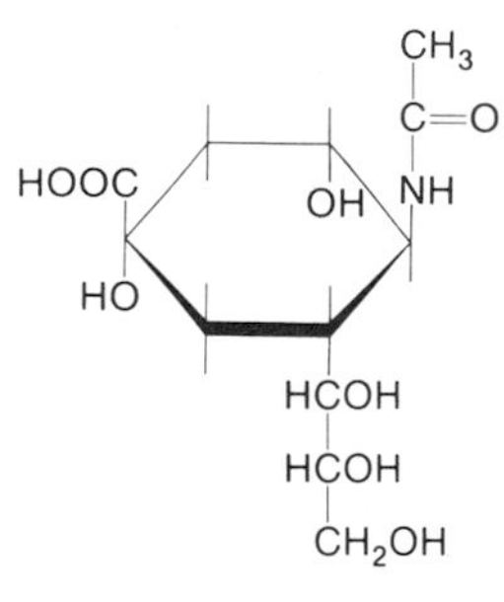

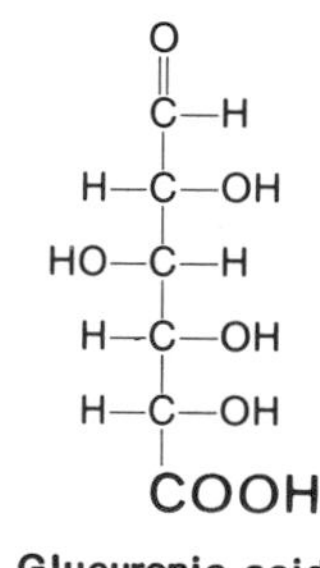

pathway, which is an alternate pathway for the oxidation of glucose 6-phosphate. The pathway and enzymes involved are shown in Figure 6.9.

a. The end-product of this pathway in humans, D-xylulose, is phosphorylated by a *kinase* to D-xylulose 5-phosphate, which can enter the hexose monophosphate pathway and produce the glycolytic intermediates glyceraldehyde 3-phosphate and fructose 6-phosphate (see p. 146). Thus, excess glucuronic acid can be used to produce energy by means of glycolysis or can be converted into glycogen by gluconeogenesis and glycogenesis.

b. A deficiency of *L-xylulose reductase* causes the rare genetic disorder ***essential pentosuria*** (Figure 6.9).

c. The uronic acid pathway also provides a mechanism by which dietary D-xylitol can enter the central metabolic pathways.

B. Formation of UDP-glucuronic acid

1. The active form of glucuronic acid that donates the sugar in various reactions is UDP-glucuronic acid, which is produced by the oxidation of UDP-glucose (Figure 6.10).

Study Questions

Choose the ONE best answer:

6.8 N-Acetylneuraminic acid arises biologically from the condensation of which one of the following pairs of compounds?

A. Erythrose and N-acetylxylosamine
B. Erythrose and N-acetylribosamine
C. Pyruvate and N-acetylglucosamine
D. Glyceraldehyde 3-phosphate and N-acetylglucosamine
E. Phosphoenolpyruvate and N-acetylmannosamine

6.9 Which one of the following statements about an individual with hereditary pentosuria is INCORRECT?

A. Dietary xylitol can be metabolized by the liver.
B. Most dietary glucuronic acid will be converted to pentoses, which will be found in the urine.
C. The patient will be unable to synthesize inositol and will require it in the diet.
D. The patient's ability to synthesize glucuronylated bilirubin will not be impaired.
E. A normal supply of ribose required for the biosynthesis of nucleic acids will be provided by the hexose monophosphate pathway.

6.10 Biosynthesis of glucuronic acid requires the

A. oxidation of UDP-glucose.
B. oxidation of glucose 6-phosphate.
C. oxidation of 6-phosphogluconate.
D. oxidation of glucose.
E. reduction of sorbitol.

VI. SORBITOL METABOLISM

A. Sources and metabolic fates of sorbitol

1. Although most sugars are rapidly phosphorylated following their entry into cells, *aldose reductase (NADPH-linked sorbitol de-*

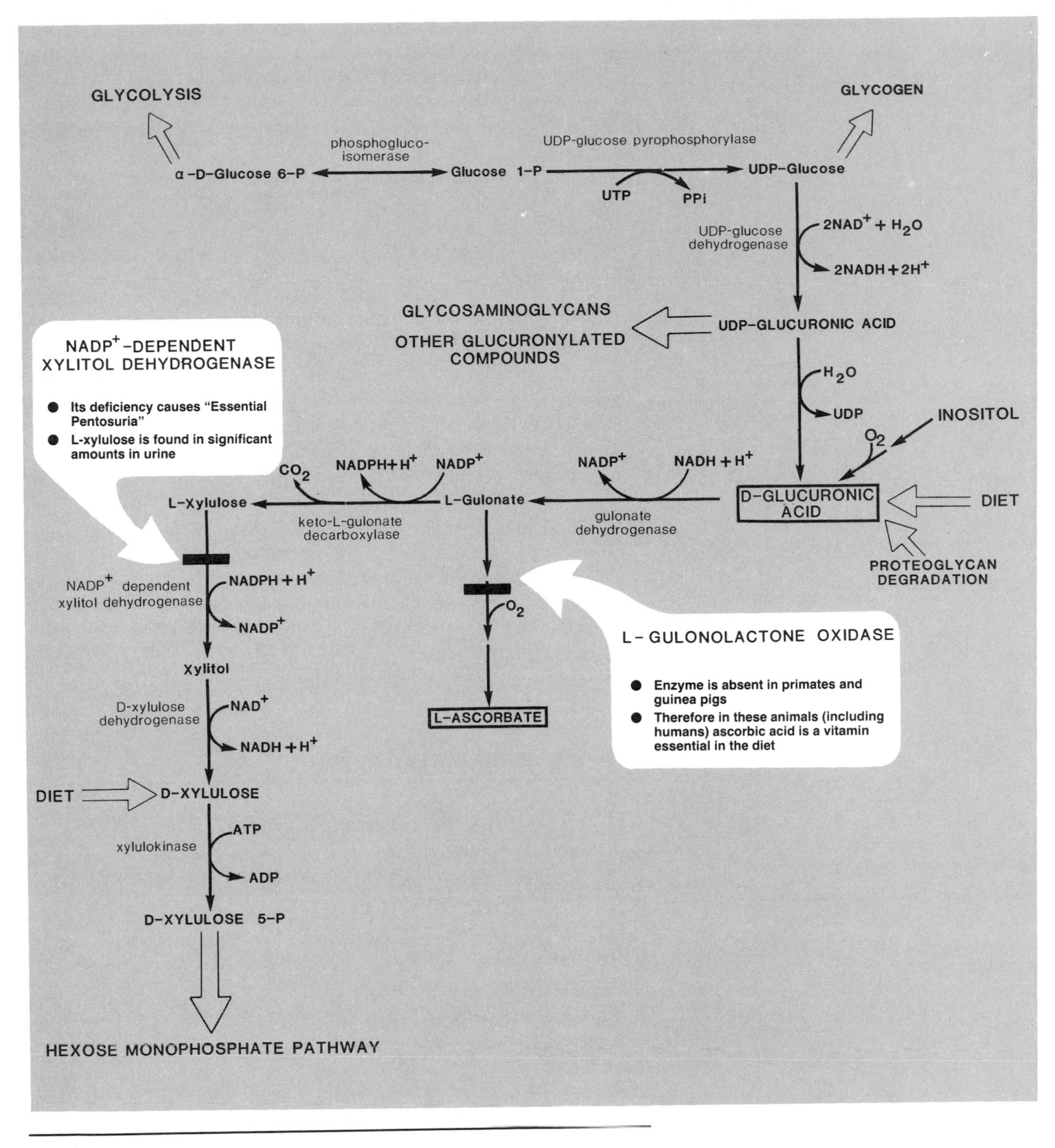

Figure 6.9
Uronic acid pathway.

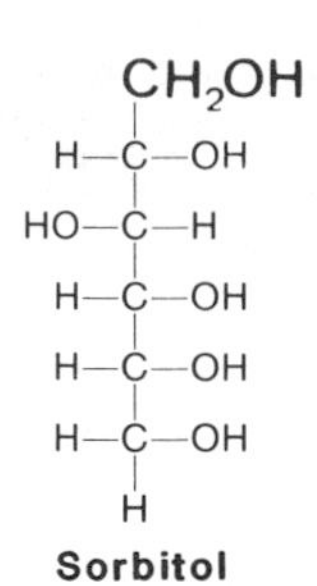

hydrogenase) can alternatively reduce glucose to produce sorbitol. This enzyme is found in significant concentrations in the epithelium of the lens, the Schwann cells of peripheral nerves, the papillae in the kidney, and the cells of the seminal vesicles.

2. In liver and seminal vesicle cells there is a second enzyme, *sorbitol dehydrogenase* (NADH-linked), that can oxidize the sorbitol, producing fructose (Figure 6.11).
3. The two-reaction pathway from glucose to fructose by means of sorbitol in the seminal vesicles is an important source of fructose for sperm cells, in which fructose is the preferred carbohydrate energy source.

B. The effect of hyperglycemia on sorbitol metabolism

1. Because insulin is not required for entry of glucose into the cells listed above, large amounts of glucose may enter these cells during times of hyperglycemia, for example, as seen in ***diabetes***.
2. Elevated intracellular glucose will cause a significant increase in the amount of sorbitol produced, which, unlike glucose, cannot pass freely through cell membranes and therefore remains trapped inside the cell (Figure 6.11).
3. Because *sorbitol dehydrogenase* is absent in the lens and nerve cells, and because the *aldose reductase* equilibrium lies far to the right, sorbitol will accumulate in these cells, causing strong osmotic effects and therefore cell swelling owing to water retention. Many of the physiologic and pathologic alterations associated with diabetes can be attributed to this phenomenon, including cataract formation, peripheral neuropathy, and vascular problems leading to atherosclerosis, nephropathy, and retinopathy.

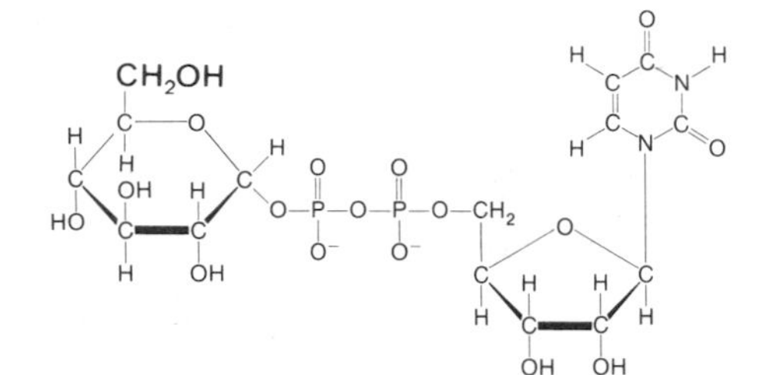

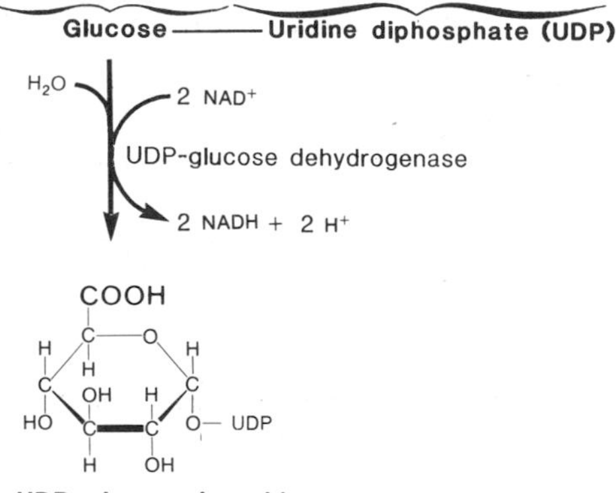

Figure 6.10
Oxidation of UDP-glucose to UDP-glucuronic acid.

VII. LACTOSE METABOLISM

A. Structure and dietary sources of lactose

1. Lactose is a ***disaccharide,*** whose structure consists of a molecule of β-galactose attached by a 1→4 linkage to glucose. Therefore, lactose is β-galactosyl-1,4-glucose.
2. Lactose, known as "milk sugar," is produced by the mammary glands of most but not all mammals. Therefore, milk and other dairy products are the primary dietary sources of lactose.

B. Synthesis and degradation of lactose

1. Lactose is synthesized by *lactose synthase* (*UDP-galactose:glucose galactosyl transferase*), which transfers galactose from UDP-galactose to glucose, releasing UDP (Figure 6.12). This enzyme is composed of two proteins, A and B.
2. *Protein A* is a *β-D-galactosyl transferase* and is found in a number of body tissues. In tissues other than the lactating mammary gland, this enzyme transfers galactose from UDP-galactose to N-acetyl-D-glucosamine, forming the same β-(1→4) linkage as is found in lactose and producing N-acetyllactosamine (allolactose).
3. Protein B is found only in lactating mammary glands. It is ***α-lactalbumin*** and is found in large quantities in milk.

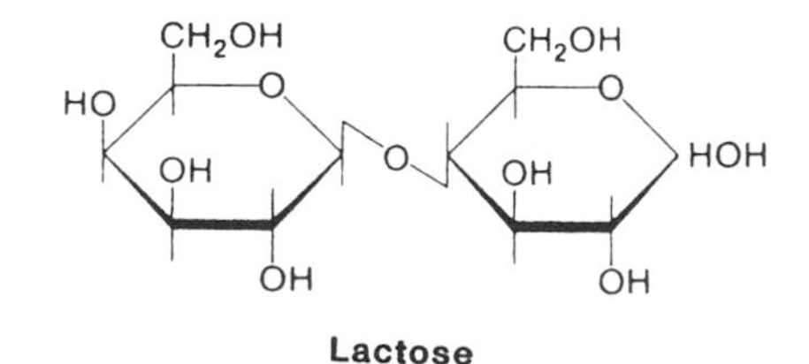

4. The degradation of lactose in the intestine was discussed on p. 52.

C. Hormonal control of lactose synthesis

1. Before and during pregnancy, the mammary gland synthesizes N-acetyllactosamine. During pregnancy, ***progesterone*** inhibits the synthesis of protein B.
2. After birth, progesterone levels drop significantly, stimulating the synthesis of ***prolactin***. α-Lactalbumin synthesis is stimulated by prolactin. The resulting regulatory protein B forms a complex with the enzyme, *protein A,* changing the specificity of that *transferase* so that lactose is now produced.

VIII. SUCROSE AND MALTOSE METABOLISM

A. Sucrose

1. Sucrose is synthesized in the leaves of plants and serves as a transportable form of carbohydrate that nourishes the rest of the plant.
2. Sucrose contains both ***glucose*** and ***fructose***. Unlike lactose, however, the two monosaccharides are attached through a glycosidic bond between their two anomeric carbons, that is, carbon #1 of glucose attached to carbon #2 of fructose, forming α-D-glucopyranosyl-(1→2)-β-D-fructofuranoside. (The fructose has, in effect, been "flipped over.")
3. Sucrose is therefore a ***nonreducing sugar,*** since neither anomeric carbon is free (unlike lactose, in which the anomeric carbon of glucose is not attached to anything else and therefore is a reducing sugar that can undergo mutarotation [see p. 47 for a discussion of this process]).

B. Maltose

1. Maltose (α-D-glucopyranosyl-(1→4)-β-D-glucopyranose) is obtained primarily from ingestion of beer and the digestion of dietary starches by *α-amylase* (see p. 51). It is a reducing sugar and therefore can undergo mutarotation.
2. ***Isomaltose,*** which is also obtained from the digestion of the branch points of starches such as glycogen, is also a disaccharide containing two glucose molecules. In this case, however, the bond is between carbon #1 of one glucose and carbon #6 of the second glucose.

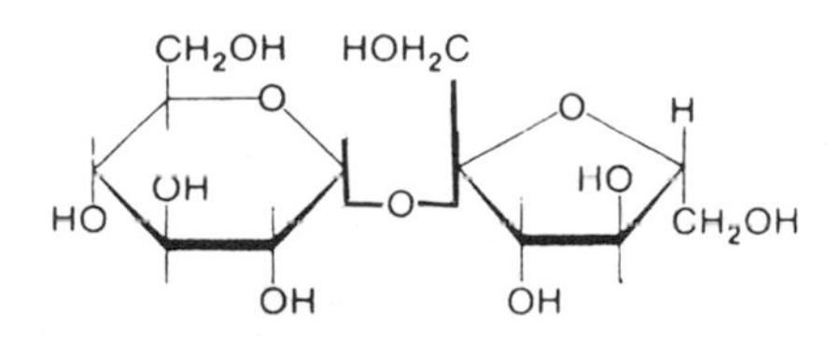

Sucrose

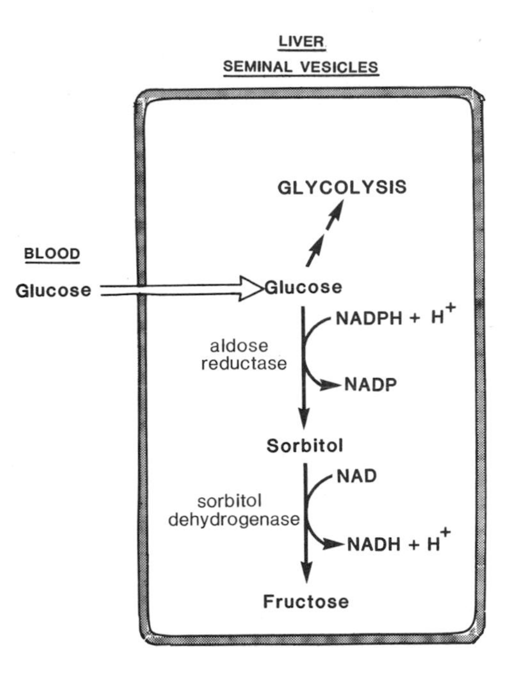

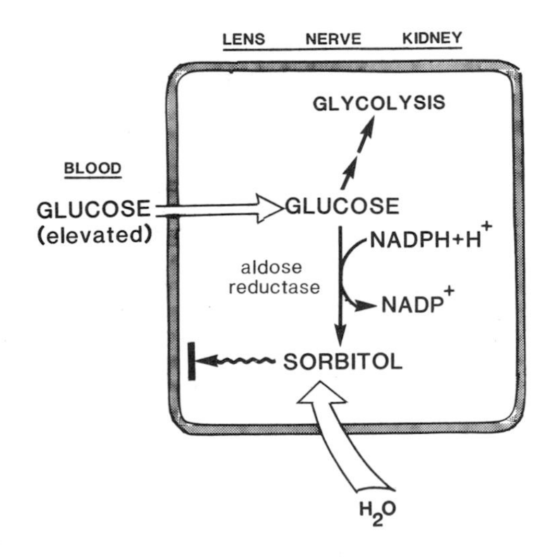

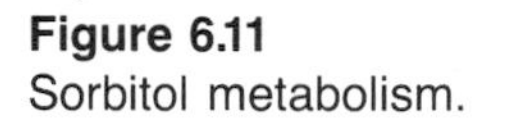

Figure 6.11
Sorbitol metabolism.

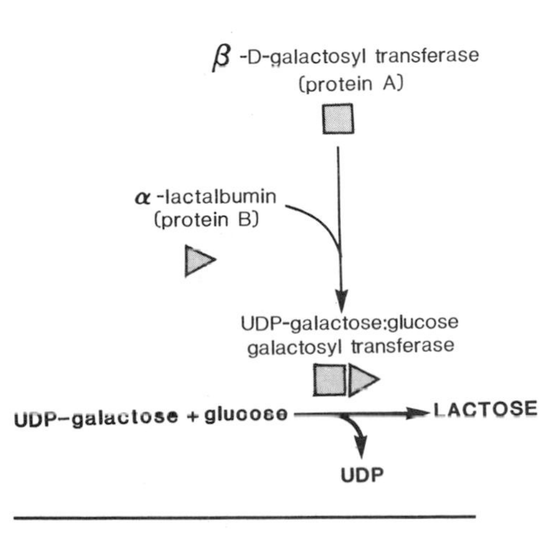

Figure 6.12
Lactose synthesis.

Study Questions

Choose the ONE best answer:

6.11 A major contributing factor to cataract formation in diabetes may be the accumulation of sorbitol in the lens. For that to occur, glucose has to interact with

A. glucose oxidase.
B. NADPH-dependent aldose reductase.
C. glucokinase.
D. hexokinase and glucose 6-phosphate dehydrogenase.
E. hexokinase and phosphoglucoisomerase.

6.12 In lactose biosynthesis, an immediate precursor for lactose is

A. UDP-glucose.
B. UDP-galactose.
C. galactose 1-phosphate.
D. glucose 1-phosphate.
E. galactose.

6.13 No lactose is metabolized after its intravenous injection into a rat; however, ingestion of lactose leads to rapid metabolism of galactose. The difference in these results is due to

A. the absence of lactase in the serum.
B. the absence of hepatic galactokinase.
C. the presence of maltase in the serum.
D. the presence of lactase in the intestine.
E. a combination of A and D above.

6.14 Which one of the following statements is NOT correct about lactose?

A. It can undergo mutarotation.
B. It is a reducing sugar.
C. It is hydrolyzed by β-galactosidase to glucose and galactose.
D. It is synthesized in the mammary gland by galactosyl transferase.
E. It can be converted into sucrose by epimerization of its galactose residue, so that the two disaccharides are freely interchangeable.

Questions 6.15–6.17
For each of the disaccharides listed below, choose the monosaccharides of which it is composed:
A. Fructose only
B. Glucose only
C. Glucose and fructose
D. Glucose and galactose
E. Fructose and galactose

6.15 Sucrose

6.16 Lactose

6.17 Maltose

Glycogen Metabolism

7

I. OVERVIEW

A constant source of blood glucose is an absolute requirement for human life. Glucose is the preferred energy source of the brain and is the required energy source for cells with few or no mitochondria, such as mature erythrocytes. Glucose is also essential as an energy source in exercising muscle, where it serves as the substrate for the pathway of anaerobic glycolysis.

Glucose can be supplied to the body from several different dietary sources, such as starch and the disaccharides lactose, maltose, and sucrose (Figure 7.1). Carbon skeletons of other monosaccharides (e.g., fructose, galactose, mannose), amino acid carbon skeletons (those classified as glucogenic; see p. 239), and small carbohydrates (e.g., glycerol and glyceraldehyde) are also precursors of glucose. These compounds enter intermediary metabolism and can eventually be converted into glucose by the pathway of gluconeogenesis. (This pathway is described on p. 125.)

Dietary intake of glucose and glucose precursors is sporadic, however, and is not always a reliable source of blood glucose. Therefore, the body has developed mechanisms for storing a supply of glucose in the form of glycogen. When glycogen stores are depleted, the body then synthesizes glucose *de novo,* using amino acids from the body's proteins as the primary source of carbons for the gluconeogenic pathway.

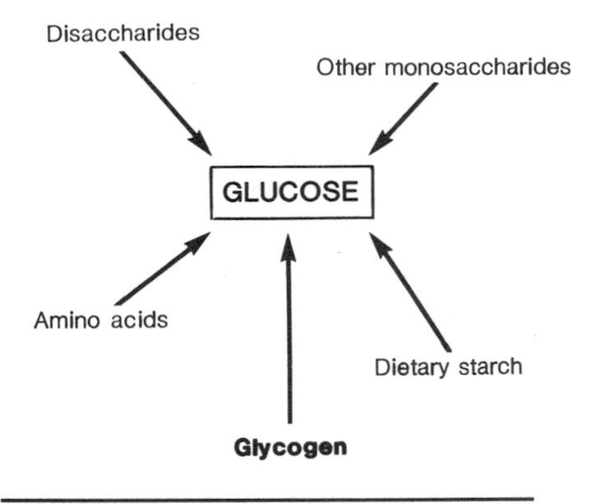

Figure 7.1
Sources of glucose.

II. STRUCTURE AND FUNCTION OF GLYCOGEN

A. Location and function of glycogen

1. The main stores of glycogen in the body are found in the ***skeletal muscle*** and ***liver***. Approximately 400 g of glycogen make up 1% to 2% of the fresh weight of resting muscle, and approximately 100 g of glycogen makes up 6% to 10% of the fresh weight of a well-fed liver. What limits the production of glycogen in the liver and muscle to these amounts is unknown. In some ***glycogen storage diseases*** (summarized in Figures 7.4 and 7.5), however, the amount of glycogen in liver and muscle can be significantly higher.
2. The function of muscle glycogen is to serve as a fuel reserve for the synthesis of ATP during muscle contraction. The function of liver glycogen is to maintain blood glucose concentration,

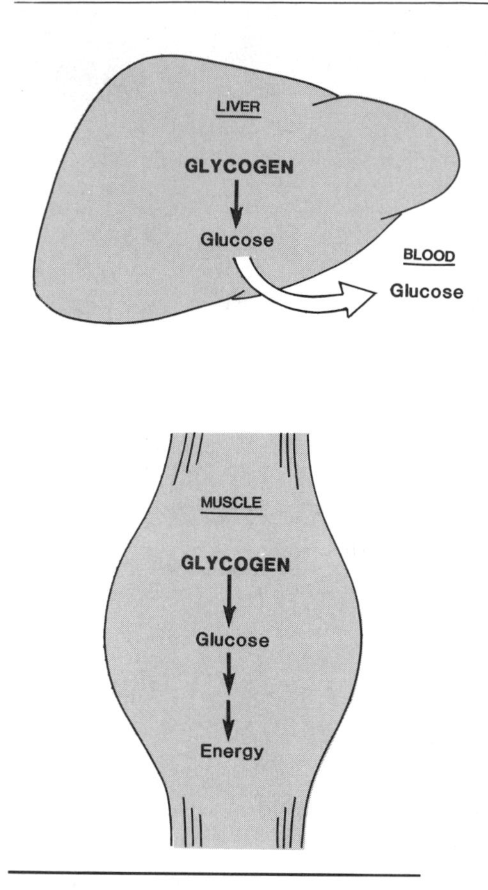

Figure 7.2
Functions of muscle and liver glycogen.

particularly during the early stages of a fast (see p. 285 and Figure 7.2).

3. A single molecule of glycogen can have a molecular weight up to 10^8. These molecules exist in discrete ***cytoplasmic granules*** that contain most of the enzymes necessary for glycogen synthesis and degradation.

B. Chemical structure of glycogen

1. Structurally, glycogen is a branched-chain homopolysaccharide made exclusively from α-D-glucose (Figure 7.3).
2. The primary glycosidic bond is an α-1→4 linkage (Figure 7.3).
3. After every 8 to 10 glucosyl residues there is a branch. At each branch point the branching chain is attached by an α-1→6 linkage.

III. SYNTHESIS OF GLYCOGEN

A. Synthesis of UDP-glucose

1. Glucose attached to uridine diphosphate (UDP) is the source of the glucosyl residues that are contributed to the growing glycogen molecule. UDP-glucose is synthesized by the following reactions (summarized in Figure 7.4):
   a. Glucose 6-phosphate is converted to glucose 1-phosphate by *phosphoglucomutase*. Glucose 1,6-bisphosphate is an obligatory intermediate in this reaction.
   b. Glucose 1-phosphate reacts with UTP to form UDP-glucose

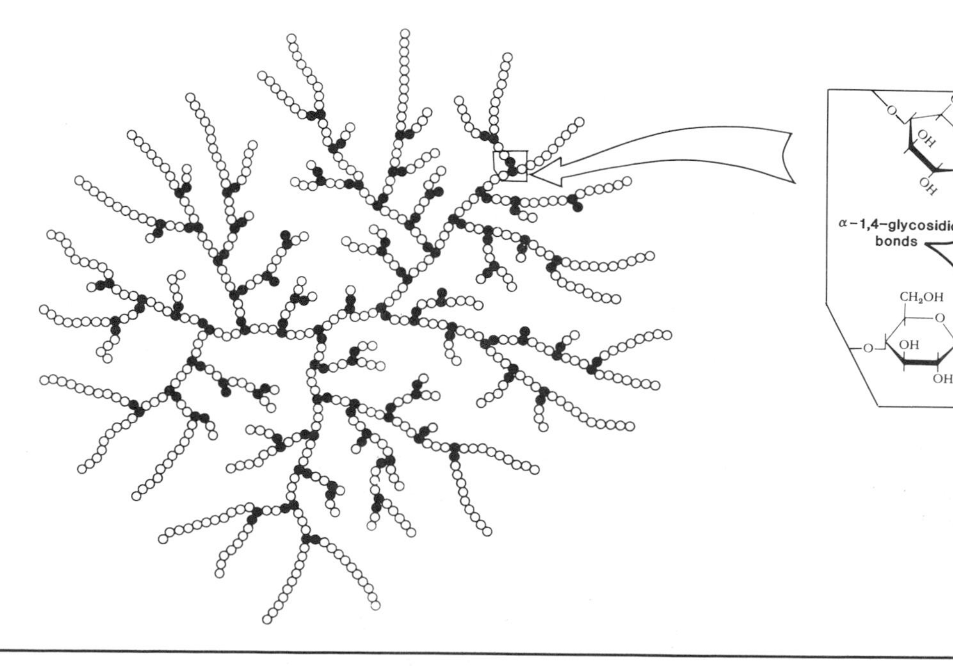

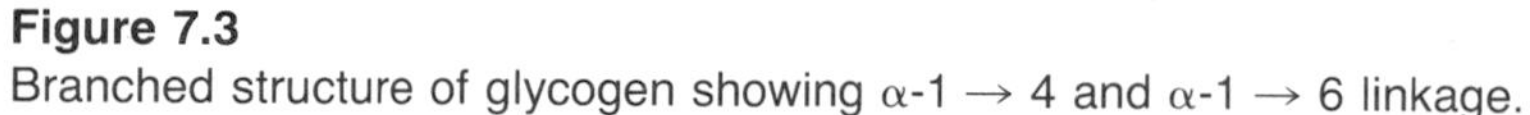

Figure 7.3
Branched structure of glycogen showing α-1 → 4 and α-1 → 6 linkage.

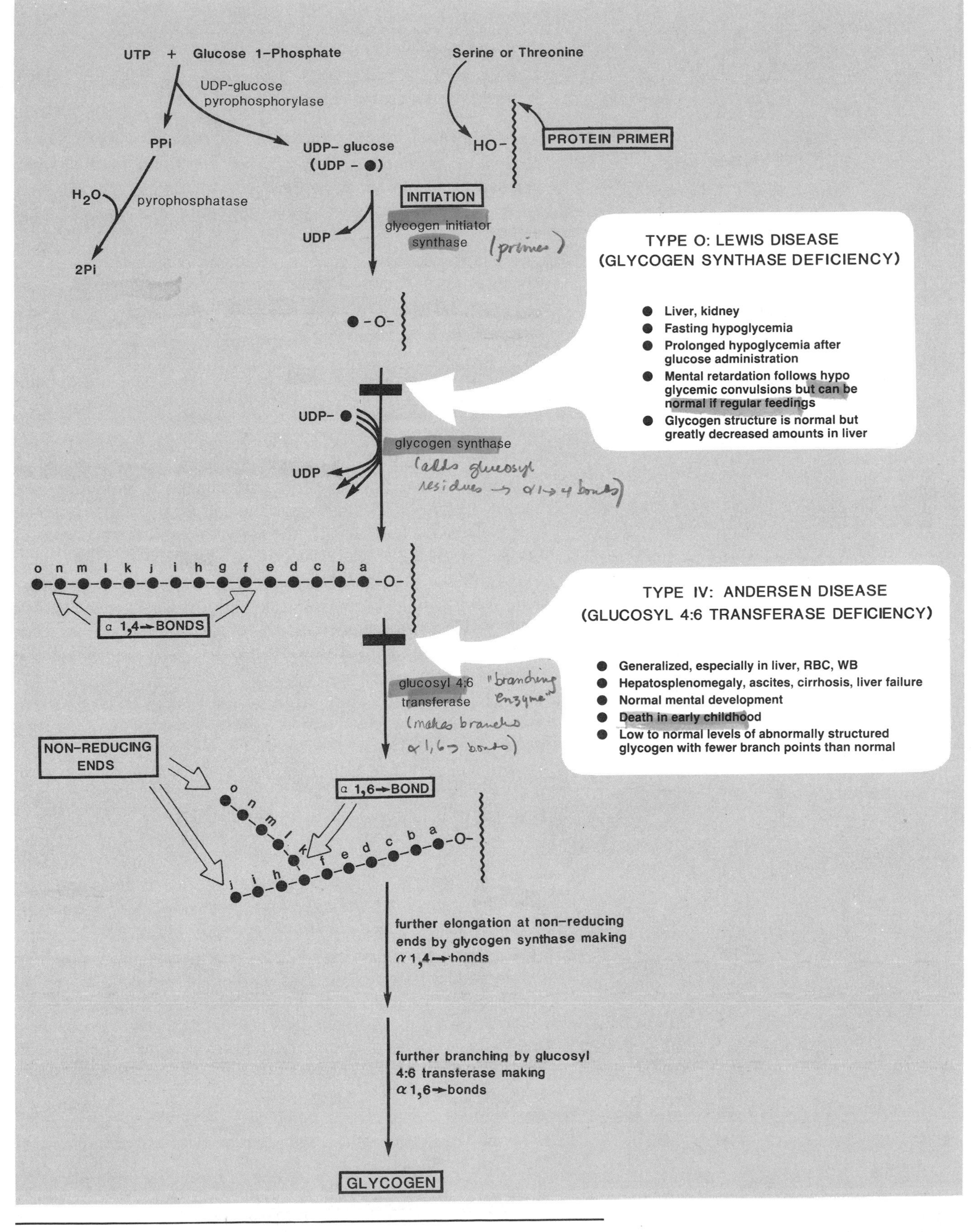

Figure 7.4
Glycogen synthesis.

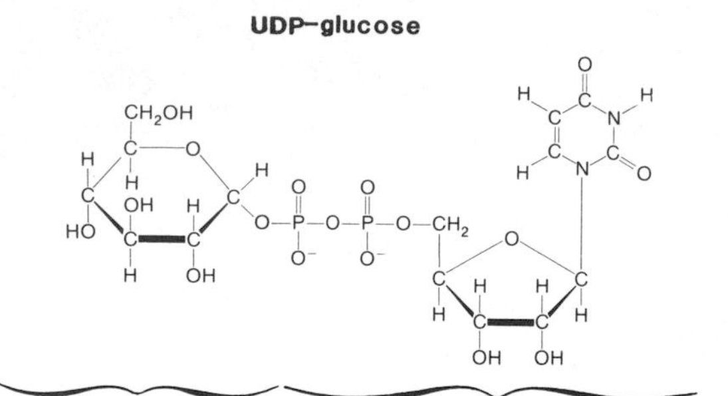

plus pyrophosphate (PP_i). The immediate hydrolysis of PP_i to two inorganic phosphates (catalyzed by *pyrophosphatase*) ensures that the reaction will progress in the direction of UDP-glucose production.

B. A primer is required for glycogen synthesis

1. Free glucose cannot accept a molecule of glucose from UDP-glucose to initiate chain synthesis. A fragment of glycogen can serve as a primer in cells whose glycogen stores are not totally depleted.
2. In the absence of a glycogen fragment, a specific protein can serve as an acceptor of glucose residues, the hydroxyl groups of the serine and threonine side-chains serving as sites where glucosyl units can be attached. The enzyme that can transfer the first molecules of glucose from UDP-glucose to the protein is *glycogen initiator synthetase*.

C. Elongation of glycogen chains

1. Elongation of the glycogen chain involves the transfer of glucose from UDP-glucose to the ***nonreducing end*** of the growing chain, forming a new glycosidic bond between the hydroxyl group of carbon #1 of the activated sugar and carbon #4 of the accepting glucosyl residue (Figure 7.4). The enzyme responsible for making the α-1$\rightarrow$4 linkages in glycogen is *glycogen synthase* (also called *glucosyltransferase*).
2. If no other synthetic enzyme acted on the chain, the resulting structure would be a linear molecule of glucosyl residues attached by α-1$\rightarrow$4 linkages. Such a compound is found in fruits and is called amylose.
3. The UDP released when the new α-1$\rightarrow$4 glycosidic bond is made can be converted back to UTP by the enzyme *nucleoside diphosphokinase* (UDP + ATP$\rightarrow$UTP + ADP).

D. Creating branches in glycogen

1. Unlike amylose, which is an unbranched polysaccharide, glycogen has branches located approximately 8 glucosyl residues apart on each chain, resulting in a highly branched, treelike structure. The branches are made through the activity of the "branching enzyme" *glucosyl 4:6 transferase* (*amylo-α-(1,4)-α-(1,6)-transglycosylase*).
2. This enzyme transfers a chain of 5 to 8 glucosyl residues from the nonreducing end of the glycogen chain (breaking an α-1$\rightarrow$4 bond) to another residue on the chain where it attaches the two sections by an α-1$\rightarrow$6 linkage. The resulting new nonreducing end as well as the old nonreducing end from which the 5 to 8 residues were removed can now be further elongated by *glycogen synthase* (Figure 7.4).
3. After further elongation of these two ends has occurred, their terminal 5 to 8 glycosyl residues can be removed and utilized to make further branches.
4. Branches have two important functions: First, branching results in increased solubility of the glycogen molecule; and second,

branching increases the number of nonreducing ends to which new glucosyl residues can be added (and, as described later, from which these residues can be removed), thereby greatly accelerating the rate at which glycogen synthesis and degradation can occur.

5. A summary of glycogen synthesis is shown in Figure 7.4.

IV. DEGRADATION OF GLYCOGEN

The degradative pathway responsible for the mobilization of stored glycogen in the liver and skeletal muscle is not a simple reversal of the synthetic reactions. Instead, a second, independent set of enzymes is required. When glycogen is degraded the primary product is glucose 1-phosphate. In addition, free glucose is released from each α-1$\rightarrow$6 linkage.

A. Shortening of chains

1. The first enzyme of the degradative pathway, *glycogen phosphorylase,* cleaves the α-1$\rightarrow$4 glycosidic bonds between the glucosyl residues at the nonreducing ends of the glycogen chains by simple phosphorolysis (Figure 7.6).
2. This enzyme is an ***exo****glucosidase* and sequentially degrades the glycogen chains at their nonreducing ends until four glucosyl units remain on each chain before the branch point. The resulting structure is called a ***limit dextrin,*** and the *phosphorylase* cannot degrade this structure any further.

B. Removal of branches

1. Branches are removed through the two enzymatic activities of the ***debranching enzyme*** (Figure 7.5):
   a. First, *glucosyl 4:4 transferase (amylo-α-(1,4):α-(1,4)-glucan transferase)* activity removes the outer 3 of the 4 glucosyl residues attached at a branch and transfers them to the nonreducing end of another chain. (Thus an α-1$\rightarrow$4 bond is broken, and an α-1$\rightarrow$4 bond is made.)
   b. Next, the single glucose residue attached in an α-1$\rightarrow$6 linkage is then removed hydrolytically by the *α-amylo-(1:6)-glucosidase* activity of the "debranching enzyme," releasing free glucose. The glucosyl chain is now available again for degradation by *glycogen phosphorylase* until four glucosyl units from the next branch are reached.
2. A summary of the steps in glycogen degradation is shown in Figure 7.5.

C. Lysosomal degradation of glycogen

1. Approximately 1% to 3% of cellular glycogen is being continuously degraded by the lysosomal enzyme *α-glucosidase (acid maltase).*
2. A deficiency of this enzyme causes the accumulation of glycogen in vacuoles in the cytoplasm, resulting in glycogen storage disease type II (Pompe's disease; see Figure 7.5). A summary of the steps in glycogen degradation is shown in Figure 7.5.

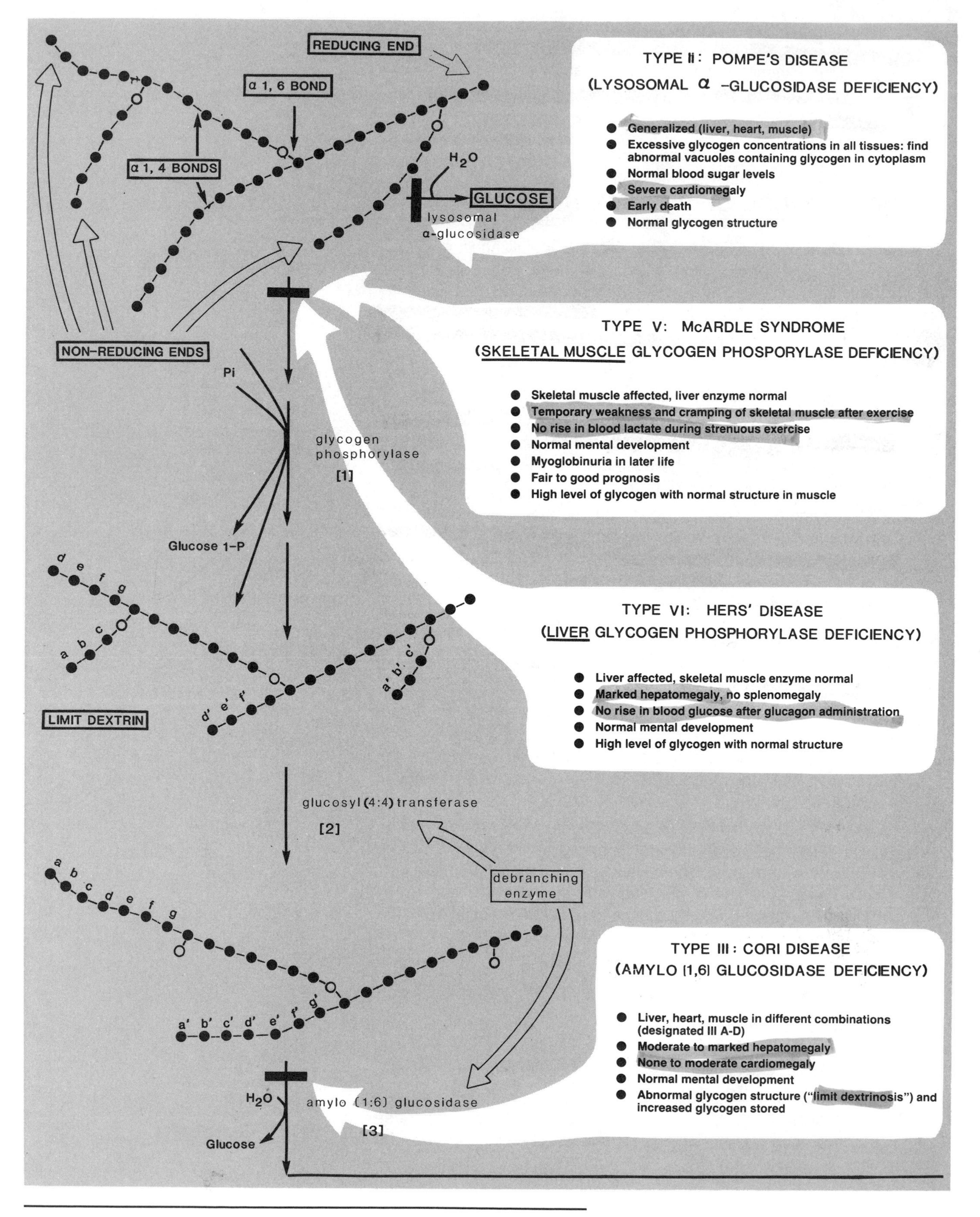

Figure 7.5
Glycogen degradation.

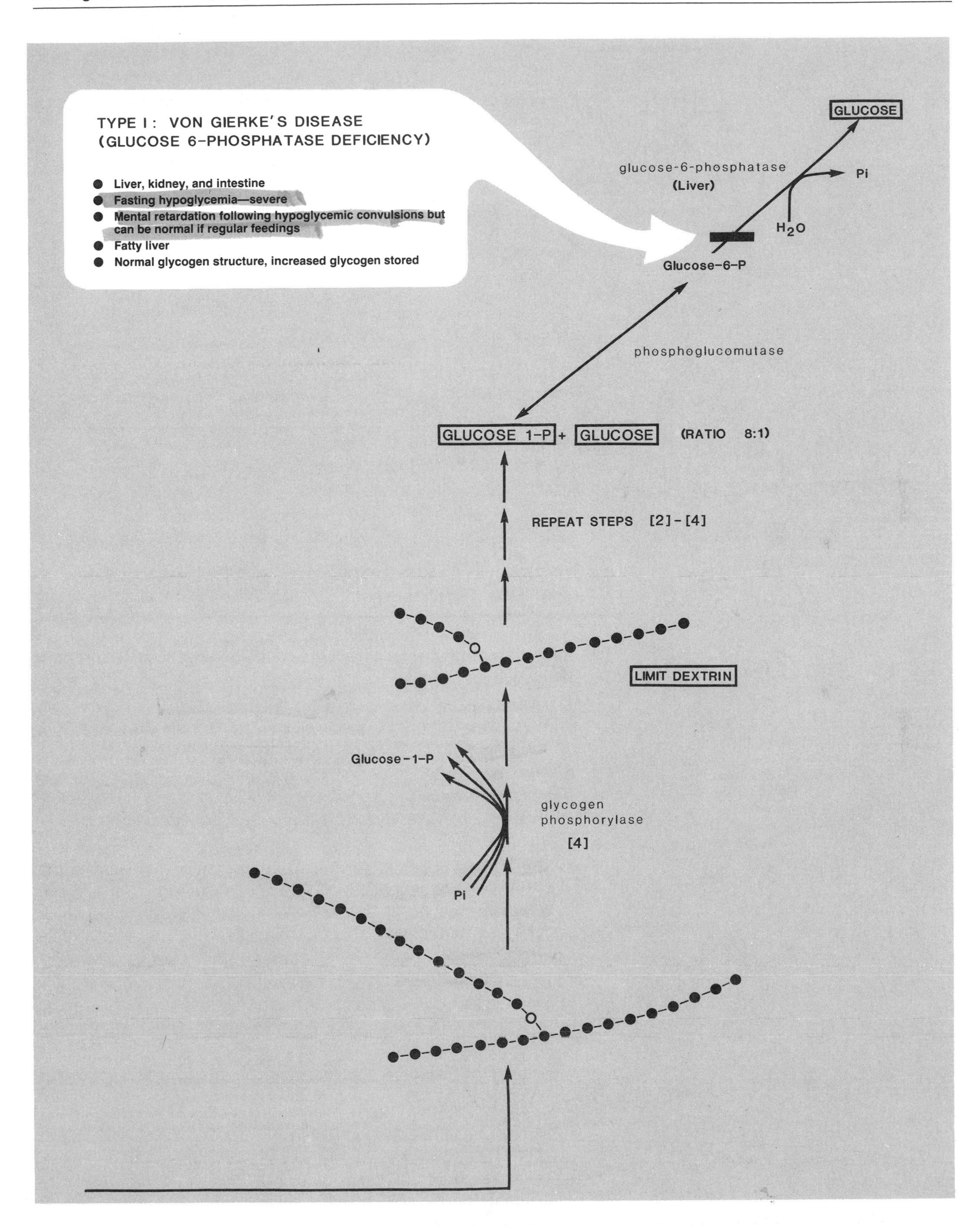
TYPE I: VON GIERKE'S DISEASE
(GLUCOSE 6-PHOSPHATASE DEFICIENCY)
Liver, kidney, and intestine
Fasting hypoglycemia—severe
Mental retardation following hypoglycemic convulsions but can be normal if regular feedings
Fatty liver
Normal glycogen structure, increased glycogen stored
GLUCOSE
glucose-6-phosphatase
(Liver)
Pi
H_2O
Glucose-6-P
phosphoglucomutase
GLUCOSE 1-P + GLUCOSE
(RATIO 8:1)
REPEAT STEPS [2]-[4]
LIMIT DEXTRIN
Glucose-1-P
glycogen phosphorylase
[4]
Pi

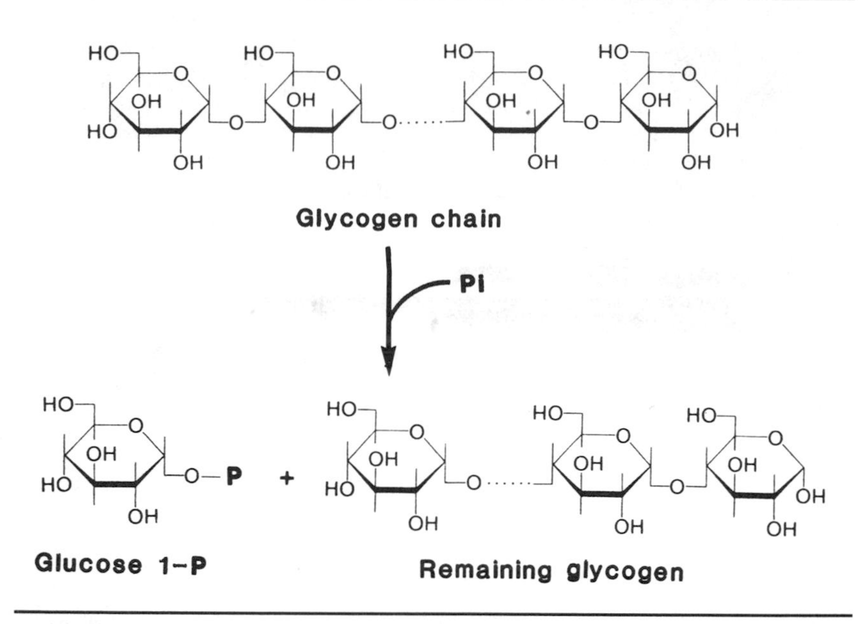

Figure 7.6
Cleavage of the α-1 → 4-glycosidic bond.

V. REGULATION OF GLYCOGEN SYNTHESIS AND DEGRADATION

A. Inhibition of glycogen synthesis by a 3′-5′-cyclic AMP-directed pathway.

1. The regulated enzyme is *glycogen synthase.* It exists in two forms: the I form that is active, and the D form that is inactive. The I form is not phosphorylated, but the D form is.
2. The I form of *glycogen synthase* is converted to the D form and therefore inactivated by phosphorylation at a number of sites. This process is catalyzed by a group of *protein kinases,* one of which is cAMP-dependent.
3. The binding of hormones such as glucagon and epinephrine to the hepatocyte receptors, or of epinephrine to the muscle cell receptors, results in the activation of *adenyl cyclase,* which catalyzes the synthesis of cAMP (Figure 7.8). The cAMP activates *protein kinase,* which phosphorylates and therefore ***inactivates*** *glycogen synthase.*
4. *Glycogen synthase D* can be transformed back to *synthase I* by *protein phosphatase,* which removes the phosphate groups hydrolytically.
5. See Figure 7.8 for a summary of the regulation of glycogen synthesis.

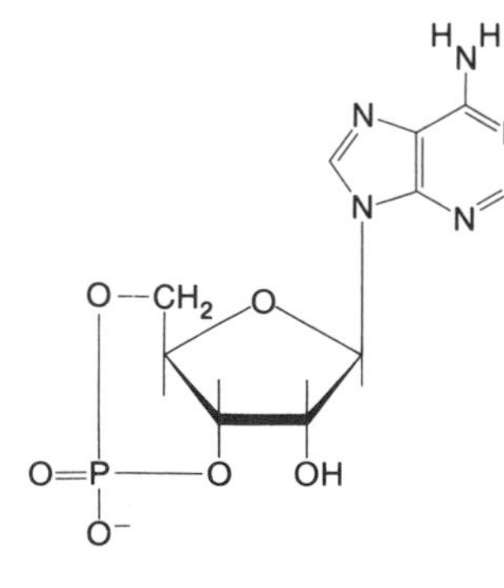

B. Activation of glycogen degradation by a 3′-5′-cyclic AMP-directed pathway.

1. The binding of hormones such as ***glucagon*** or ***epinephrine*** to receptors on the cell surface of hepatocytes and adipocytes, or

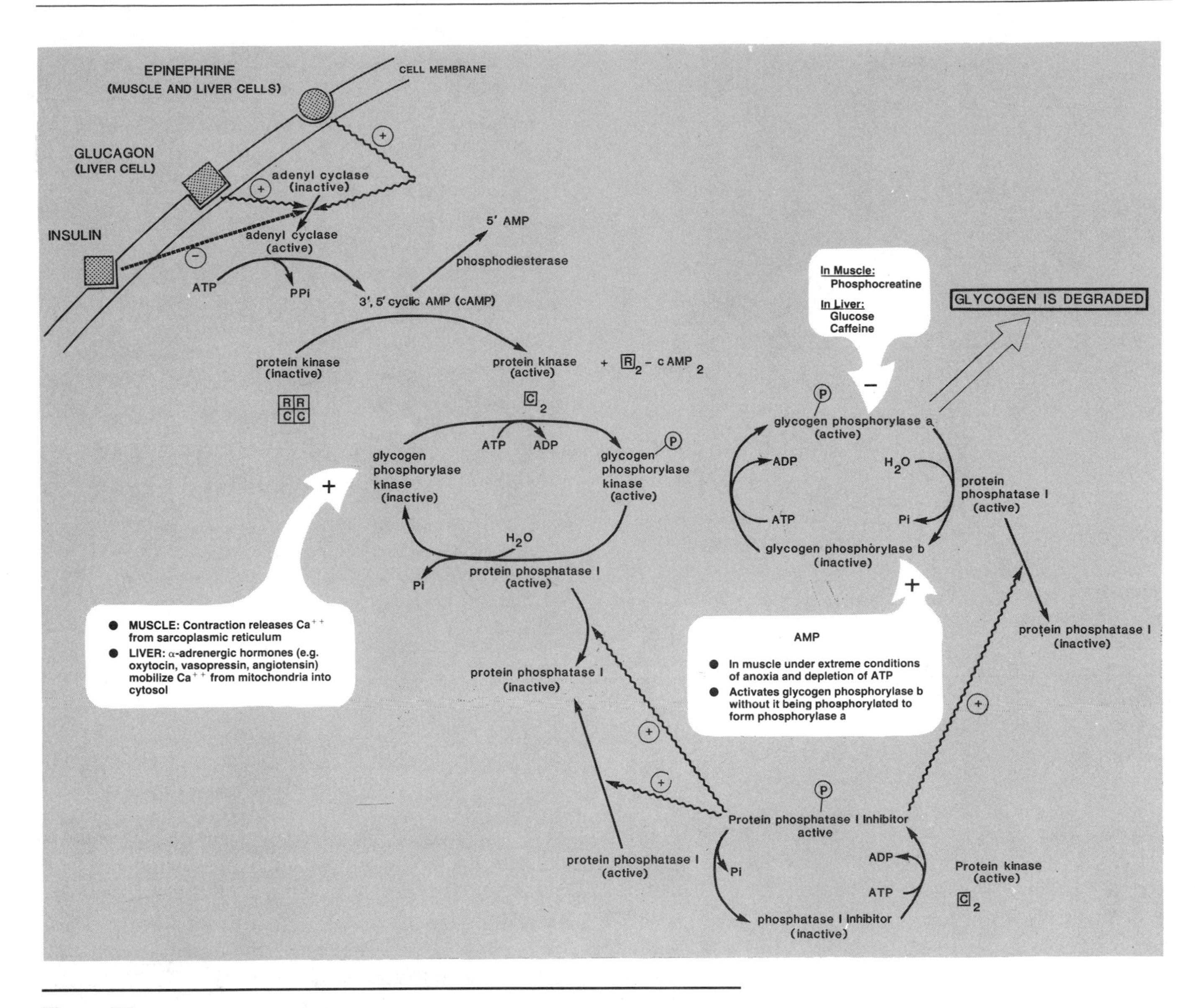

Figure 7.7
Regulation of glycogen degradation.

of epinephrine to muscle cells, results in the activation of membrane-associated, intracellular *adenyl cyclase* (Figure 7.7). This enzyme catalyzes the synthesis of ***3′-5′-cyclic AMP*** (cAMP) from ATP.

$$\text{ATP} \rightarrow \text{cAMP} + \text{PP}_i$$

a. (Note: cAMP is continuously degraded to 5′-AMP by *phosphodiesterase,* and therefore in the absence of hormonal stimulus rapidly disappears from the cell.)

2. cAMP activates *protein kinase*. This enzyme is a tetramer, having two regulatory subunits (R) and two catalytic subunits (C). cAMP binds to the regulatory subunits, releasing C_2, which has catalytic activity. When cAMP is removed, the inactive tetramer is formed again.

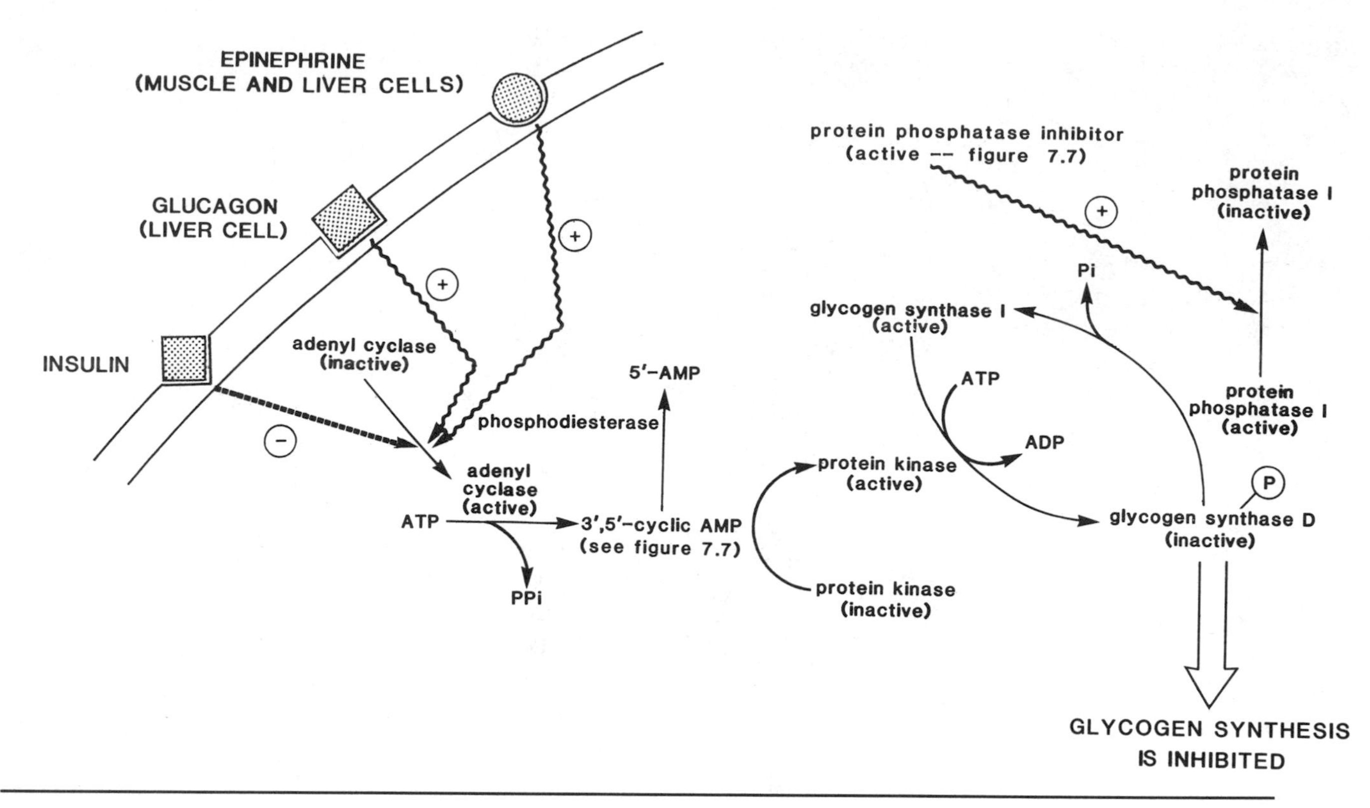

Figure 7.8
Regulation of glycogen synthesis.

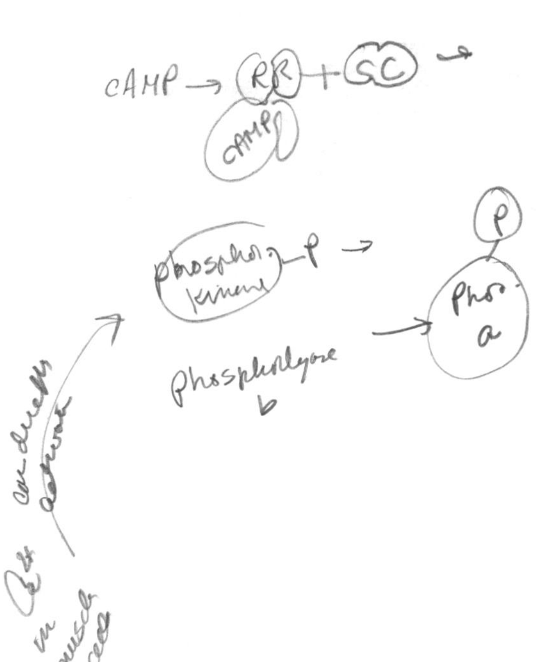

3. Active *protein kinase* phosphorylates the enzyme *phosphorylase kinase,* resulting in its activation. The phosphorylated enzyme can be inactivated by the hydrolytic removal of its phosphate by *protein phosphatase.*

4. Active *phosphorylase kinase* phosphorylates *glycogen phosphorylase b,* converting it into the active *glycogen phosphorylase a,* which then begins glycogen breakdown. *Phosphorylase a* is reconverted to *phosphorylase b* by the hydrolytic removal of its phosphate by *protein phosphatase.*

5. Summary: What is observed, then, is a cascade of reactions that result in glycogen degradation. The purpose of the large number of sequential steps is the ***amplification*** of the effect of the hormonal signal. For example, a few hormone molecules binding to their receptors result in a number of *protein kinase* molecules being activated, which can each activate many *phosphorylase kinase* molecules, finally causing a large number of active *glycogen phosphorylase a* molecules to degrade glycogen.

6. See Figure 7.7 for a summary of the steps in the regulation of glycogen degradation.

C. Additional activation of glycogen degradation in the muscle by calcium and AMP

1. During muscle contraction there is a rapid and urgent need for ATP, the energy for which is supplied by the stored muscle

glycogen as the source of glucose. Nerve impulses cause membrane depolarization, which in turn promotes Ca^{++} release from the sarcoplasmic reticulum into the sarcoplasm of muscle cells. Ca^{++} binds to calmodulin—a subunit of *phosphorylase kinase*—and activates this enzyme without the need for its phosphorylation by *protein kinase* (see Figure 7.7).

2. Muscle *glycogen phosphorylase b* is enzymatically active in the presence of high AMP concentration. A high concentration of AMP is seen in the muscle only under extreme conditions of anoxia and ATP depletion. AMP binds to *phosphorylase b,* causing its activation without phosphorylation (Figure 7.7).

D. Summary of the regulation of glycogen synthesis and degradation

1. Glycogen synthesis and degradation are regulated by the same hormonal signals: Elevated insulin results in overall increased glycogen synthesis; elevated glucagon (or epinephrine) causes increased glycogen degradation.
   a. Cyclic AMP levels in cells increase in response to hormonal stimuli, for example, glucagon and epinephrine in the liver and epinephrine in the muscle. cAMP levels decrease in the presence of insulin.
   b. Key enzymes are phosphorylated by a family of *kinases,* some of which are cAMP-dependent.
   c. The phosphorylation of an enzyme causes a conformational change that affects the active site. This can either greatly increase the catalytic activity of some enzymes or decrease it for others.
   d. The added phosphate groups can be removed hydrolytically by *phosphatases,* and therefore the action of *phosphatases* always opposes that of the *kinases*. If the *kinases* have greater activity than the *phosphatases,* then more of the regulated enzyme will be in the phosphorylated mode, and vice versa.

VI. GLYCOGEN STORAGE DISEASES

A. These are a group of diseases that result from a defect in a step of glycogen synthesis or degradation. They all result in either formation of glycogen that has an abnormal structure or accumulation of excessive amounts of glycogen in specific tissues.

B. A particular enzyme may be defective in a single tissue such as the liver, or may be more generalized, affecting muscle, kidney, intestine, and myocardium. The severity of the disease may range from fatal in infancy to mild disorders that are not life-threatening. Some glycogen storage diseases are illustrated in Figures 7.4 and 7.5.

Study Questions

Choose the ONE best answer:

7.1 An abnormal, poorly branched glycogen was isolated from the liver of a patient with type IV glycogen storage disease. The deficiency is most probably in

A. phosphorylase kinase.
B. glycogen phosphorylase a.
C. protein kinase.
D. amylo-α-(1,6)-glucosidase.
E. amylo-α-(1,4):α-(1,6)-transglycosylase.

7.2 Epinephrine and glucagon have the following effects on glycogen metabolism in the liver:

A. The net synthesis of glycogen is increased.
B. Glycogen phosphorylase is activated, whereas glycogen synthase is inactivated.
C. Both glycogen phosphorylase and glycogen synthase are activated but at markedly different rates.
D. Glycogen phosphorylase is inactivated, whereas glycogen synthase is activated.
E. Cyclic AMP-dependent protein kinase is activated, whereas phosphorylase kinase is inactivated.

7.3 In the muscle, a sudden elevation of the Ca^{++} concentration will cause

A. activation of cyclic AMP-dependent protein kinase.
B. dissociation of cyclic AMP-dependent protein kinase into catalytic and regulatory subunits.
C. inactivation of phosphorylase kinase owing to the action of a protein phosphatase.
D. conversion of glycogen phosphorylase b to phosphorylase a.
E. conversion of cyclic AMP to AMP by phosphodiesterase.

7.4 Muscle glycogen cannot contribute directly to blood glucose levels because

A. muscle glycogen cannot be converted to glucose 6-phosphate.
B. muscle lacks glucose 6-phosphate phosphatase.
C. muscle contains no glucokinase.
D. muscle contains no glycogen phosphorylase.
E. muscle lacks phosphoglucoisomerase.

7.5 In the liver, a significant increase in the activities of protein phosphatase(s) that act on the enzymes responsible for glycogen synthesis and degradation will most probably lead to

A. increased rate of glycogen synthesis and decreased rate of degradation.
B. decreased rate of glycogen synthesis and increased rate of degradation.
C. increased rate of glycogen synthesis and increased rate of degradation.
D. decreased rate of glycogen synthesis and decreased rate of degradation.
E. no net change in the rates of either synthesis or degradation of glycogen.

7.6 How does 3′,5′-cyclic AMP increase the rate of glycogenolysis?

A. It promotes the formation of a phosphorylated form of glycogen phosphorylase.
B. It serves as a cofactor for glycogen phosphorylase.
C. It serves as a precursor of 5′-AMP, which is a cofactor for glycogen phosphorylase.
D. It furnishes phosphate for the phosphorolysis of glycogen.
E. It serves as a potential source of ATP.

7.7 Which of the following conditions would exist in a mutant tissue culture line derived from ***liver*** that is unable to synthesize 3′,5′-cyclic AMP?

A. An abnormally low cellular content of glycogen
B. A high phosphorylase a/phosphorylase b ratio
C. An increased level of protein kinase activity after incubating the cells with glucagon
D. Little effect of glucose 6-phosphate on the activity of glycogen synthase
E. Increased phosphodiesterase activity

7.8 The laboratory report on a patient with glycogen storage disease was as follows: fasting blood glucose, 45 mg/dl; blood glucose after epinephrine infusion, 41 mg/dl; blood glucose after oral fructose administration, 95 mg/dl; blood lactate in the resting condition, 18 mg/dl; blood lactate after exercise, 39 mg/dl. Glycogen from both liver and muscle was structurally normal. The laboratory results suggest an absence of

A. liver and muscle α-(1,6)-glucosidase.
B. liver glycogen synthase.
C. muscle phosphorylase.
D. liver fructokinase.
E. liver glucose 6-phosphatase.

Glycosaminoglycans

8

I. OVERVIEW

Glycosaminoglycans are large complexes of ***negatively charged*** carbohydrate chains generally associated with a small amount of protein. These compounds have the special ability to bind large amounts of water, thereby producing the gel-like matrix that forms the basis of the body's ***ground substance. Connective tissue,*** found in skin, tendons, cartilage, ligaments, and the matrix of bone, comprises insoluble protein fibers distributed in the ground substance. The character of connective tissue is dependent to a large extent on the relative proportions of the ground substance and embedded fibrous proteins. For example, cartilage is rich in ground substance, whereas tendon is composed primarily of fibers. The viscous, lubricating properties of ***mucous secretions*** also result from an aqueous solution of glycosaminoglycans, a fact that led to the original naming of these compounds, ***mucopolysaccharides***. An additional example of specialized ground substance is the ***synovial fluid*** that serves as a lubricant in joints, tendon sheaths, and bursa (Figure 8.1).

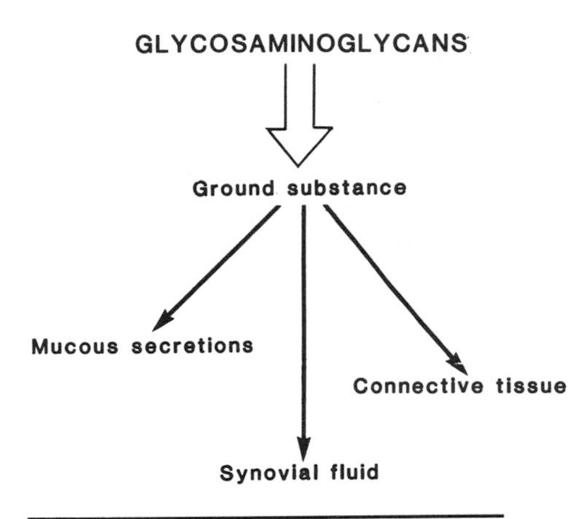

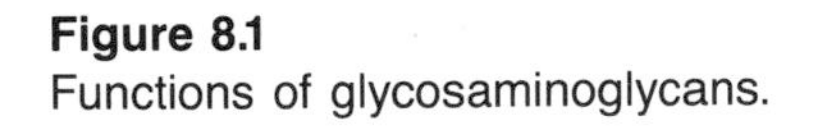
Figure 8.1
Functions of glycosaminoglycans.

II. STRUCTURE AND FUNCTION OF GLYCOSAMINOGLYCANS

A. Carbohydrate components of glycosaminoglycans

1. The carbohydrate component of glycosaminoglycans is a long, unbranched heteropolysaccharide, generally comprising a ***repeating disaccharide unit,*** [amino sugar – acidic sugar]$_n$.
2. The amino sugar is either D-glucosamine or D-galactosamine, in which the amino group is usually but not always acetylated. The amino sugar may also be sulfated on carbon #4 or 6, or a nonacetylated nitrogen (Figure 8.2)
3. The acidic sugar is either D-glucuronic acid or its C-5 epimer, L-iduronic acid. These sugars contain carboxyl groups that are negatively charged at physiologic pH and, together with the sulfate groups, give the glycosaminoglycans their strongly negative (acidic) nature.
   a. Because of the large number of negative charges, these heteropolysaccharide chains tend to be extended in solution and repel each other while at the same time are surrounded by a shell of water molecules. When brought together, they

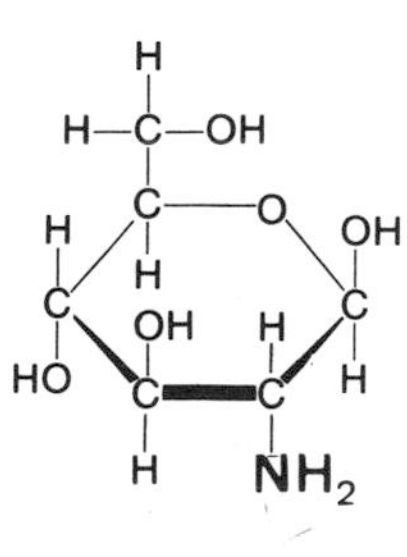

Glucosamine

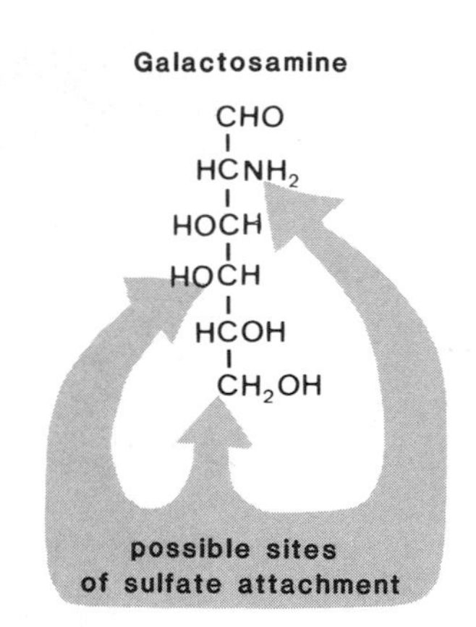

Figure 8.2
Structure and possible sulfation sites of D-galactosamine.

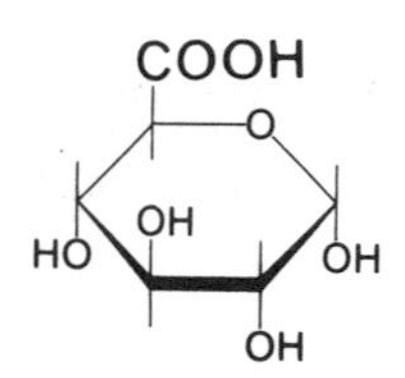

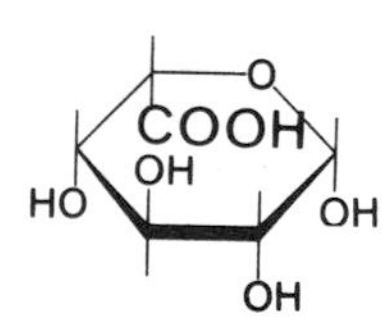

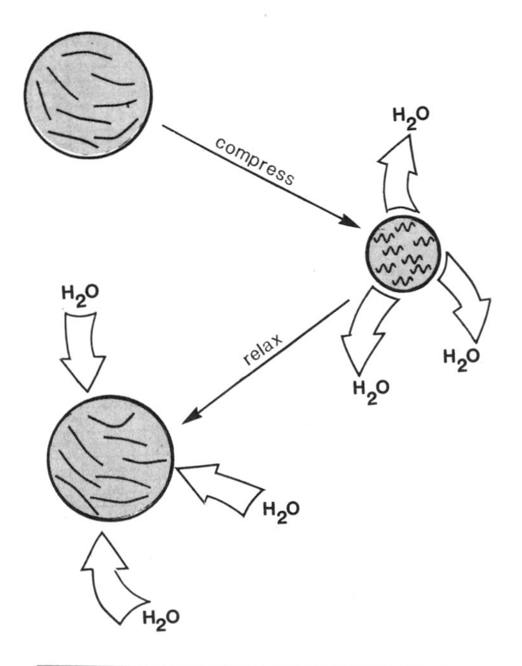

Figure 8.3
Resilience of glycosaminoglycans.

"slip" past each other, much as two magnets with the same polarity seem to slip past each other. This produces the "slippery" consistency of mucous secretions and synovial fluid.

b. When a solution of glycosaminoglycans is compressed, the water will be "squeezed out" and the glycosaminoglycans forced to occupy a smaller volume. However, when the compression is released, the glycosaminoglycans will spring back to their original, hydrated volume owing to the repulsion of their negative charges. This property contributes the resilience observed in synovial fluid and the vitreous humor of the eye (Figure 8.3).

c. The structure and distribution of the glycosaminoglycans is illustrated in Figure 8.4.

B. Protein components of glycosaminoglycans

1. All of the glycosaminoglycan polysaccharide chains, with the exception of hyaluronic acid, are found covalently attached to protein, forming ***proteoglycan monomers***.
2. A proteoglycan monomer found in cartilage consists of a ***core protein*** to which the linear carbohydrate chains are covalently attached. These carbohydrate chains, which may number more than 100, extend out from the core protein and remain separated from each other because of the repulsion of their extensive negative charges. The resulting structure resembles a "bottle brush" (Figure 8.5). In the case of cartilage proteoglycan, the species of glycosaminoglycans include chondroitin sulfate and keratan sulfate.
3. The linkage between the carbohydrate chain and the protein is generally through a trihexose (galactose-galactose-xylose) on the end of the carbohydrate and a serine residue of the protein. A glycosidic bond is formed between the xylose and the hydroxyl group of the serine (Figure 8.6).
4. The proteoglycan monomers associate with a molecule of hyaluronic acid to form ***proteoglycan aggregates***. The association is not covalent but is primarily through ionic interactions between the core protein and the hyaluronic acid. The association is stabilized by additional small proteins called ***link proteins*** (Figure 8.7).

C. Classification of glycosaminoglycans

1. There are six major classes of glycosaminoglycans. They are classified according to their monomer compositions, type of glycosidic linkages, and degree and location of their sulfate units.
2. Figure 8.4 illustrates their composition and general distribution.

III. SYNTHESIS OF GLYCOSAMINOGLYCANS

The polysaccharide chains are elongated by the sequential addition of alternating acidic and amino sugars, donated by their UDP-derivatives. The reactions are catalyzed by a family of specific transferases. (The synthesis of UDP-N-acetylglucosamine, UDP-N-acetylgalactosamine, and UDP-glucuronic acid was discussed on p. 60.) The synthesis of

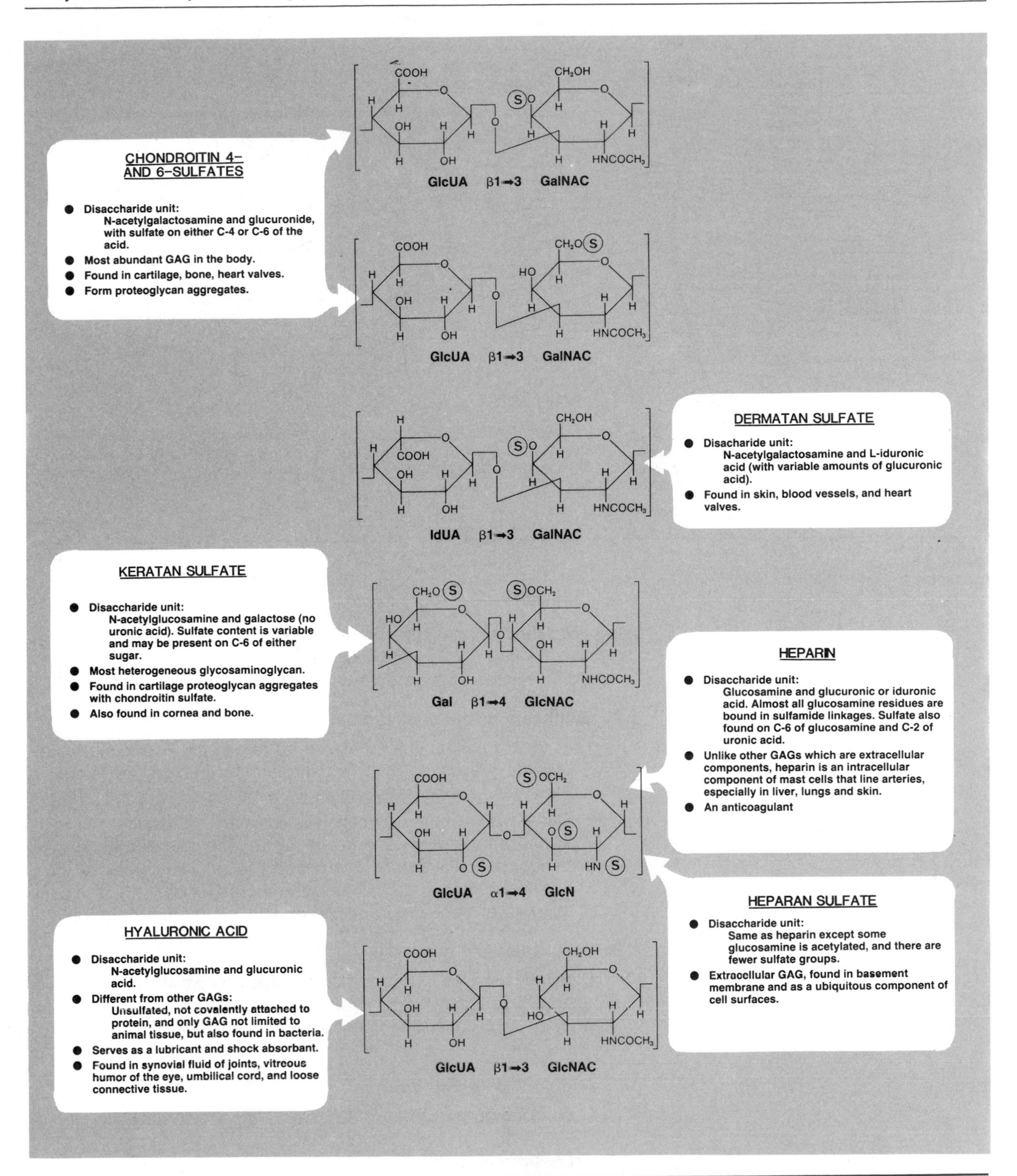

Figure 8.4
Structure and distribution of glycosaminoglycans. Sulfate group (S) are shown in all possible positions.

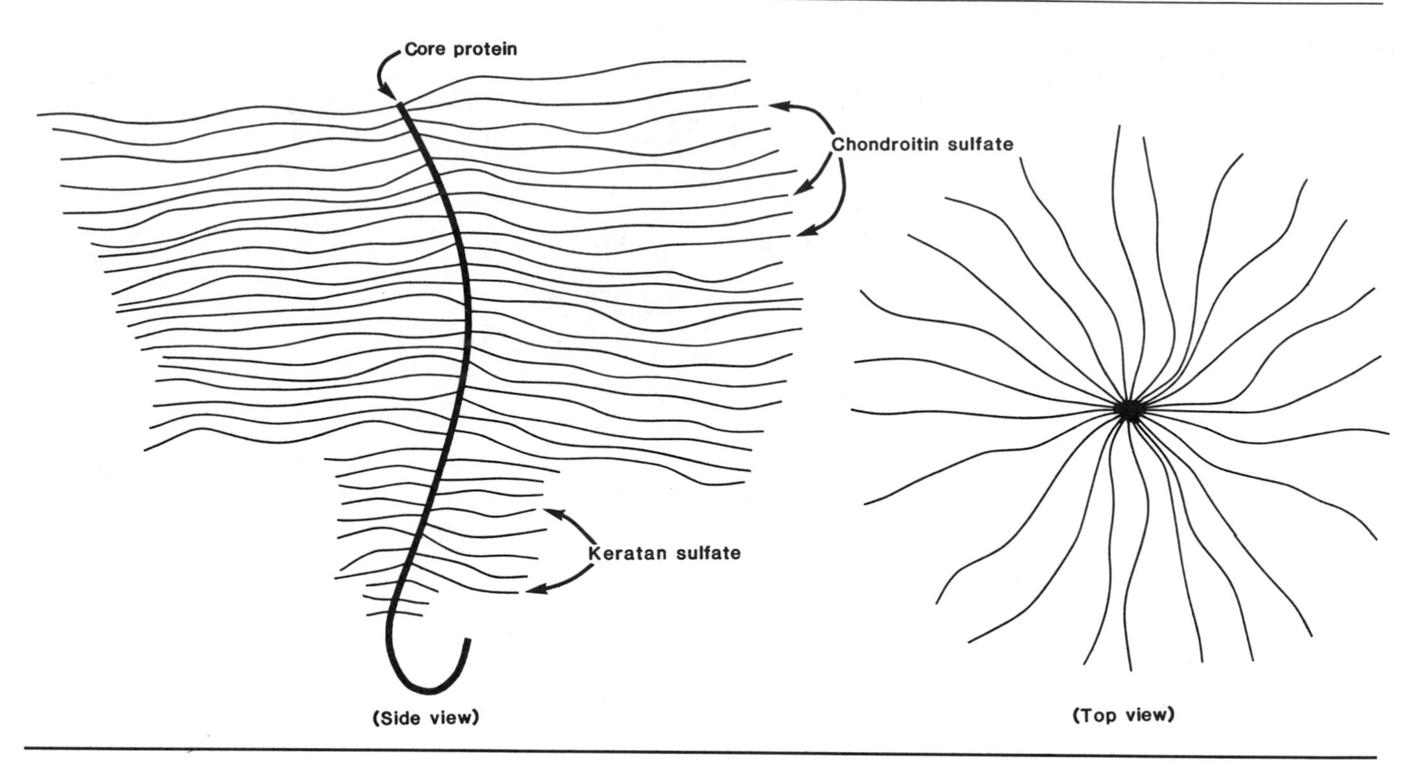

Figure 8.5
"Bottle-brush" model of a proteoglycan monomer.

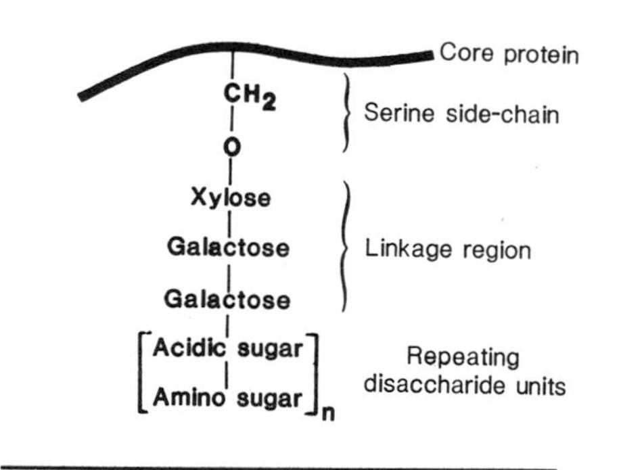

Figure 8.6
Linkage region of glycosaminoglycans.

the glycosaminoglycans is similar to that of glycogen except that the glycosaminoglycans are produced for export from the cell. Their synthesis occurs, therefore, in the endoplasmic reticulum and the Golgi apparatus.

A. Synthesis of the core protein

1. The core protein is synthesized on and enters the rough endoplasmic reticulum (ER). The protein is then glycosylated by membrane-bound transferases as it moves through the ER.
2. Carbohydrate chain formation is initiated by the transfer of a xylose from UDP-xylose to the hydroxyl group of a serine (or threonine), catalyzed by *xylosyltransferase*. Two galactose molecules are then added, completing the trihexose linkage region, followed by sequential addition of acidic and amino sugars.

B. L-Iduronic acid synthesis

1. Synthesis of the L-iduronic acid residues occurs ***after*** D-glucuronic acid has already been incorporated into the carbohydrate chain. *Uronosyl 5-epimerase* causes the epimerization of the D- to the L-sugar.

C. Addition of sulfate groups

1. Sulfation of the carbohydrate chain also occurs after the monosaccharide has been incorporated into the growing carbohydrate chain.
2. The source of the sulfate is ***3′-phosphoadenosyl-5′-phosphosulfate*** (PAPS). Sulfotransferases cause the sulfation of the carbohydrate chain at specific sites.

D. An example of the synthesis of a glycosaminoglycan, chondroitin sulfate, is shown in Figure 8.8.

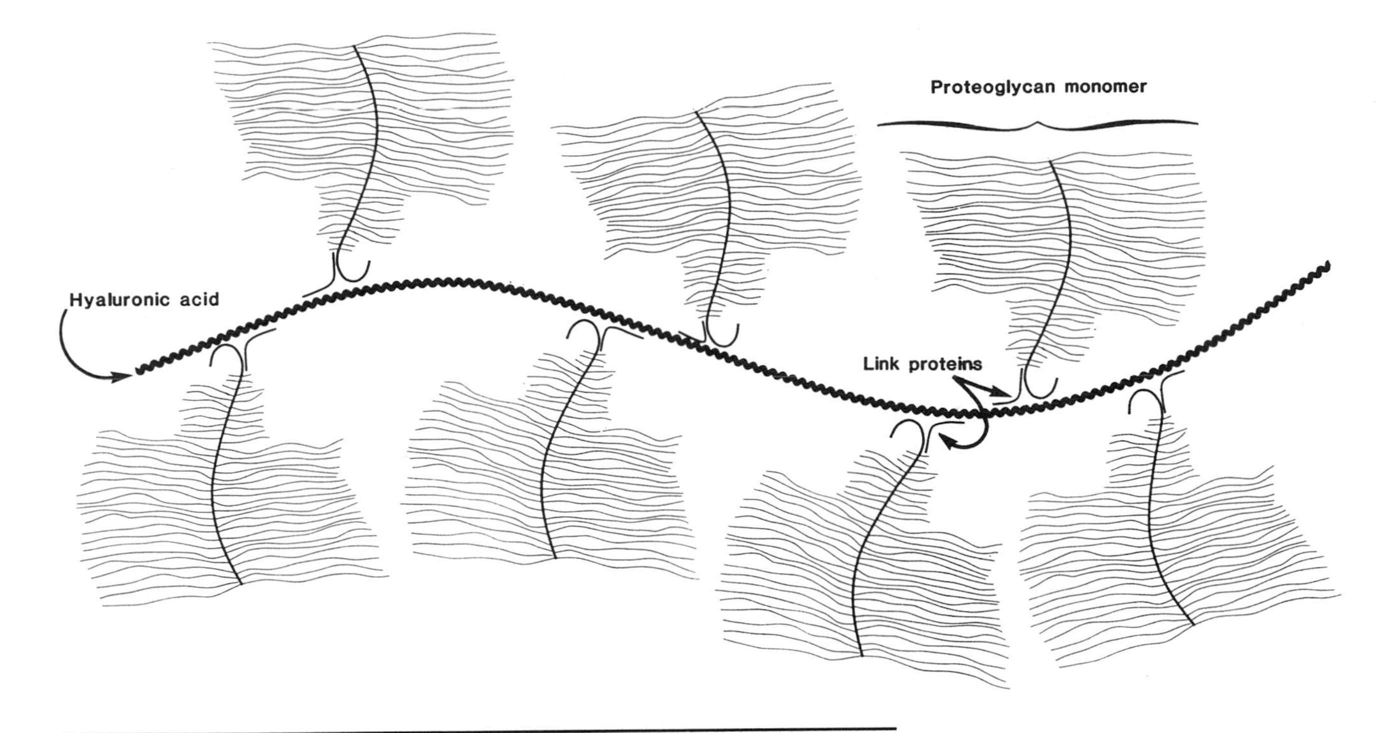

Figure 8.7
Proteoglycan aggregates.

IV. DEGRADATION OF GLYCOSAMINOGLYCANS

Glycosaminoglycans are degraded in ***lysosomes***. Lysosomes are found in all eukaryotic cells and contain hydrolytic enzymes whose maximum activity occurs at a pH of approximately 5. (Therefore, as a group, they are called *acid hydrolases*.) The low pH optimum is a protective mechanism that prevents the enzymes from destroying the cell should leakage into the cytoplasm—where the pH is neutral—occur.

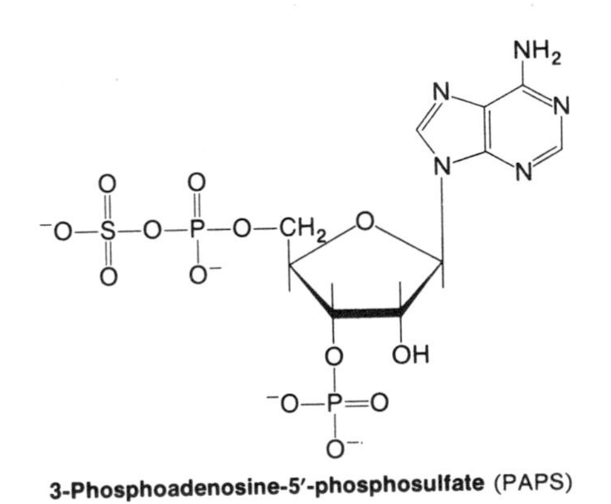

3-Phosphoadenosine-5′-phosphosulfate (PAPS)

With the exception of keratan sulfate, which has a half-life of greater than 120 days, the glycosaminoglycans have a relatively short half-life, ranging from about 3 days for hyaluronic acid to 10 days for chondroitin and dermatan sulfates.

A. Lysosomal degradation of glycosaminoglycans

1. The lysosomal degradation of these compounds requires a large number of hydrolytic enzymes for complete digestion.
   a. Note: Because glycosaminoglycans are ***extracellular*** compounds, a cell must engulf them by an invagination of the cell membrane, forming a vacuole inside of which are the glycosaminoglycans to be degraded. This vacuole can fuse with a lysosome, resulting in a single digestive vacuole ("secondary lysosome") in which the glycosaminoglycans are efficiently degraded. This process is illustrated in Figure 8.9.
2. Degradation of glycosaminoglycans occurs sequentially, the last group added during synthesis being the first group removed during degradation. Examples of these enzymes and the bonds they hydrolyze are shown in Figure 8.10.

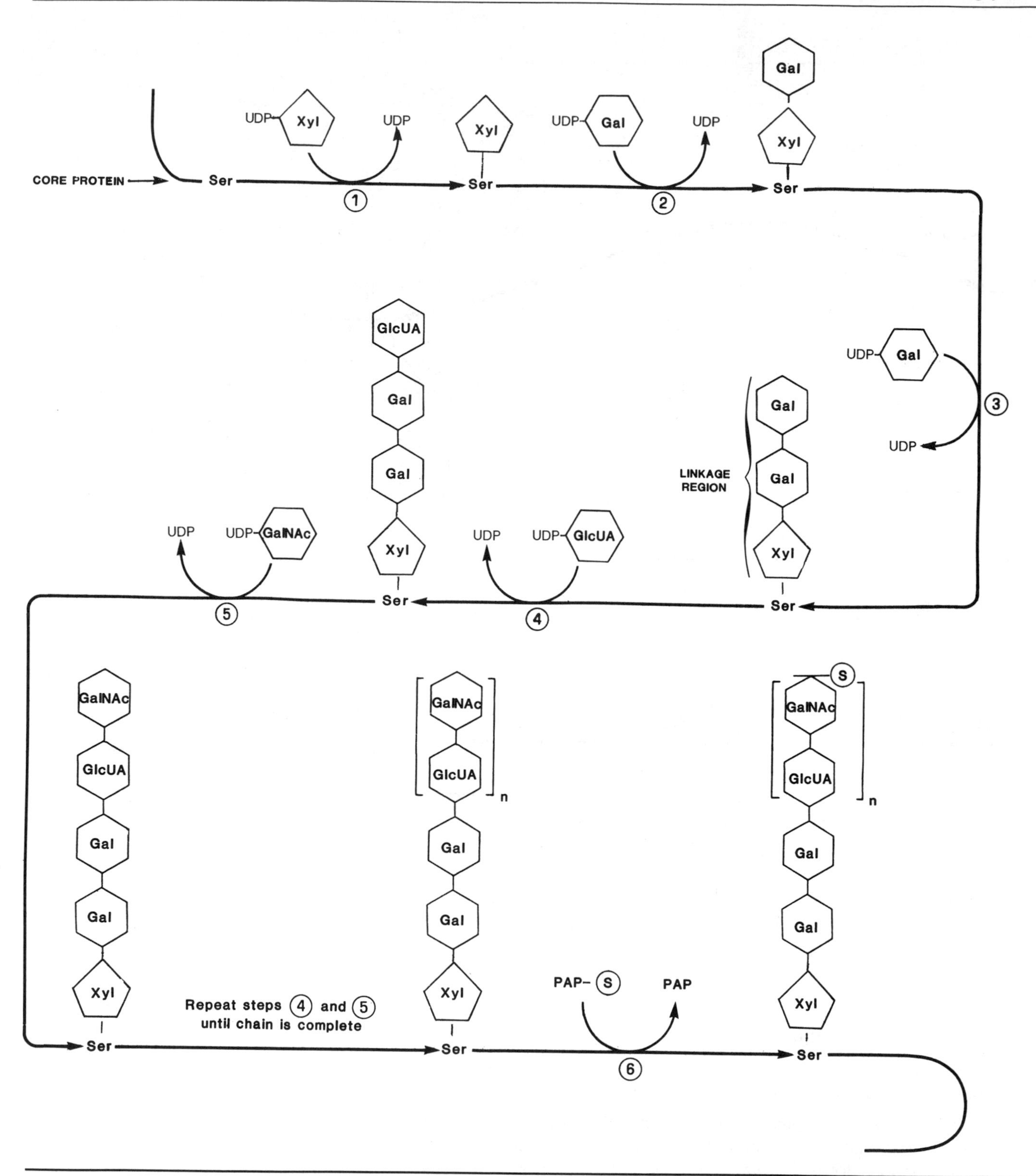

Figure 8.8
Synthesis of chondroitin sulfate.

V. MUCOPOLYSACCHARIDOSES

The mucopolysaccharidoses are hereditary disorders that are clinically progressive and characterized by accumulation of glycosaminoglycans in various tissues. The tissues most affected are those that normally produce the largest quantity of a particular glycosaminoglycan species.

A. Characteristics of this group of diseases

1. Mucopolysaccharidoses result from a deficiency of one of the lysosomal, hydrolytic enzymes normally involved in the degradation of one or more of the ***glycosaminoglycans***.
2. The diseases also result in the presence of oligosaccharides in the urine. These are due to incomplete degradation of glycosaminoglycans and can be used to identify the specific mucopolysaccharidosis. Diagnosis is confirmed by measuring the level of the lysosomal hydrolytic enzyme in cells such as fibroblasts.
3. All of the deficiencies are autosomal and recessively inherited except Hunter syndrome, which is X-linked. Prenatal diagnosis for these deficiencies is possible.
4. Children who are homozygous for one of the mucopolysaccharidoses are apparently normal at birth, then gradually deteriorate. In severe cases, death occurs in childhood. No effective therapy exists at present.
5. A summary of the mucopolysaccharidoses resulting from the deficiencies of enzymes required for the degradation of heparan sulfate is shown in Figure 8.10.

B. Additional disorders resulting from a lack of these lysosomal enzymes

1. Some of the lysosomal enzymes required for the degradation of glycosaminoglycans also participate in the degradation of lipids and glycoproteins. Therefore an individual suffering from a mucopolysaccharidosis may also have a lipidosis or glycoprotein-oligosaccharidosis.

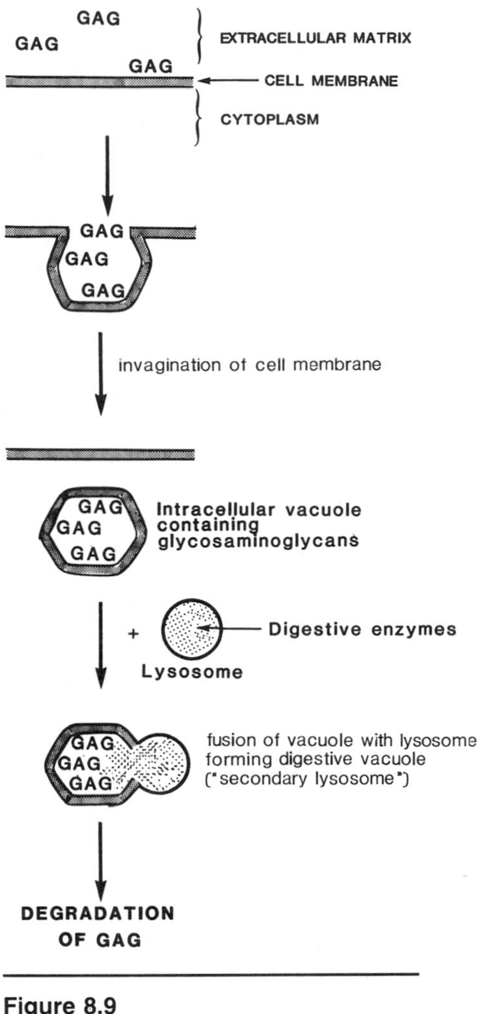

Figure 8.9
Formation of a "digestive vacuole."

Study Questions

Choose the ONE best answer:

8.1 Mucopolysaccharidoses are inherited storage diseases. They are caused by

A. an increased rate of synthesis of proteoglycans.
B. the synthesis of polysaccharides with an altered structure.
C. defects in the degradation of proteoglycans.
D. the synthesis of abnormally small amounts of protein cores.
E. an insufficient amount of proteolytic enzymes.

8.2 Mucopolysaccharidoses are a family of diseases characterized by each of the following ***EXCEPT***

A. elevated urinary excretion of oligosaccharides containing glucuronic acid.
B. elevated urinary excretion of oligosaccharides containing hexosamine.
C. tissue accumulation of glycosaminoglycans.
D. deficiency in lysosomal enzymes.
E. elevated urinary excretion of hyaluronic acid.

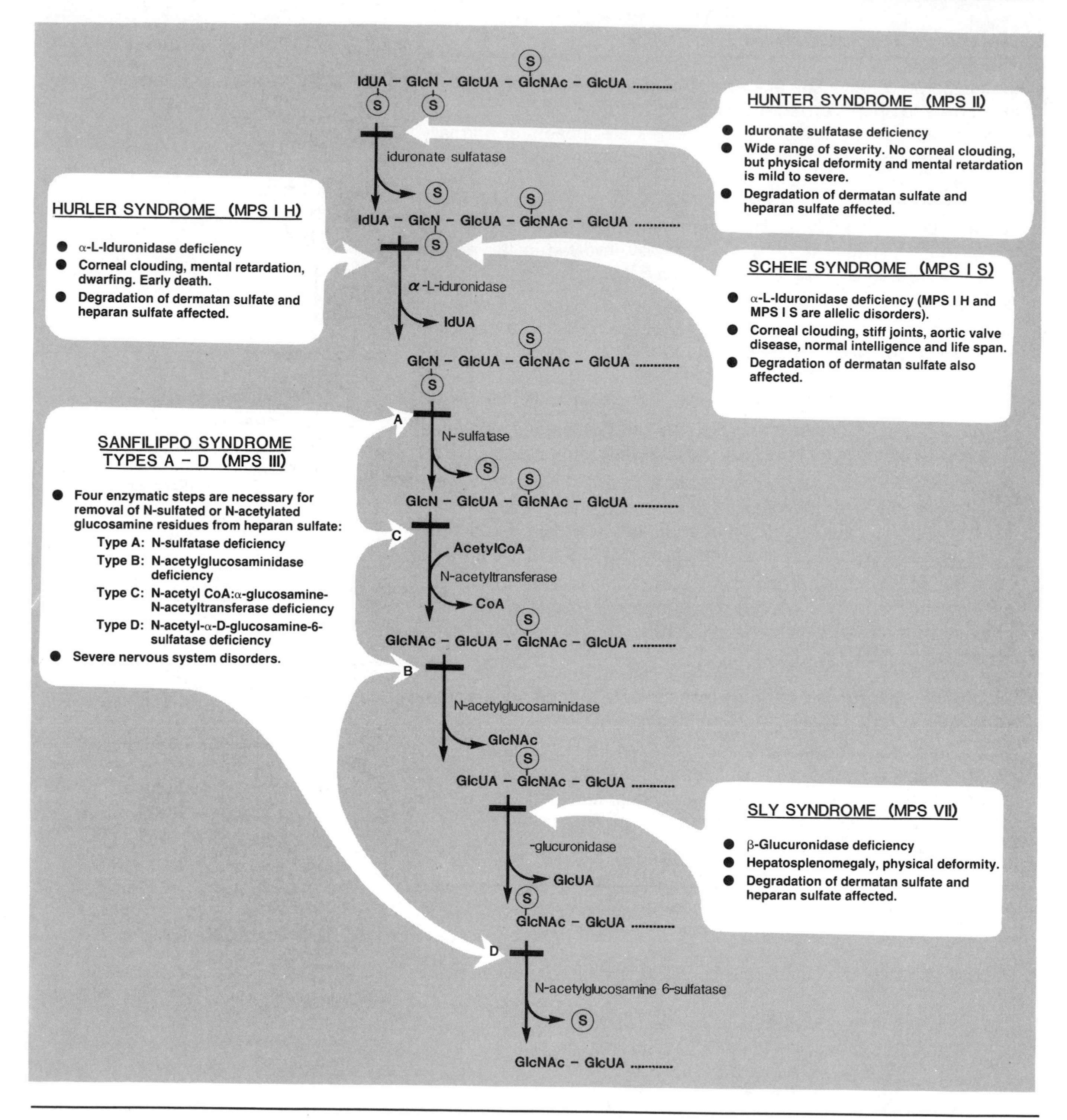

Figure 8.10
Degradation of the glycosaminoglycan heparan sulfate.

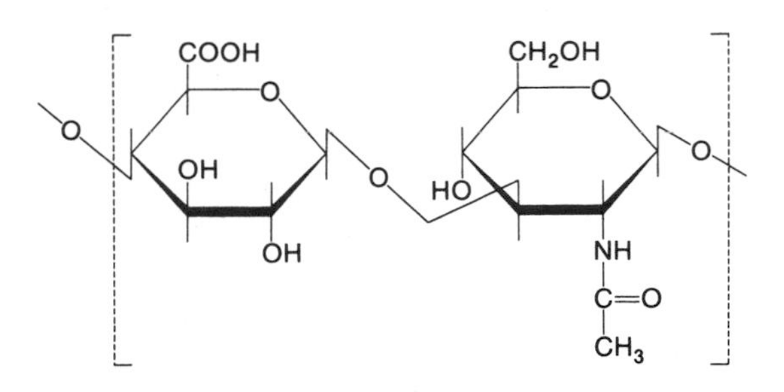

8.3 The polymeric substance shown above belongs to a group of compounds known as

A. amylose.
B. amylopectin.
C. glycogen.
D. proteoglycan.
E. keratin.

8.4 The substance shown above is

A. lactose.
B. hyaluronic acid.
C. heparin.
D. N-acetylneuraminic acid.
E. sucrose.

8.5 The component monosaccharides shown above are

A. gluconic acid and N-acetyl glucosamine.
B. N-acetyl glucosamine and N-acetylneuraminic acid.
C. glucuronic acid and N-acetylneuraminic acid.
D. gluconic acid and N-acetylneuraminic acid.
E. glucuronic acid and N-acetylglucosamine.

8.6 This compound is of particular functional importance in

A. blood clotting.
B. synovial fluid.
C. liver cells.
D. mast cells.
E. skin.

8.7 The predominant proteoglycan in cartilage is

A. keratin sulfate.
B. dermatan sulfate.
C. chondroitin sulfate.
D. heparan sulfate.
E. heparin.

Answer A if 1, 2, and 3 are correct
B if 1 and 3 are correct
C if 2 and 4 are correct
D if only 4 is correct
E if all are correct

8.8 Which of the following statements about proteoglycans is(are) CORRECT?

1. In proteoglycans, a carbohydrate chain is linked to a protein through a unique linkage region that contains xylosyl and galactosyl residues.
2. Proteoglycans are generally composed of a disaccharide repeating unit containing an acidic and an amino sugar.
3. The iduronic acid of dermatan sulfate is synthesized by an epimerase that acts on a glucuronic acid residue in the polysaccharide.
4. Sulfation of the proteoglycan occurs after monosaccharides have already been incorporated into the carbohydrate chain.

Glycoproteins

9

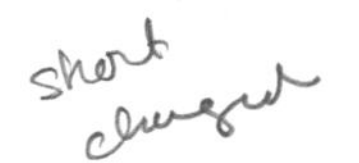

I. OVERVIEW

Glycoproteins are proteins to which oligosaccharides are covalently attached. They differ from the glycosaminoglycans in that the length of the carbohydrate chain is relatively short (usually two to ten sugar residues in length) in the glycoproteins, whereas it can be very long in the glycosaminoglycans (see p. 81). The glycoprotein carbohydrate chains are often branched instead of linear and may be negatively charged.

Glycoproteins participate in a broad range of cellular phenomena, including cell surface recognition (by other cells, hormones, viruses), cell surface antigenicity such as the blood group antigens, as a component of the extracellular matrix, and as a component of the mucins of the gastrointestinal and urogenital tracts, where they act as protective biological lubricants (Figure 9.1).

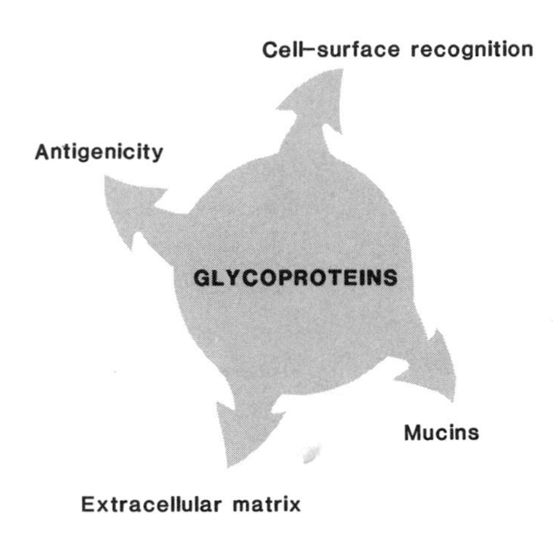

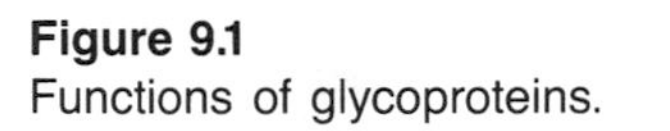

Figure 9.1
Functions of glycoproteins.

II. STRUCTURE OF GLYCOPROTEINS

A. Composition of the carbohydrate portion of glycoproteins

1. The oligosaccharide components of glycoproteins are generally branched heteropolymers composed primarily of D-hexoses, with the addition in some cases of N-acetylneuraminic acid (NANA)—a nine carbon, acidic monosaccharide (see p. 61)—and L-fucose, a 6-deoxyhexose.

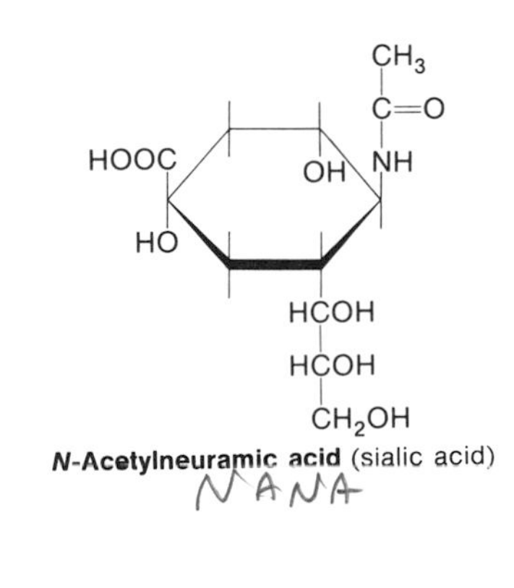

***N*-Acetylneuramic acid** (sialic acid)

B. Structure of link between carbohydrate and protein

1. The oligosaccharide may be attached to the protein either through an N- or an O-glycosidic link (see p. 49). In the former case, the sugar chain is attached to the amide group of an asparagine side-chain, and in the latter case, to a hydroxyl group of either a serine or threonine R-group. (Note: In the case of collagen, there is an O-glycosidic linkage between galactose or glucose and a hydroxyl group of hydroxylysine.)
2. The N-linked oligosaccharides fall into two broad classes: ***complex oligosaccharides*** and ***high-mannose oligosaccharides***. Both contain the same ***core pentasaccharide*** as is shown in Figure 9.2, but the complex oligosaccharides contain a diverse group of additional sugars, whereas the high mannose oligosaccharides contain primarily mannose.

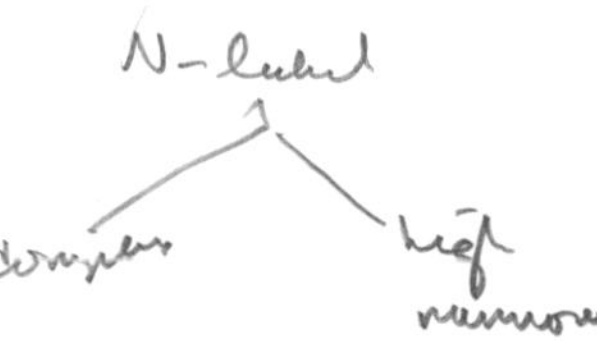

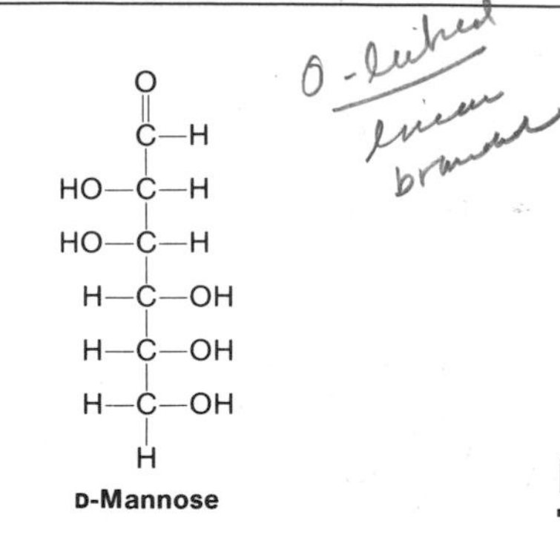

3. The O-linked oligosaccharides may have one or more of a wide variety of sugars arranged in either a linear or a branched configuration.
4. A glycoprotein may contain only one type of glycosidic linkage or may have both O- and N-linked oligosaccharides within the same molecule.

III. SYNTHESIS OF GLYCOPROTEINS

A. Building blocks of glycoproteins

1. The building blocks of the glycoproteins are ***sugar nucleotides***. These include UDP-glucose, UDP-galactose, UDP-N-acetylglucosamine, and UDP-N-acetylgalactosamine, whose syntheses are described on p. 58. In addition, GDP-mannose, GDP-L-fucose (which is synthesized from GDP-mannose), and CMP-N-acetylneuraminic acid (whose synthesis is also described on p. 61) may donate sugars to the growing chain. When NANA is present, the oligosaccharide will have a negative charge at physiologic pH.

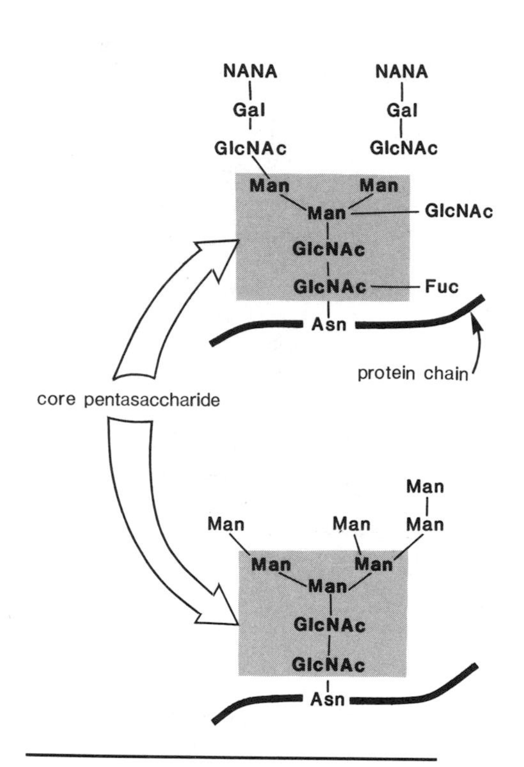

Figure 9.2
Complex (top) and high-mannose (bottom) oligosaccharides.

B. Synthesis of O-linked glycosides

1. The synthesis of the O-linked glycosides is very similar to that of the glycosaminoglycans (see p. 82). First, the protein to which the oligosaccharides are to be attached is synthesized on the rough endoplasmic reticulum and extruded into the ER (see p. 383). Glycosylation begins immediately.
2. The glycosyl transferases responsible for synthesizing the oligosaccharides are bound to the membranes of the rough or smooth ER or the Golgi apparatus. These transferases must act in a very specific order, without using a template like those required for DNA, RNA, and protein synthesis (Unit 7), but rather by recognizing the actual structure of the growing oligosaccharide as the appropriate substrate.
3. Sugars are added to the growing oligosaccharide as the protein moves from the endoplasmic reticulum to the Golgi. There, those glycoproteins that are to be secreted from the cell will remain free in the lumen, whereas those that are to become components of the cell membrane become integrated into the Golgi membrane, their carbohydrate portions oriented toward the lumen.
4. Secretory vesicles are formed that move into the cytoplasm and fuse with the cell membrane, releasing the free glycoproteins and adding the membrane of the vesicle to the cell membrane. The attached glycoproteins are thus oriented with the carbohydrate portion on the outside of the cell.

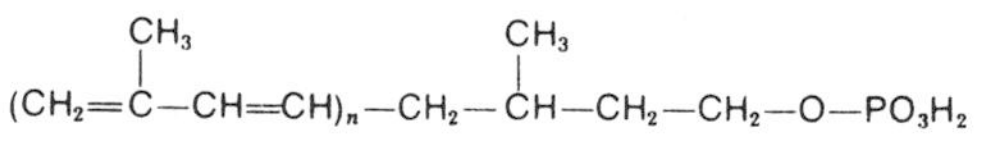

C. Synthesis of the N-linked glycosides

1. The synthesis of N-linked glycoproteins has additional processing steps and requires the participation of a lipid, dolichol (Figure 9.3).
2. First, as with the O-linked glycosides, protein is synthesized on the rough ER and enters the ER where it begins to be glycosylated.
3. The protein does not become glycosylated with individual sugars at this stage of glycoprotein synthesis, but rather a lipid-linked oligosaccharide is first constructed that consists of ***dolichol*** (a lipid

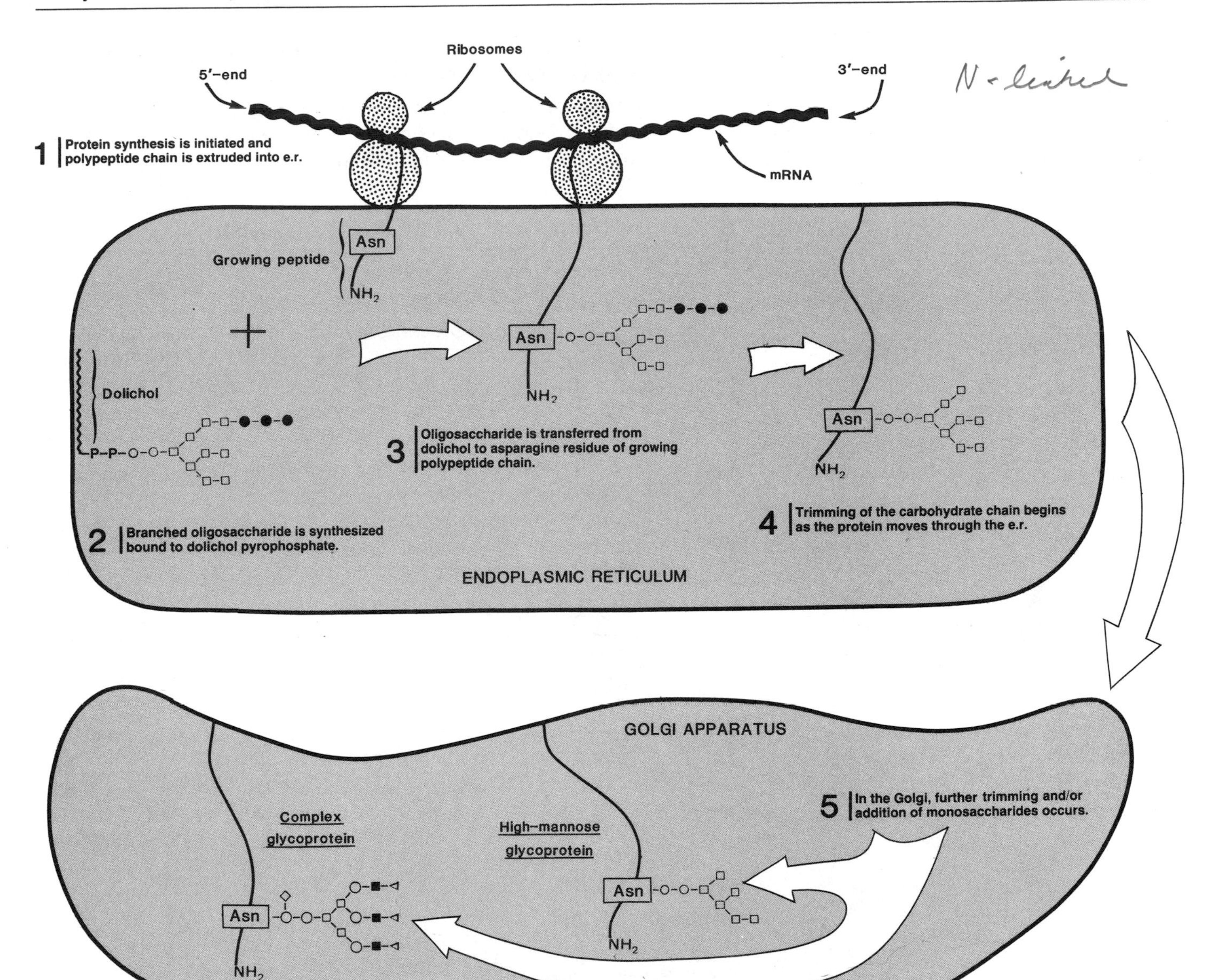

Figure 9.3
Synthesis of glycoproteins.

more than 100 carbons in length) attached to an oligosaccharide containing N-acetylglucosamine, mannose, and glucose.

4. The first sugars to be added by the membrane-bound *glycosyl transferases* are N-acetylglucosamine, mannose, and glucose.
5. The oligosaccharide is transferred from the dolichol to an asparagine side group of the protein by a *protein-oligosaccharyl transferase* present in the endoplasmic reticulum.
6. After incorporation into the protein, the N-linked oligosaccharide is processed by the removal of specific mannose and glucose residues as the glycoprotein moves through the smooth ER.
7. Finally, the oligosaccharide chains are completed by addition of a variety of sugars, producing a ***complex glycoprotein,*** or are not

N-linked

oligo saccaride chain linked to dolichol then transferred to asp residue processed further, leaving branched mannose-containing chains in a ***high-mannose glycoprotein*** (see Figure 9.2).

8. The ultimate fate of the N-linked glycoproteins is the same as that of the O-linked—either they are released by the cell, or they become part of the cell membrane.

IV. DEGRADATION OF GLYCOPROTEINS

A. Glycoproteins are degraded in lysosomes

1. Degradation of glycoproteins is very similar to that of the glycosaminoglycans (see p. 85). The ***lysosomal, hydrolytic enzymes*** are each generally specific for the removal of one component of the glycoprotein. They are mostly ***exoenzymes*** and remove their respective groups in a ***sequential*** series of reactions. If any one is missing, degradation of the glycoprotein by the other exoenzymes cannot continue.
2. A group of genetic diseases called the ***glycoprotein storage diseases*** (oligosaccharidoses), caused by a deficiency of one of the degradative enzymes, result in accumulation of partially digested glycoproteins and oligosaccharides in cells.

Study Questions

Choose the ONE best answer:

9.1 The presence of the following compound in the urine of a patient suggests a deficiency in which one of the enzymes listed below?

```
        Sulfate            Sulfate
        |                  |
GlcUA—GalNac—GlcUA—GalNAc
```

A. Galactosidase
B. Sulfatase
C. Glucuronidase
D. Mannosidase
E. Glucosidase

9.2 Which one of the following is ***NOT*** a common feature of the carbohydrate structure in N-linked and O-linked glycoproteins?

A. They may contain N-acetylneuraminic acid.
B. They may contain glucose.
C. Their degradation *in vivo* involves action of lysosomal enzymes.
D. Their synthesis involves participation of a lipid carrier.
E. They are synthesized in the endoplasmic reticulum and the Golgi apparatus.

9.3 The synthesis of the carbohydrate portion of glycoproteins

A. is catalyzed by specific enzymes, each of which synthesizes a specific glycosidic bond in a determined sequence.
B. is a process catalyzed by the action of specific glycosidic hydrolases present in most cells.
C. is usually initiated by the addition of N-acetylneuraminic acid.
D. is initiated at a glutamine or methionine residue on the protein.
E. produces an oligosaccharide with a reducing end belonging to the last monosaccharide added.

Bioenergetics and Oxidative Phosphorylation

10

I. OVERVIEW OF BIOENERGETICS

Bioenergetics deals with the release, storage, and use of energy in biological systems. The study of bioenergetics provides a measure of the energetic feasibility of a chemical reaction and can therefore allow one to predict whether a reaction will take place and the extent to which it will occur.

Bioenergetics is concerned only with the initial and final energy states of reaction components, not with the mechanism of the process or how much time is needed for the chemical change to take place. For example, consider the magnitude of the loss of potential energy when the boulder moves downhill, as is shown in Figure 10.1. The energy released is the same whether the rock falls directly from the top (path a) or rolls down by a series of drops (path b). In each case, the initial and final energy states are the same, even though two different pathways or mechanisms of descent are used. Further, the energy loss of the rock omits any consideration of time; the magnitude of the loss is the same if the trip down the mountain is fast or slow. (Of course, this model ignores any loss of energy caused by rolling friction.) In short, bioenergetics predicts whether a process is possible, and kinetics measures how fast it occurs.

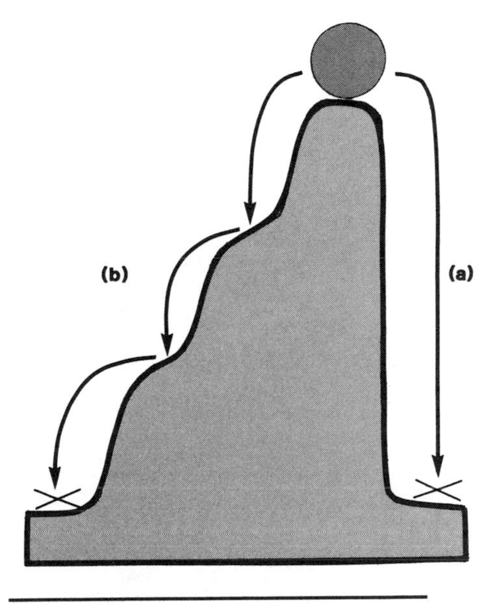

Figure 10.1
Model of energy loss by a boulder rolling downhill using two different pathways.

II. THERMODYNAMICS

The direction and extent to which a chemical reaction will proceed is determined by the degree to which two factors change during the reaction. These two factors are ***enthalpy*** (a measure of the heat content of the reactants and products) and ***entropy*** (a measure of their randomness or disorder). Neither of these thermodynamic quantities by itself is sufficient to determine whether a chemical reaction will go spontaneously in the direction it is written. However, when combined mathematically, enthalapy and entropy can be used to derive a third quantity, ***free energy,*** which directly predicts the direction in which a reaction will go spontaneously.

A. Enthalpy

1. A change in heat content is one of the two fundamental factors that influence whether a process is energetically favorable and

can proceed in a given direction. Heat is the most common form of energy encountered with biochemical reactions, since other forms of energy, such as kinetic, radiant, and electrical energy, all tend to change ultimately into heat energy. (It should be noted that these interconversions between the various forms of energy neither create nor destroy energy; therefore, the total energy of the universe remains constant. This is the ***First Law of Thermodynamics.***)

2. The change in enthalpy, ΔH, that occurs during a reaction is measured by observing the heat produced or absorbed by the reaction (at constant pressure). A reaction is called ***exothermic*** if heat is produced as a result of the reaction (ΔH is negative). It is called ***endothermic*** if heat is absorbed (ΔH is positive).
3. Heat changes are measured in a ***calorimeter.*** The unit of heat energy is a ***calorie*** and is defined as the amount of energy required, in the form of heat, to raise the temperature of 1 g of water from 15° to 16°C. (Its abbreviation is "cal.") A ***kilocalorie*** (abbreviated kcal or Cal) is equal to 1000 cal.
4. Many reactions that occur spontaneously show a negative ΔH, that is, give off heat. However, this is not universally true. Some reactions that occur quite readily (such as the dissolving of ammonium sulfate in water) have a positive ΔH, that is, the solution becomes cool owing to the uptake of heat. Thus, the sign or magnitude of ΔH is not sufficient to predict the direction of a reaction.
5. Each organic compound has a characteristic ***heat of combustion,*** which is defined as the number of kilocalories of heat given off (i.e., ΔH) as one mole of the substance is burned completely at the expense of molecular oxygen (i.e., is completely oxidized).
   a. For example, one mole of glucose completely oxidized to CO_2 and H_2O produces 673,000 cal. This is equivalent to 3.74 kcal/g of glucose. A more highly reduced compound such as triacylglycerol (see p. 159) produces 9.3 kcal/g when fully oxidized. This energy, if captured as heat, could be used, for example, to produce steam that could do work.
   b. The human body, however, is isothermal (i.e., it does not change temperature under normal conditions); therefore, heat is not a useful form of energy for performing biological work.

B. Entropy

1. The change in entropy, ΔS, during a chemical reaction is the second fundamental factor that influences whether that reaction is energetically favorable and can proceed in a given direction. Entropy of a system is a measure of its "disorder" or "randomness." For example, ice has a high degree of order (or low entropy) because the molecules are rigidly arranged in a crystalline lattice. This contrasts with liquid water, which has higher entropy because the water molecules can move independently. The transition from ice to liquid water shows an increase in entropy, and ΔS is positive. Conversely, reactions in which the products are more ordered than the reactants have a negative ΔS.
2. The ***Second Law of Thermodynamics*** states that all physical and chemical processes proceed in such a direction that the ***entropy***

(randomness) of the universe increases to the maximum possible; at that point, no further change occurs and equilibrium is established. For example, suppose pure water is layered over a concentrated solution of salt (Figure 10.2). The salt molecules will diffuse into the water, leading to an increase in the randomness of the population of salt molecules. As the disorder increases, entropy increases. Ultimately, the salt molecules will be randomly distributed throughout the solvent in a uniform concentration, and the system will be in equilibrium.

3. Some reactions that occur spontaneously show a negative ΔS, whereas others have a positive ΔS. Thus, the sign or magnitude of ΔS is not sufficient to predict the direction of a reaction.

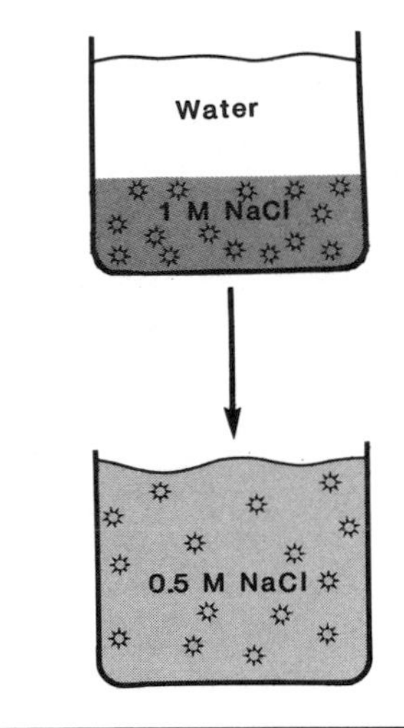

Figure 10.2
Increased randomization of salt molecules after addition of water to a 1 M solution of sodium chloride.

C. Free energy

1. The change in free energy, ΔG, is that part of the total energy of the reaction components available to do work at a constant pressure and temperature.
2. Under conditions of constant temperature, pressure, and volume (characteristic of the living cell), entropy, enthalpy, and free energy are related by the equation

$$\Delta G = \Delta H - T\Delta S$$

where ΔG is the change in free energy
ΔH is the change in heat energy (enthalpy)
ΔS is the change in entropy
T is the absolute temperature in degrees Kelvin (°K): °K = °C + 273

3. Just as the entropy proceeds to a maximum as a reaction approaches equilibrium, the free energy proceeds to a minimum (i.e., entropy gets larger and free energy gets smaller).

III. DETERMINANTS OF THE DIRECTION OF A CHEMICAL REACTION

A. The free energy change, ΔG

1. The change in free energy, ΔG, can be used to predict the direction of a reaction at constant temperature and pressure. Consider the reaction

$$A \rightleftarrows B$$

a. If $\Delta G < 0$ (i.e., is a negative number), there will be a net loss of energy, and the reaction will go spontaneously as written, that is, A will be converted into B (Figure 10.3).

b. If $\Delta G > 0$ (i.e., is a positive number), there will be a net gain of energy, and the reaction will not go spontaneously as written; energy must then be added to the system to make the reaction go in the direction of B.

c. If $\Delta G = 0$, the reaction is at equilibrium.

2. When a reaction is proceeding spontaneously, that is, free energy is being lost, the reaction will continue until ΔG reaches zero and equilibrium is established.

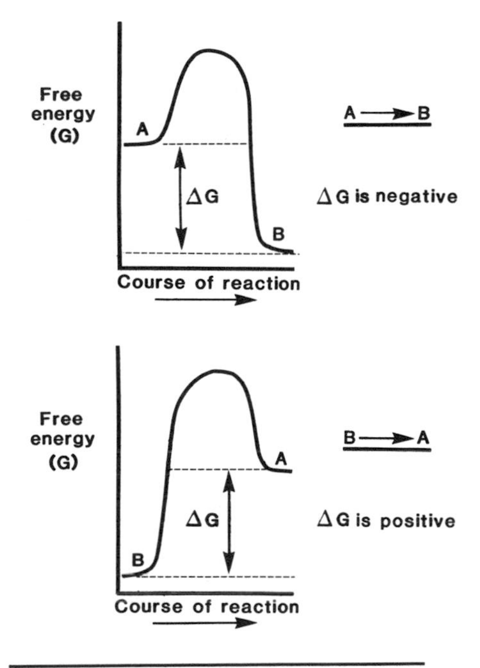

Figure 10.3
Change in free energy (ΔG) during a reaction. *(Top)* The product has a lower free energy (G) than does the substrate. *(Bottom)* The product has a higher free energy than does the substrate.

3. The free energy of the forward reaction ($A \rightarrow B$) is equal in magnitude but opposite in sign to that of the back reaction ($B \rightarrow A$). For example, if the ΔG of the forward reaction is -5 kcal/mole, then that of the back reaction is $+5$ kcal/mole.
4. The free energy change, ΔG, of the reaction $A + B \rightleftarrows C + D$ depends on the concentrations of the reactants and products. At constant temperature and pressure the following relation can be derived:

$$\Delta G = \Delta G^\circ + RT \ln \frac{[C][D]}{[A][B]}$$

where ΔG° is the ***standard free energy change***

R is the gas constant (1.987 cal/mole degree)

T is the absolute temperature (°K)

[A], [B], [C], and [D] are the actual concentrations of the substrates and products.

5. ΔG can be altered by changing the concentration of reactants or products, or both, so that reactions can be made to go either as written (where ΔG is negative) or in the reverse direction (where ΔG is positive).

B. Standard free energy change, ΔG°

1. ΔG° is called the ***standard*** free energy change because it is equal to the free energy change, ΔG, under standard conditions, that is when all reactants and products are kept at 1 M concentrations. Under these conditions, the natural logarithm (ln) of the ratio of products to reactants will be zero [ln(1) = 0], and therefore the equation shown above will become

$$\Delta G = \Delta G^\circ + 0$$

2. Under standard conditions, ΔG° can be used to predict the direction a reaction will go, because, under these conditions, ΔG° is equal to ΔG. However, ΔG° cannot predict the direction a reaction will go under normal, physiologic conditions, since it is composed solely of constants (R, T, and K_{eq}, see section C. below) and is therefore not altered by changes in product or substrate concentrations.

C. The relationship between ΔG° and K_{eq}

1. In a chemical reaction, for example, $A + B \rightleftarrows C + D$, a point of equilibrium is reached at which no further ***net*** chemical change takes place, that is, A and B are being converted to C and D as fast as C and D are being converted to A and B. In this state, the ***ratio*** of the concentrations of the products ([C][D]) to the concentrations of the substrates ([A][B]) will be constant, regardless of the actual concentrations of the four compounds:

$$K_{eq} = \frac{[C]_{eq}[D]_{eq}}{[A]_{eq}[B]_{eq}}$$

where K_{eq} is the equilibrium constant, and $[A]_{eq}$, $[B]_{eq}$, $[C]_{eq}$, and $[D]_{eq}$ are the concentrations of compounds A, B, C, and D at equilibrium.

2. If the reaction $A + B \rightleftarrows C + D$ is allowed to go to equilibrium at constant temperature and pressure, then at equilibrium the overall free energy change (ΔG) will be zero. Therefore,

$$\Delta G = 0 = \Delta G^\circ + RT \ln \frac{[C]_{eq}[D]_{eq}}{[A]_{eq}[B]_{eq}}$$

where $[A]_{eq}$, $[B]_{eq}$, $[C]_{eq}$, and $[D]_{eq}$ are the equilibrium concentrations of reactants and products, and their ratio as shown above is the K_{eq}.

Thus: $\Delta G^\circ = -RT \ln K_{eq}$

If $K_{eq} = 1$, then $\Delta G^\circ = 0$

If $K_{eq} > 1$, then $\Delta G^\circ < 0$

If $K_{eq} < 1$, then $\Delta G^\circ > 0$

3. A small change in the ΔG° results in a large change in the equilibrium constant (K_{eq}) (Figure 10.4). This is due, of course, to the fact that ΔG° is proportional to the logarithm of the K_{eq}.

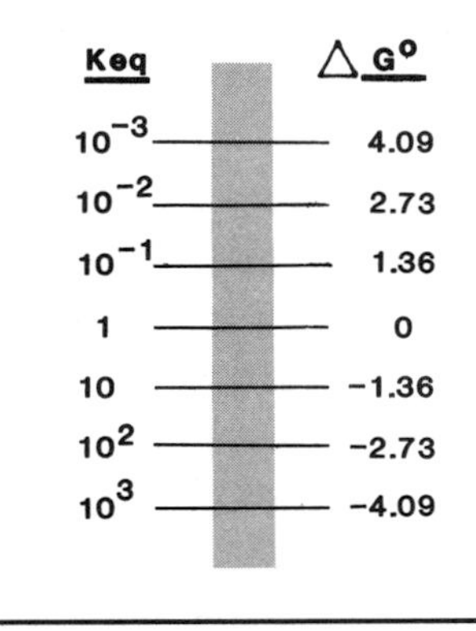

Figure 10.4
The numerical relation between standard free energy changes (ΔG°) and their corresponding equilibrium constants.

D. ΔG°s are additive

1. The standard free energy changes (ΔG°) are additive in any sequence of consecutive reactions, as are the free energy changes (ΔG).

e.g. Glucose + ATP → glucose 6-P + ADP	ΔG° =	−4000 cal
Glucose 6-P → fructose 6-P	ΔG° =	+400 cal
so: Glucose + ATP → fructose 6-P + ADP	ΔG° =	−3600 cal

2. This additive property of free energy changes is very important in biochemical pathways through which substrates must pass in a particular direction (e.g., A→B→C→D→...): As long as the ***sum*** of the ΔG's of the individual reactions is negative, the pathway can potentially proceed as written even if some of the individual component reactions of the pathway have positive ΔG's. The actual rate of the reactions will, of course, depend on the activity of the enzymes that catalyze the reactions (see p. 36).

3. Some of the reactions in a pathway may, in fact, be far from equilibrium, with the pathway in ***steady-state,*** that is, with all enzymes operating at the same velocity and the concentrations of the intermediates defined as "***steady-state concentrations***" (see p. 38).

IV. ATP AS ENERGY CARRIER

A. Chemical reactions are coupled through common intermediates.

1. Two chemical reactions have a ***common intermediate*** when they occur sequentially so that the product of the first reaction is the substrate for the second:

e.g. given the reactions A + B → C + D
and D + X → Y + Z

Here D is the common intermediate.

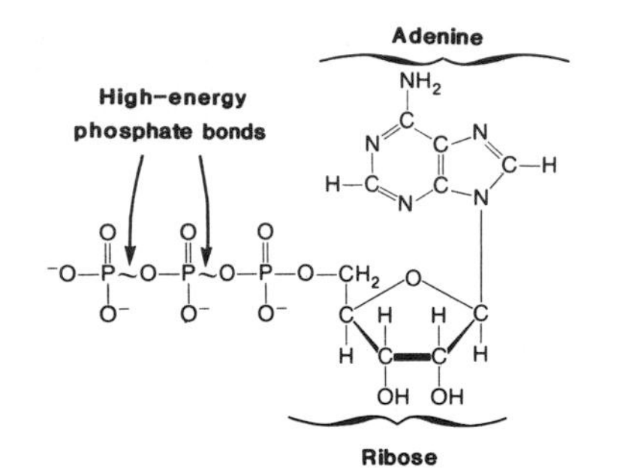

Figure 10.5
Adenosine triphosphate.

2. Because humans are isothermal, the only way in which energy can be transferred between two chemical reactions is for them to have a common intermediate that links them. In the example given above, D could be a carrier of chemical energy between the two reactions.
3. Adenosine triphosphate (ATP) serves as a carrier of chemical energy between high-energy phosphate donors and low-energy phosphate acceptors because it is a common intermediate in both energy-delivering and energy-requiring reactions of the cell (Figure 10.6).

B. The energy carried by ATP is stored in its two terminal phosphate groups

1. ATP is composed of a molecule of adenosine to which three phosphate groups are attached (Figure 10.5). If one phosphate is removed, ADP (adenosine diphosphate) is produced; if two phosphates are removed, AMP (adenosine monophosphate) results.
2. At physiologic pH, ATP is highly negatively charged, having a total of three or four negative charges on its phosphates. ATP therefore forms stable complexes with Mg^{++} and Mn^{++}.

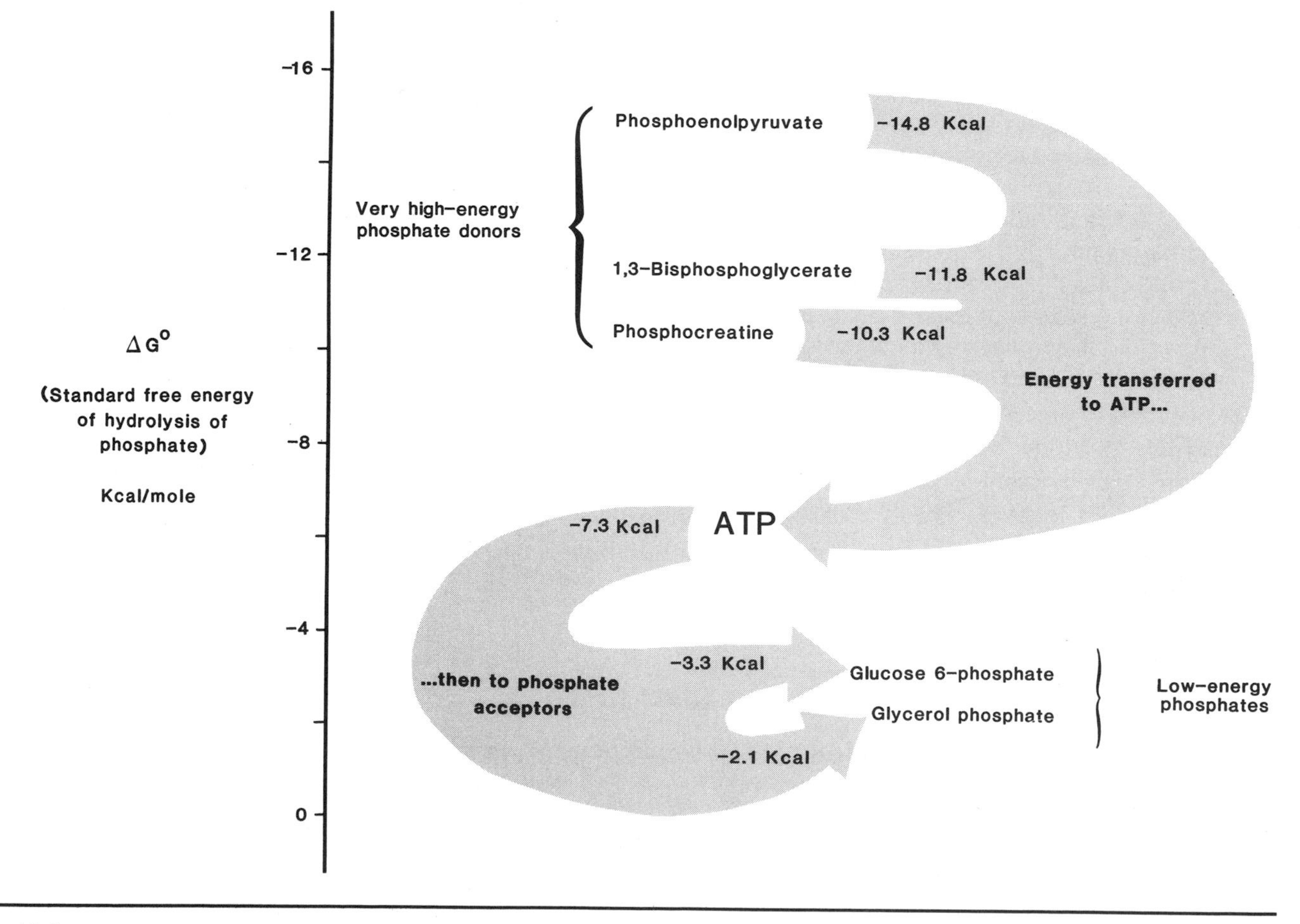

Figure 10.6
ATP carries energy between high- and low-energy compounds.

3. The standard free energy of hydrolysis, ΔG°, is approximately −7300 cal/mole for each of the two terminal phosphate groups. Because of this large, negative ΔG°, ATP is called a ***high-energy phosphate compound***.
4. Compounds exist that contain phosphates with an energy higher than that of ATP. These very high-energy compounds include phosphoenolpyruvate (see p. 116), 1,3-biphosphoglycerate (see p. 114), and phosphocreatine (see p. 260), all of which have a standard free energy of hydrolysis of greater than −10,000 cal.
5. Other phosphate-containing compounds have low-energy phosphates, which have standard free energies of hydrolysis of less than −4000 cal. These include glucose 6-phosphate (see p. 111), glycerol 3-phosphate (see p. 167), and AMP.
6. ATP thus occupies an intermediate position on the bioenergetic scale of phosphate-containing compounds. ADP can serve as an acceptor of phosphate groups from cellular phosphates containing higher-energy phosphates. ATP can donate these phosphates to compounds in the cell forming phosphates of lower energy (Figure 10.6). There are no enzymes in cells that can transfer phosphate groups directly from very high-energy donors to low-energy acceptors without their first being transferred to ATP.

Phosphoenolpyruvate

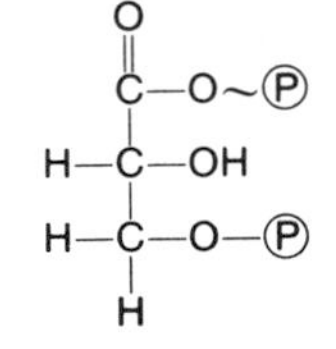

1,3-Bisphosphoglycerate

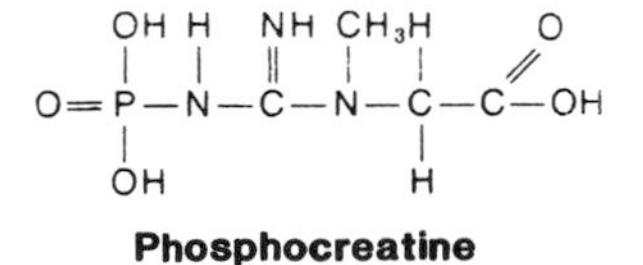

Phosphocreatine

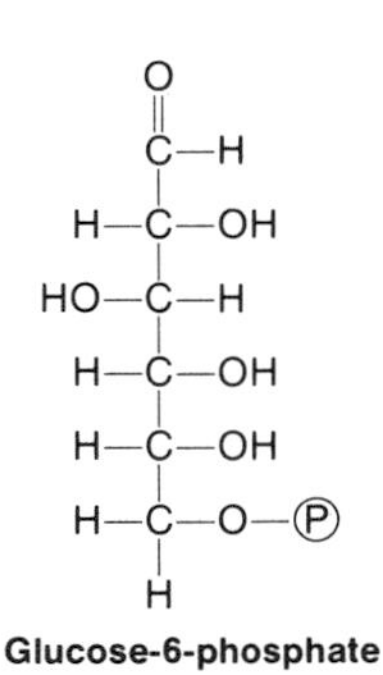

Glucose-6-phosphate

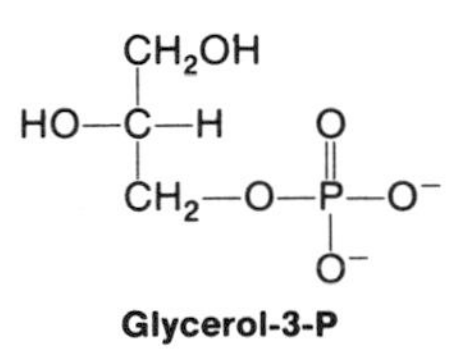

Glycerol-3-P

Study Questions

Choose the ONE best answer:

10.1 The free energy change, ΔG,

A. is directly proportional to the standard free energy change, ΔG°.
B. is equal to zero at equilibrium.
C. can be calculated only when the reactants and products are present at 1 M concentrations.
D. will indicate the rate and direction of the reaction, if you also know the standard free energy change and the concentrations of products and reactants.
E. is equal to $-RT \ln K_{eq}$.

10.2 Under standard conditions (i.e., where all reactants and products are present at 1 M concentrations),

A. the free energy change, ΔG, is equal to 0.
B. the standard free energy change, ΔG°, is equal to 0.
C. the free energy change, ΔG, is equal to the standard free energy change, ΔG°.
D. K_{eq} is equal to 1.
E. K_{eq} is equal to 0.

10.3 Consider the following reaction:

$$\text{Fructose 6-P} + P_i \rightarrow \text{fructose 1,6-bisphosphate} + H_2O$$

This reaction has an equilibrium constant (K_{eq}) of 0.001 at pH 7, where T = 25°C = 298°K, R = 1.98 cal/mole·degree. (The ln of a number is equal to 2.303 log of the number)

The standard free energy change, ΔG°, for this reaction is equal to approximately

A. +4.0 kcal/mole.
B. −4.0 kcal/mole.
C. +2.0 kcal/mole.

D. −2.0 kcal/mole.
E. none of the above.

10.4 The complete oxidation of one mole of glucose results in the release of about 700,000 calories of free energy. If this process is coupled to ATP biosynthesis from ADP + P_i with approximately 40% efficiency, the number of moles of ATP that could be produced under standard conditions would be approximately

A. 2.
B. 7.
C. 20.
D. 40.
E. 100.

10.5 Under physiologic conditions, each of the following contains a high-energy phosphate group EXCEPT

A. ATP.
B. ADP.
C. AMP.
D. phosphoenolpyruvate.
E. phosphocreatine.

Answer A if 1, 2, and 3 are correct
B if 1 and 3 are correct
C if 2 and 4 are correct
D if only 4 is correct
E if all are correct

10.6 Given the following sequence of reactions where the components A through D are present at steady-state concentrations and where X is present in an inexhaustible reservoir:

$$X \rightarrow A \rightleftarrows B \rightleftarrows C \rightleftarrows D \rightarrow \text{products}$$

Which of the following statements about that pathway is(are) correct?

1. If the observed concentration ratio of [B]/[A] equals the equilibrium constant for the reaction $A \rightleftarrows B$, the overall pathway would be at equilibrium and no products would be made.
2. None of the individual reactions could be rate-limiting unless its $\Delta G°$ was equal to zero.
3. The reactant A could not be converted to D unless the sum of all of the $\Delta G°$ values for the individual reactions of A to D is negative.
4. The $\Delta G°$ for the conversion of A to D is equal to the sum of the $\Delta G°$ values for each individual reaction.

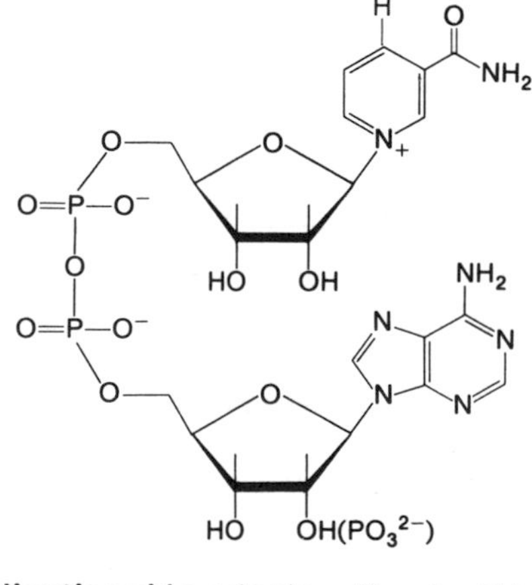

Nicotinamide adenine dinucleotide (NAD^+)

V. ELECTRON TRANSPORT CHAIN AND OXIDATIVE PHOSPHORYLATION

A number of reactions in cells result in the transfer of hydrogen atoms, consisting of a proton (H^+) and an electron from a substrate to a hydrogen acceptor. For example, in each revolution of the TCA cycle (see p. 138) there are four dehydrogenation steps: three that produce an oxidized substrate plus reduced nicotinamide adenine dinucleotide (NADH), and one that produces oxidized substrate plus reduced flavin adenine dinucleotide ($FADH_2$). These reduced cofactors can, in turn, each donate a pair of electrons to a specialized set of electron carriers, collectively called the ***electron transport chain***. The electrons are passed from one member of this chain to the next, ultimately reaching the end of the chain where they combine with oxygen and protons to form water. This requirement for oxygen results in the additional naming of the electron transport process the "respiratory chain" and accounts for the greatest portion of the body's requirement for oxygen.

The respiratory chain is the final common pathway by which all electrons derived from different fuels of the body flow to oxygen. As they are passed down the electron transport chain they lose much of their free energy. Part of this energy can be captured and stored by the production of ATP from ADP and inorganic phosphate (P_i). This process is called ***oxidative phosphorylation***. The remainder of the free energy is lost as heat.

Electron transport and oxidative phosphorylation proceed continuously in all cells of the body that contain mitochondria. (Mature red and white blood cells lack mitochondria.)

A. Composition of the electron transport chain

1. The components of the electron transport chain are located in the inner mitochondrial membrane. Although the outer mitochondrial membrane is freely permeable to most ions and small molecules, the ***inner*** mitochondrial membrane is a specialized structure ***impermeable*** to most small ions, including H^+, Na^+, and K^+, small molecules such as ATP, ADP, and pyruvate, and larger molecules (Figure 10.7). Specialized carriers or transport systems are required to move ions or molecules across this membrane.
2. The inner mitochondrial membrane is highly convoluted (Figure 10.8). The convolutions are called ***christae*** and serve to greatly increase the surface area of the membrane.
3. *ATP synthetase complexes,* referred to as "inner membrane particles," are attached to the inner surface of the mitochondrial membrane. They appear as spheres that protrude into the mitochondrial matrix.
4. The mitochondrial matrix is a gel-like solution that contains nearly all of the dehydrogenases responsible for the oxidation of pyruvate and amino acids (by the TCA cycle, p. 133), and of fatty acids (by β-oxidation, p. 171). In addition, it contains NAD^+ and FAD (the oxidized forms of these two cofactors, which are required as hydrogen acceptors), and ADP and P_i, which are used to produce ATP.

B. Reactions of the electron transport chain

1. With the single exception of coenzyme Q, all of the members of this chain are associated with protein. The protein may function as an enzyme, as is the case with the various dehydrogenases, may contain iron either as part of an ***iron-sulfur center*** or coordinated with a porphyrin ring, as in the cytochromes, or may contain copper, as in cytochrome a_3.
2. In the first step of the electron transport chain, NAD^+ is reduced to NADH by one of a number of dehydrogenases, each of which removes two hydrogen atoms from its substrate. (For examples of these reactions, see the discussion of the dehydrogenases found in the TCA cycle, p. 137.) Both electrons but only one proton (i.e., a hydride ion, $:H^-$) are transferred to the NAD^+, forming NADH plus a free proton, H^+, which is released into the medium.
3. The free proton plus the hydride ion carried by NADH are next transferred to *NADH dehydrogenase,* an enzyme complex embed-

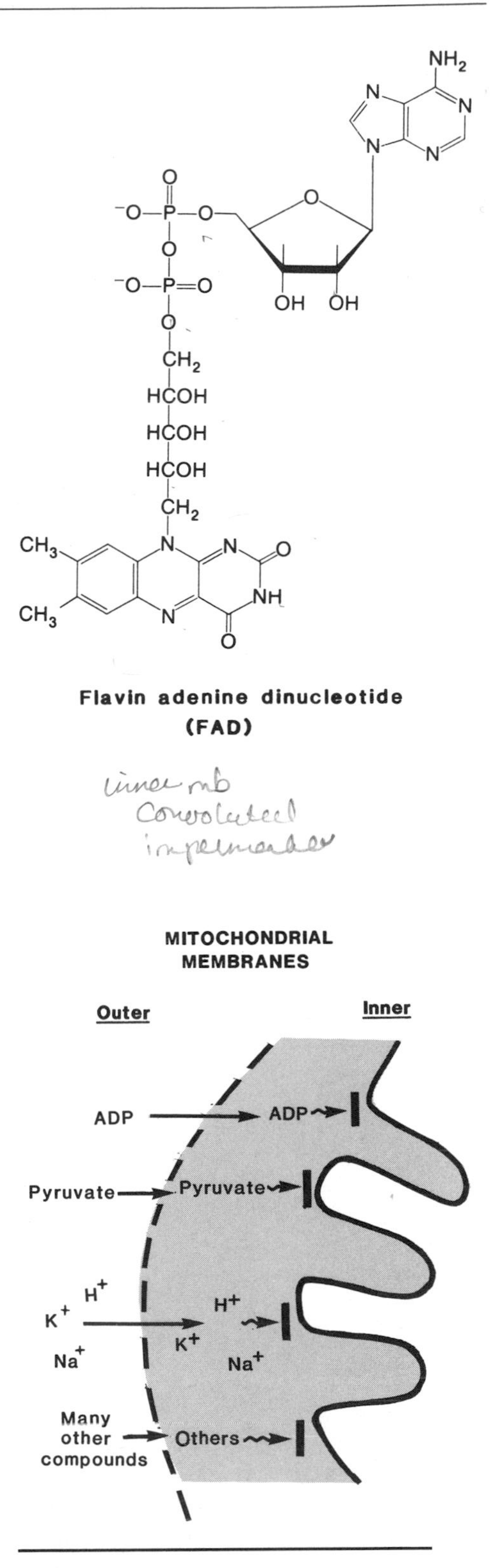

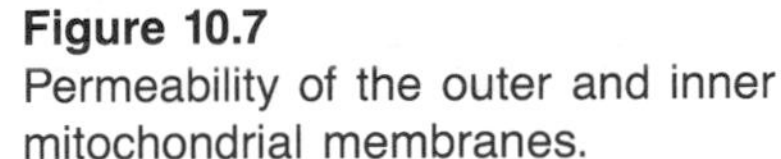

Figure 10.7
Permeability of the outer and inner mitochondrial membranes.

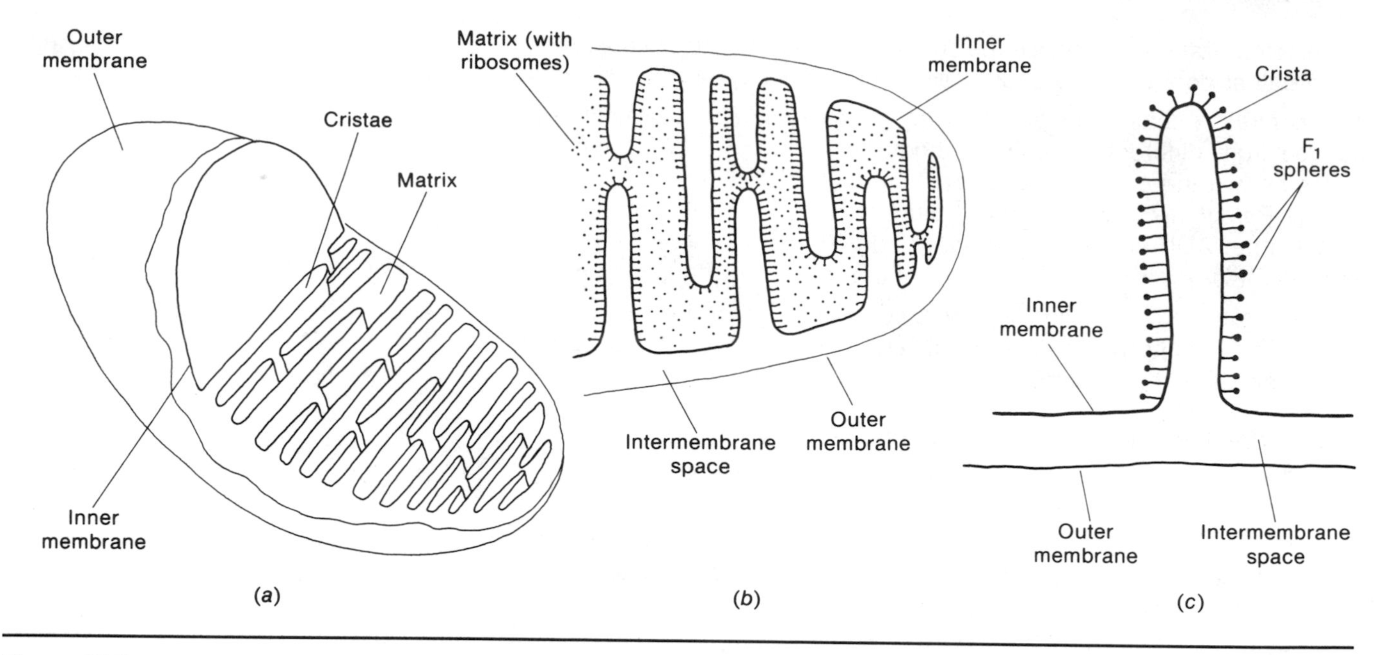

Figure 10.8
Stylized version of the mitochondrion and its components. (*a*) Cross-section of a mitochondrion showing involuted inner membrane (*b*) Detail showing relation between matrix and mitochondrial membrane (*c*) Single crista illustrating location of *ATPase* (F_1 spheres).

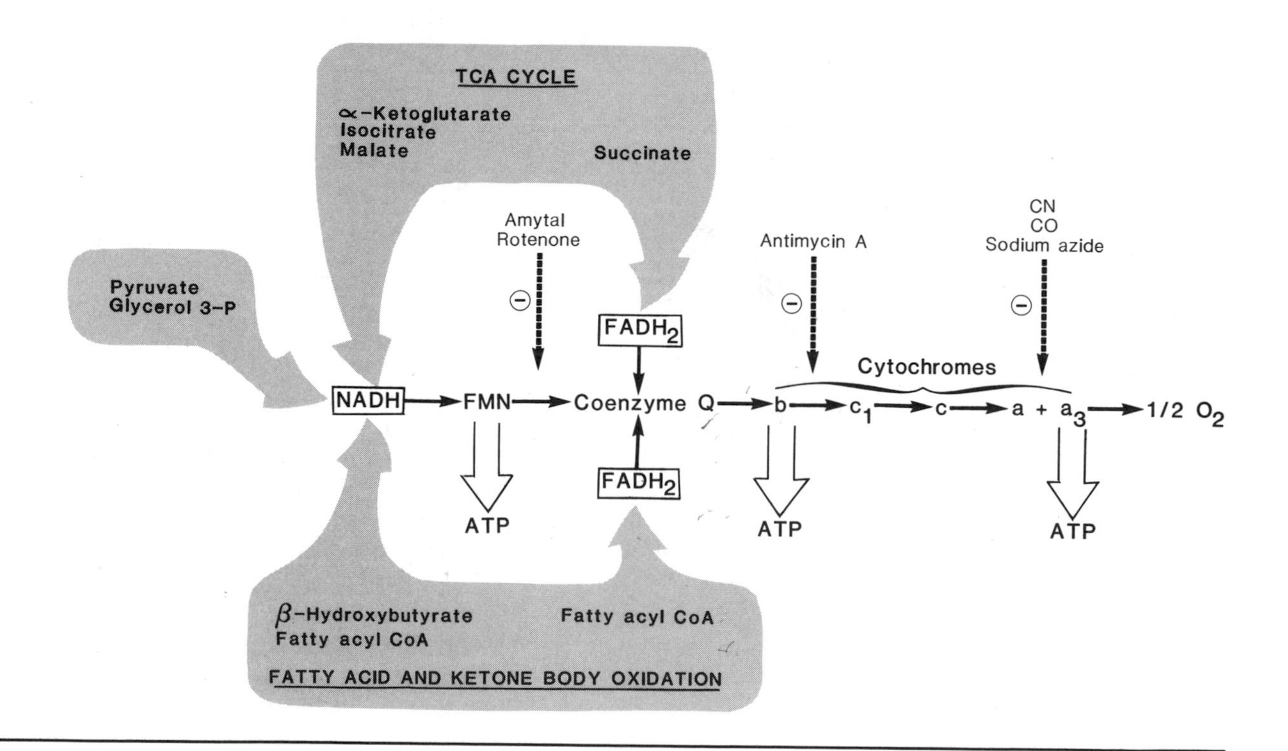

Figure 10.9
Electron transport chain illustrating components and site-specific inhibitors. The sources of reducing equivalents (NADH, $FADH_2$) are shown in their reduced forms. The components of the electron transport chain are shown in their oxidized forms, ready to accept hydrogen atoms or electrons. The substrates of dehydrogenases that produce NADH and FADH, are shaded gray.

ded in the inner mitochondrial membrane. This complex has as a cofactor a tightly bound molecule of flavin mononucleotide (FMN, a cofactor structurally related to FAD) that accepts the two hydrogen atoms, becoming $FMNH_2$. *NADH dehydrogenase* also contains several iron atoms paired with sulfur atoms to make ***iron-sulfur centers.*** These are necessary for the transfer of the hydrogen atoms to the next member of the chain, ***ubiquinone*** (known as coenzyme Q).

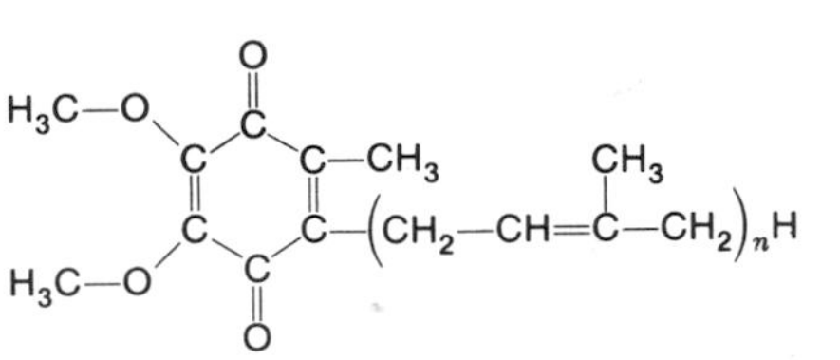

Coenzyme Q (ubiquinone)

4. Coenzyme Q is a quinone derivative with a long isoprenoid tail. It is also called ubiquinone because it is ubiquitous in biological systems. Coenzyme Q can accept hydrogen atoms both from $FMNH_2$ and from $FADH_2$, which is produced by dehydrogenases such as *succinate dehydrogenase* (see p. 138) and the dehydrogenase that participates in fatty acid degradation (see p. 171), as well as by the action of the glycerol phosphate shuttle.
5. The remaining members of the electron transport chain are ***cytochromes.*** Each of these proteins contains a heme group made of a ***porphyrin ring*** containing an atom of iron (see p. 255). Unlike the heme groups of hemoglobin, the cytochrome iron atom is reversibly converted from its ferric (Fe^{+3}) to its ferrous (Fe^{+2}) form as a normal part of its function as a reversible carrier of electrons. Electrons are passed down the chain from coenzyme Q to cytochromes b, c_1, c, and a + a_3 (Figure 10.9).

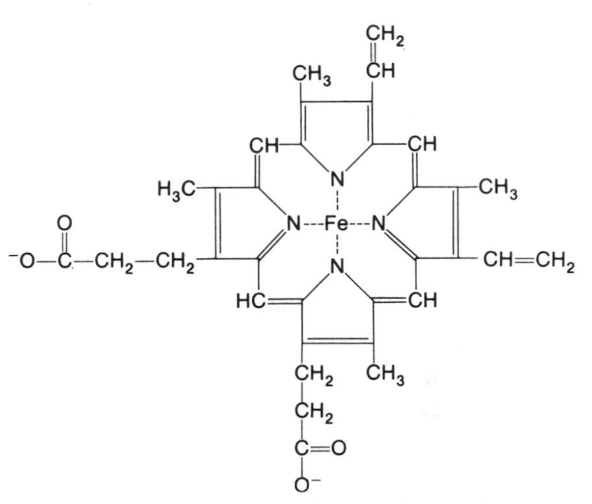

Heme group of cytochrome b

6. **Cytochrome a_3** is the only cytochrome in which the heme iron has a free ligand that can react directly with molecular oxygen. It is at this site that the transported electrons, molecular oxygen, and free protons are brought together to produce water (Figure 10.9). Cytochrome a_3 also contains bound ***copper atoms,*** which are required for this complex reaction to occur.
7. Specific ***inhibitors*** of electron transport have been identified and are illustrated in Figure 10.9. These compounds prevent the passage of electrons by binding to a component of the chain, blocking the oxidation/reduction reaction. Therefore, all electron carriers ***before*** the block will be fully ***reduced,*** whereas those occurring ***after*** the block will be ***oxidized*** (Figure 10.10).

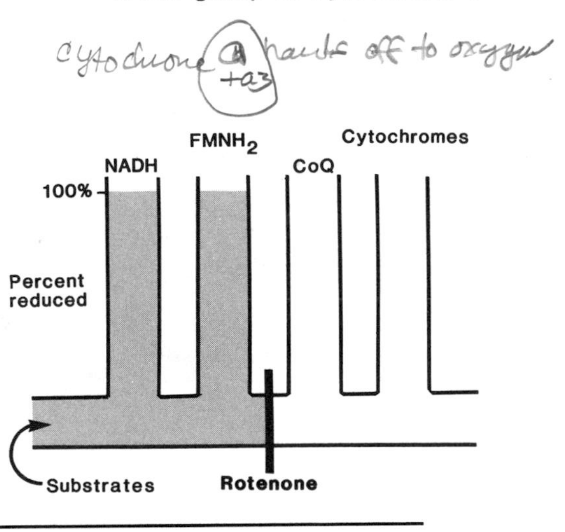

Figure 10.10
Hydraulic model illustrating the oxidized or reduced state of electron transport chain components in the presence of the site-specific inhibitor rotenone.

C. Release of free energy during electron transport

1. Free energy is released as electrons are transferred along the electron transport chain. Electrons are transferred from an electron donor (reducing agent or reductant) to an electron acceptor (oxidizing agent or oxidant). These electrons can be transferred in different forms, for example, as hydride ions ($:H^-$) to NAD^+, as hydrogen atoms to FMN, coenzyme Q, and FAD, or as pure electrons to cytochromes.
2. When a compound loses an electron (i.e., serves as a reductant), the structure that is left behind becomes capable of accepting an electron (i.e., serving as an oxidant):

e.g. cytochrome b (Fe^{++}) + cytochrome c_1 (Fe^{+++}) →
reductant X ***oxidant Y***

cytochrome b (Fe^{+++}) + cytochrome c_1 (Fe^{++})
oxidant X′ ***reductant Y′***

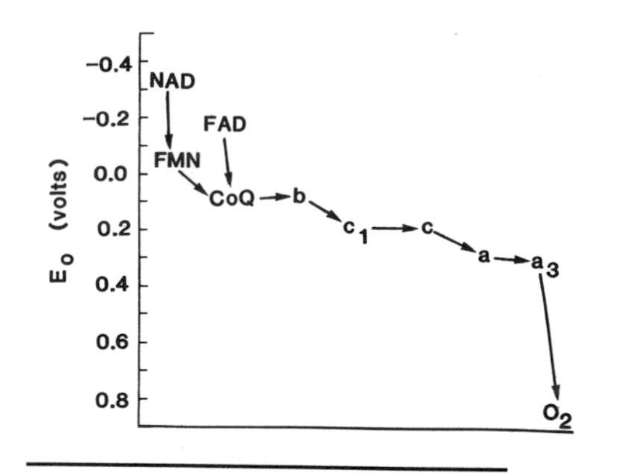

Figure 10.11
E_o values for some members of the electron transport chain.

Reductant X and oxidant X′ are termed a "redox" pair, as are reductant Y′ and oxidant Y. Pairs differ in their tendency to lose electrons. This tendency is a characteristic of a particular redox pair and can be quantitatively specified by a constant, the ***standard reduction potential***, E_o, with units in volts.

3. The standard reduction potentials of various redox pairs can be put into a table, ranging from the most negative E_o to the most positive. The more ***negative*** the standard reduction potential of a redox pair, the greater is the tendency of the reductant member of that pair to lose electrons. The more ***positive*** the E_o, the greater is the tendency of the oxidant member of that pair to ***accept*** electrons. Therefore, electrons will flow from the pair with the more negative E_o to that with the more positive E_o. The E_o values for some members of the electron transport chain are shown in Figure 10.11.

4. Free energy declines as electrons are transferred along the electron transport chain. This decline is related directly to the magnitude of the change in E_o that accompanies that transfer:

$$\Delta G^\circ = -n\mathcal{F}\Delta E_o$$

where n = number of electrons transferred (1 for a cytochrome, 2 for NADH, $FADH_2$, and coenzyme Q)

$\mathcal{F}$ = Faraday constant (23,062 cal/v·mole)

ΔE_o = E_o of the electron accepting pair minus the E_o of the electron donating pair

ΔG_o = change in the standard free energy

e.g. Calculate the ΔG° for the reaction

$$NADH + H^+ + \tfrac{1}{2}O_2 \rightarrow NAD^+ + H_2O$$

(E_o for $NADH/NAD^+ = -0.32$ v, E_o for $H_2O/O_2 = +0.82$ v)

Therefore, $\Delta G^\circ = -2(23{,}062)\ (+0.82 - [-0.32]) = 52{,}580$ cal/pair of electrons transferred

a. The standard free energy of hydrolysis of the terminal phosphate group of ATP is −7300 cal (see p. 101). Therefore, in order to add a phosphate molecule to ADP it would be necessary to put +7300 cal into the system. The transport of a pair of electrons from NADH to oxygen by means of the electron transport chain produces +52,580 cal (from calculation above), and therefore plenty of energy is made available to produce 3 ATP from 3 ADP and 3 P_i (3 × 7,300 = 21,900 cal). The remaining calories are released as heat.

b. The large, negative, free energy change produced by the passage of a pair of electrons from NADH, through the chain, to oxygen is divided over a number of electron transfers, three of which provide enough energy to theoretically produce one ATP (see Figure 10.9).

D. Mitchell's chemiosmotic hypothesis

1. Mitchell's chemiosmotic hypothesis explains how the free energy generated by the transport of electrons by the electron transport chain is used to produce ATP from ADP + P_i.

2. The members of the electron transport chain are arrayed asymmetrically in the inner mitochondrial membrane, forming loops as shown in Figure 10.12. Mitchell's hypothesis states that these loops consist of alternating hydrogen atom and electron carriers that transfer protons (H^+) from the mitochondrial matrix to the cytoplasmic side of the inner mitochondrial membrane. This process creates across the mitochondrial membrane both an electrical gradient (with more positive charges on the ***outside*** of the membrane than on the inside) and a pH gradient (the outside of the membrane at a lower pH than the inside). The energy inherent in this dual gradient is sufficient to drive ATP synthesis.

3. *ATP synthetase* is the enzyme complex that synthesizes ATP, using the energy provided by the electron transport chain. (Note: It is also called *ATPase* because it hydrolyzes ATP to ADP and inorganic phosphate when isolated from the inner mitochondrial membrane.) Mitchell's chemiosmotic hypothesis proposes that after protons have been transferred to the cytoplasmic side of the inner mitochondrial membrane, they can reenter the mitochondrial matrix by passing through a channel in the *ATP synthetase* molecule, resulting at the same time in the synthesis of ATP from ADP + P_i.

   a. ***Oligomycin,*** a drug that binds to the stalk of the *ATP synthetase*, closes the H^+ channel and prevents the reentry of protons into the mitochondrial matrix (Figure 10.13). Because the pH and electrical gradients cannot be dissipated in the presence of this drug, electron transport will also stop owing to the difficulty of pumping any more protons against the steep gradients. Electron transport and phosphorylation are therefore said to be ***tightly coupled processes***—if one is turned off, the other will also cease.

   b. Electron transport and phosphorylation can be ***uncoupled*** by compounds that ***increase the permeability*** of the inner mitochondrial membrane to protons. An example of an ***uncoupling agent*** is ***2,4-dinitrophenol***, which allows electron transport to proceed at a rapid rate without establishing a proton gradient. The energy produced by the transport of electrons is released as heat rather than being used to synthesize ATP.

4. The inner mitochondrial membrane requires specialized carriers to transport ADP and P_i from the cytoplasm (where ATP is used and converted to ADP in many energy-requiring reactions) into the mitochondria, where ATP can be resynthesized. Two specific transport systems are required: translocase

   a. ***Adenine nucleotide carrier*** transports one molecule of ADP from the cytoplasm into the mitochondria, while at the same time exporting one ATP from the mitochondria back into the cytoplasm (Figure 10.14). This carrier is strongly inhibited by the plant toxin ***atractyloside,*** resulting in a depletion of the intramitochondrial ADP pool and therefore a cessation of ATP production.

   b. A phosphate carrier is responsible for transporting inorganic phosphate from the cytoplasm to the mitochondria.

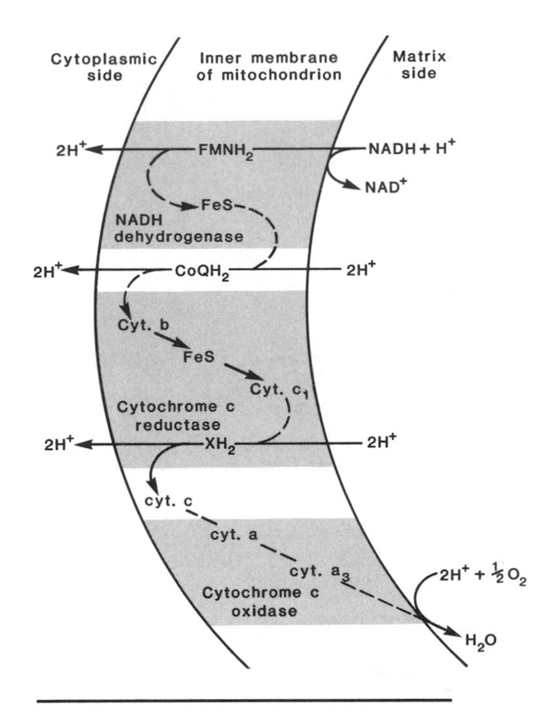

Figure 10.12
Vectorial arrangement across the inner mitochondrial membrane of electron transport chain members creating both a pH and an electrical gradient.

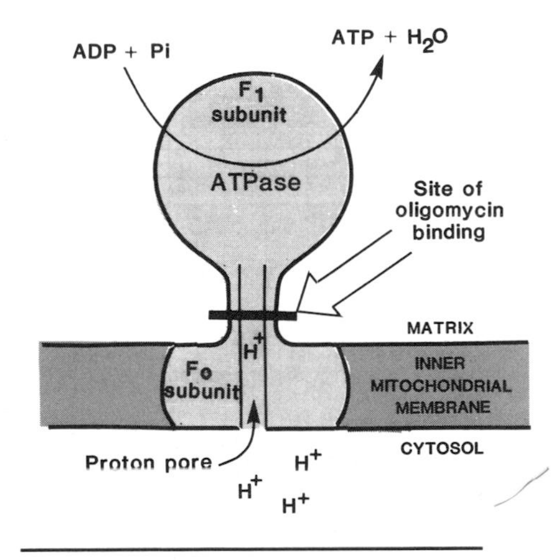

Figure 10.13
Closing of the H^+ channel of *ATP synthetase* by oligomycin.

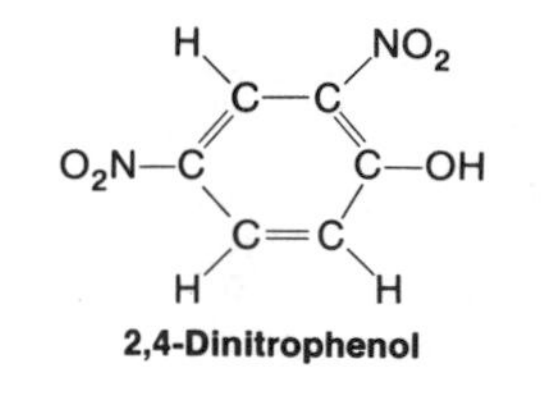

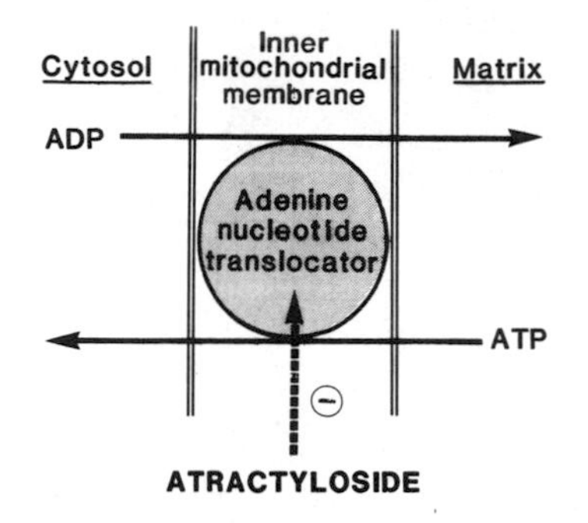

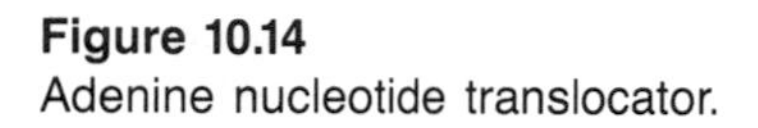

Figure 10.14
Adenine nucleotide translocator.

Study Questions

Choose the ONE best answer

10.7 An uncoupler of oxidative phosphorylation such as dinitrophenol

A. inhibits respiration and ATP synthesis.
B. allows electron transport to proceed without ATP synthesis.
C. inhibits respiration without impairment of ATP synthesis.
D. specifically inhibits cytochrome b.
E. acts as a competitive inhibitor of NAD^+-requiring reactions in the mitochondrion.

10.8 In an intact mitochondrial suspension, rotenone or amytal inhibits the oxidation of malate to oxaloacetate but not that of succinate to fumarate. The reason why these two agents have this discriminatory effect is because they

A. restrict the flow of electrons between NADH and coenzyme Q.
B. prevent mitochondria from accumulating calcium.
C. inhibit the ATP synthesizing complex.
D. compete with ATP in substrate level phosphorylation reactions.
E. make the inner mitochondrial membrane permeable to protons.

10.9 Which one of the statements listed below about the enzymic complex that carries out the synthesis of ATP during oxidative phosphorylation is INCORRECT?

A. It is located on the matrix side of the inner mitochondrial membrane.
B. It is inhibited by oligomycin.
C. It contains a proton channel.
D. It can exhibit ATPase activity.
E. It can bind molecular oxygen.

Answer A if 1, 2, and 3 are correct
B if 1 and 3 are correct
C if 2 and 4 are correct
D if only 4 is correct
E if all are correct

10.10 Which of the following statements correctly completes the sentence "NADH dehydrogenase. . . ."

1. . . . contains FMN and iron/sulfur centers.
2. . . . has a standard reduction potential (E_o) less positive than that of cytochrome c.
3. . . . is oxidized by coenzyme Q.
4. . . . is inhibited directly by oligomycin.

10.11 According to the Mitchell chemiosmotic hypothesis for oxidative phosphorylation, which of the following statements is(are) CORRECT?

1. The cytoplasmic side of the inner mitochondrial membrane becomes positively charged with respect to the matrix as respiration occurs in normal functioning mitochondria.
2. ATP formation in mitochondria is accompanied by movement of protons from the cytoplasmic to the matrix side of the inner mitochondrial membrane.
3. The electron transport chain consists of loops of alternating hydrogen and electron carriers.
4. The inner mitochondrial membrane must be permeable to protons in order to build up a proton gradient.

10.12 Which of the following statements about mitochondria is(are) CORRECT?

1. Calcium ions can diffuse freely across the inner mitochondrial membrane.
2. The outer mitochondrial membrane is permeable to most small molecules, whereas the inner membrane is impermeable to most.
3. The matrix is a protein-rich gel that contains the enzymes involved in oxidation/reduction reactions.
4. The inner mitochondrial membrane is folded into cristae so as to increase its surface area.

10.13 From the known effects of 2,4-dinitrophenol on the process of oxidative phosphorylation, one may infer that its administration might cause which of the following physiologic manifestations?

1. Muscle weakness or general fatigue owing to a deficiency in ATP synthesis.
2. Weight loss owing to an increased catabolism of carbohydrate, lipid, and protein reserves to generate ATP by way of substrate level phosphorylation.
3. Fever, since the energy from respiration would be converted to heat instead of being used for the formation of ATP.
4. Increased need for oxygen by the body, and therefore an increased rate of breathing.

10.14 Given the following reaction

$$\text{Succinate} + \text{FAD} \rightleftarrows \text{Fumarate} + \text{FADH}_2$$

where the standard reduction potential, E_o for succinate/fumarate is -0.03 v and the E_o for $FADH_2$/FAD is -0.06 v, which of the following statements is(are) CORRECT?

1. There would be a net production of fumarate under standard conditions.
2. Under standard conditions, the overall ΔG would be less than $\Delta G°$.
3. Since the reduction potential for $FADH_2$/FAD is lower than that for succinate/fumarate, $FADH_2$ could not be used as a reducing agent in the mitochondria.
4. The $\Delta G°$ for the conversion of succinate to fumarate would be $(+0.03)(n)(\mathcal{F})$, where n is the number of electrons transferred to FAD and $\mathcal{F}$ is the Faraday constant.

Glycolysis

11

I. OVERVIEW

The glycolytic pathway is used by all tissues for the breakdown of glucose, providing energy and building blocks for synthetic reactions. Glycolysis is at the hub of carbohydrate metabolism because virtually all sugars (whether arising from the diet or from catabolic reactions in the body) ultimately can be converted to glucose (Figure 11.1). Three of the reactions of glycolysis are physiologically irreversible and are regulated by the energy and synthetic needs of the cell. Pyruvate is the end-product of glycolysis in tissues with mitochondria and an adequate supply of oxygen (Figure 11.2). This series of ten reactions, called ***aerobic glycolysis,*** sets the stage for the oxidative decarboxylation of pyruvate to acetyl CoA, a major fuel of the citric acid cycle. Alternatively, under anaerobic conditions, pyruvate can be reduced by NADH to form lactate (Figure 11.2). This occurs when the rate of NADH formation exceeds the oxidative capacity of the cell. The conversion of glucose to lactate by ***anaerobic glycolysis*** allows the continued production of ATP in tissues that lack mitochondria (e.g., red blood cells) or in cells that are deprived of sufficient oxygen.

II. REACTIONS OF GLYCOLYSIS

A. Phosphorylation of glucose

1. The irreversible phosphorylation reaction, shown in Figure 11.3, effectively traps glucose in a form that does not diffuse out of the cell, since phosphorylated sugar molecules do not readily penetrate cell membranes without specific carriers. This commits glucose to further metabolism in the cell.
2. In all tissues the phosphorylation of glucose is catalyzed by *hexokinase*, one of three ***regulatory enzymes*** of glycolysis (see also *phosphofructokinase* and *pyruvate kinase*).
   a. *Hexokinase* is inhibited by the reaction product, glucose 6-phosphate, that accumulates when further metabolism of this hexose phosphate is reduced, for example, by a high ATP/ADP ratio.
   b. *Hexokinase* has a low K_m (and therefore a high affinity) for glucose (see p. 38). This allows the efficient phosphorylation and subsequent metabolism of glucose even when the tissue concentrations of the sugar are low (Figure 11.4).

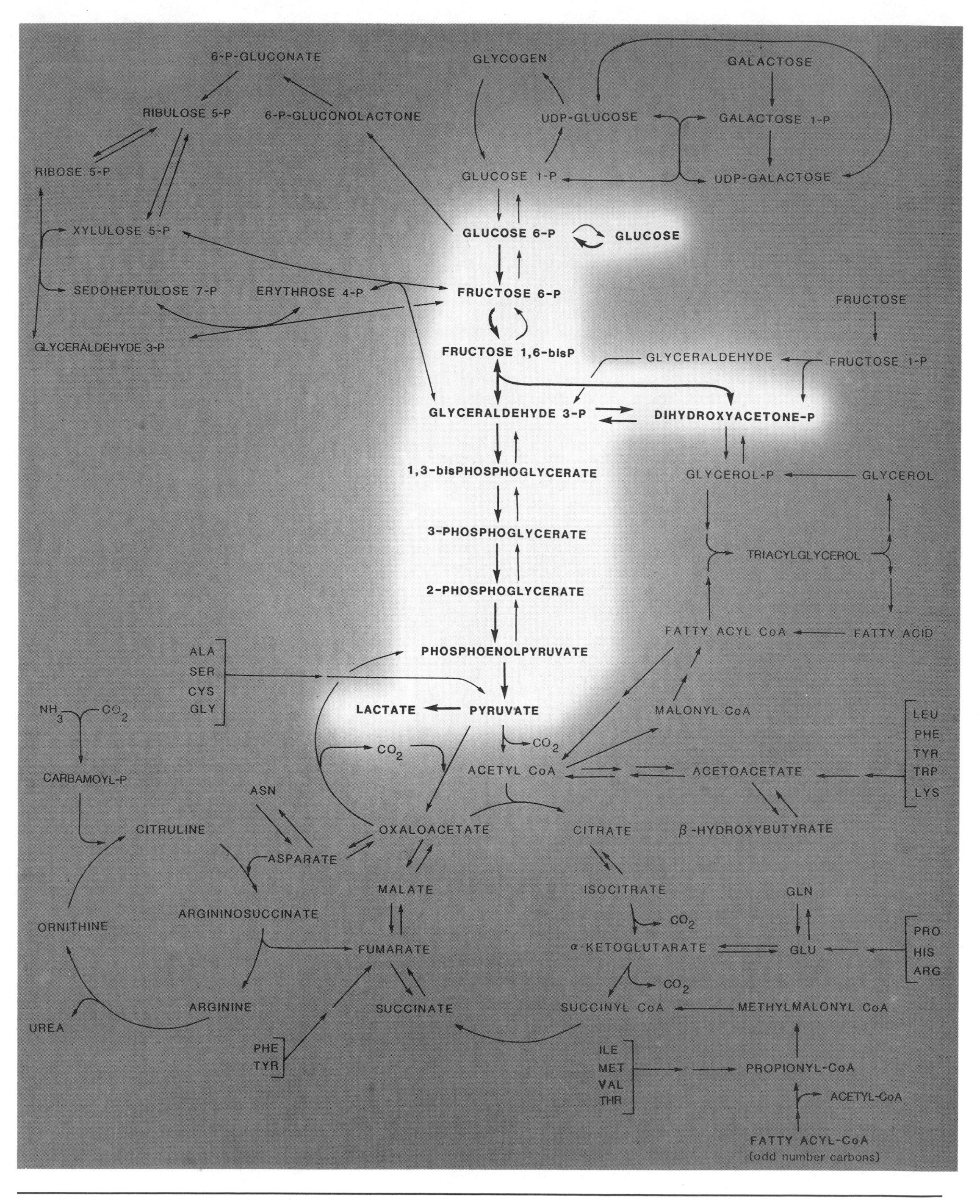

Figure 11.1
Important reactions of intermediary metabolism with the reactions of glycosis highlighted.

c. *Hexokinase,* however, has a low V_{max} for glucose and therefore cannot phosphorylate large quantities of glucose (Figure 11.4).

d. *Hexokinase* has a broad specificity and can phosphorylate several hexoses in addition to glucose.

3. Liver has an additional enzyme, *glucokinase,* that phosphorylates only glucose.

a. Because *glucokinase* has a high K_m, it functions only when the intracellular concentration of glucose is elevated. This occurs during the brief period after consumption of a carbohydrate-rich meal, when high levels of glucose are delivered to the liver by means of the portal vein. (Blood glucose equilibrates rapidly across the membrane of the hepatocyte.)

b. *Glucokinase* has a high V_m, allowing the liver to remove effectively this flood of glucose from the portal blood. This prevents large amounts of glucose from entering the circulation after a carbohydrate-rich meal, and thus minimizes hyperglycemia during the absorptive period.

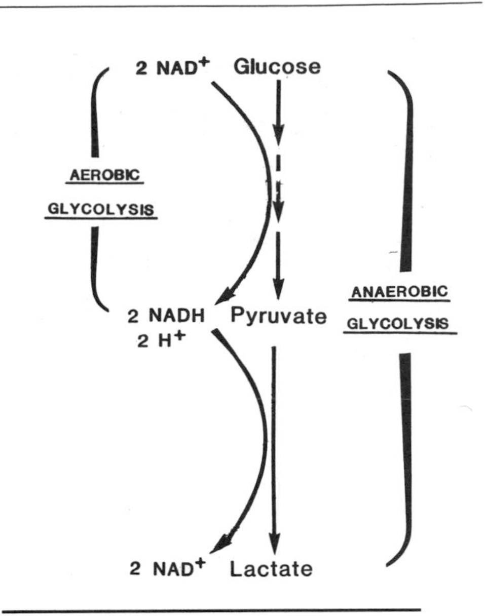

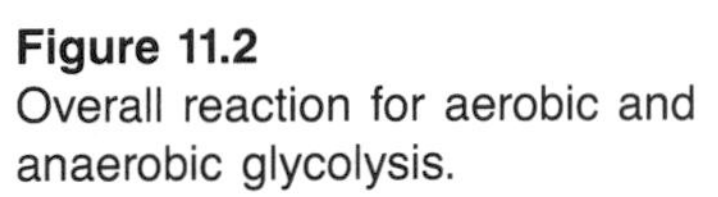
Figure 11.2
Overall reaction for aerobic and anaerobic glycolysis.

TABLE 11.1: PROPERTIES OF HEXOKINASE AND GLUCOKINASE

	Hexokinase	*Glucokinase*
Tissue Distribution	Most tissues	Liver only
K_m	Low (0.1 mM = 2 mg%*)	High (10 mM = 200 mg%*)
V_m	Low	High
Substrate Specificity	D-glucose Other hexoses	D-glucose only
Inhibition by Glucose 6-Phosphate	Yes	No

*mg% = milligrams glucose per 100 ml plasma; normal fasting blood glucose is 70-90 mg%, or about 5 mM.

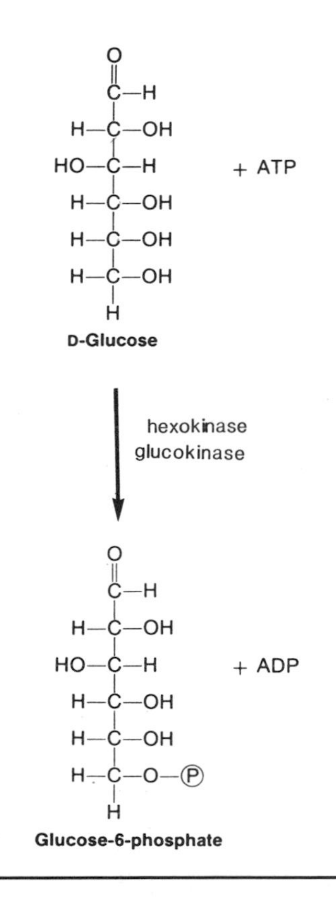

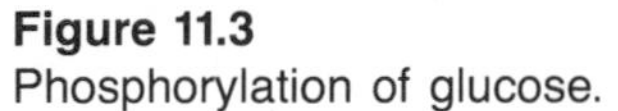
Figure 11.3
Phosphorylation of glucose.

B. Isomerization of glucose 6-phosphate

1. The isomerization of glucose 6-phosphate (an aldose sugar) to fructose 6-phosphate (a ketose sugar) is catalyzed by *phosphoglucose isomerase* (Figure 11.5). The reaction is readily reversible and is not a rate-limiting or regulated step in glycolysis.

C. Phosphorylation of fructose 6-phosphate

1. The irreversible phosphorylation reaction, catalyzed by *phosphofructokinase I* (PFK I), is the most important ***control point*** of glycolysis (Figure 11.6). Within the cell the PFK I reaction is the ***rate-limiting step*** in the glycolytic breakdown of glucose. The rate of PFK I is controlled by the concentrations of the substrates ATP and fructose 6-phosphate. Enzyme activity is also altered by a large series of regulatory substances (effectors or modulators) described below.

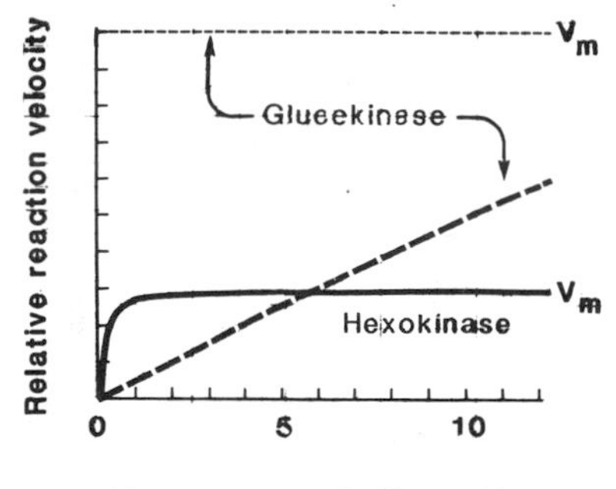

Figure 11.4
Effect of glucose concentration on the rate of phosphorylation catalyzed by *hexokinase* and *glucokinase*.

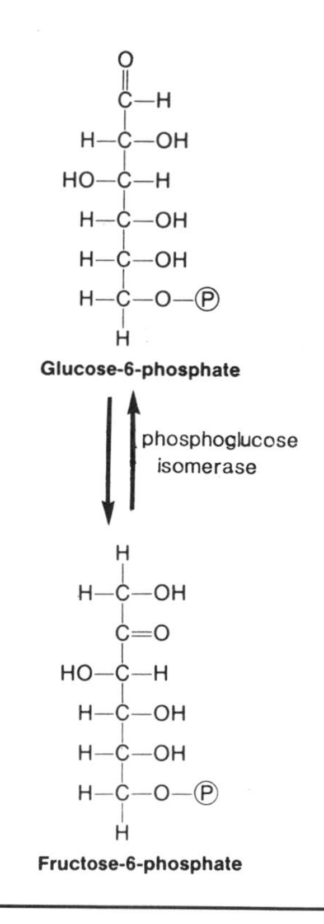

Figure 11.5
Conversion of glucose 6-phosphate to fructose 6-phosphate.

2. PFK I is ***inhibited*** allosterically by elevated levels of ATP or citrate, which signal that the cell has adequate energy stores.
3. PFK I is ***activated*** allosterically by high concentrations of AMP, which signal that the cell's energy stores are depleted.
4. ***Fructose 2,6-bisphosphate*** is the most potent ***activator*** of PFK I. This unusual compound also acts as an inhibitor of *fructose 1,6-bisphosphatase* (see p. 127).
   a. Fructose 2,6-bisphosphate is formed by *phosphofructokinase II* (PFK II), an enzyme different from *phosphofructokinase I*. Fructose 2,6-bisphosphate is converted back to fructose 6-phosphate by a specific *fructose 2,6-bisphosphatase* (Figure 11.7).
   b. Elevated levels of glucagon (see p. 268), such as those observed during starvation, decrease the intracellular concentration of hepatic fructose 2,6-bisphosphate. This results in a decrease in the overall rate of glycolysis and an increase in the overall rate of gluconeogenesis (see p. 129).
   c. Decreased levels of glucagon, such as observed after ingestion of a carbohydrate-rich meal, cause an increase in fructose 2,6-bisphosphate and in the rate of glycolysis. Fructose 2,6-bisphosphate thus acts as an intracellular signal indicating that glucose is abundant.

D. Cleavage of fructose 1,6-bisphosphate

1. *Aldolase A* cleaves fructose 1,6-bisphosphate to dihydroxyacetone phosphate and glyceraldehyde 3-phosphate (Figure 11.8). The reaction is reversible and is not subject to regulation.

E. Isomerization of dihydroxyacetone phosphate

1. *Triose phosphate isomerase* catalyzes the reversible interconversion of dihydroxyacetone phosphate and glyceraldehyde 3-phosphate (Figure 11.9). Dihydroxyacetone phosphate cannot proceed further on the direct pathway of glycolysis and must be isomerized to glyceraldehyde 3-phosphate for further metabolism in the glycolytic sequence.
2. This isomerization results in the production of ***two*** molecules of glyceraldehyde phosphate from the cleavage products of fructose 1,6-bisphosphate.
3. Dihydroxyacetone phosphate, glyceraldehyde 3-phosphate, and the remaining compounds in the glycolytic pathway are trioses.

F. Oxidation of glyceraldehyde 3-phosphate

1. The conversion of glyceraldehyde 3-phosphate to 1,3-diphosphoglycerate by *glyceraldehyde 3-phosphate dehydrogenase* is the first oxidation-reduction reaction of glycolysis (Figure 11.10). Because there is only a limited amount of NAD^+ in the cell, the NADH formed in this reaction must be reoxidized back to NAD^+ for glycolysis to continue. Two major mechanisms for oxidizing NADH are (a) the NADH-linked conversion of pyruvate to lactate and (b) oxidation by the respiratory chain.
2. The oxidation of the aldehyde group of glyceraldehyde 3-phos-

phate to a carboxyl group is coupled to the attachment of P_i to the carboxyl group. The high-energy phosphate group at carbon 1 of 1,3-diphosphoglycerate conserves much of the free energy produced by the oxidation of glyceraldehyde 3-phosphate. The formation of 1,3-diphosphoglycerate is an example of ***substrate-level phosphorylation*** in which the production of a high-energy phosphate is coupled to the conversion of substrate to product, instead of resulting from oxidative phosphorylation (see p. 102). The energy trapped in this new high-energy phosphate will be used to drive the synthesis of ATP in the next reaction of glycolysis.

3. 1,3-Diphosphoglycerate can be converted to ***2,3-diphosphoglycerate*** (2,3-DPG) by the action of a mutase. 2,3-DPG, which is found only in trace amounts in most cells, is present at high concentrations in red blood cells (see p. 26). 2,3-DPG is hydrolyzed by a phosphatase to 3-phosphoglycerate, which is also an intermediate in glycolysis.

G. Formation of ATP from 1,3-diphosphoglycerate and ADP

1. The high-energy phosphate group of 1,3-diphosphoglycerate is used to synthesize ATP from ADP in a reaction catalyzed by *phosphoglycerate kinase* (Figure 11.11). Unlike most other kinases, this reaction is reversible.
2. Two molecules of 1,3-diphosphoglycerate are formed from each glucose molecule. This kinase reaction, therefore, yields two ATP and, in effect, replaces the two ATP consumed in the earlier formation of glucose 6-phosphate and fructose 1,6-bisphosphate.

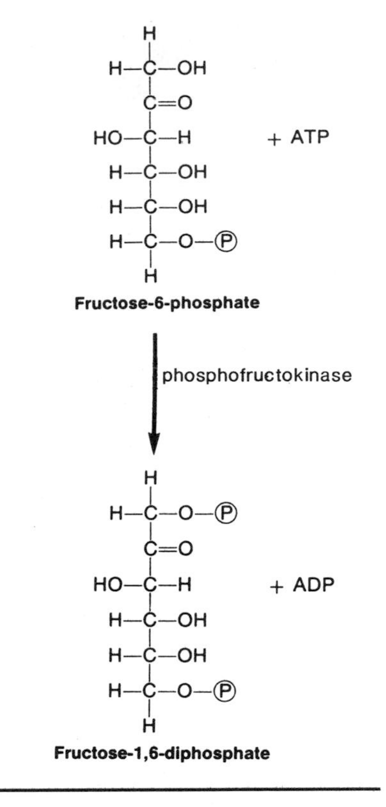

Figure 11.6
Phosphorylation of fructose 6-phosphate.

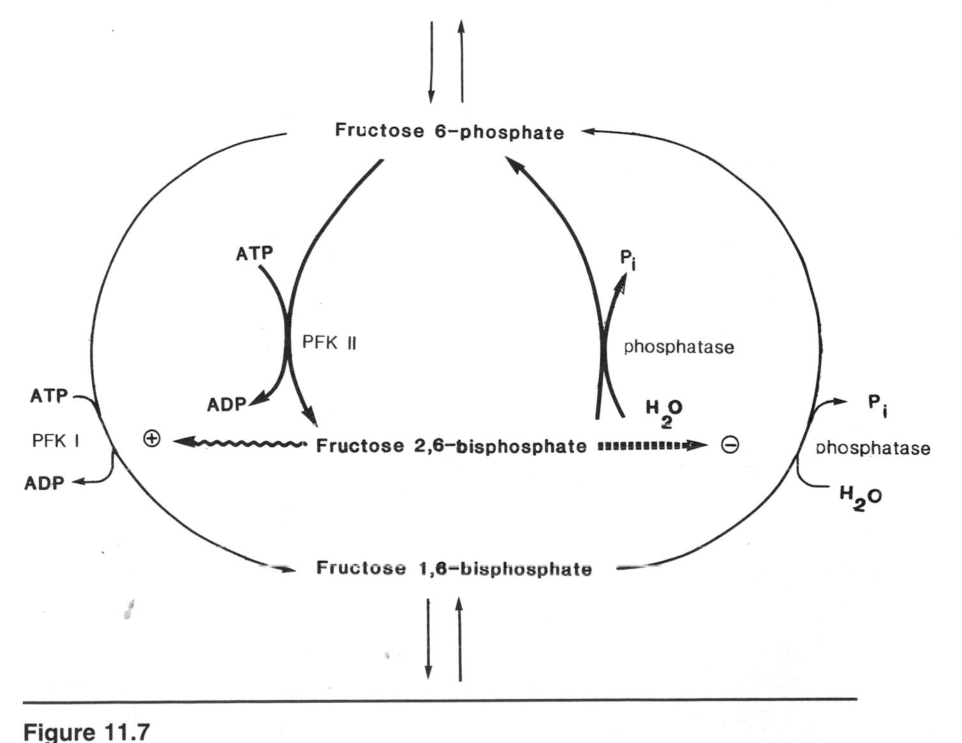

Figure 11.7
Formation, degradation, and regulatory effects of fructose 2,6-bisphosphate.

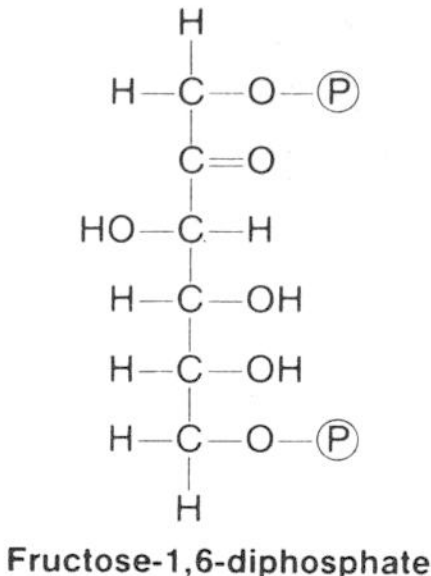

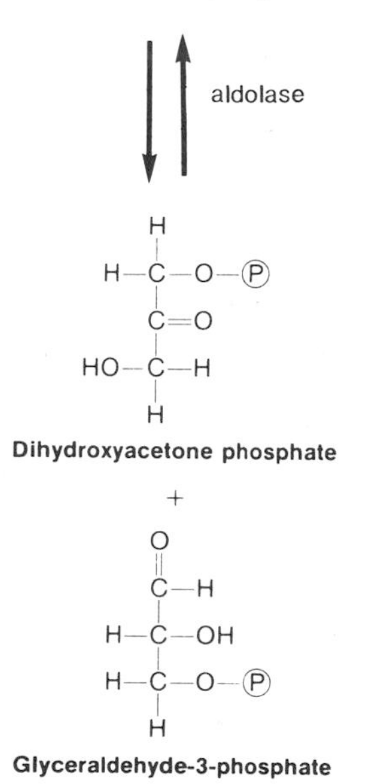

Figure 11.8
Cleavage of fructose 1,6-bisphosphate.

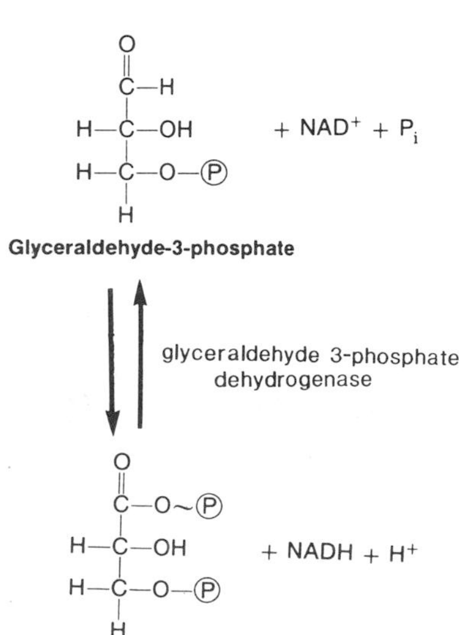

Figure 11.10
Conversion of glyceraldehyde 3-phosphate to 1,3-diphosphoglycerate.

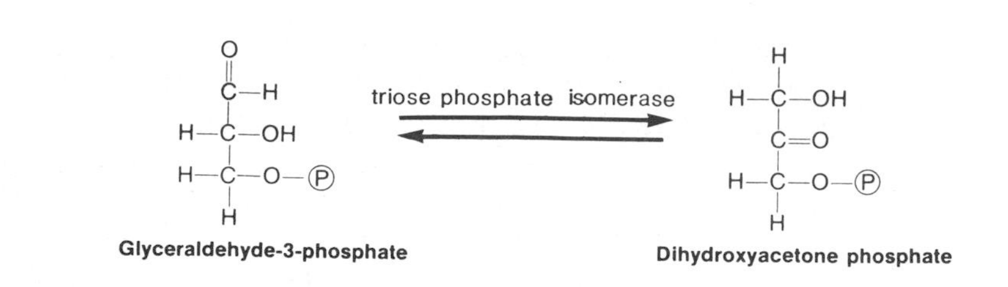

Figure 11.9
Isomerization of dihydroxyacetone phosphate.

H. Shift of the phosphate group from carbon 3 to carbon 2

1. The shift of the phosphate group from carbon #3 to carbon #2 catalyzed by *phosphoglyceromutase* is freely reversible (Figure 11.12).

I. Dehydration of 2-phosphoglycerate

1. The dehydration of 2-phosphoglycerate catalyzed by *enolase* redistributes the energy within the 2-phosphoglycerate molecule, resulting in the formation of phosphoenolpyruvate (PEP), which contains a high-energy enol phosphate (Figure 11.12).
2. The reaction is reversible despite the high-energy nature of the product.

J. Formation of pyruvate

1. The equilibrium of the reaction catalyzed by *pyruvate kinase* is far to the right, favoring the formation of ATP (Figure 11.13).
2. *Pyruvate kinase* is activated by fructose 1,6-bisphosphate, the product of the *phosphofructokinase* reaction. This type of feed-forward (instead of the more usual feed-back) regulation has the effect of linking the two kinase activities: Increases in *phosphofructokinase*, resulting in elevated levels of fructose 1,6-bisphosphate, will activate *pyruvate kinase.*
3. *Pyruvate kinase* is also subject to covalent modulation:
   a. Phosphorylation by a *cAMP-dependent protein kinase* leads to inactivation of *pyruvate kinase.* When blood glucose levels are low, elevated glucagon increases the intracellular levels of cAMP, which favors the phosphorylation and inactivation of *pyruvate kinase* (see p. 129). Therefore PEP cannot continue in glycolysis but instead enters the gluconeogenesis pathway. This in part explains the observed inhibition of hepatic glycolysis and stimulation of gluconeogenesis by glucagon.
   b. Dephosphorylation by a *phosphoprotein phosphatase* results in reactivation of the enzyme.
4. ***Pyruvate kinase deficiency***: This genetic deficiency of *pyruvate kinase* in the erythrocyte leads to hemolytic anemia (excessive erythrocyte destruction). Almost all individuals with PK deficiency have a mutant enzyme that shows abnormal properties, most often altered kinetics.
   a. The normal mature erythrocyte has no mitochondria and is completely dependent on glycolysis for its production of ATP.

b. Patients' red blood cells typically have 5% to 25% of normal *pyruvate kinase* activity, and hence the rate of glycolysis in these cells is severely decreased.

c. The anemia observed in PK-deficiency may be a consequence of the reduced rate of glycolysis. The rate of ATP synthesis is thought to be inadequate to meet the energy needs of the cell and to maintain the structural integrity of the erythrocyte.

d. The inability of the red blood cell to maintain its membrane leads to changes in the shape of the cell and ultimately to phagocytosis by the cells of the reticuloendothelial system, particularly macrophages of the spleen.

e. The premature death and lysis of the red blood cell result in hemolytic anemia.

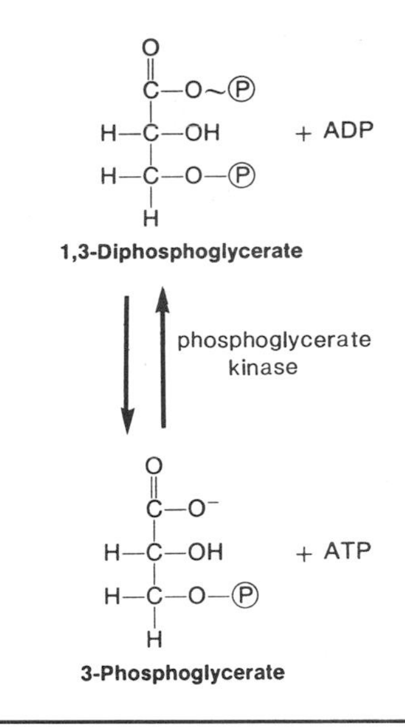

Figure 11.11
Formation of ATP from 1,3-diphosphoglycerate and ADP.

K. Reduction of pyruvate to lactate

1. Lactate, formed by the action of *lactate dehydrogenase*, is the final product of anaerobic glycolysis in eukaryotic cells (Figure 11.14). The formation of lactate is the major fate for pyruvate in red blood cells that lack mitochondria, and therefore do not have the enzymes of the TCA cycle.

2. In exercising skeletal muscle, NADH production (by the *glyceraldehyde 3-phosphate dehydrogenase* reaction and by the three NAD^+-linked dehydrogenase reactions of the citric acid cycle) exceeds the oxidative capacity of the respiratory chain, resulting in an elevated $NADH/NAD^+$ ratio that favors reduction of pyruvate to lactate. Therefore, during intense exercise, lactate accumulates in the muscle, causing a drop in the intracellular pH, potentially resulting in cramps. Much of this lactate eventually diffuses from the muscle cells into the blood stream.

3. The direction of the *lactate dehydrogenase* reaction depends on the relative intracellular concentrations of pyruvate and lactate and on the ratio of $NADH/NAD^+$ in the cell. For example, in tissues such as liver and heart, the ratio of $NADH/NAD^+$ is lower than that in exercising muscle. These tissues can oxidize lactate (obtained from the blood) to pyruvate. In the liver, pyruvate is either converted to glucose by gluconeogenesis (see p. 125) or oxidized in the TCA cycle. Heart muscle exclusively oxidizes lactate to CO_2 and H_2O by means of the citric acid cycle. Figure 11.15 summarizes the reactions of glycolysis.

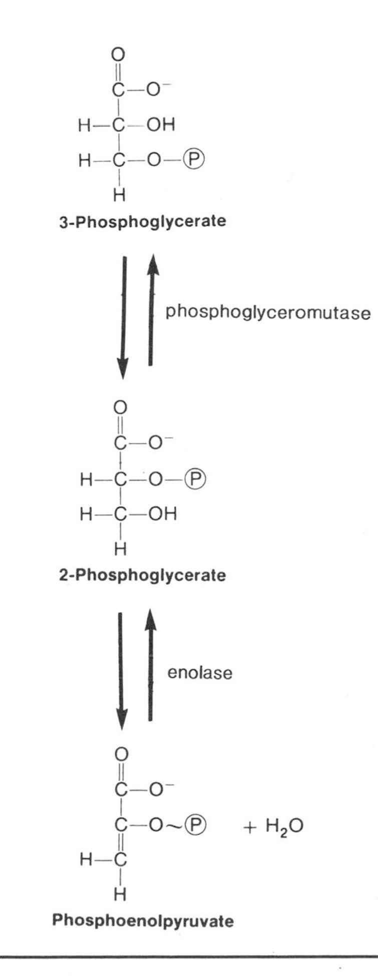

Figure 11.12
Reactions catalyzed by *phosphoglyceromutase* and *enolase*.

III. ALTERNATE FATES OF PYRUVATE

A. The oxidative decarboxylation of pyruvate

1. The oxidative decarboxylation of pyruvate by *pyruvate dehydrogenase* is an important pathway in tissues with a high oxidative capacity, such as cardiac muscle (Figure 11.16).

2. *Pyruvate dehydrogenase* irreversibly converts pyruvate, the end-product of glycolysis, into acetyl-CoA, a major fuel for the citric acid cycle (see p. 133) and the building block for fatty acid synthesis (see p. 161).

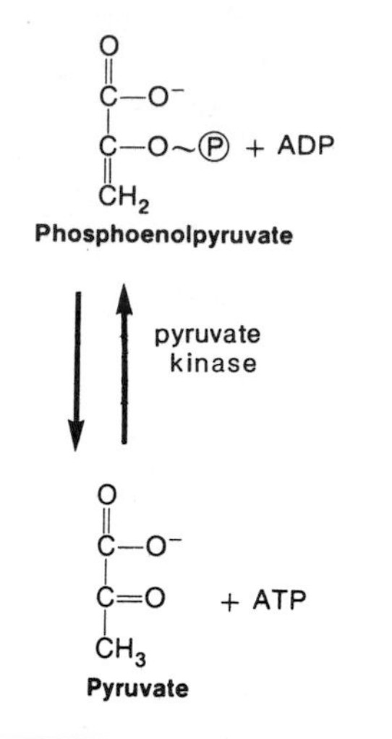

Figure 11.13
Formation of pyruvate.

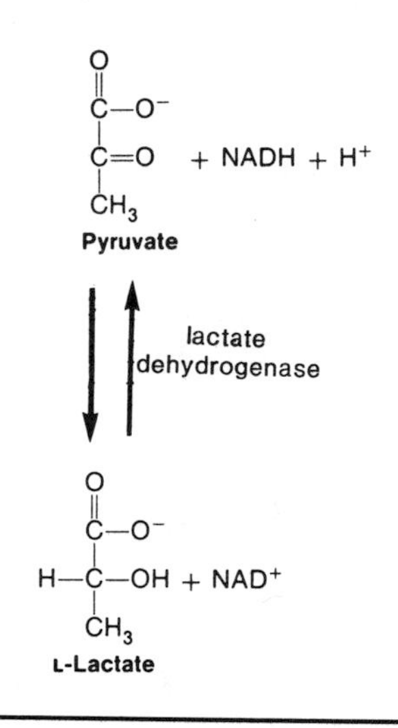

Figure 11.14
Reduction of pyruvate.

B. Carboxylation of pyruvate to oxaloacetate

1. The carboxylation of pyruvate to oxaloacetate (OAA) by *pyruvate carboxylase* is a ***biotin-dependent*** reaction (Figure 11.16). This reaction is important because it both replenishes the citric acid cycle intermediates and provides substrate for gluconeogenesis (see p. 125).

C. Reduction of pyruvate to ethanol (microorganisms):

1. The conversion of pyruvate to ethanol occurs by the two reactions summarized in Figure 11.16 and shown in detail in Figure 11.17.
2. The decarboxylation of pyruvate by *pyruvate decarboxylase* occurs in yeast and certain microorganisms but ***not*** in humans. The enzyme contains ***thiamine pyrophosphate*** as a cofactor and catalyzes a reaction similar to that described for *pyruvate dehydrogenase* (see p. 133).

IV. OXIDATION OF ETHANOL IN HUMANS

A. Alcohol is a significant source of calories in many individuals. The metabolism of ethanol yields acetate by means of a pathway composed of two oxidation reactions (Figure 11.18).

1. ***Formation of acetaldehyde:*** The first oxidation in the metabolism of ethanol occurs primarily in the liver and is catalyzed by *alcohol dehydrogenase* (Figure 11.18). Some acetaldehyde is formed by a microsomal ethanol oxidizing system (MEOS) involving NADPH, O_2, and cytochrome P_{450} (see p. 146). This oxidative system is also used to inactive drugs such as pentobarbital.
2. ***Formation of acetate:*** Acetaldehyde, the reaction product of ethanol oxidation, is further oxidized to acetate by the enzyme *aldehyde dehydrogenase,* also found in the liver. The metabolism of ethanol is summarized in Figure 11.18.

V. ENERGY YIELD OF GLYCOLYSIS

A. Anaerobic glycolysis

Overall reaction:

$$\text{Glucose} + 2P_i + 2\text{ADP} \rightarrow 2\ \text{lactate} + 2\text{ATP} + 2H_2O$$

1. A net of two molecules of ATP is generated for each molecule of glucose converted to lactate, as is shown in the reactions summarized in Table 11.2.
2. Anaerobic glycolysis, although releasing only a small fraction of the energy contained in the glucose molecule, is a valuable source of energy under the following conditions:
   a. when oxygen supply is limited, as in muscle during intensive exercise.
   b. in tissues with few or no mitochondria, such as the medulla of the kidney, mature erythrocytes, and leukocytes.

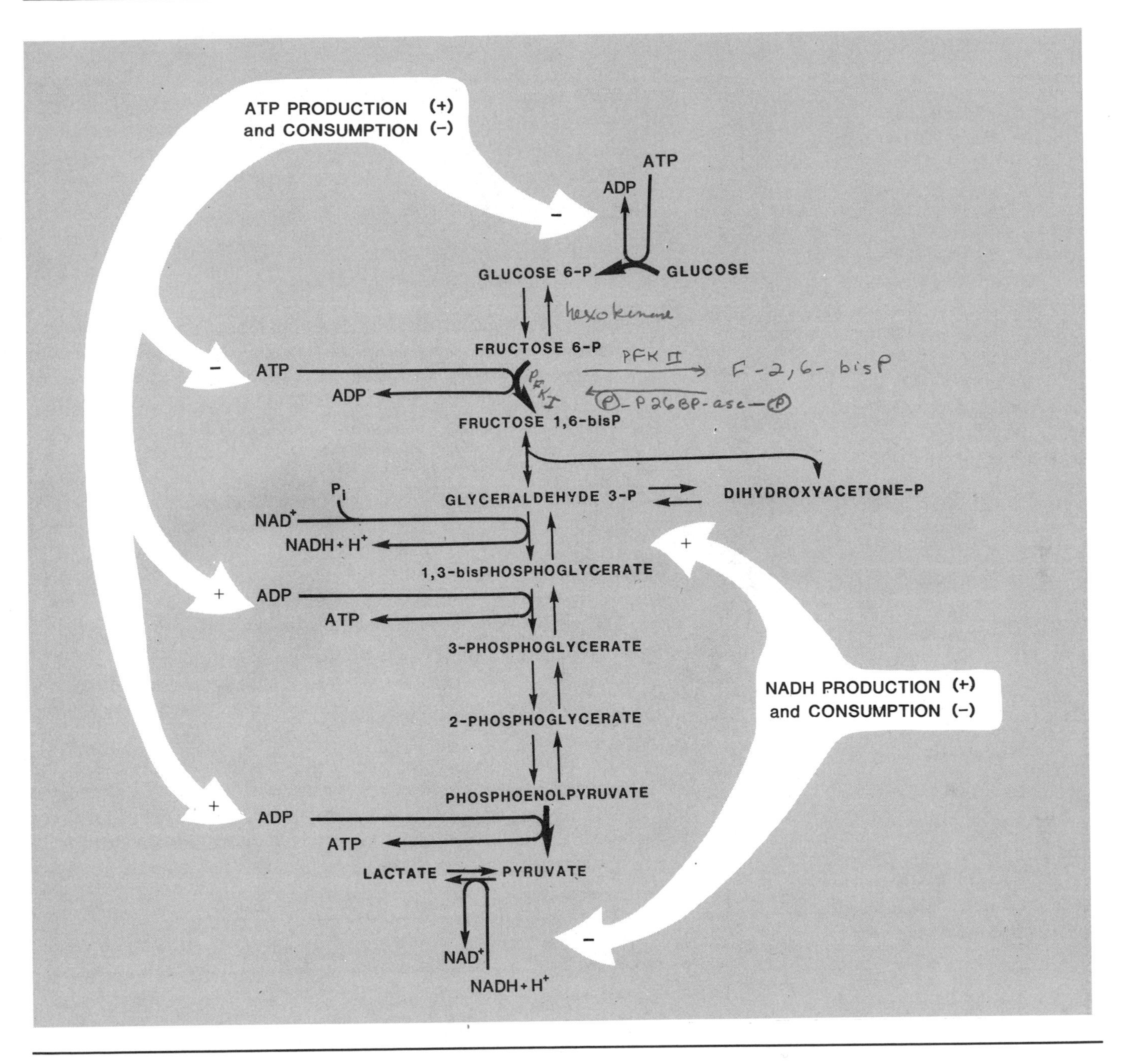

Figure 11.15
Summary of anaerobic glycolysis. Reactions involving the production or consumption of ATP or NADH are highlighted. The irreversible reactions of glycolysis are shown with thick reaction arrows.

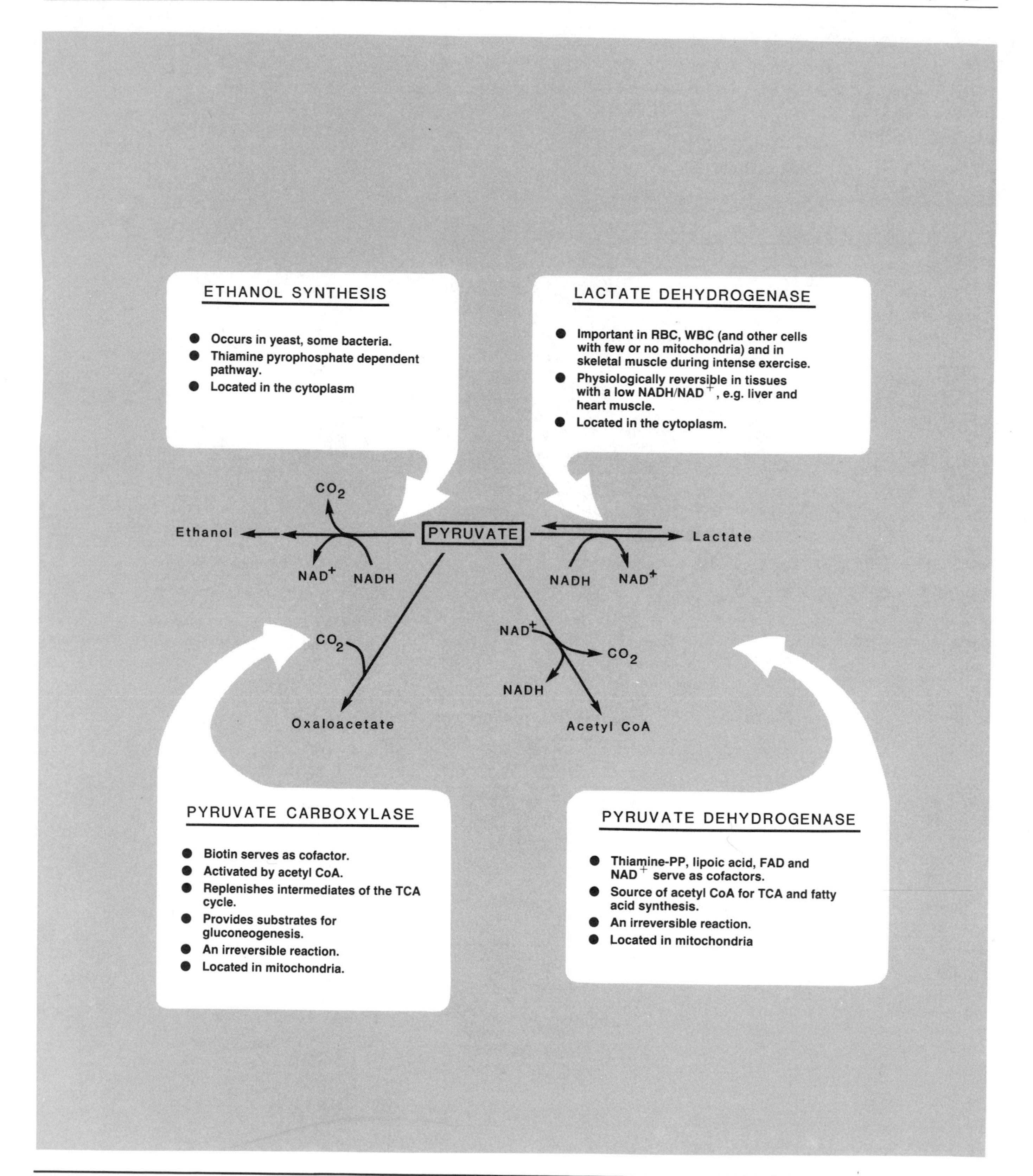

Figure 11.16
Summary of the metabolic fates of pyruvate.

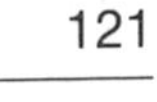

TABLE 11.2 FORMATION AND CONSUMPTION OF ATP IN ANAEROBIC GLYCOLYSIS

Reaction	Change in ATP per Glucose Consumed
Glucose → Glucose 6-phosphate	−1
Fructose 6-phosphate → Fructose 1,6-bisphosphate	−1
(2) 1,3-diphosphoglycerate → (2) 3-phosphoglycerate	+2
(2) Phosphoenolpyruvate → (2) Pyruvate	+2
Net:	+2ATP

3. In anaerobic glycolysis there is no net production or consumption of NADH; the NADH formed by *glyceraldehyde 3-phosphate dehydrogenase* is used by *lactate dehydrogenase* to reduce pyruvate to lactate (Table 11.3). Two trioses are produced for each glucose molecule metabolized.

TABLE 11.3 FORMATION AND CONSUMPTION OF NADH ATP IN ANAEROBIC GLYCOLYSIS

Reaction	Changes in NADH per glucose consumed
(2) glyceraldehyde 3-phosphate → (2) 1,3-diphosphoglycerate	+2
(2) pyruvate → (2) lactate	−2
net:	0 NADH

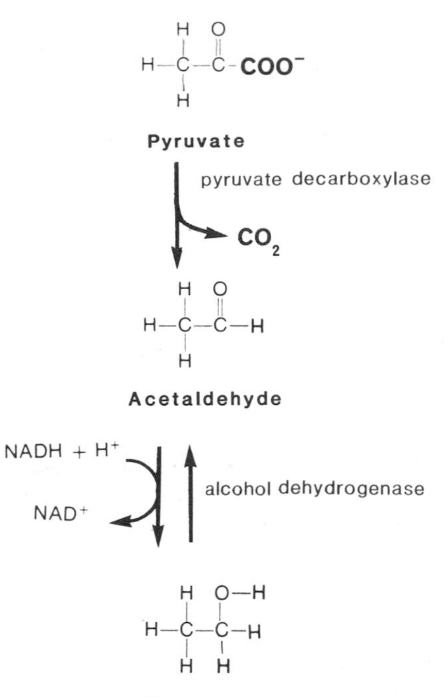

Figure 11.17
Reduction of pyruvate to ethanol (microorganisms).

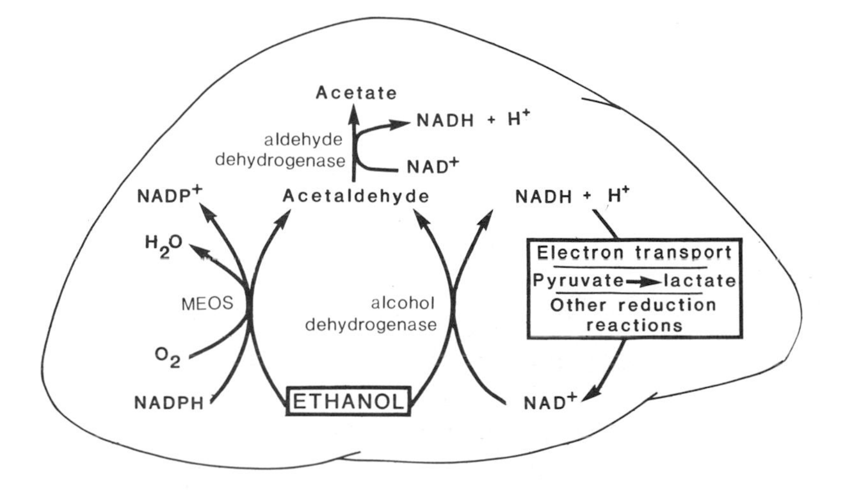

Figure 11.18
Summary of ethanol metabolism.

B. Aerobic glycolysis

Overall reaction:

$$\text{glucose} + 2P_i + 2NAD^+ + 2ADP \rightarrow$$
$$2\text{ pyruvate} + 2ATP + 2NADH + 2H^+ + H_2O$$

1. The direct formation and the consumption of ATP are the same as in anaerobic glycolysis, that is, a net gain of 2 ATP per molecule of glucose.
2. Two moles of NADH are produced per mole of glucose. Ongoing aerobic glycolysis requires the oxidation of most of this NADH by the respiratory chain.

TABLE 11.4 FORMATION OF ATP IN AEROBIC GLYCOLYSIS

Reaction			Change in ATP per glucose consumed
glucose	→	(2) pyruvate	+2
(substrate level phosphorylations described for anaerobic glycolysis, p. 115)			
(2) NADH	→	(2) NAD^+	+6*
(oxidation by election transport chain resulting in 3ATP generated per mole of NADH oxidized, p. 105)			
		net:	+8 ATP per glucose oxidized

*Controversy exists as to the number of ATP molecules produced from the oxidation of cytoplasmic NADH. For purpose of illustration, a value of 3 ATP per NADH oxidized is used in Table 11.4.

Study Questions

Answer A if 1, 2, and 3 are correct
B if 1 and 3 are correct
C if 2 and 4 are correct
D if only 4 is correct
E if all are correct

11.1 Glucokinase

1. is widely distributed and occurs in most mammalian tissues.
2. has a high K_m for glucose, and hence is important in the phosphorylation of glucose primarily after ingestion of a carbohydrate-rich meal.
3. is inhibited by glucose 6-phosphate.
4. is specific for the phosphorylation of glucose.

11.2 The reaction catalyzed by phosphofructokinase

1. is inhibited by high concentrations of ATP and citrate.
2. uses fructose 1-phosphate as substrate.
3. is an important control point in the glycolytic pathway.
4. is near equilibrium in most tissues.

11.3 Compared to the resting state, vigorously contracting muscle shows

1. increased lactate formation.
2. increases oxidation of pyruvate to CO_2 and water.
3. an increased $NADH/NAD^+$ ratio.
4. increased conversion of pyruvate to acetaldehyde.

11.4 Under anoxic (low oxygen concentration) conditions, glycolysis in muscle becomes more rapid because of an increase in the intracellular concentration of

1. NAD^+.
2. ATP.
3. glycogen.
4. AMP.

11.5 The rate of glycolysis is controlled in part by inhibition of

1. hexokinase by glucose 6-phosphate.
2. phosphofructokinase by citrate.
3. phosphofructokinase by ATP.
4. glucokinase by ATP.

Choose the ONE best answer

11.6 The conversion of glucose 6-phosphate to lactate in the glycolytic pathway is accompanied by a net gain of

A. one mole of ATP.
B. two moles of ATP.
C. three moles of ATP.
D. one mole of NADH.
E. none of the above.

11.7 During strenuous exercise, the NADH formed in the glyceraldehyde 3-phosphate dehydrogenase reaction in skeletal muscle must be reoxidized to NAD^+ if glycolysis is to continue. The most important reaction involved in the reoxidation of NADH is

A. oxaloacetate $\rightarrow$ malate.
B. pyruvate $\rightarrow$ lactate.
C. dihydroxyacetone phosphate $\rightarrow$ glycerol phosphate.
D. isocitrate $\rightarrow$ α-ketoglutarate.
E. glucose 6-phosphate $\rightarrow$ fructose 6-phosphate.

11.8 In pyruvate kinase deficiency, hemolysis of red cells occurs primarily because of increased intracellular levels of

A. lactate.
B. pyruvate.
C. the ratio of ADP to ATP.
D. 2,3-diphosphoglycerate.
E. fructose 1,6-bisphosphate.

Gluconeogenesis

12

I. OVERVIEW

Some tissues, such as the brain, red blood cells, and exercising muscle, require a continuing supply of glucose as a metabolic fuel. Liver glycogen can meet these needs only for 10 to 18 hours without dietary carbohydrate. During a prolonged fast, hepatic glycogen stores are depleted and glucose is formed from precursors such as lactate, pyruvate, glycerol (derived from the backbone of triglyceride), and α-ketoacids (derived from amino acid catabolism). The formation of glucose does not occur by a simple reversal of glycolysis, since the overall equilibrium of glycolysis strongly favors pyruvate formation. Instead, glucose is synthesized by a special pathway, ***gluconeogenesis***. Although gluconeogenesis uses eight of the reactions of glycolysis, it substitutes four new reactions for the three glycolytic steps that are physiologically irreversible (Figure 12.1). These reactions, unique to gluconeogenesis, couple the hydrolysis of ATP or phosphate esters to the synthesis of glucose. As a result the equilibrium of the gluconeogenic pathway favors the synthesis of glucose. Gluconeogenesis occurs primarily in the liver. The kidney plays a minor role in gluconeogenesis except in prolonged starvation, when it becomes a major glucose-producing organ. Figure 12.1 shows the relationship of gluconeogenesis to other important reactions of intermediary metabolism.

II. REACTIONS UNIQUE TO GLUCONEOGENESIS

Eight of the 11 reactions of glycolysis are reversible and are used in the synthesis of glucose from lactate or pyruvate. However, three of the glycolytic reactions are irreversible and must be circumvented by alternate reactions that energetically favor the synthesis of glucose. These reactions, unique to gluconeogenesis, are summarized in Table 12.1 and described below.

A. Carboxylation of pyruvate

1. The first "roadblock" to overcome in the synthesis of glucose from pyruvate is the conversion of pyruvate to phosphoenolpyruvate (PEP) by *pyruvate kinase*. Pyruvate is first carboxylated by *pyruvate carboxylase* to oxaloacetate (OAA). (OAA is then converted to PEP by the action of *PEP-carboxykinase*, (see Figure 12.4).

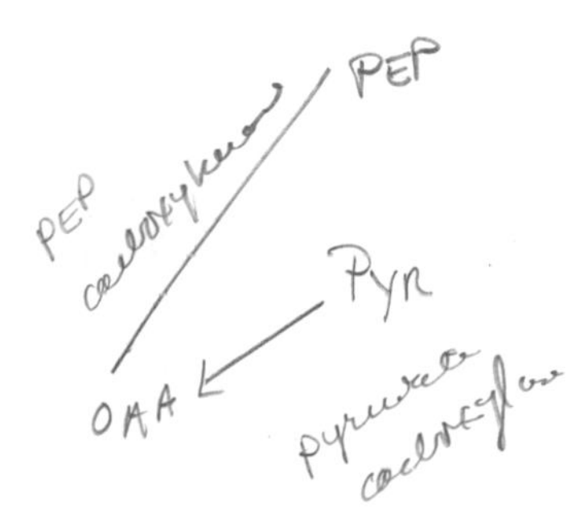

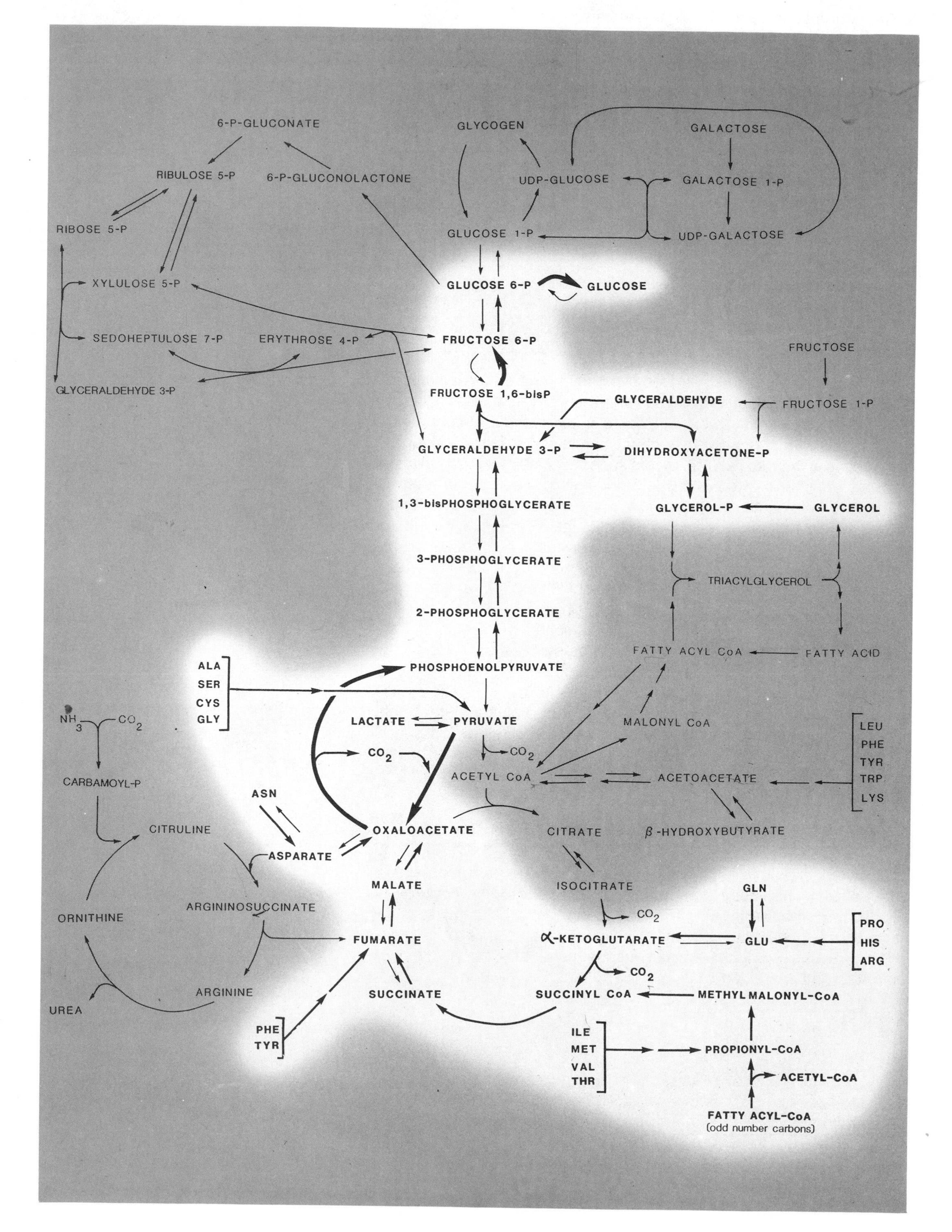

6-P-GLUCONATE
RIBULOSE 5-P
6-P-GLUCONOLACTONE
RIBOSE 5-P
XYLULOSE 5-P
SEDOHEPTULOSE 7-P
ERYTHROSE 4-P
GLYCERALDEHYDE 3-P
GLYCOGEN
UDP-GLUCOSE
GALACTOSE
GALACTOSE 1-P
UDP-GALACTOSE
GLUCOSE 1-P
GLUCOSE 6-P
GLUCOSE
FRUCTOSE 6-P
FRUCTOSE
FRUCTOSE 1,6-bisP
GLYCERALDEHYDE
FRUCTOSE 1-P
GLYCERALDEHYDE 3-P
DIHYDROXYACETONE-P
1,3-bisPHOSPHOGLYCERATE
GLYCEROL-P
GLYCEROL
3-PHOSPHOGLYCERATE
TRIACYLGLYCEROL
2-PHOSPHOGLYCERATE
FATTY ACYL CoA
FATTY ACID
ALA
SER
CYS
GLY
PHOSPHOENOLPYRUVATE
NH_3
CO_2
LACTATE
PYRUVATE
MALONYL CoA
LEU
PHE
TYR
TRP
LYS
CO_2
CO_2
CARBAMOYL-P
ACETYL CoA
ACETOACETATE
ASN
CITRULINE
OXALOACETATE
CITRATE
β-HYDROXYBUTYRATE
ASPARATE
MALATE
ISOCITRATE
GLN
ARGININOSUCCINATE
ORNITHINE
CO_2
PRO
HIS
ARG
FUMARATE
α-KETOGLUTARATE
GLU
CO_2
ARGININE
SUCCINATE
SUCCINYL CoA
METHYL MALONYL-CoA
UREA
PHE
TYR
ILE
MET
VAL
THR
PROPIONYL-CoA
ACETYL-CoA
FATTY ACYL-CoA
(odd number carbons)

2. *Pyruvate carboxylase* contains biotin, which is covalently bound to the enzyme through an ε-amino group of lysine (Figure 12.2). Cleavage of the high-energy phosphate of ATP drives the formation of an enzyme-biotin-CO_2 intermediate. This high-energy complex subsequently carboxylates pyruvate to form oxaloacetate.
3. *Pyruvate carboxylase* is found in the mitochondria of liver and kidney cells but not muscle.
4. *Pyruvate carboxylase* is ***allosterically activated by acetyl-CoA***. Elevated levels of acetyl CoA may signal one of several metabolic states in which the increased synthesis of oxaloacetate is required. For example, this state may occur during starvation when OAA is used for the synthesis of glucose by gluconeogenesis. The carboxylation of pyruvate also functions to replenish the TCA cycle intermediates that may become depleted owing to the synthetic needs of the cell.

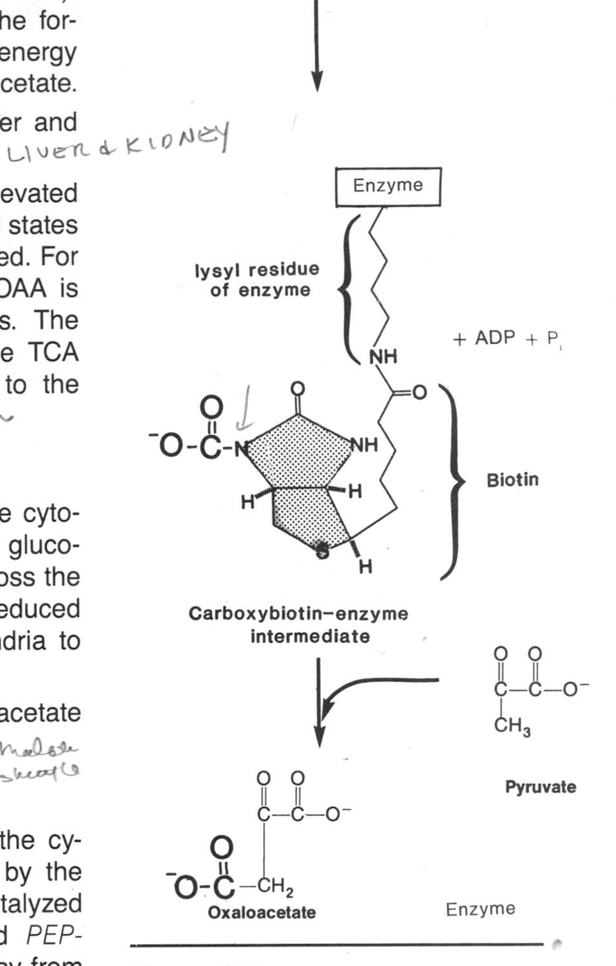

Figure 12.2
Activation and tranfer of CO_2 by *pyruvate carboxylase.*

B. Transport of oxaloacetate to the cytoplasm

1. Oxaloacetate, formed in the mitochondria, must enter the cytoplasmic portion of the cell where the other enzymes of gluconeogenesis are located. However, oxaloacetate cannot cross the inner mitochondrial membrane directly; it must first be reduced to malate, which can be transported from the mitochondria to cytoplasm (Figure 12.3).
2. In the cytoplasm, malate is reoxidized to oxaloacetate (Figure 12.3).

C. Decarboxylation of cytoplasmic oxaloacetate

1. Oxaloacetate is decarboxylated and phosphorylated in the cytoplasm by *PEP-carboxykinase*. The reaction is driven by the hydrolysis of GTP (Figure 12.4). The overall reaction catalyzed by the combined action of *pyruvate carboxylase* and *PEP-carboxykinase* provides an energetically favorable pathway from pyruvate to PEP.
2. Once formed, PEP enters the reversed reactions of glycolysis until it reaches fructose 1,6-bisphosphate.

D. Dephosphorylation of fructose 1,6-bisphosphate

1. The hydrolysis of fructose 1,6-bisphosphate by *fructose 1,6-bisphosphatase* bypasses the irreversible *phosphofructokinase* reaction. This hydrolysis provides an energetically favorable pathway for the formation of fructose 6-phosphate (Figure 12.5).
2. *Fructose 1,6-bisphosphatase* is inhibited by elevated levels of AMP, which signal an "energy poor" state in the cell. Conversely, high levels of ATP and low concentrations of AMP lead to a stimulation of gluconeogenesis.
3. *Fructose 1,6-bisphosphatase* is inhibited by fructose 2,6-bisphosphate, an allosteric modifier whose concentration is influenced by the levels of circulating glucagon (see p. 114).

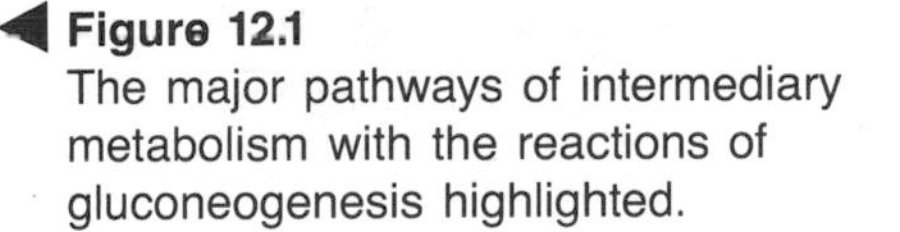

◀ **Figure 12.1**
The major pathways of intermediary metabolism with the reactions of gluconeogenesis highlighted.

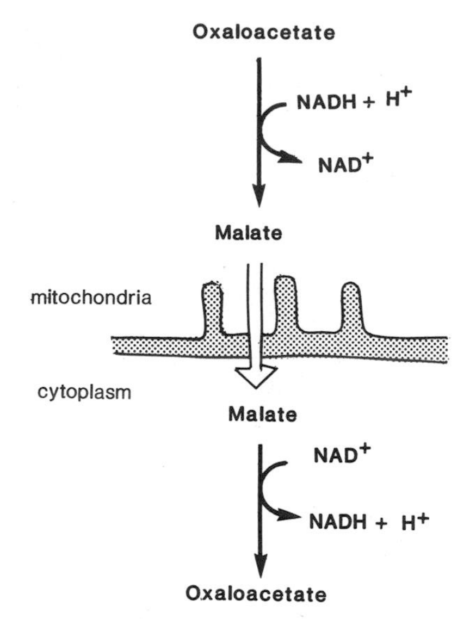

Figure 12.3
Transport of oxaloacetate from the mitochondria to the cytoplasm.

4. *Fructose 1,6-bisphosphatase* is found in liver and kidney.

E. Dephosphorylation of glucose 6-phosphate

1. The hydrolysis of glucose 6-phosphate by *glucose 6-phosphatase* bypasses the irreversible *hexokinase* reaction. This hydrolysis provides an energetically favorable pathway for the formation of free glucose (Figure 12.6).
2. *Glucose 6-phosphatase*, like *pyruvate carboxylase*, occurs in liver and kidney but is absent in muscle. Thus, muscle cannot synthesize glucose by gluconeogenesis; further, glucose 6-phosphate derived from muscle glycogen cannot be dephosphorylated to yield free glucose.
3. Type I glycogen storage disease (see p. 77) results from an inherited deficiency of *glucose 6-phosphatase* (see Figure 7.5).

F. Summary of the reactions common to glycolysis and gluconeogenesis

1. The eight reversible reactions of glycolysis are shown in regular type in Table 12.1. The four reactions unique to gluconeogenesis are printed in bold type.
2. In gluconeogenesis, the equilibria of the eight reversible reactions are pushed in favor of glucose synthesis as a result of the essentially irreversible formation of PEP, fructose 6-phosphate, and glucose catalyzed by the gluconeogenic enzymes.

G. Energy cost of gluconeogenesis

1. The stoichiometry of gluconeogenesis couples the cleavage of six high-energy phosphate bonds with the formation of each molecule of glucose as tabulated in Table 12.1:

TABLE 12.1 CONSUMPTION OF ATP AND NADH IN ANAEROBIC GLUCONEOGENESIS

Reaction		Change in ATP/ Glucose
(2) pyruvate	→ ***(2) oxaloacetate***	***−2***
(2) oxaloacetate	→ ***(2) phosphoenolpyruvate***	***−2 (GTP)***
(2) phosphoenolpyruvate	→ (2) 2-phosphoglycerate	0
(2) 2-phosphoglycerate	→ (2) 3-phosphoglycerate	0
(2) 3-phosphoglycerate	→ (2) 1,3-diphosphoglycerate	−2
(2) 1,3-diphosphoglycerate	→ (2) glyceraldehyde 3-phosphate	0
glyceraldehyde 3-phosphate	→ dihydroxyacetone phosphate	0
glyceraldehyde 3-phosphate + dihydroxyacetone phosphate	→ fructose 1,6-bisphosphate	0
fructose 1,6-bisphosphate	→ ***fructose 6-phosphate***	***0***
fructose 6-phosphate	→ glucose 6-phosphate	0
glucose 6-phosphate	→ ***glucose***	***0***

Summary: 2 pyruvate + 4ATP + 2GTP + 2NADH + $2H^+$ → glucose + $2NAD^+$ + 4ADP + 2GDP + $6P_i$

III. SUBSTRATES FOR GLUCONEOGENESIS

A. ***Gluconeogenic precursors are molecules that can give rise to a net synthesis of glucose.*** They include all the intermediates of glycolysis and the citric acid cycle. Glycerol, lactate, and the α-ketoacids obtained from the deamination of glycogenic amino acids are the most important gluconeogenic precursors.

1. Glycerol is released during the hydrolysis of triacylglycerols in adipose tissue (see p. 171) and is delivered by the blood to the liver. Glycerol is phosphorylated to glycerol phosphate, which is oxidized to dihydroxyacetone phosphate, an intermediate of glycolysis (see Figure 12.1).
2. Lactate is released into the blood by cells that lack mitochondria, such as red blood cells, and by exercising skeletal muscle. In the Cori cycle, blood-borne glucose is converted by exercising muscle to lactate, which diffuses into the blood. This lactate is taken up by the liver and converted to glucose, which is released back into the circulation (Figure 12.7).
3. α-Ketoacids, such as pyruvate, oxaloacetate, and α-ketoglutarate, are derived from the metabolism of glycogenic amino acids (see p. 239). These gluconeogenic substances can enter the citric acid cycle and form oxaloacetate, a direct precursor of pyruvate.

B. ***Acetyl CoA and compounds that give rise to acetyl CoA (e.g., acetoacetate and ketogenic amino acids) cannot give rise to a net synthesis of glucose.*** This is due to the irreversible nature of *pyruvate dehydrogenase*, which converts pyruvate to acetyl CoA (see p. 125).

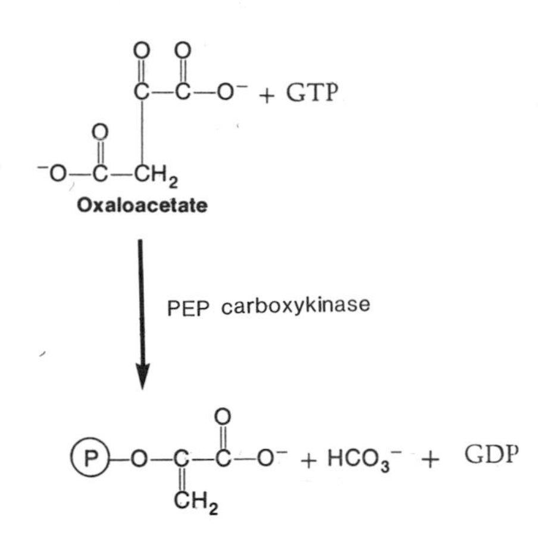

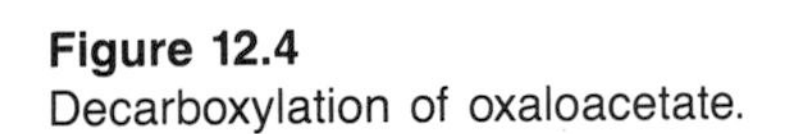

Figure 12.4
Decarboxylation of oxaloacetate.

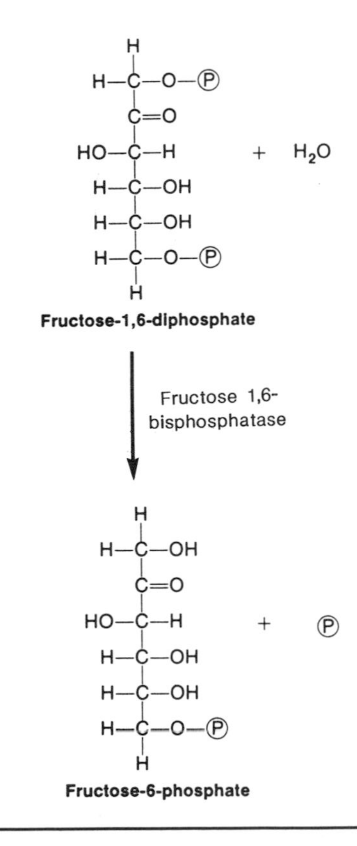

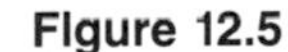

Figure 12.5
Dephosphorylation of fructose 1,6-bisphosphate.

IV. REGULATION OF GLUCONEOGENESIS

The minute to minute regulation of gluconeogenesis is determined primarily by the circulating levels of glucagon and by the availability of gluconeogenic substrates. In addition, slow adaptive changes in the amount of enzyme activity result from an alteration in the rate of enzyme synthesis or degradation, or both.

A. ***Glucagon:*** Glucagon is a pancreatic hormone (see p. 268) that stimulates gluconeogenesis by two mechanisms (Figure 12.8).

1. ***Changes in allosteric effectors.*** Glucagon lowers the level of fructose 2,6-bisphosphate, resulting in activation of *fructose 1,6-bisphosphatase* and inhibition of phosphofructokinase (Figure 12.8).
2. ***Covalent modification of enzyme activity.*** Glucagon, by an elevation in cAMP levels and *protein kinase* activity, stimulates the conversion of *pyruvate kinase* to its inactive (phosphorylated) form. This decreases the conversion of PEP to pyruvate, which has the effect of diverting PEP to the synthesis of glucose (Figure 12.8).

B. ***Substrate availability:*** The availability of gluconeogenic precursors, particularly glucogenic amino acids, markedly influences the rate of hepatic glucose synthesis. Decreased levels of insulin favor mobi-

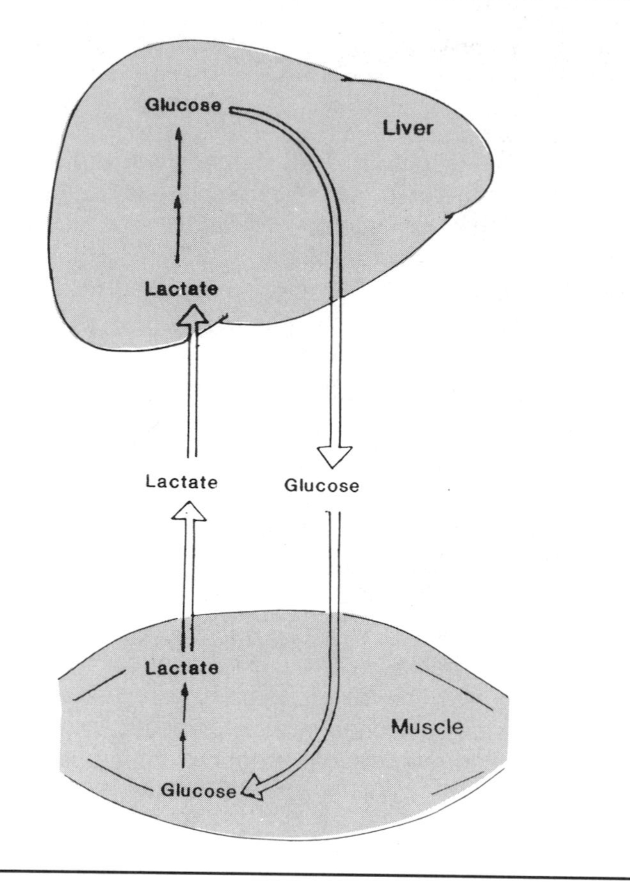

Figure 12.7
The Cori cycle.

O
‖
C—H
H—C—OH
HO—C—H   + H_2O
H—C—OH
H—C—OH
H—C—O—Ⓟ
H
Glucose-6-phosphate

↓ Glucose 6-phosphatase

O
‖
C—H
H—C—OH
HO—C—H   + P_i
H—C—OH
H—C—OH
H—C—OH
H
D-Glucose

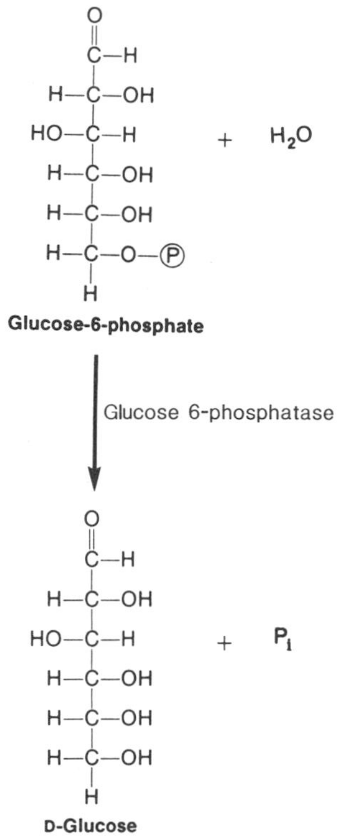

Figure 12.6
Dephosphorylation of glucose 6-phosphate.

lization of amino acids from muscle protein and provide the carbon skeletons for gluconeogenesis.

C. ***Allosteric activation by acetyl CoA:*** Allosteric activation of hepatic *pyruvate carboxylase* by acetyl CoA occurs during starvation. As a result of excessive lipolysis in adipose tissue, the liver is flooded with fatty acids. The rate of formation of acetyl CoA by β-oxidation of these fatty acids exceeds the capacity of the liver to oxidize it to CO_2 and H_2O. As a result, acetyl CoA accumulates and leads to an activation of *pyruvate carboxylase.*

Study Questions

Choose the ONE best answer

12.1 The synthesis of glucose from pyruvate by gluconeogenesis

A. occurs exclusively in the cytoplasm.
B. is inhibited by elevated levels of glucagon.
C. requires the participation of biotin.
D. involves lactate as an intermediate.
E. requires the oxidation/reduction of FAD.

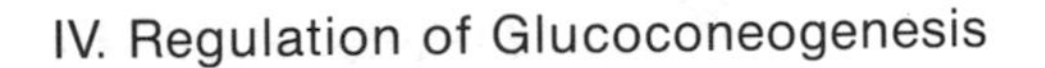

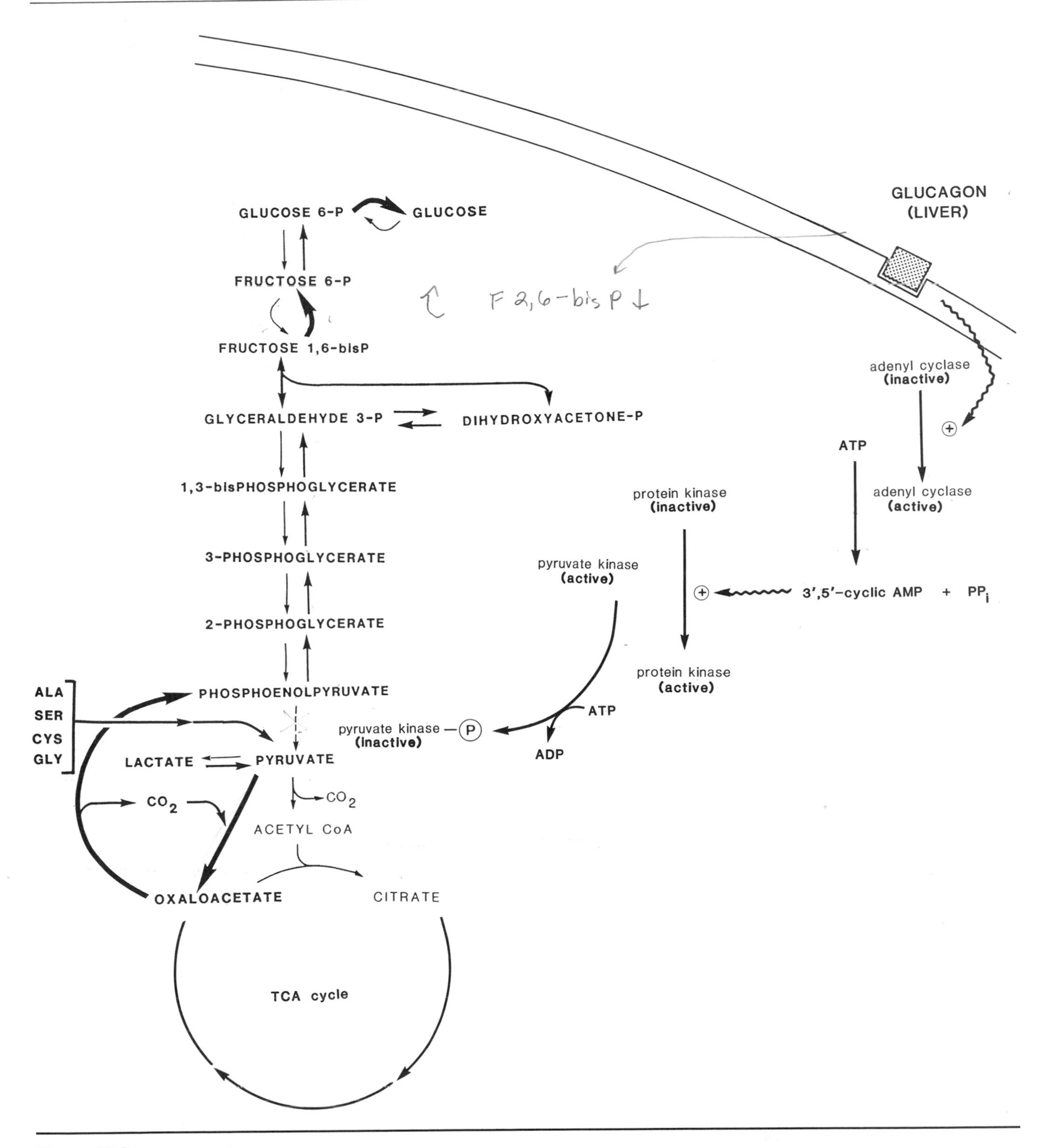

Figure 12.8
Effects of glucagon and allosteric modulators on gluconeogenesis.

12.2 Which one of the following is NOT a characteristic of gluconeogenesis?

A. It requires energy in the form of ATP or GTP.
B. It is important in maintaining blood glucose during the normal overnight fast.
C. It uses carbon skeletons provided by degradation of amino acids.
D. It consists of the reactions of glycolysis functioning in the reverse direction.
E. It involves the enzyme fructose 1,6-bisphosphatase.

12.3 Which one of the following reactions is unique to gluconeogenesis?

A. Lactate → pyruvate
B. Phosphoenolpyruvate (PEP) → pyruvate
C. Oxaloacetate → phosphoenolpyruvate
D. Glucose 6-phosphate → fructose 6-phosphate
E. 1,3-Diphosphoglycerate → 3-phosphoglycerate

12.4 Which of the following compounds CANNOT give rise to the net synthesis of glucose?

A. Lactate
B. Glycerol
C. α-Ketoglutarate
D. Oxaloacetate
E. Acetyl-CoA

Citric Acid Cycle

13

I. OVERVIEW

The citric acid cycle (also called the ***Krebs cycle*** or the ***tricarboxylic acid cycle***) oxidizes acetyl CoA to CO_2 and H_2O. Acetyl CoA is obtained from the metabolism of fuel molecules such as amino acids, fatty acids,and carbohydrates (Figure 13.1). The oxidation of acetyl CoA accounts for about two thirds of the total oxygen consumption and ATP production in most animals, including man. The citric acid cycle is also important in the formation of glucose from the carbon skeletons of amino acids and provides building blocks for other biosynthetic reactions. The citric acid cycle occurs totally in the mitochondrial matrix.

II. REACTIONS OF THE CITRIC ACID CYCLE

A. The oxidative decarboxylation of pyruvate

1. *Pyruvate dehydrogenase* is a multi-enzyme complex located in the mitochondrial matrix. It converts pyruvate, the end-product of aerobic glycolysis, into acetyl CoA, a major fuel for the citric acid cycle (Figure 13.2). The irreversibility of the reaction precludes the formation of pyruvate from acetyl CoA and is why glucose cannot be formed from acetyl CoA in gluconeogenesis (see p. 129). Strictly speaking, *pyruvate dehydrogenase* is not part of the citric acid cycle proper but is a major source of acetyl CoA—the two-carbon substrate for the cycle.
2. The *pyruvate dehydrogenase* complex is an unusual arrangement of three enzymes: *decarboxylase, dihydrolipoyl transacetylase,* and *dihydrolipoyl dehydrogenase*. Each of these enzymes catalyzes a part of the overall reaction. Their physical association facilitates linking the reactions together in proper sequence without the release of intermediates.
3. The *pyruvate dehydrogenase* complex also contains five cofactors that act as carriers or oxidants for the intermediates of the reaction shown in Figure 13.3.

Enzymes	***Cofactors***
decarboxylase (E_1)	thiamine pyrophosphate
dihydrolipoly transacetylase (E_2)	lipoic acid
dihydrolipoyl dehydrogenase (E_3)	FAD, NAD^+, CoA

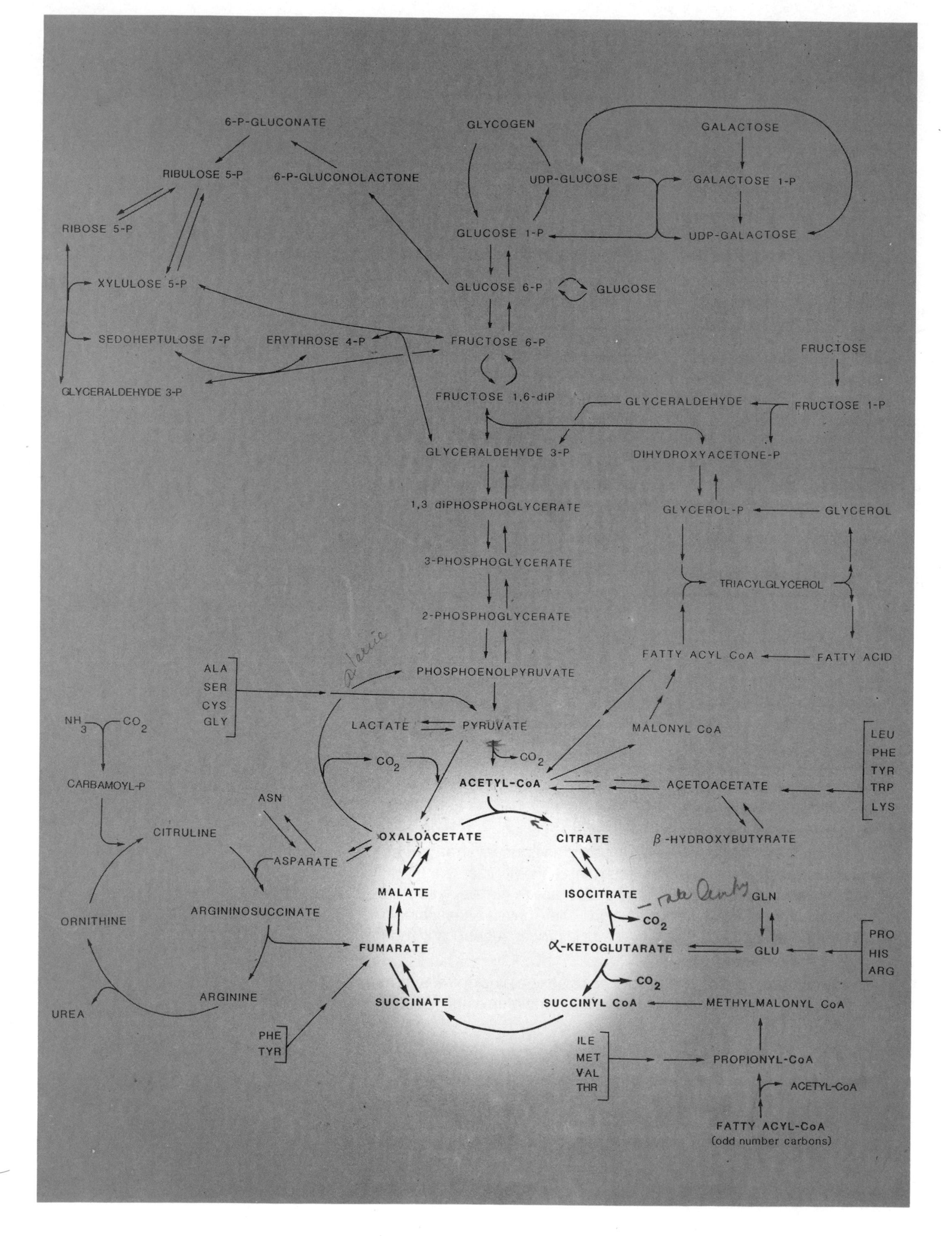

6-P-GLUCONATE
GLYCOGEN
GALACTOSE
RIBULOSE 5-P
6-P-GLUCONOLACTONE
UDP-GLUCOSE
GALACTOSE 1-P
RIBOSE 5-P
GLUCOSE 1-P
UDP-GALACTOSE
XYLULOSE 5-P
GLUCOSE 6-P
GLUCOSE
SEDOHEPTULOSE 7-P
ERYTHROSE 4-P
FRUCTOSE 6-P
FRUCTOSE
GLYCERALDEHYDE 3-P
FRUCTOSE 1,6-diP
GLYCERALDEHYDE
FRUCTOSE 1-P
GLYCERALDEHYDE 3-P
DIHYDROXYACETONE-P
1,3 diPHOSPHOGLYCERATE
GLYCEROL-P
GLYCEROL
3-PHOSPHOGLYCERATE
TRIACYLGLYCEROL
2-PHOSPHOGLYCERATE
FATTY ACYL CoA
FATTY ACID
ALA
SER
CYS
GLY
PHOSPHOENOLPYRUVATE
NH_3
CO_2
LACTATE
PYRUVATE
MALONYL CoA
LEU
PHE
TYR
TRP
LYS
CO_2
CO_2
CARBAMOYL-P
ACETYL-CoA
ACETOACETATE
ASN
CITRULINE
OXALOACETATE
CITRATE
β-HYDROXYBUTYRATE
ASPARATE
MALATE
ISOCITRATE
GLN
ORNITHINE
ARGININOSUCCINATE
CO_2
PRO
HIS
ARG
FUMARATE
α-KETOGLUTARATE
GLU
CO_2
ARGININE
UREA
SUCCINATE
SUCCINYL CoA
METHYLMALONYL CoA
PHE
TYR
ILE
MET
VAL
THR
PROPIONYL-CoA
ACETYL-CoA
FATTY ACYL-CoA
(odd number carbons)

4. *Pyruvate dehydrogenase* is regulated by two mechanisms (Figure 13.4):
   a. ***Product inhibition***: The enzyme is inhibited by acetyl CoA, which accumulates when it is being produced faster than it can be oxidized by the citric acid cycle. The enzyme is also inhibited by elevated levels of NADH, which occur when the electron transport chain is overloaded.
   b. ***Covalent modification:*** *Pyruvate dehydrogenase* exists in two forms: an active, nonphosphorylated form and an inactive, phosphorylated form (Figure 13.4). Phosphorylated and non-phosphorylated *pyruvate dehydrogenase* can be interconverted by two separate enzymes: a kinase and a phosphatase. The kinase is activated by an increase in the ratio of acetyl CoA/CoA or NADH/NAD^+. An increase in the ratio of ADP/ATP, which signals increased demand for energy production, inhibits the kinase and allows the phosphatase to produce more of the active, nonphosphorylated enzyme.

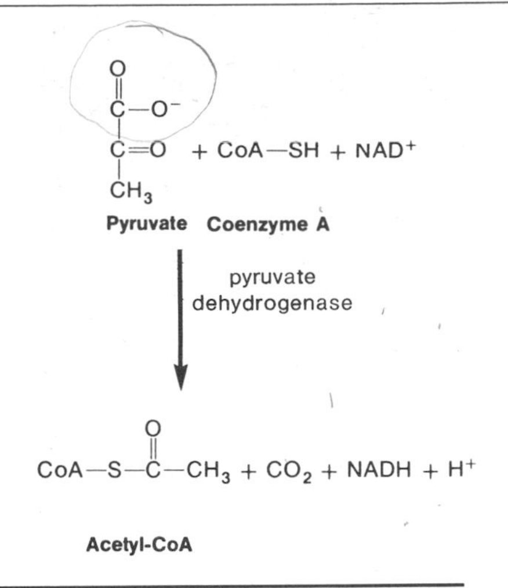

Figure 13.2
Oxidative decarboxylation of pyruvate.

B. The condensation of acetyl CoA and oxaloacetate to form citrate

1. The condensation of acetyl CoA and oxaloacetate is catalyzed by *citrate synthase* (Figure 13.5). This aldol condensation has an equilibrium far in the direction of citrate synthesis.
2. The reaction uses an intermediate of the citric acid cycle (oxaloacetate) and produces another intermediate of the cycle (citrate). Thus, the entry of acetyl CoA into the citric acid cycle does not lead to the ***net*** production or consumption of cycle intermediates.
3. *Citrate synthase* is inhibited by various compounds such as ATP, NADH, succinyl CoA, and acyl-CoA derivatives of fatty acids. The rate of the reaction is also determined by the availability of the substrates.
4. Citrate, in addition to being an intermediate in the citric acid cycle, has other functions:
   a. Citrate provides a source of acetyl CoA for the cytoplasmic synthesis of fatty acids (see p. 162).
   b. Citrate inhibits *phosphofructokinase,* the rate-setting enzyme of glycolysis (see p. 114), and activates *acetyl CoA carboxylase* the rate-limiting enzyme of fatty acid synthesis (see p. 162).

C. Isomerization of citrate

1. Citrate is isomerized to ***isocitrate*** by a dehydration step followed by a hydration step. Cis-aconitate occurs as an enzyme-bound intermediate (Figure 13.6).

D. Oxidation and decarboxylation of isocitrate

1. *Isocitrate dehydrogenase* catalyzes the irreversible oxidative decarboxylation of isocitrate, yielding the first of three NADH molecules produced by the cycle, and the first release of CO_2

Figure 13.1
Major pathways of intermediary metabolism with the reactions of citric acid cycle highlighted.

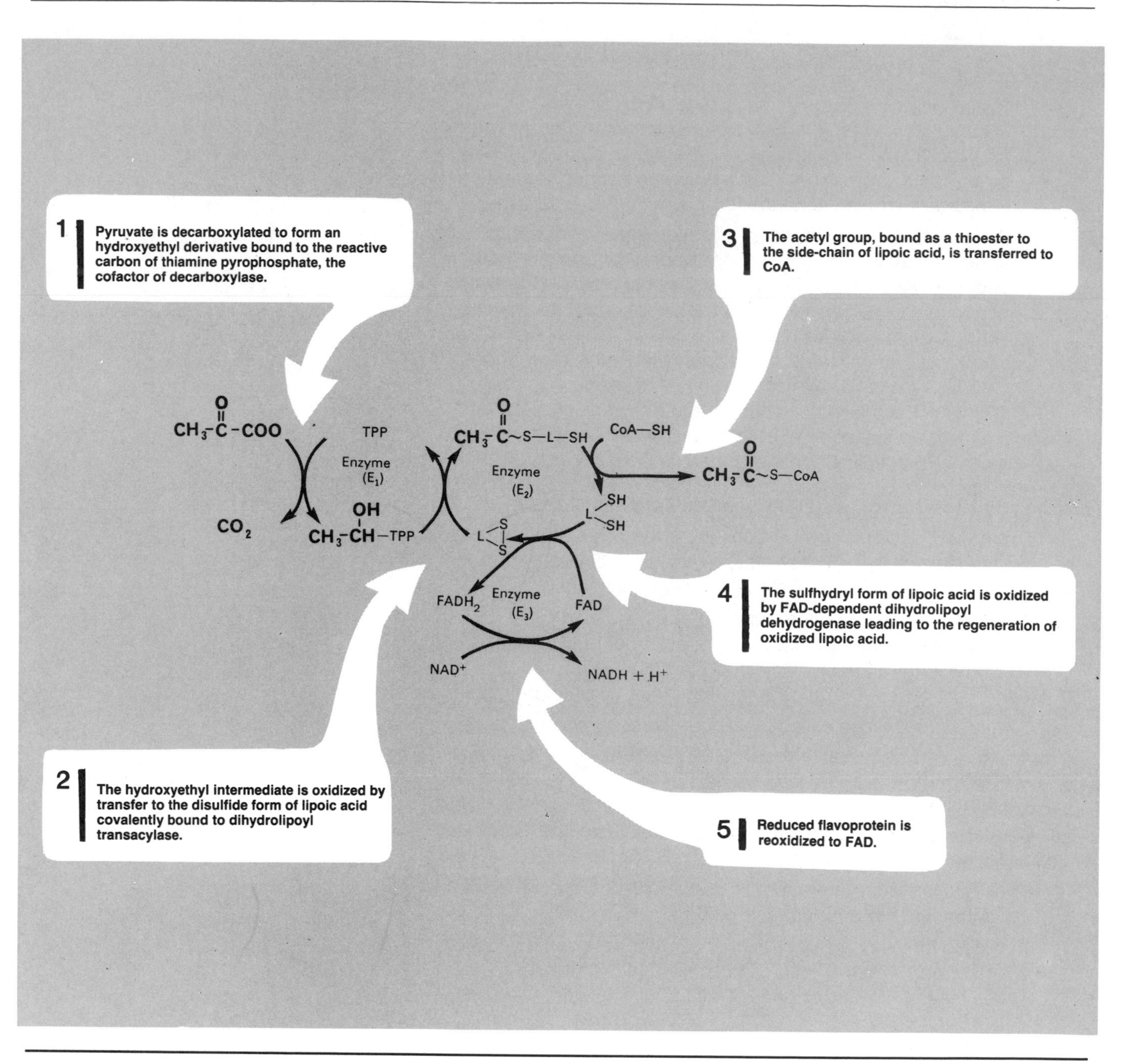

Figure 13.3
Mechanism of *pyruvate dehydrogenase.*

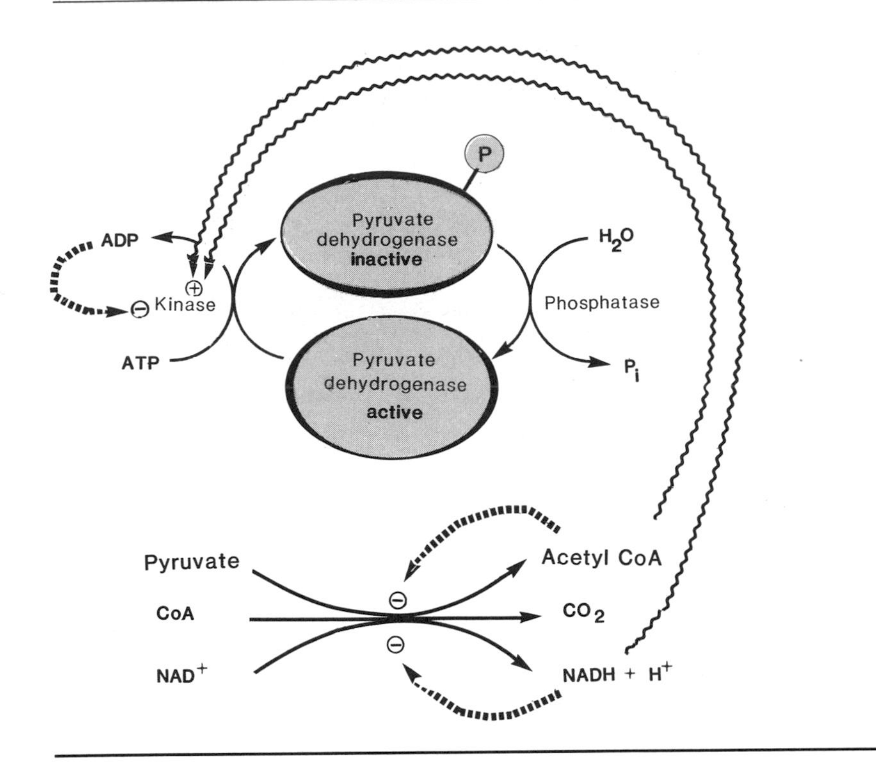

Figure 13.4
Regulation of *pyruvate dehydrogenase.*

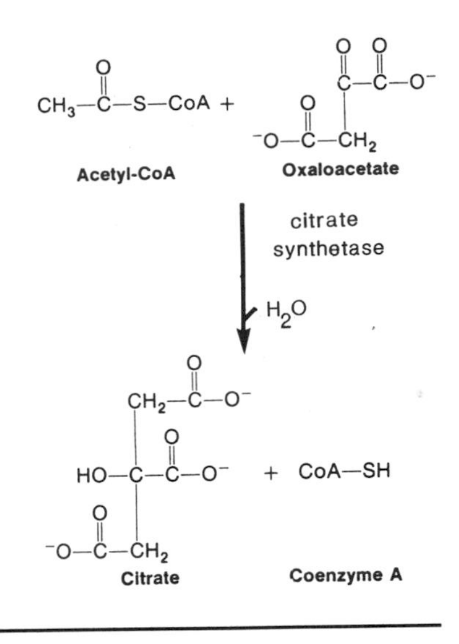

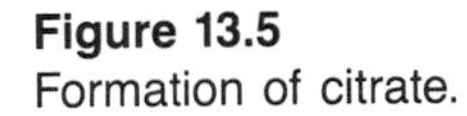

Figure 13.5
Formation of citrate.

(Figure 13.7). This is one of the rate-limiting steps of the citric acid cycle.

2. The enzyme is activated by ADP. Elevated levels of mitochondrial ADP signal a need for the generation of more high-energy phosphate (ATP).
3. The enzyme is inhibited by ATP and NADH, which are elevated when the cell has abundant energy stores.

E. Oxidative decarboxylation of α-ketoglutarate

1. The conversion of α-ketoglutarate to succinyl CoA is catalyzed by the *α-ketoglutarate dehydrogenase complex* (Figure 13.8). The mechanism of this oxidative decarboxylation is similar to that used for the conversion of pyruvate to acetyl CoA.
2. The cofactors required are thiamine pyrophosphate, lipoic acid, FAD, NAD^+, and CoA. Each functions in the catalytic mechanism in a way analogous to that described for *pyruvate dehydrogenase* (see p. 133).
3. The enzyme is inhibited by ATP, GTP, NADH, and succinyl CoA but is not regulated by phosphorylation/dephosphorylation reactions as described for *pyruvate dehydrogenase.*
4. The reaction releases the second CO_2 and produces the second NADH in the cycle. The equilibrium of the reaction is far in the direction of succinyl CoA, a high-energy thioester similar to acetyl CoA.

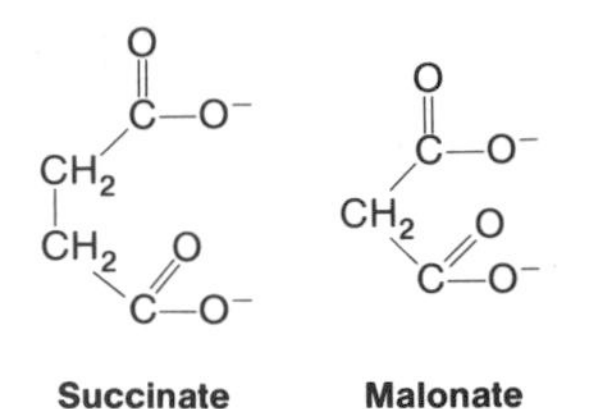

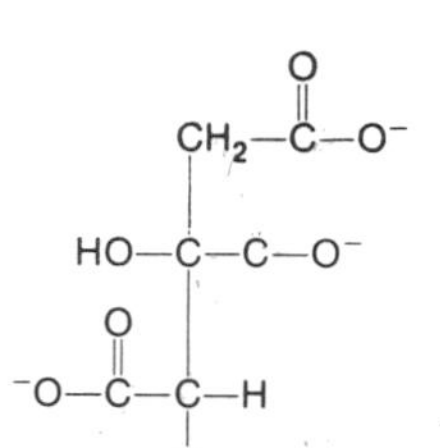

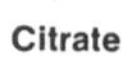

aconitase

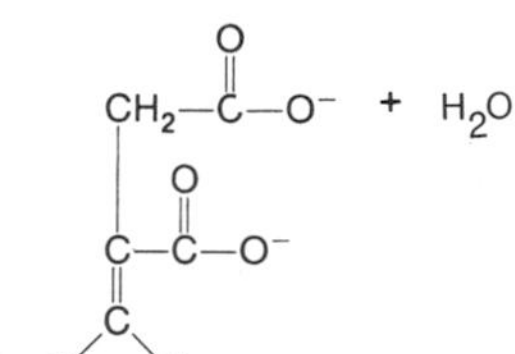

aconitase

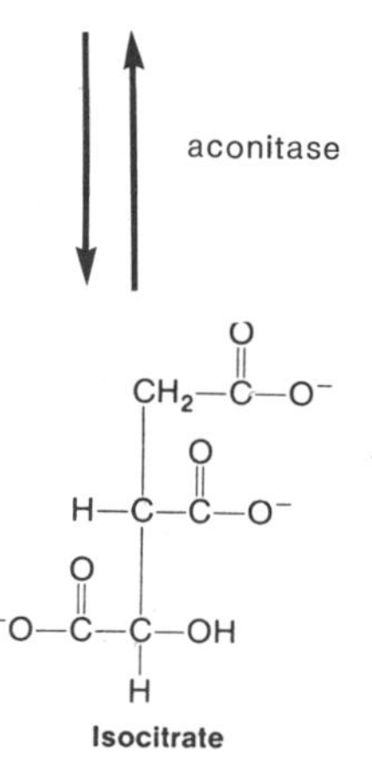

Figure 13.6
Isomerization of citrate.

F. Cleavage of succinyl CoA

1. *Succinate thiokinase* catalyzes the cleavage of the high-energy thioester bond of succinyl CoA (Figure 13.9). This reaction is coupled to the phosphorylation of GDP to GTP. The energy content of GTP is the same as that of ATP, and the two nucleotides are interconvertible by the *nucleoside diphosphate kinase* reaction:

$$\mathrm{GTP} + \mathrm{ADP} \overset{\textit{nucleoside diphosphate kinase}}{\rightleftarrows} \mathrm{GDP} + \mathrm{ATP}$$

2. This is an example of ***substrate-level phosphorylation*** in which the production of high-energy phosphate is coupled to the conversion of substrate to product, rather than resulting from oxidative phosphorylation (see p. 115).
3. Succinyl CoA is also formed from fatty acids with an odd number of carbon atoms and from the metabolism of branched-chain amino acids (see p. 244).

G. Oxidation of succinate

1. Succinate is oxidized to fumarate in the *succinate dehydrogenase* reaction, producing the reduced cofactor $FADH_2$ (Figure 13.10).
2. FAD, rather than NAD^+, is the electron acceptor, since the reducing power of succinate is not sufficient to reduce NAD^+ (see p. 105).
3. Malonate, a dicarboxylic acid that is a structural analogue of succinate, competitively inhibits *succinate dehydrogenase.*

H. Hydration of fumarate

1. Fumarate is hydrated to malate in a freely reversible reaction catalyzed by *fumarase* (Figure 13.11).

I. Oxidation of malate

1. Malate is oxidized to oxaloacetate in a reaction catalyzed by *malate dehydrogenase* (Figure 13.12).
2. This reaction produces the third and final NADH of the cycle. Figure 13.13 summarizes the reactions of the citric acid cycle.

III. STOICHIOMETRY OF THE CYCLE

$$\text{Acetyl CoA} + 3\,NAD^+ + FAD + GDP + P_i + 2H_2O \rightarrow$$
$$2CO_2 + 3\,NADH + FADH_2 + GTP + 3H^+ + CoA$$

A. Summary of reactions

1. Two carbon atoms enter the cycle as acetyl CoA and leave as CO_2.
2. The citric acid cycle does not involve the net consumption or production of oxaloacetate or any other intermediate of the cycle.
3. Four pairs of electrons are transferred during one turn of the cycle: three pairs of electrons reducing NAD^+ to NADH, and one pair reducing FAD to $FADH_2$.

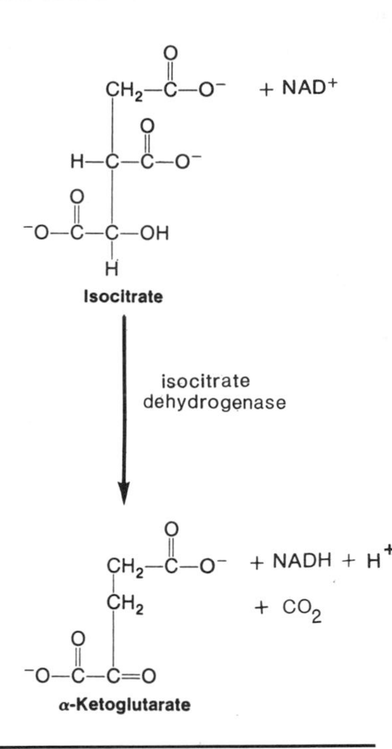

Figure 13.7
Oxidation and decarboxylation of isocitrate.

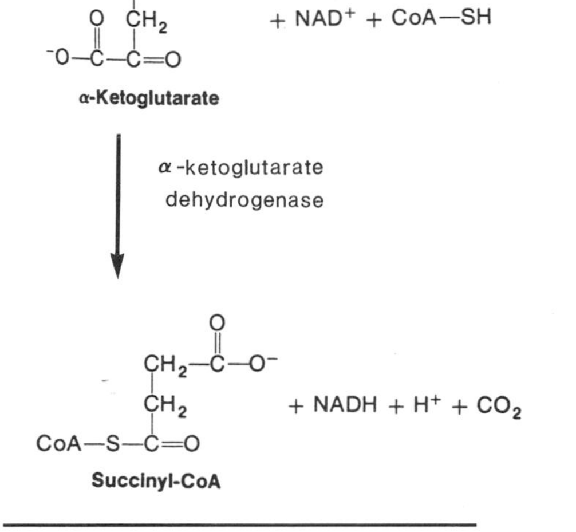

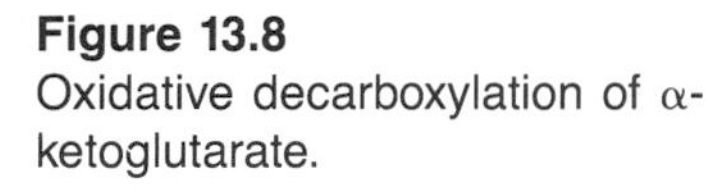
Figure 13.8
Oxidative decarboxylation of α-ketoglutarate.

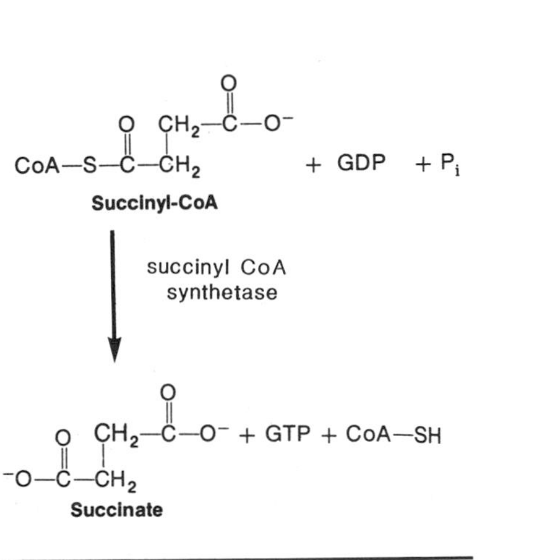

Figure 13.9
Cleavage of succinyl CoA.

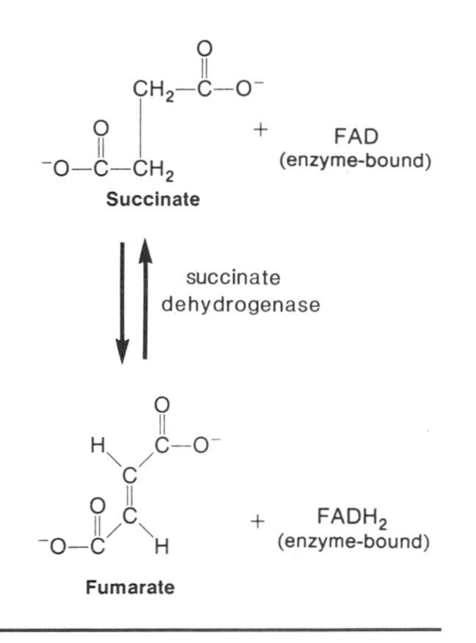

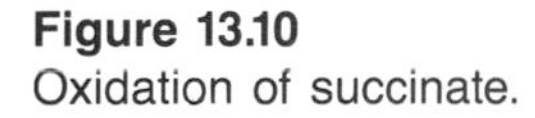
Figure 13.10
Oxidation of succinate.

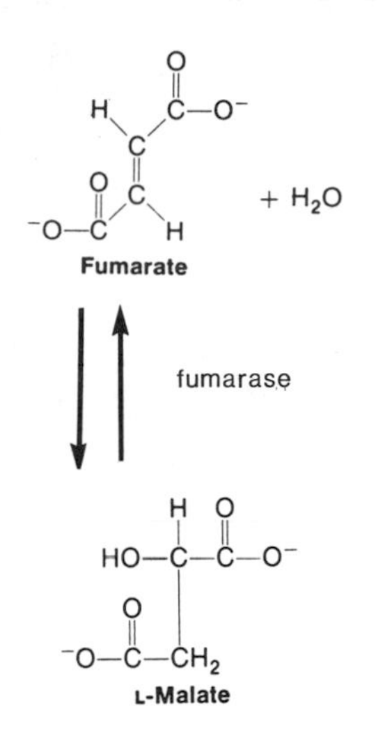

Figure 13.11
Hydration of fumarate.

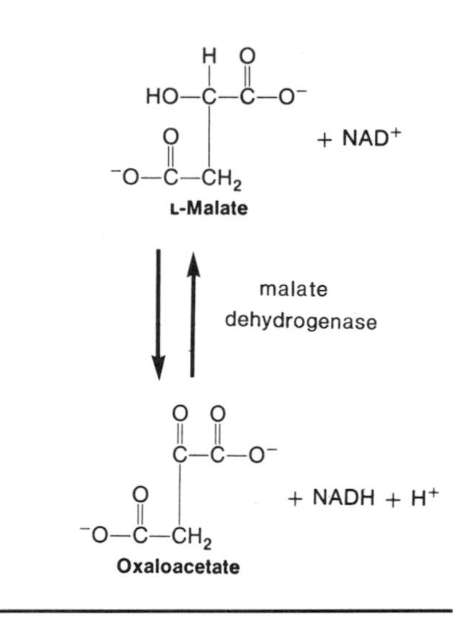

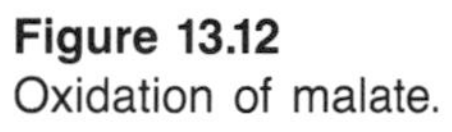

Figure 13.12
Oxidation of malate.

B. The oxidation of one NADH by the electron transport chain (see p. 106) leads to the formation of three ATP, whereas the oxidation of $FADH_2$ yields two ATP. Thus, the total yield of ATP from the oxidation of one acetyl CoA is

reaction	number of ATP produced
3NADH → $3NAD^+$	9
$FADH_2$ → FAD	2
GDP + P_i → GTP	1
	12 ATP/acetyl CoA oxidized

IV. REGULATION OF THE CYCLE

A. Regulation by activation and inhibition of enzyme activities

In contrast to glycolysis, which is regulated primarily by *phosphofructokinase,* the citric acid cycle is controlled by regulation of several enzyme activities. The most important of these regulated enzymes are *citrate synthase, isocitrate dehydrogenase,* and *α-ketoglutarate dehydrogenase,* which were described on p. 135.

B. Regulation by the availability of ADP

1. Energy consumption within the cell caused by muscular contraction, biosynthetic reactions, or other energy-consuming processes, results in the hydrolysis of ATP to ADP and P_i.
2. The resulting increase in the concentration of ADP accelerates the rate of those reactions that use ADP to generate ATP, most important of which is oxidative phosphorylation.
3. The production of ATP increases until it matches the rate of ATP consumption by energy-requiring reactions.
4. If ADP (or P_i) is present in limiting concentrations, the formation of ATP by oxidative phosphorylation will decrease owing to the lack of phosphate acceptor (ADP) or inorganic phosphate (P_i). The rate of oxidative phosphorylation is therefore proportional to $[ADP][P_i]/[ATP]$. This is known as ***respiratory control*** of energy production.
5. The oxidation of NADH and $FADH_2$ by the respiratory chain will also stop if ADP is limiting because the processes of oxidation and phosphorylation are tightly coupled and must occur simultaneously (see p. 107). As NADH and $FADH_2$ accumulate, the oxidized forms of the cofactors, NAD^+ and FAD, will become depleted, causing the oxidation of acetyl CoA by the citric acid cycle to be inhibited owing to a lack of oxidized cofactors. Thus, a decline in the concentration of ADP, which signals that the energy stores of the cell are full (*i.e.,* ATP levels high), triggers a series of events that ultimately decrease the activity of the citric acid cycle.

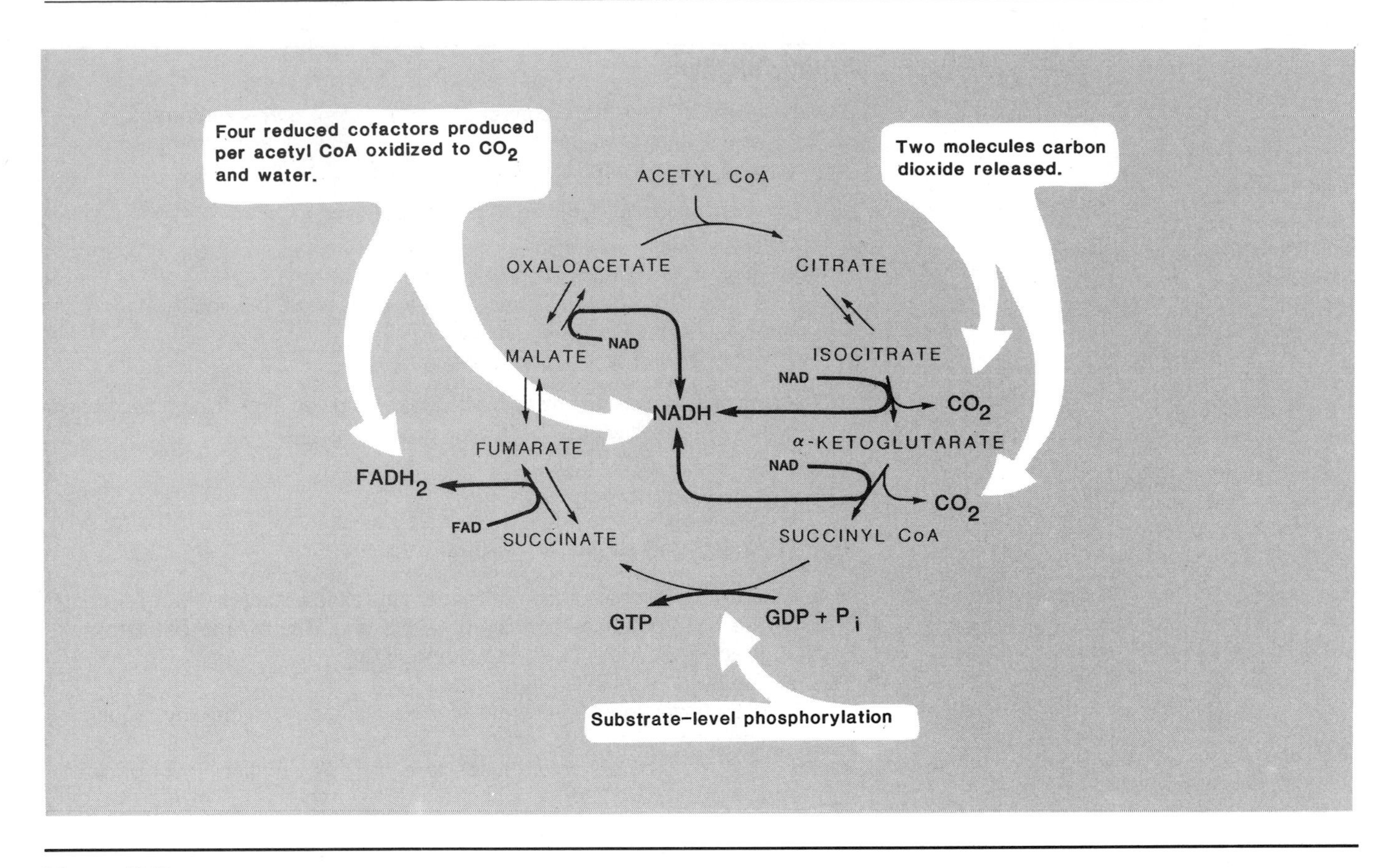

Figure 13.13
Reactions of the citric acid cycle.

Study Questions

Answer A if 1, 2, and 3 are correct
B if 1 and 3 are correct
C if 2 and 4 are correct
D if only 4 is correct
E if all are correct

13.1 The conversion of pyruvate to acetyl-CoA and CO_2
1. is essentially irreversible.
2. involves the participation of lipoic acid.
3. is inhibited when pyruvate dehydrogenase is phosphorylated by a protein kinase in the presence of ATP.
4. involves the participation of biotin.

13.2 Which of the following enzymic activities would you expect to be decreased in thiamine deficiency?
1. Pyruvate carboxylase
2. Isocitrate dehydrogenase
3. Fumarase
4. α-Ketoglutarate dehydrogenase

13.3 Which of the following statements about the citric acid cycle is(are) correct?
1. The cycle produces 3 moles of NADH and 1 mole of $FADH_2$ per mole of acetyl CoA oxidized to CO_2 and H_2O.
2. The cycle is inhibited by malate.
3. The conversion of isocitrate to α-ketoglutarate is the key regulatory step in the citric acid cycle.
4. The oxidation of acetate leads to a net consumption (loss) of oxalo-acetate.

Choose the ONE best answer

13.4 The conversion of 1 mole of isocitrate to 1 mole of succinate by the citric acid cycle results in the formation of how many moles of high-energy phosphate?
A. 3
B. 5
C. 6
D. 7
E. 8

13.5 Entry of acetyl CoA into the citric acid cycle is decreased when
A. the ratio of ATP/ADP is low.
B. NADH is rapidly oxidized through the respiratory chain.
C. the ratio of NAD^+/NADH is high.
D. the concentration of AMP is high.
E. the GTP/GDP ratio is high.

Hexose Monophosphate Pathway

14

I. OVERVIEW

The hexose monophosphate pathway (HMP; also called the pentose phosphate pathway) consists of three irreversible oxidative reactions followed by a series of reversible sugar-phosphate interconversions (Figure 14.1). No ATP is directly consumed or produced in the cycle. Carbon #1 of glucose 6-phosphate is released as CO_2, and two NADPHs are produced for each glucose 6-phosphate that enters the pathway as a product of the oxidation steps. Unlike glycolysis or the citric acid cycle in which the direction of the reactions is well defined, the interconversion reactions of the hexose monophosphate pathway (HMP) can function in several different combinations. The direction of the pathway at any given time is determined by the supply of and demand for intermediates in the cycle. The HMP pathway occurs in the ***cytoplasm*** of the cell. The pathway is particularly important in tissues such as adipose, liver, and mammary gland, which are active in the biosynthesis of fatty acids, and in the adrenal cortex, which is active in the NADPH-dependent synthesis of steroids. The HMP pathway provides a major portion of the cell's NADPH, which functions as a biochemical reductant (*e.g.* the reduction of oxidized glutathione) and in microsomal oxidations (*e.g.,* cytochrome P_{450} system, see p. 146). The HMP pathway also produces ribose-phosphate, required for the biosynthesis of nucleotides, and provides a mechanism for the metabolic use of 5-carbon sugars ingested as food.

II. OXIDATIVE REACTIONS

The oxidative portion of the HMP pathway consists of three reactions that lead to the formation of ribulose 5-phosphate, CO_2 and two molecules of NADPH.

A. Dehydrogenation of glucose 6-phosphate

1. *Glucose 6-phosphate dehydrogenase* (G6PD) catalyzes an irreversible oxidation that is specific for ***NADP***$^+$, rather than NAD^+, as cofactor (Figure 14.2).

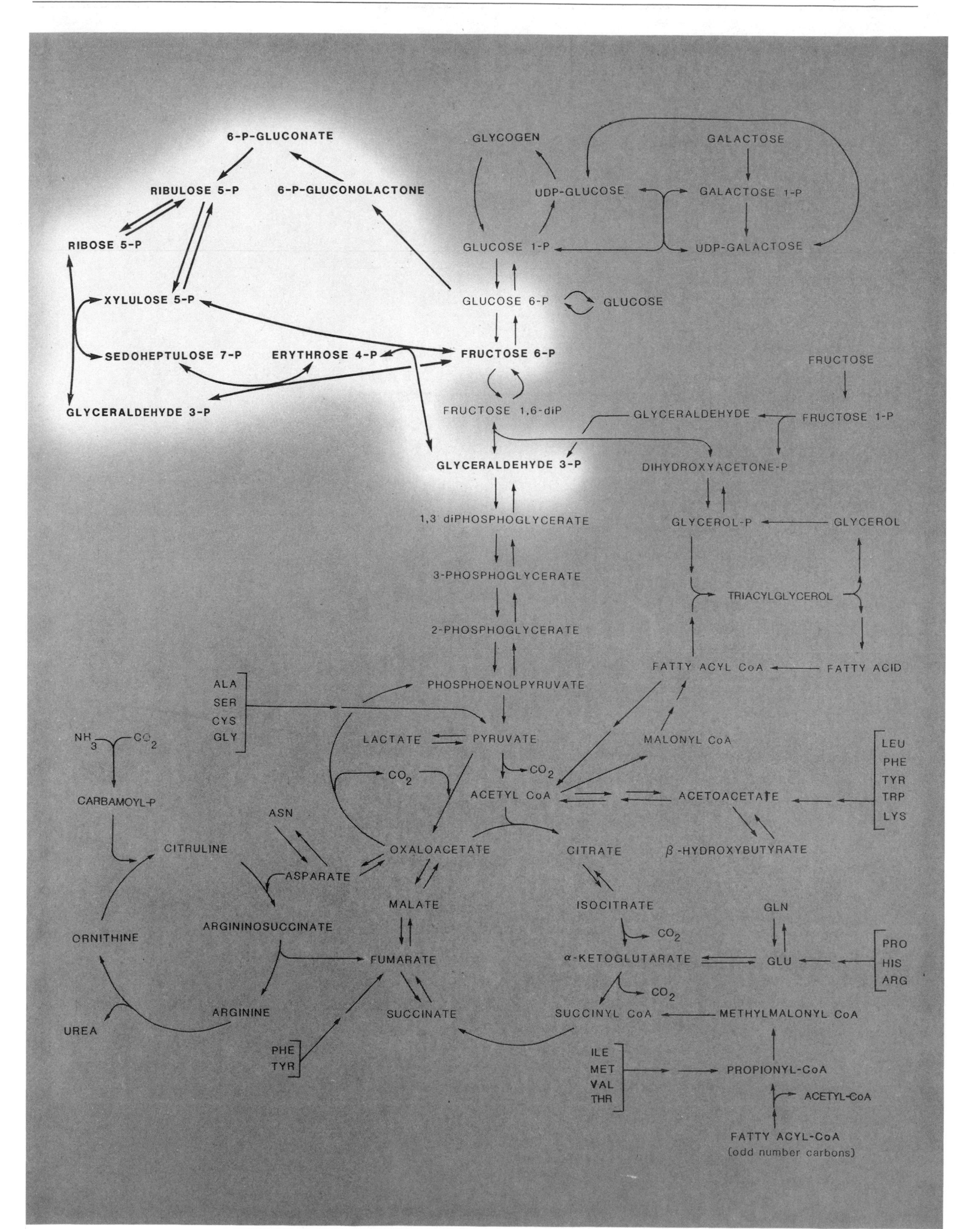
6-P-GLUCONATE
RIBULOSE 5-P
6-P-GLUCONOLACTONE
RIBOSE 5-P
XYLULOSE 5-P
SEDOHEPTULOSE 7-P
ERYTHROSE 4-P
GLYCERALDEHYDE 3-P
GLYCOGEN
GALACTOSE
UDP-GLUCOSE
GALACTOSE 1-P
GLUCOSE 1-P
UDP-GALACTOSE
GLUCOSE 6-P
GLUCOSE
FRUCTOSE 6-P
FRUCTOSE
FRUCTOSE 1,6-diP
GLYCERALDEHYDE
FRUCTOSE 1-P
GLYCERALDEHYDE 3-P
DIHYDROXYACETONE-P
1,3 diPHOSPHOGLYCERATE
GLYCEROL-P
GLYCEROL
3-PHOSPHOGLYCERATE
TRIACYLGLYCEROL
2-PHOSPHOGLYCERATE
FATTY ACYL CoA
FATTY ACID
ALA
SER
CYS
GLY
PHOSPHOENOLPYRUVATE
NH_3
CO_2
LACTATE
PYRUVATE
MALONYL CoA
LEU
PHE
TYR
TRP
LYS
CO_2
CO_2
ACETYL CoA
ACETOACETATE
CARBAMOYL-P
ASN
CITRULINE
OXALOACETATE
CITRATE
β-HYDROXYBUTYRATE
ASPARATE
MALATE
ISOCITRATE
GLN
ORNITHINE
ARGININOSUCCINATE
CO_2
FUMARATE
α-KETOGLUTARATE
GLU
PRO
HIS
ARG
CO_2
ARGININE
SUCCINATE
SUCCINYL CoA
METHYLMALONYL CoA
UREA
PHE
TYR
ILE
MET
VAL
THR
PROPIONYL-CoA
ACETYL-CoA
FATTY ACYL-CoA
(odd number carbons)

2. The major biological control of the HMP pathway occurs at this first oxidative step. G6PD is strongly inhibited by the reaction product NADPH. The ratio of $NADP^+$/NADPH is the major factor controlling the cycle.
3. The inhibition of *glucose 6-phosphate dehydrogenase* by NADPH is reversed by oxidized glutathione through a mechanism that does not involve oxidation. This is critical under normal physiologic conditions, when the concentration of NADPH in the cell is usually much higher than that of $NADP^+$.

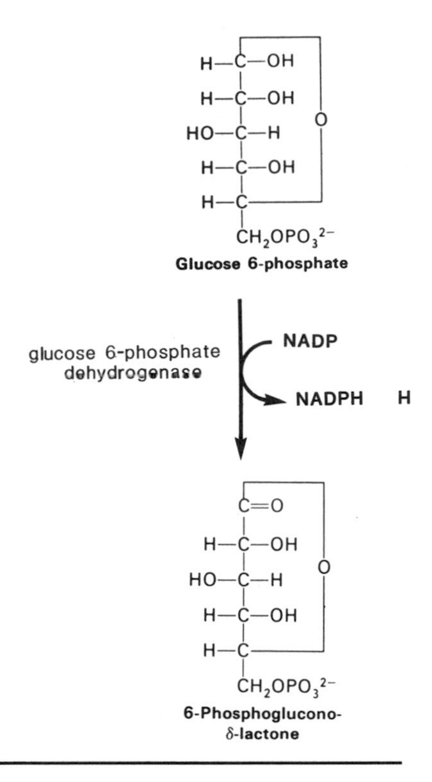

Figure 14.2
Dehydrogenation of glucose 6-phosphate.

B. Glucose 6-phosphate dehydrogenase (G6PD) deficiency

1. In erythrocytes, the HMP pathway is important because it provides NADPH for the reduction of oxidized glutathione (Figure 14.3):

$$\text{G—S—S—G} + \text{NADPH H}^+ \xrightarrow{\textit{glutathione reductase}} \text{2G—SH} + \text{NADP}^+$$

oxidized glutathione → reduced glutathione

Erythrocytes deficient in G6PD have an impaired ability to reduce $NADP^+$ to NADPH, and hence glutathione remains largely in the oxidized form. This, in turn, can lead to the accumulation of hydrogen peroxide and destruction of the erythrocyte.

2. Hydrogen peroxide is a toxic substance that, if allowed to accumulate in the erythrocyte, results in the oxidation of hemoglobin to methemoglobin and also causes damage to the cell membrane. One function of reduced glutathione is to remove hydrogen peroxide, H_2O_2:

$$\text{2G—SH} + H_2O_2 \xrightarrow{\textit{glutathione peroxidase}} \text{G—S—S—G} + H_2O$$

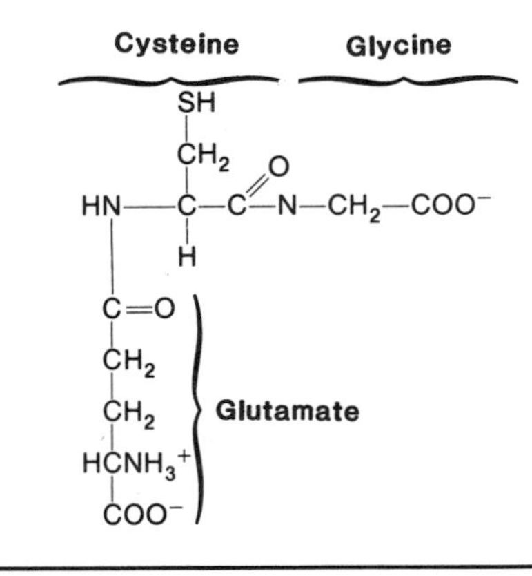

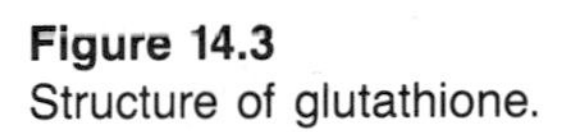

Figure 14.3
Structure of glutathione.

3. ***Glucose 6-phosphate dehydrogenase deficiency:*** An inherited enzyme deficiency, glucose 6-phosphate dehydrogenase deficiency represents a family of diseases. Mutations in the gene for G6PD may lead to the production of an altered enzyme with decreased catalytic activity, decreased stability, or altered binding affinity for $NADP^+$, NADPH, or glucose 6-phosphate. More than 80 variants of the enzyme have been described, and at least 100 million people have a partial deficiency of the enzyme. Individuals with the most commonly encountered deficiency in G6PD (Type A^-) are without symptoms under normal conditions; however, they show a ***hemolytic anemia*** when certain oxidants (*e.g.*, the antimalarial drug primaquine) are administered or during periods of stress (*e.g.*, the occurrence of an infection). The anemia induced by oxidizing compounds such as primaquine probably results from the formation of peroxides during the metabolism of the drug, causing an oxidation of glutathione. Individuals with a deficiency in *glucose 6-phosphate dehydrogenase* have a lowered capacity to form NADPH. Hence glutathione, which would normally be

◀ **Figure 14.1**
Major pathways of intermediary metabolism with the reactions of hexose monophosphate pathway highlighted.

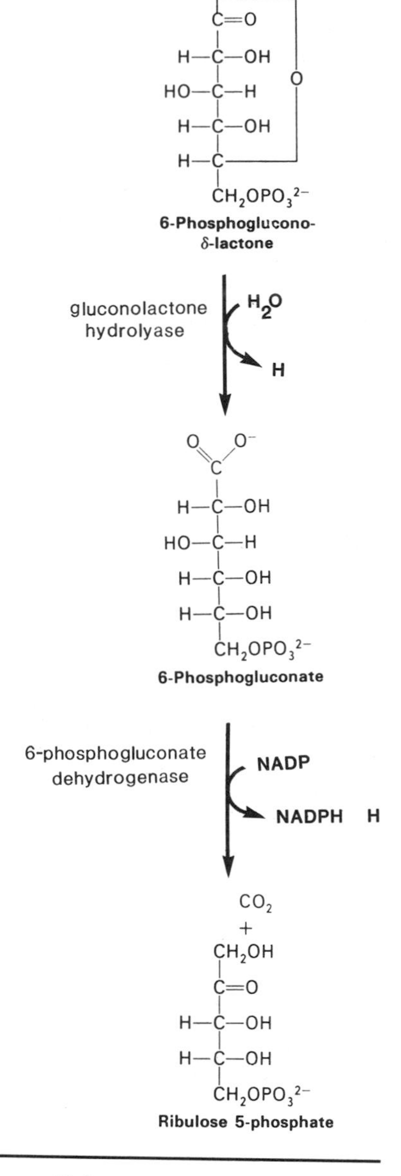

Figure 14.4
Hydrolysis of 6-phosphogluconolactone and formation of ribulose 5-p.

reduced by NADPH, remains predominantly in its oxidized form. A deficiency of reduced glutathione leads to alterations in the cell membrane and ultimately to red cell lysis and anemia. Thus, the HMP pathway of the erythrocytes is adequate under normal circumstances, but in response to stress the pathway fails to generate enough NADPH.

C. Hydrolysis of 6-phosphogluconolactone and formation of ribulose 5-phosphate

1. 6-Phosphogluconolactone is hydrolyzed by *gluconolactone hydrolyase*. The reaction is irreversible and is not rate-limiting (Figure 14.4).
2. The oxidative decarboxylation of 6-phosphogluconate is catalyzed by *6-phosphogluconate dehydrogenase*. This irreversible reaction produces a pentose sugar phosphate (ribulose 5-phosphate), CO_2 (from carbon #1 of glucose), and a second mole of NADPH.

III. NONOXIDATIVE REACTIONS

A. The nonoxidative reactions of the pentose phosphate pathway allow the ribulose 5-phosphate (produced by the oxidative portion of the pathway) to be converted either to ribose 5-phosphate (needed for nucleotide synthesis; p. 345) or to intermediates of glycolysis, such as fructose 6-phosphate and glyceraldehyde 3-phosphate (Figure 14.5).

B. In tissues in which the demand for pentoses is greater than the need for NADPH, the nonoxidative reactions can provide the biosynthesis of ribose 5-phosphate from fructose 6-phosphate in the ***absence*** of the oxidative steps (Figure 14.5).

C. The only cofactor required in the nonoxidative pathway is ***thiamine pyrophosphate,*** which is the prosthetic group of *transketolase* (see p. 311).

IV. USES OF NADPH

A. Reduction of glutathione

1. Glutathione is a tripeptide-thiol with the structure shown in Figure 14.3. Glutathione is present at high concentrations in most cells, where it serves several important functions:
   a. Oxidation of hydrogen peroxide (see p. 145).
   b. Protection of lipids against auto-oxidation.
   c. Amino acid transport in the γ-glutamyl cycle (see p. 227).

B. Cytochrome P_{450} system

1. A supply of NADPH is critical for the liver *microsomal cytochrome P_{450} mono-oxygenase* system (Figure 14.6). This is the major pathway for the hydroxylation of aromatic and aliphatic compounds, such as steroids, alcohol, and many drugs.

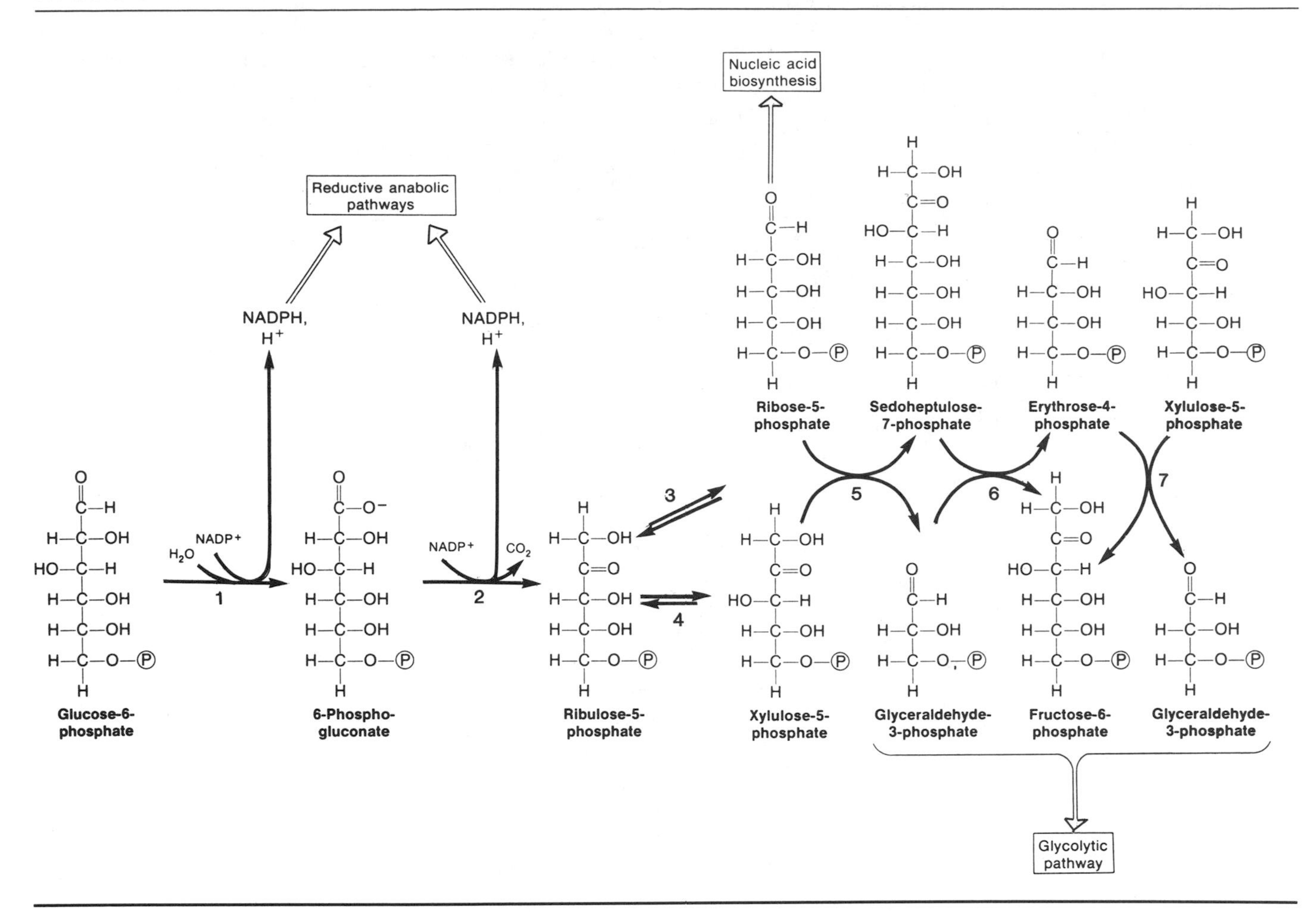

Figure 14.5
Reactions of the hexose monophosphate pathways. Enzymes numbered above are (1) glucose 6-phosphate dehydrogenase and gluconolactone hydrolyase, (2) 6-phosphogluconate dehydrogenase, (3) phosphopentose isomerase, (4) phosphopentose epimerase, (5) transketolase (cofactor thiamine pyrophosphate), (6) transaldolase, (7) transketolase (cofactor thiamine pyrophosphate).

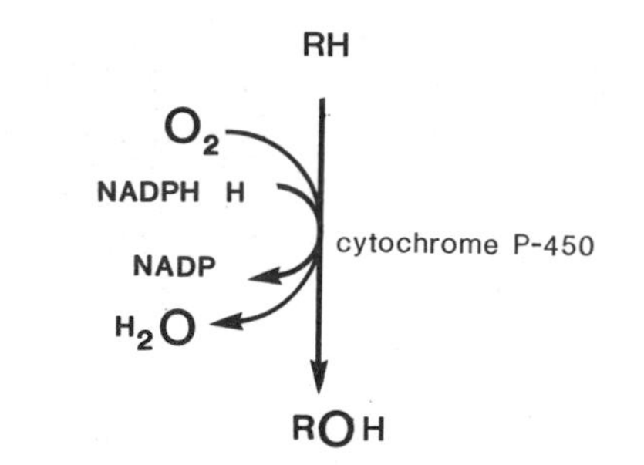

Figure 14.6
Microsomal cytochrome P_{450} monooxygenase system.

2. These oxidations also serve to detoxify drug and foreign compounds and to convert them into forms more readily excreted through the kidney.
3. Large quantities of NADPH are used in the biosynthesis of fatty acids (see p. 165) and steroids (see p. 200).

Study Questions

Choose the ONE best answer

14.1 Which one of the following is NOT characteristic of the hexose monophosphate pathway?

A. It produces CO_2.
B. It uses $NADP^+$ as a cofactor.
C. It requires ATP for phosphorylation.
D. It produces ribose 5-phosphate.
E. It involves the breakage and formation of C—C bonds.

14.2 Which one of the following reactions does NOT consume NADPH?

A. Reduction of oxidized glutathione (G—S—S—G)
B. Synthesis of steroids
C. Conversion of glucose 6-phosphate to 6-phosphogluconolactone
D. Microsomal hydroxylation with the cytochrome P_{450} oxygenase system
E. Fatty acid synthesis

14.3 Glutathione functions in erythrocytes largely to

A. produce NADPH.
B. reduce methemoglobin to hemoglobin.
C. produce NADH.
D. reduce pyruvate to lactate.
E. reduce oxidizing agents such as H_2O_2.

14.4 Which one of the following metabolites is not directly produced in the hexose monophosphate pathway?

A. Fructose 6-phosphate
B. Dihydroxyacetone phosphate
C. CO_2
D. Erythrose 4-phosphate
E. Gluconolactone 6-phosphate

UNIT IV: *Lipid Metabolism*

Metabolism of Dietary Lipids

15

I. OVERVIEW

Lipids are a heterogeneous group of water-insoluble (hydrophobic) organic molecules that can be extracted from tissues by nonpolar solvents (Figure 15.1). Because of their insolubility in aqueous solutions, body lipids are generally found either compartmentalized, as in the case of membrane-associated lipids and droplets of triacylglycerols in adipocytes, or transported throughout the body in association with protein as lipoprotein particles. These particles include the chylomicrons, very low-density lipoproteins (VLDL), low-density lipoproteins (LDL), and high-density lipoproteins (HDL).

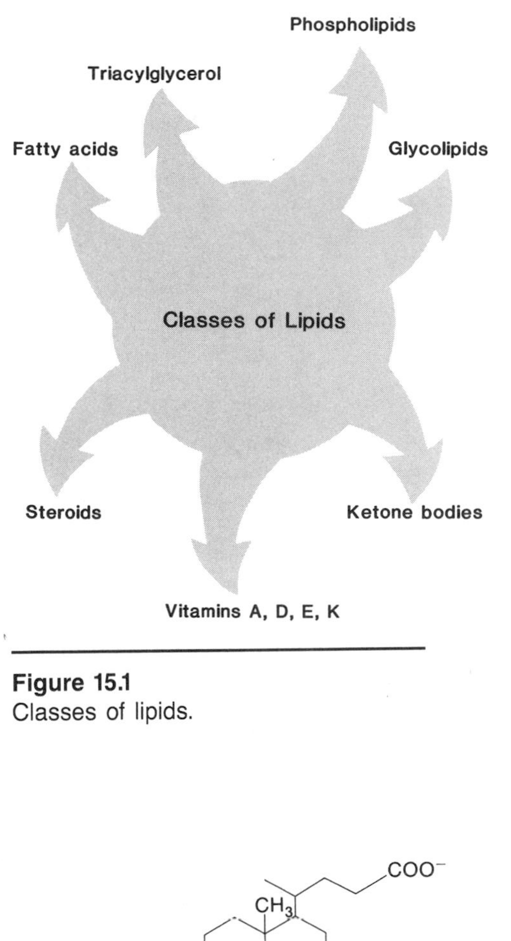

Figure 15.1
Classes of lipids.

II. DIGESTION, ABSORPTION, SECRETION, AND USE OF DIETARY LIPIDS

A. Limited processing of dietary lipid in mouth and stomach

1. Dietary lipids are not digested to any extent in either the mouth or the stomach, but rather progress more or less intact to the small intestine (Figure 15.2).

B. Emulsification of dietary fat in the small intestine

1. In the duodenum, the critical process of emulsification of the dietary lipids occurs. Because these compounds are practically insoluble in water, the enzymatic hydrolysis of lipids can occur only on the surface of a lipid droplet, that is, at the interface between the lipid droplet and the surrounding aqueous solution. The purpose of emulsification is to increase the surface area of the lipid droplets, thereby increasing the area on which the digestive enzymes can act effectively.
2. This emulsification is accomplished by two complementary mechanisms: use of the ***detergent*** properties of the bile salts, and ***mechanical mixing*** due to peristalsis.
   a. ***Bile salts*** are derivatives of cholesterol and consist of a sterol ring to which a molecule of glycine or taurine is covalently attached. These emulsifying agents can interact both with the lipid particles and the aqueous duodenal contents, thereby stabilizing the particles as they become smaller and preventing

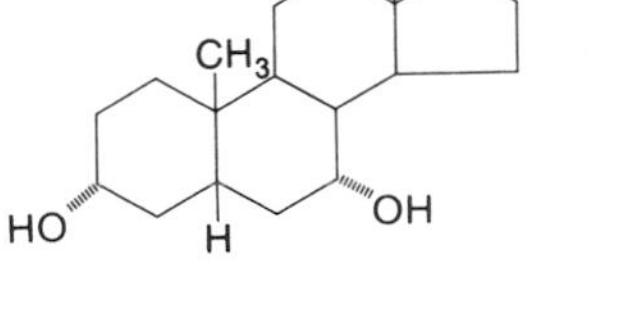

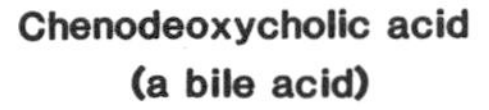

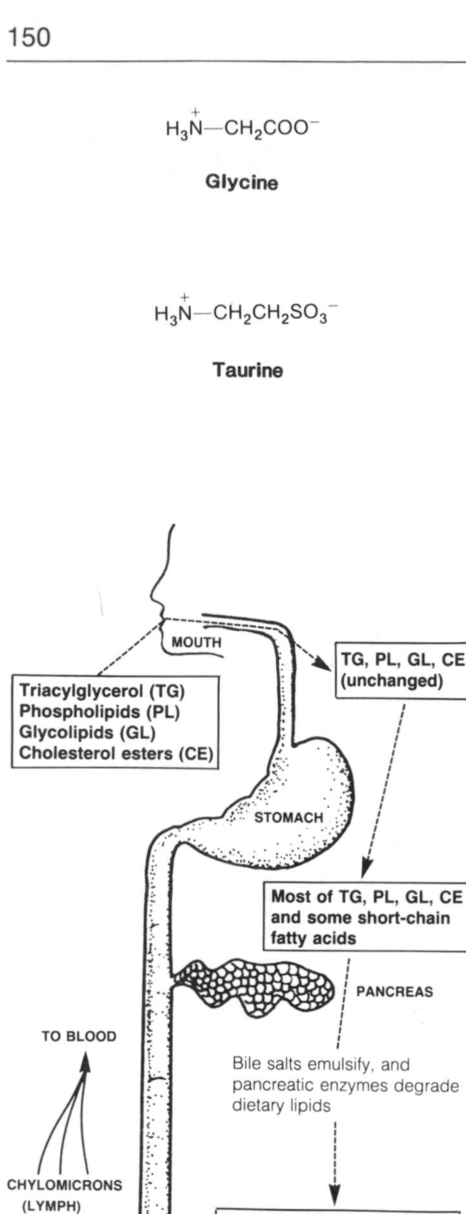

Figure 15.2
Overview of lipid digestion.

them from coalescing. A more complete discussion of the metabolism of bile salts is given on p. 204.

C. Enzymatic degradation of dietary lipids by pancreatic enzymes in the small intestine.

1. ***Hormonal control of lipid digestion:***

   a. The hydrolytic enzymes used to degrade dietary lipids in the small intestine are supplied by the pancreas in the pancreatic juice. Their release is ***hormonally controlled*** (Figure 15.3). Cells in the jejunum and lower duodenum produce a hormone, ***cholecystokinin*** (pancreozymin), in response to the stimulation from fats and partially digested proteins that enter these areas. This hormone acts both on the gallbladder (causing it to contract and release bile) and on the exocrine cells of the pancreas, resulting in the release of pancreatic enzymes. It also causes decreased gastric motility, resulting in a slower release of the gastric contents into the small intestine.

   b. The same intestinal cells produce a second hormone, ***secretin,*** in response to the low pH of the chyme entering the intestine. Secretin causes the pancreas to release a watery solution rich in bicarbonate that helps neutralize the pH of the intestinal contents, bringing it to the appropriate pH for enzymatic digestive activity.

2. ***Triacylglycerol degradation:***

   a. Triacylglycerol molecules are too large to be taken up efficiently by the mucosal cells of the intestinal villae. They are therefore acted upon by an esterase, *pancreatic lipase*, which preferentially removes the fatty acids at carbons #1 and 3. The primary products of hydrolysis are a mixture of ***2-monoacylglycerol*** (formerly called 2-monoglyceride) and free fatty acids (Figure 15.4) (see summary table of lipases, p. 217)

   b. A second protein, ***colipase,*** also present in pancreatic juice, helps to stabilize the *lipase* at the lipid-aqueous phase interface.

3. ***Cholesterol ester degradation:***

   a. Cholesterol esters are hydrolyzed by *cholesterol esterase* (*cholesterol ester hydrolase*), which produces cholesterol plus free fatty acids (Figure 15.5).

4. ***Phospholipid degradation:***

   a. Pancreatic juice is rich in the proenzyme of *phospholipase* A_2, which is converted in the intestine to its active form by *trypsin*. *Phospholipase* A_2 removes the fatty acid at carbon #2 of the phospholipid, leaving a ***lysophospholipid***. For example, the phospholipid lecithin (phosphatidylcholine) becomes lysolecithin (Figure 15.6).

   b. The remaining fatty acid at carbon #1 is removed by *lysophospholipase*, leaving a glycerylphosphorylbase (e.g., glycerylphosphorylcholine) that may be excreted in the feces or be further degraded and absorbed.

D. Absorption of lipids by intestinal mucosal cells

1. Free fatty acids, free cholesterol, and 2-monoacylglycerol are the primary products of dietary lipid degradation in the jejunum.

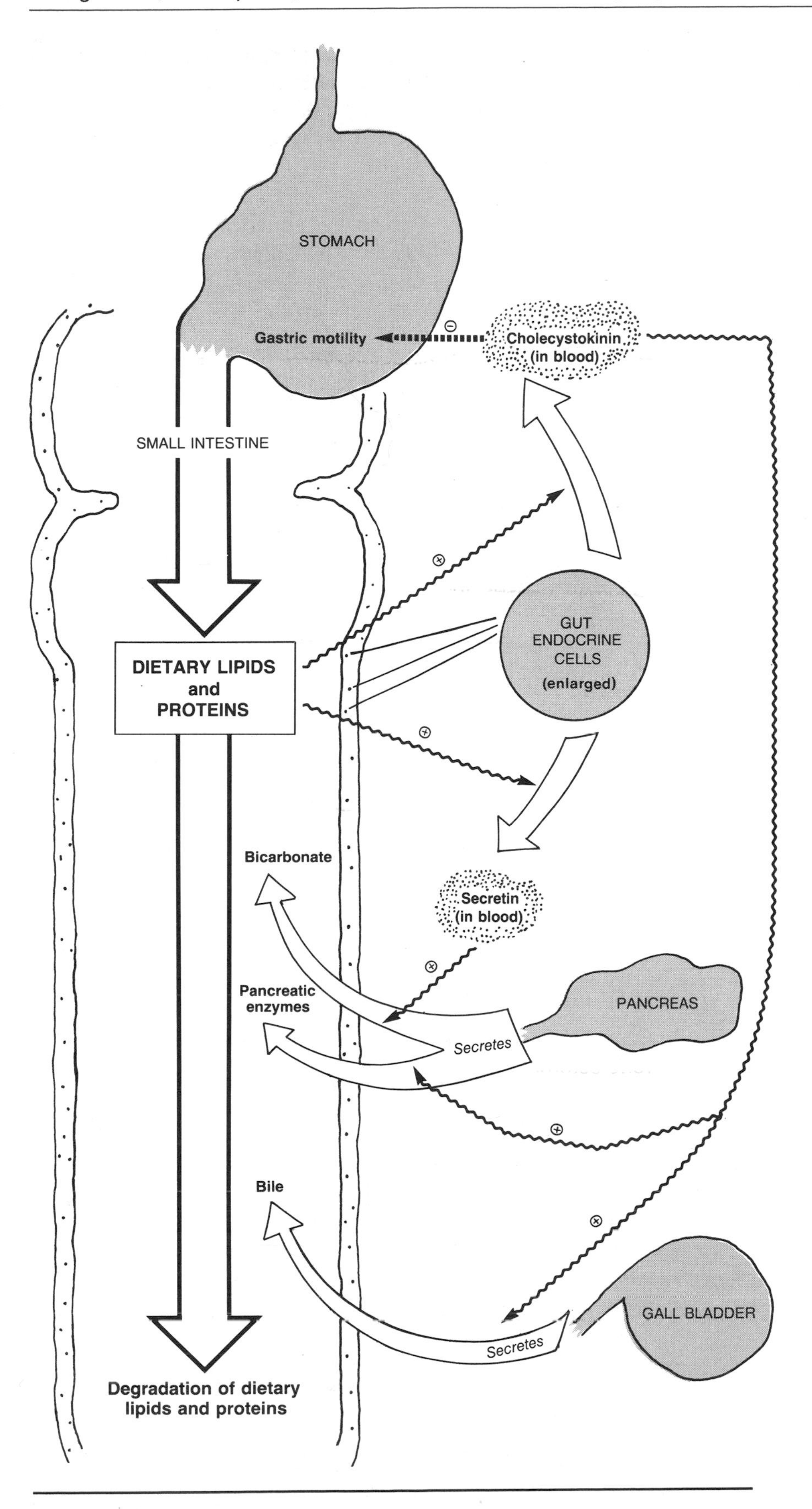

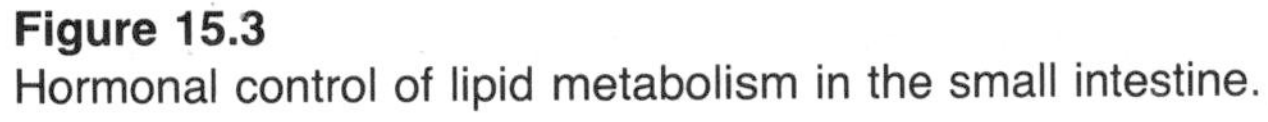

Figure 15.3
Hormonal control of lipid metabolism in the small intestine.

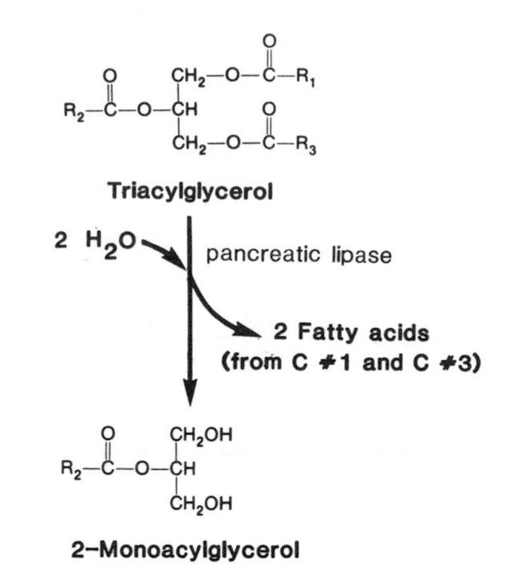

Figure 15.4
Enzymatic degradation of dietary triacylglycerol.

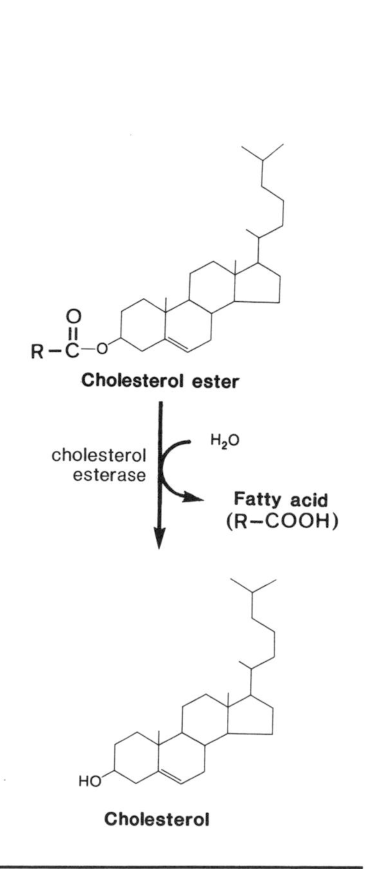

Figure 15.5
Degradation of cholesterol ester.

These, together with bile salts, form ***mixed micelles***—clusters of amphipathic lipids that coalesce with their hydrophobic groups on the inside and their hydrophilic groups on the outside of the cluster, and which are soluble in the aqueous environment of the intestinal lumen (Figure 15.7).

2. The mixed micelles approach the primary site of lipid absorption, the brush border of the intestinal mucosal cells. There, the component lipids pass through the unstirred water layer and are absorbed (Figure 15.8).
3. Fatty acids are converted into their activated form by the enzyme *fatty acyl CoA synthetase* (*thiokinase*) (Figure 15.9).
4. The 2-monoacylglycerols absorbed by the intestinal mucosal cells are converted to triacylglycerols, using the fatty acyl-CoA derivatives:

   2-monoacylglycerol + 2 fatty acyl-CoA →
   triacylglycerol + 2 Coenzyme A (CoA)

   The enzymes involved belong to a family of *acyl transferases* that recognize fatty acyl-CoA's of specific chain lengths. Virtually all of the long-chain fatty acids that enter the intestinal mucosal cells are utilized in this fashion to reform triacylglycerols.
5. A family of *fatty acyl transferases* is responsible for the reacylation of lysophospholipids and cholesterol, producing phospholipids and cholesterol esters.
6. ***Lipid malabsorption***, resulting in a loss of lipid in the feces (i.e., ***steatorrhea***), can be caused by a number of conditions (Figure 15.10), including
   a. exclusion of bile owing to severe liver dysfunction, or extrahepatic biliary obstruction or fistula.
   b. exclusion of pancreatic juice owing to obstruction of the pancreatic duct, or damage to or excision of pancreatic tissue.
   c. defect of the intestinal mucosa (including ***nontropical*** and ***tropical sprue*** in adults and ***celiac disease*** in children) in which emulsification and digestion are normal but absorption is inactive.

E. Secretion of lipids from intestinal mucosal cells

1. The newly resynthesized triacylglycerols and cholesterol esters are very hydrophobic and aggregate in aqueous solution. Therefore it is necessary that they be packaged as lipid droplets surrounded by a thin layer of protein and phospholipid. These layers stabilize the particle and increase its solubility. The protein, ***apoprotein B***, is synthesized by the intestinal mucosal cells. If this protein is not synthesized, triacylglycerol accumulates in these cells, producing the genetic disorder ***congenital abetalipoproteinemia***.
2. The presence of these particles in the lymph after a lipid-rich meal gives the lymph a milky appearance. This solution is called chyle (as opposed to ***chyme***, the name given to the semifluid mass of partially digested food that passes from the stomach to the duodenum). The small particles have therefore been named ***chylomicrons***.
3. The chylomicrons are released by exocytosis from the intestinal

mucosal cells into the intestinal lacteals (lymphatic vessels originating in the villi of the small intestine), follow the lymphatic system to the thoracic duct, and are then conveyed to the left subclavian vein where they enter the blood. (For a more extensive discussion of chylomicron structure, see p. 208.)

4. The steps in the production of chylomicrons are summarized in Figure 15.11.

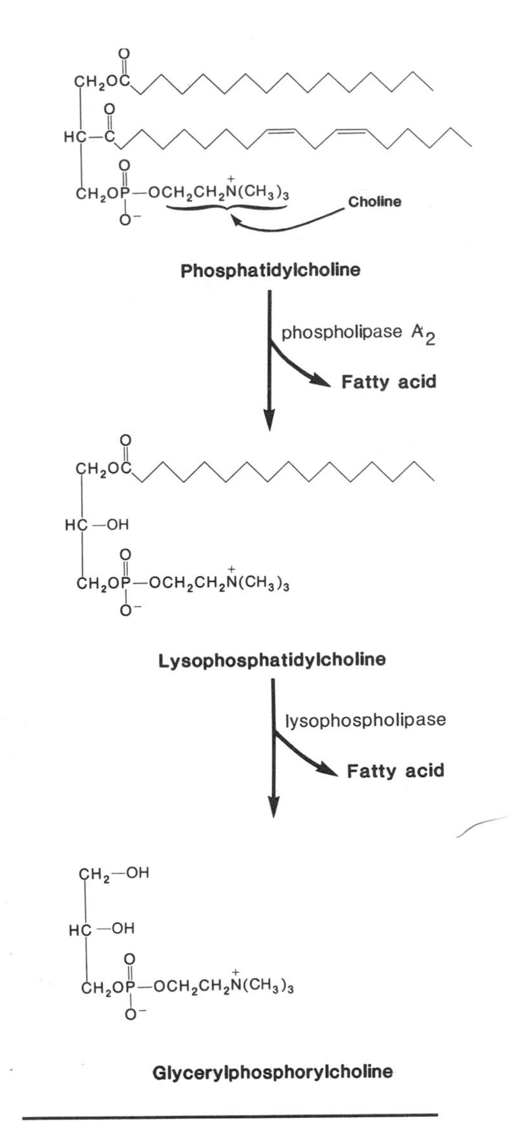

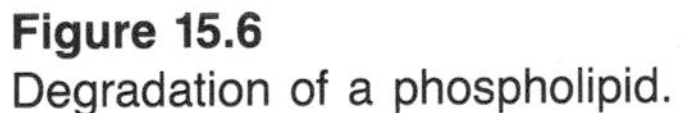

Figure 15.6
Degradation of a phospholipid.

F. Use of dietary lipids by the tissues

1. The triacylglycerol contained in the chylomicron is broken down primarily by the ***muscle*** and ***adipose tissues***, but also by the heart, lung, kidney, and liver.
2. The triacylglycerol in the circulating chylomicrons is degraded to free fatty acids and glycerol by *lipoprotein lipase*. This enzyme is synthesized primarily in the adipose tissue. It is released into the blood, where it travels to and becomes associated with the luminal surface of endothelial cells of the capillary beds of the peripheral tissues.
   a. The free fatty acids derived from the hydrolysis of triacylglycerol may directly enter adjacent muscle cells or adipocytes. Alternatively, the free fatty acids may be transported in the blood in association with serum albumin until they are taken up by cells.
   b. The glycerol that is released is used almost exclusively by the liver to produce glycerol 3-phosphate. (For a further discussion of chylomicron degradation, see p. 210.)
3. After most of the triacylglycerol has been removed, the remaining ***chylomicron remnants*** that contain cholesterol esters, phospholipid, protein, and some triacylglycerol are taken up by the liver, where they are completely degraded.
4. ***Familial lipoprotein lipase deficiency (type I hyperlipoproteinemia)*** is a rare autosomal recessive genetic disorder that results from a deficiency of the *lipoprotein lipase*. The result is massive chylomicronemia.
5. If removal of chylomicron remnants from the plasma is defective, they will accumulate in the plasma. This is seen in ***familial type III hyperlipoproteinemia*** (also called familial dysbetalipoproteinemia), which is due to a deficiency of apoprotein E (see p. 210).

G. Summary of the potential fates of the products of dietary lipid metabolism

1. Fatty acids can be oxidized by the tissues to produce energy (see p. 171).
2. Fatty acids can be taken up by tissues and reesterified to produce triglyceride, which is stored (see p. 153).
3. Glycerol can be converted by the liver to glycerol 3-phosphate, which in turn can enter glycolysis (see p. 171) or gluconeogenesis by oxidation to dihydroxyacetone phosphate (see p. 129).
4. Cholesterol and the bases of phospholipids (e.g., choline, ethanolamine) can be recycled by the body (see p. 150).

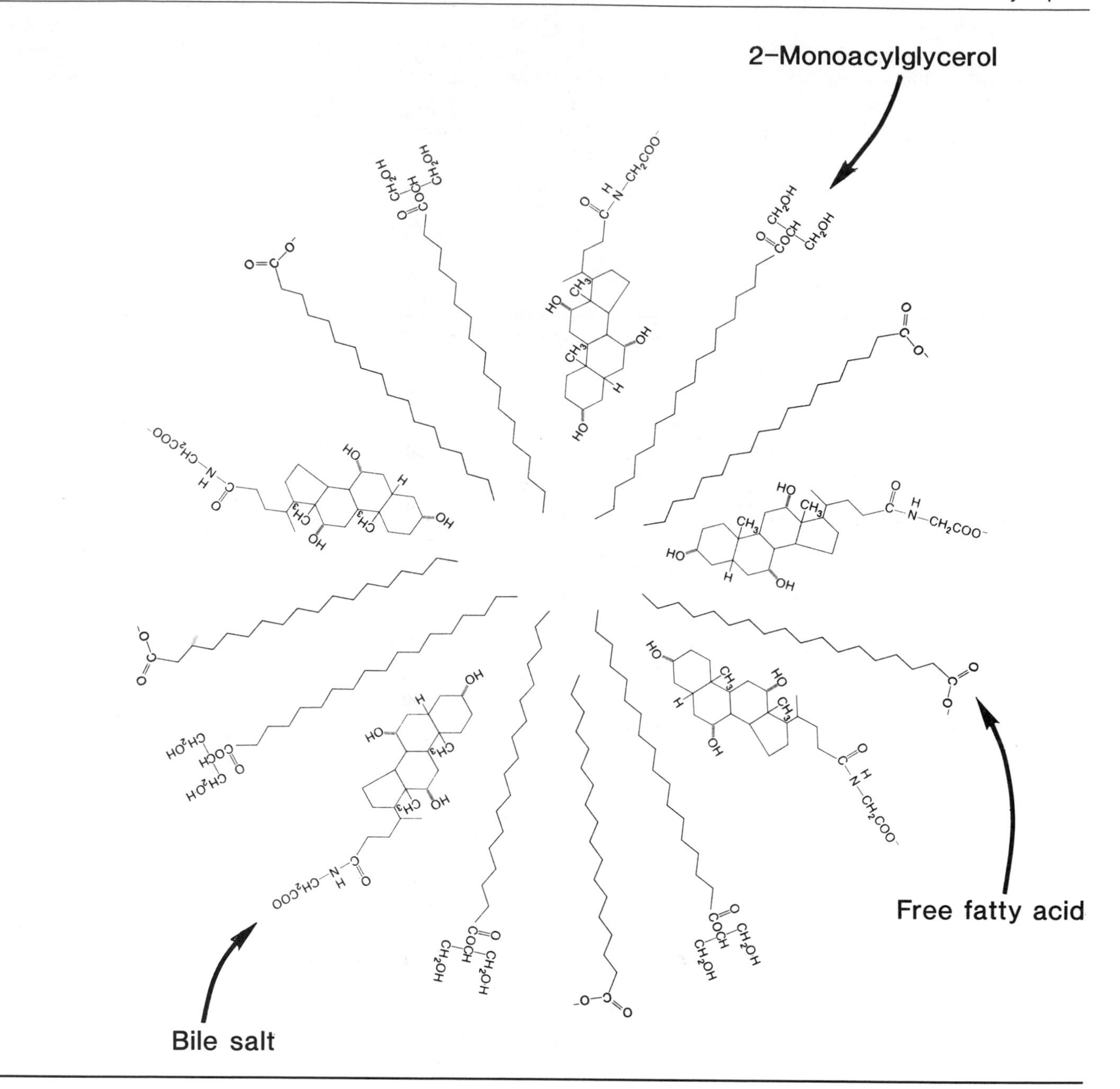

Figure 15.7
Mixed micelle containing bile salts, free fatty acids, and 2-monoacylglycerol.

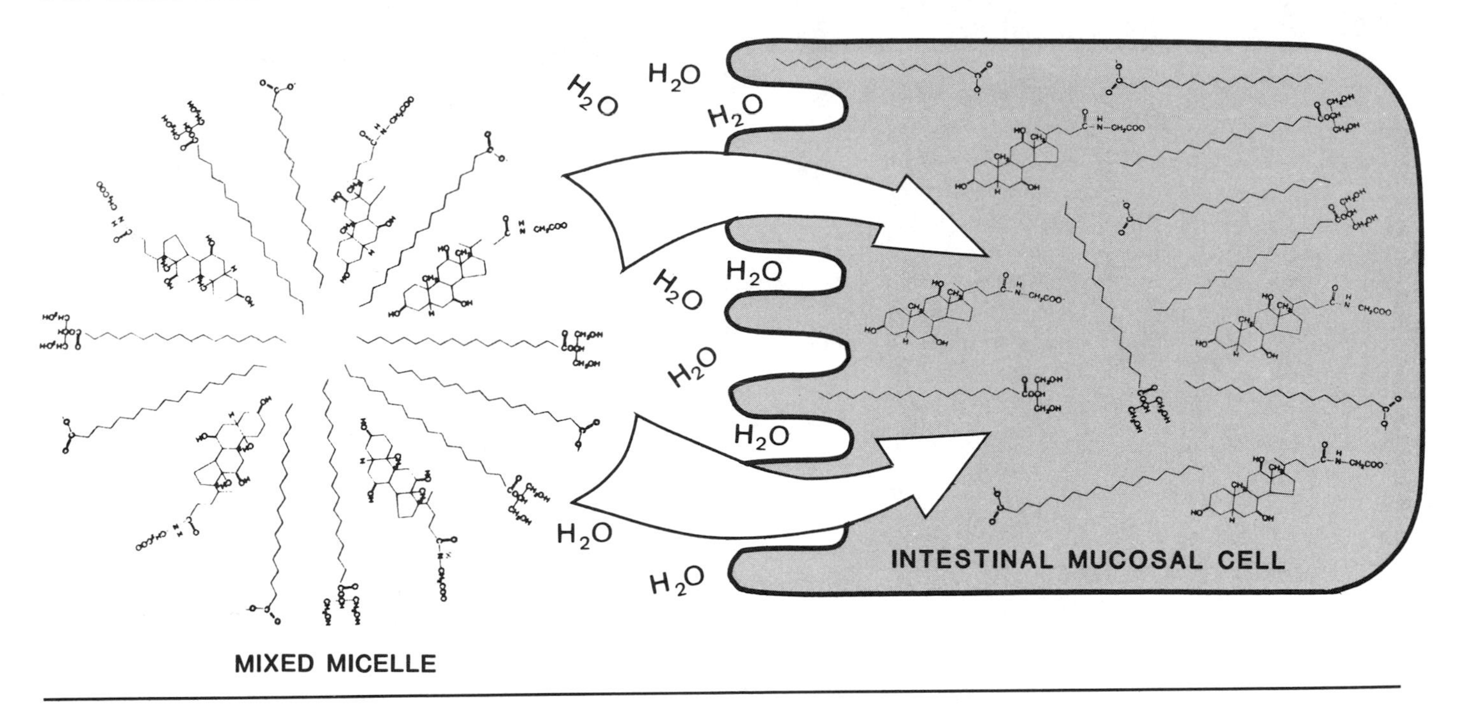

Figure 15.8
Absorption of lipids by intestinal mucosal cells.

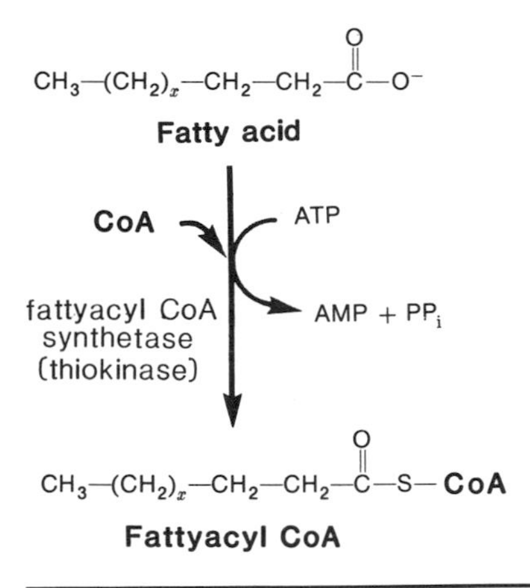

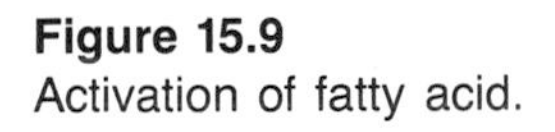

Figure 15.9
Activation of fatty acid.

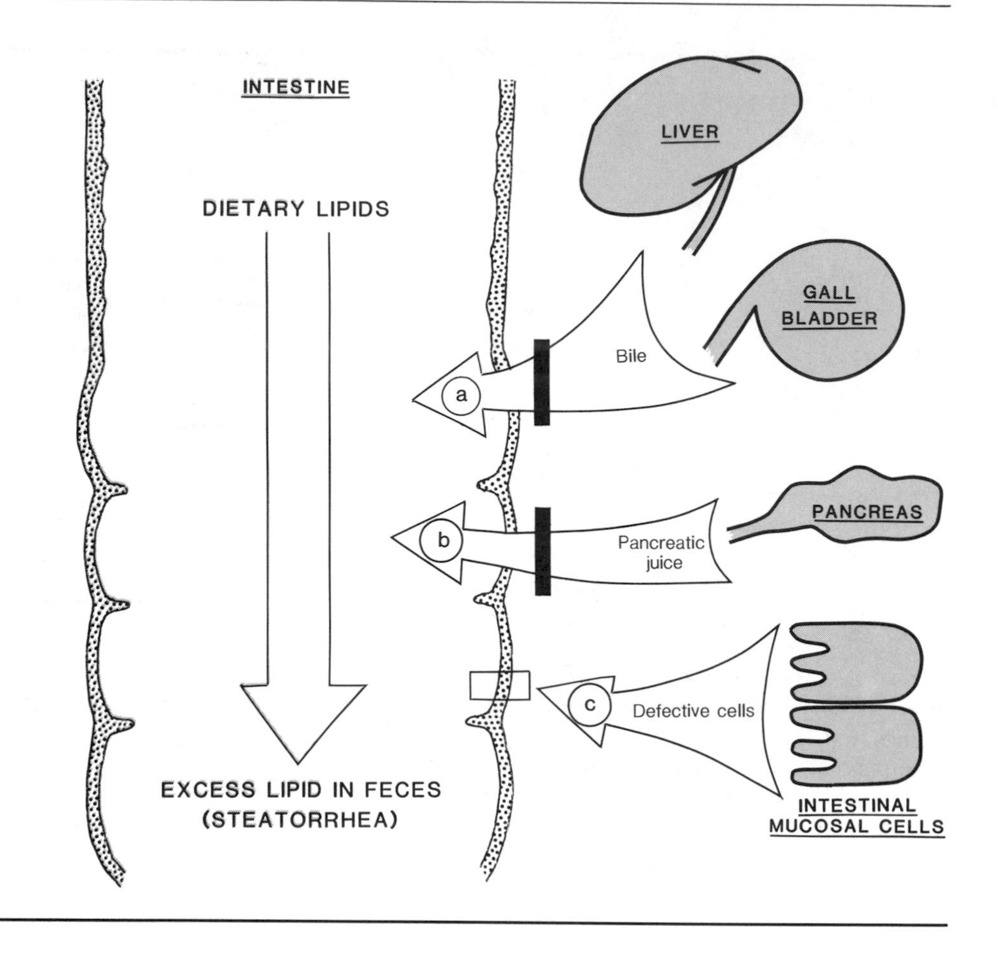

Figure 15.10
Possible causes of the steatorrhea; circled letters on the figure correspond to similarly circled citations in the text.

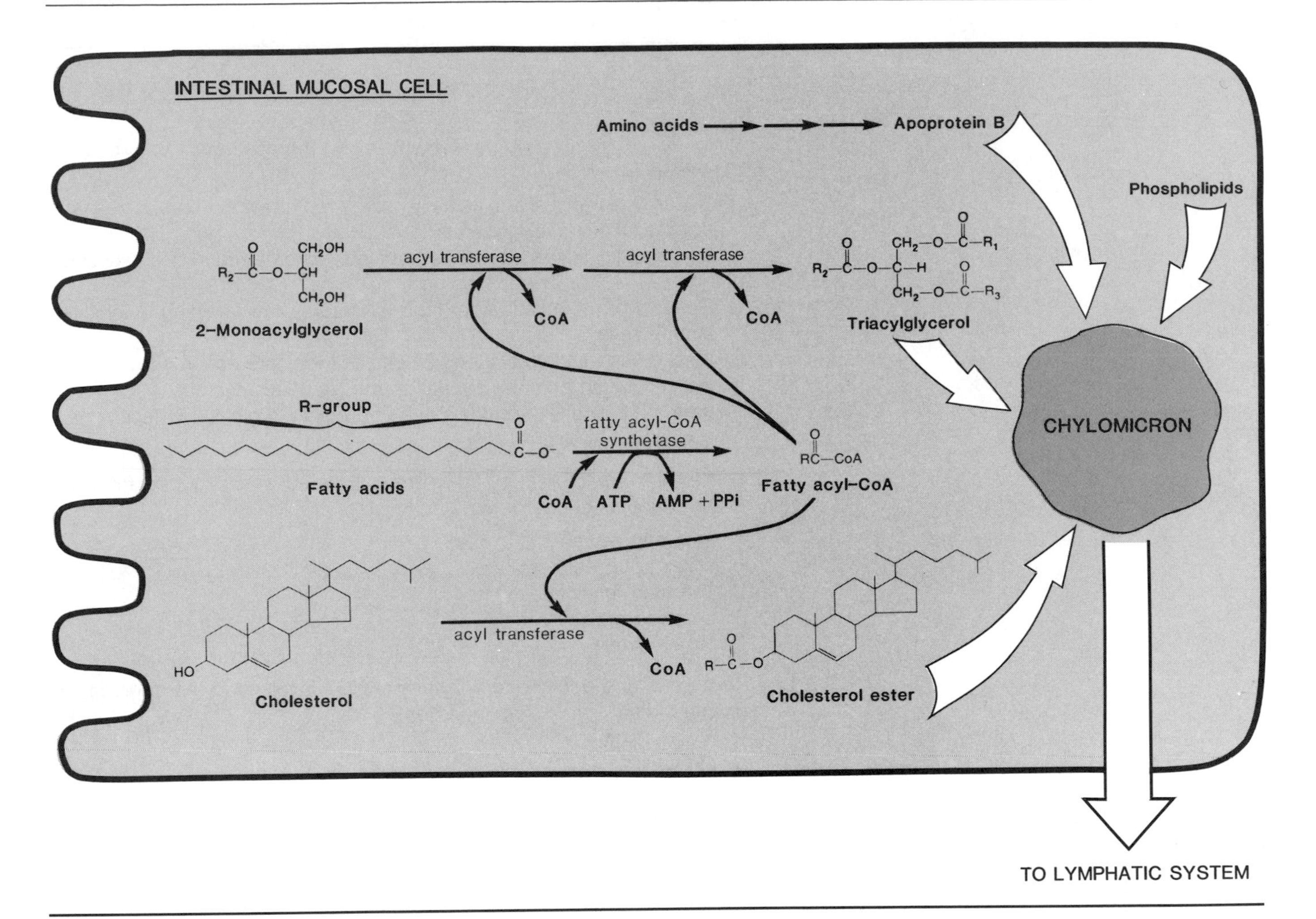

Figure 15.11
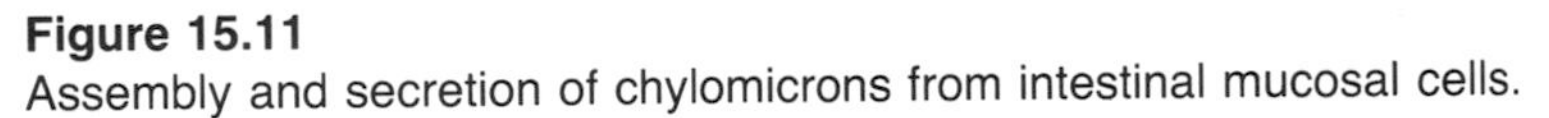
Assembly and secretion of chylomicrons from intestinal mucosal cells.

Study Questions

Choose the ONE best answer

15.1 Which one of the following statements about the absorption of lipids from the intestine is ***correct***?

A. Dietary triacylglycerol is partially hydrolyzed and absorbed as free fatty acids and monoacylglycerol.
B. Dietary triacylglycerol must be completely hydrolyzed to free fatty acids and glycerol before absorption.
C. Release of fatty acids from triacylglycerol in the intestine is inhibited by bile salts.
D. Fatty acids that contain ten carbons or fewer are absorbed and enter the circulation primarily by way of the lymphatic system.
E. Formation of chylomicrons does not require protein synthesis in the intestinal mucosa.

15.2 The form in which dietary lipids are packaged and exported from the intestinal mucosal cells is as

A. free fatty acids.
B. mixed micelles.
C. free triacylglycerol.
D. 2-monoacylglycerol.
E. chylomicrons.

15.3 Which one of the following enzymes is NOT involved in the degradation of total dietary lipid during digestion?

A. Gastric lipase
B. Pancreatic lipase
C. Lipoprotein lipase
D. Phospholipase A_2
E. Cholesterol esterase

Fatty Acid and Triacylglycerol Metabolism

16

I. OVERVIEW

Fatty acids exist in the body either as free, unesterifed fatty acids or as fatty acyl esters in more complex molecules, such as triacylglycerol. Low levels of free fatty acids occur in all tissues but can sometimes be found in substantial amounts in the plasma, particularly during starvation. Plasma free fatty acids (transported by serum albumin) can be envisioned as molecules that are "en route" from their point of origin (triacylglycerol of adipose tissue or circulating lipoproteins) to their site of consumption (most tissues). Free fatty acids can be oxidized by many tissues, such as liver and muscle, providing a source of energy. Fatty acids are also precursors of many compounds, including glycolipids, phospholipids, steroids, prostaglandins, and cholesterol esters. Fatty acids in the form of triacylglycerols serve as the major energy reserve of the body.

II. STRUCTURE OF FATTY ACIDS

A. Amphipathic properties of fatty acids

1. A fatty acid consists of a ***hydrocarbon chain*** with a terminal ***carboxyl group*** (Figure 16.1.).
2. At physiologic pH, the terminal carboxyl group (—COOH), which has a pK_a around 4.8, ionizes, becoming $—COO^-$. This anionic group has an affinity for water, giving the fatty acid its ***amphipathic*** nature (having both a hydrophilic and a hydrophobic region). However, for long-chain fatty acids the hydrophobic portion is predominant, and these molecules are highly water-insoluble and must be transported in the circulation in association with the serum protein ***albumin***.

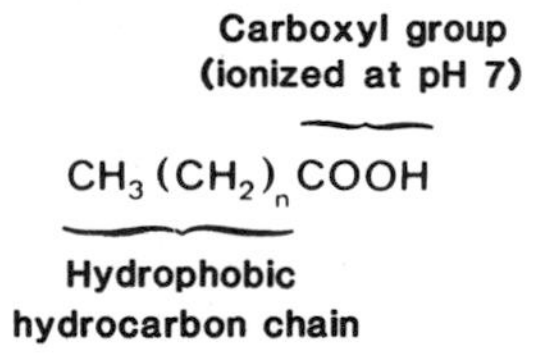

Carboxyl group (ionized at pH 7)

$CH_3(CH_2)_nCOOH$

Hydrophobic hydrocarbon chain

Figure 16.1
Structure of a fatty acid.

B. Unsaturation and chain length of fatty acids

1. The fatty acid chains may contain no double bonds, that is, be ***saturated*** (e.g., palmitic acid), or contain one or more double bonds, that is, be ***unsaturated*** (e.g., oleic acid).

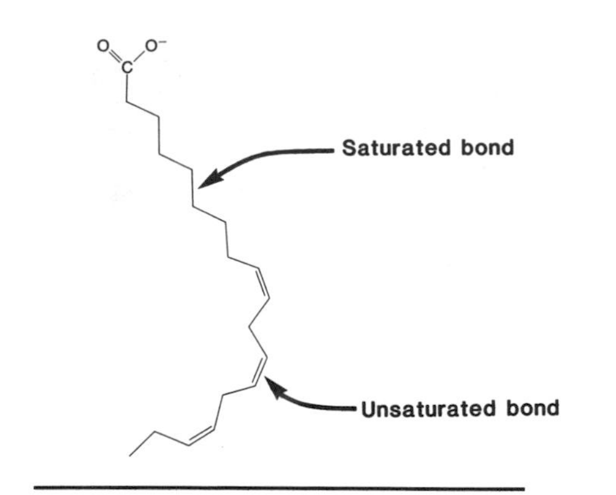

Figure 16.2
Cis double bond causes a fatty acid to "kink."

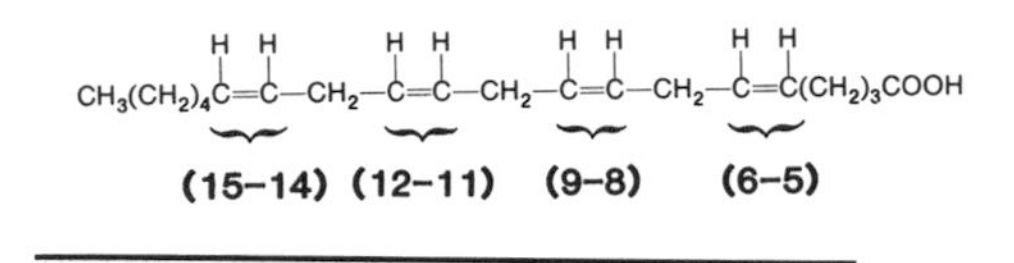

Figure 16.3
Arachidonic acid illustrating position of double bonds.

2. When double bonds are present, they are nearly always found in the ***cis*** configuration rather than in the ***trans***. The introduction of a cis double bond causes the fatty acid to "kink" at that position (Figure 16.2).
3. If the fatty acid has two or more double bonds, the bonds are always spaced at ***three carbon intervals***.
4. The common names and compositions of some fatty acids of physiologic importance are listed in Table 16.1. Note that almost all fatty acids present in mammalian tissue are of the straight-chain variety.
   a. The number written to the right of the fatty acid in Table 16.1 indicates the number of carbons in the chain and the number and position of double bonds. The carbon atoms are numbered beginning with the carboxyl carbon as C#1.

      For example, arachidonic acid, 20:4(5, 8, 11, 14) is 20 carbons long and has 4 double bonds (between carbons 5-6, 8-9, 11-12, and 14-15) (Figure 16.3).

      (Note: The carbon to which the carboxyl group is attached [C2] is also called the α-carbon, C3 is the β-carbon, and C4 is the γ-carbon. The terminal methyl group is called the ω-carbon regardless of the chain length.)
5. In general, increasing the chain length will increase the melting temperature (T_m) of a fatty acid; addition of double bonds decreases the T_m. Therefore, the presence in membrane lipids of fatty acids that contain double bonds helps maintain the fluid nature of those lipids.
6. Two fatty acids are ***essential*** in humans (see p. 301): ***linoleic acid***, the precursor of the prostaglandins, and ***linolenic acid***. Arachidonic acid becomes essential if its precursor, linoleic acid, is missing in the diet.

TABLE 16.1

Common Name	Structure	Functional Significance
Formic acid	1	
Acetic acid	2:0	
Propionic acid	3:0	
Butyric acid	4:0	Fatty acids with chain lengths of 4–10 carbons are found in significant quantities in milk
Capric acid	10:0	
Palmitic acid	16:0	Structural lipids and triglycerides primarily contain fatty acids of at least 16 carbons
Palmitoleic acid	16:1(9)	
Stearic acid	18:0	
Oleic acid	18:1(9)	
Linoleic acid	18:2(9, 12)	
Linolenic acid	18:3(9, 12, 15)	
Arachidonic acid	20:4(5, 8, 11, 14)	Precursor of prostaglandins
Lignoceric acid	24:0	
Nervonic acid	24:1(15)	Component of cerebrosides

7. More than 90% of the fatty acid found in plasma is in the form of fatty acid esters (primarily triacylglycerol, cholesterol esters, and phospholipids) contained in plasma lipoproteins (see p. 208).

Study Questions

Choose the ONE best answer

16.1 Palmitic acid

A. is one of the most abundant monounsaturated fatty acids.
B. contains a double bond at carbon number 9.
C. is a short-chain fatty acid.
D. contains more double bonds than arachidonic acid.
E. has a negative charge at pH 7.4.

16.2 Which one of the following fatty acids is not synthesized in humans?

A. Oleic acid
B. Linoleic acid
C. Palmitic acid
D. Stearic acid
E. Propionic acid

16.3 Which one of the following statements about fatty acids is ***incorrect***?

A. Almost all fatty acids found in mammalian tissues are of the straight chain variety, but branched chain fatty acids do exist in nature.
B. More than 90% of the fatty acids found in the plasma are "free," that is, are not esterified to another compound.
C. Addition of double bonds to a fatty acid chain lowers its melting temperature.
D. Linoleic acid cannot be synthesized by humans and thus must be supplied by the diet.
E. In general, the longer the chain length of a saturated fatty acid, the higher is its melting temperature.

16.4 Which one of the following compounds is obtained on complete hydrogenation (i.e., saturation) of linoleic acid?

A. Palmitic acid
B. Oleic acid
C. Myristic acid
D. Stearic acid
E. Fumaric acid

III. *DE NOVO* SYNTHESIS OF FATTY ACIDS

Fatty acid synthesis occurs in the ***cytoplasm of cells*** from many tissue types, including liver, adipose, lactating mammary glands, and, to a lesser extent, kidney. The process incorporates carbons from ***acetyl CoA*** into the growing fatty acid chain, using ***ATP*** and ***reduced nicotinamide adenine dinucleotide phosphate (NADPH)*** as cofactors. The rate of fatty acid synthesis in adipose cells is increased by insulin, which promotes the uptake of glucose by these cells.

A. Production of cytoplasmic acetyl CoA

1. The first step in fatty acid synthesis is the transfer of acetate units from mitochondrial acetyl CoA (which is produced by the oxidation of pyruvate or the degradation of fatty acids or amino acids) to the cytoplasm, forming ***cytoplasmic acetyl CoA***. The coen-

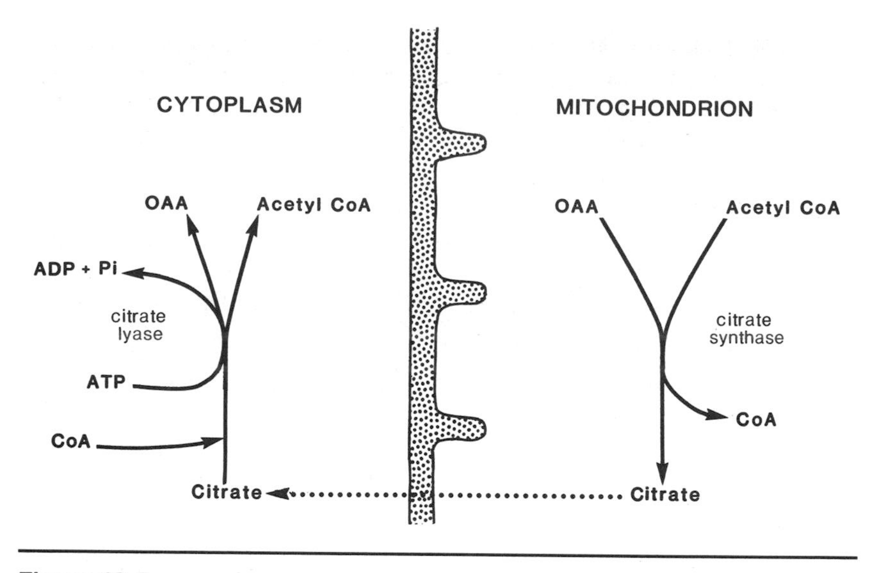

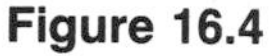

Figure 16.4
Production of cytoplasmic acetyl CoA.

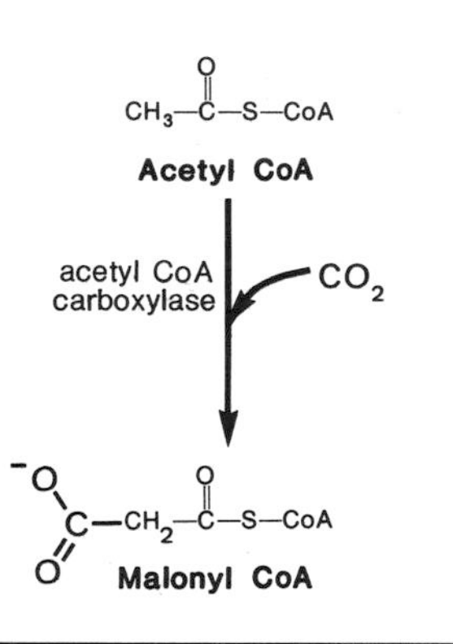

Figure 16.5
Malonyl CoA synthesis. The carboxyl group contributed by CO_2 is shown in larger print.

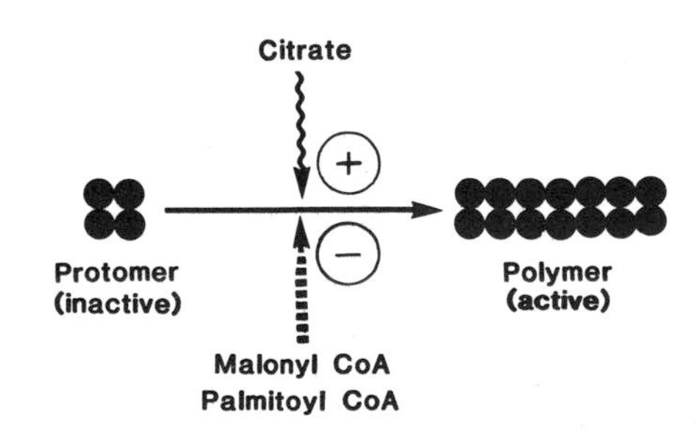

Figure 16.6
Regulation of *acetyl CoA carboxylase.*

zyme A portion of acetyl CoA, however, cannot cross the mitochondrial membrane, and only the acetyl portion is transported to the cytoplasm (in the form of citrate produced by the condensation of oxaloacetate and acetyl CoA, Figure 16.4).

2. This process of ***translocation*** of citrate from the mitochondrion to the cytoplasm occurs when the citrate concentration is high. This is observed when *isocitrate dehydrogenase* is inhibited by the presence of large amounts of ATP, causing citrate and isocitrate to accumulate (see p. 137). Because a large amount of ATP is needed for fatty acid synthesis, the related increase in both ATP and citrate enhances the opportunity for this pathway to occur.

B. Carboxylation of acetyl CoA to form malonyl CoA

1. The energy for the carbon-to-carbon condensations in fatty acid synthesis is supplied by the process of carboxylation and then decarboxylation of acetyl groups in the cytoplasm.
2. The carboxylation of acetyl CoA is catalyzed by *acetyl CoA carboxylase* (Figure 16.5) and requires ATP. The enzyme cofactor is ***biotin,*** which is covalently bound to a lysyl residue of the enzyme (see pp. 127 and 317).
3. This carboxylation is the ***regulated step*** in fatty acid synthesis: The inactive form of *acetyl CoA carboxylase* consists of a protomer made of four subunits (Figure 16.6). The enzyme is activated by citrate, which causes the protomers to polymerize. The enzyme can be inactivated by malonyl CoA (an intermediate in the pathway) or palmitoyl CoA (the end product of the pathway), which cause its depolymerization.

C. Fatty acid synthase: a multienzyme complex

1. The remaining series of reactions in fatty acid synthesis are catalyzed by a multienzyme complex. In eukaryotes this enzyme complex, *fatty acid synthase,* consists of two subunits that,

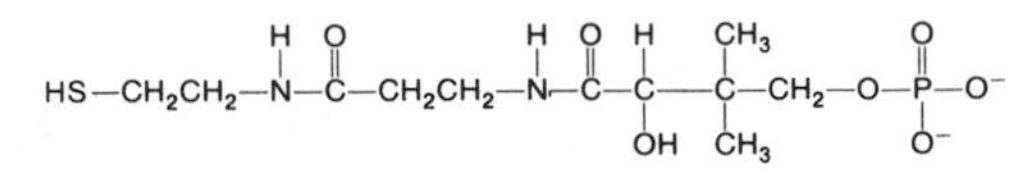

4′-Phosphopantetheine

together, have seven enzymatic acitivities. Each subunit also has a covalently attached molecule of ***4′-phosphopantetheine*** on each subunit. (Note: In *E. coli,* the protein carrying the 4′-phosphopantetheine residue is called the ***acyl carrier protein*** [ACP]. This name will be used below in the discussion of eukaryotic fatty acid synthesis.)

a. 4′-Phosphopantetheine, a derivative of the vitamin pantothenic acid (see p. 322), is also a component of coenzyme A. It carries acetyl and acyl units on its terminal thiol (—SH) group during fatty acid synthesis.

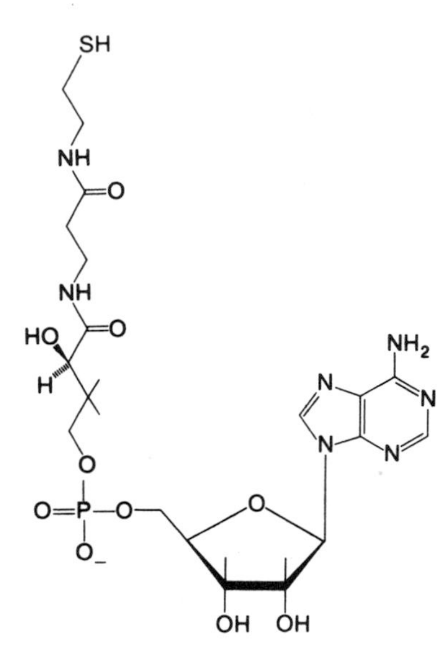

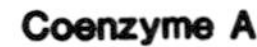

Coenzyme A

2. The reaction numbers in brackets below refer to Figure 16.7. The "enzymes" listed are actually separate enzymic activities present in the *fatty acid synthase* complex.

[1]: A molecule of acetate is transferred from acetyl CoA to the —SH group of the ACP:

Acetyl CoA + ACP—SH → acetyl—S—ACP + CoA

Enzyme: *Acetyl CoA—ACP transacylase*

[2]: Next, this two-carbon fragment is transferred to a cysteine residue on the enzyme, which acts as a temporary holding site:

Acetyl—S—ACP + enzyme—SH →
acetyl—S—enzyme + ACP—SH

[3]: The now-vacant ACP accepts a three-carbon malonate unit from malonyl CoA:

Malonyl CoA + ACP—SH → malonyl—S—ACP + CoA

Enzyme: *Malonyl—CoA—ACP—transacylase*

[4]: The acetyl group condenses with the malonyl group, in the process losing the CO_2 originally added to produce the malonyl CoA. The loss of free energy from this decarboxylation drives the reaction:

Malonyl—S—ACP + acetyl—S—enzyme →
acetoacetyl-S-ACP + CO_2

Enzyme: β-*ketoacyl-ACP synthase*

3. The next three reactions convert the β-ketoacyl group to the corresponding saturated acyl group by a pair of reductions and a dehydration step:

[5]: The keto group is converted to an alcohol:

Acetoacetyl—S—ACP + NADPH + H^+ →
β-hydroxybutyryl—ACP + $NADP^+$

Reduction using NADPH

Enzyme: β-*ketoacyl—ACP reductase*

[6]: A molecule of water is removed:

β-Hydroxybutyryl—S—ACP → crotonyl—S—ACP + H_2O

Enzyme: β-*hydroxyacyl-ACP dehydratase*

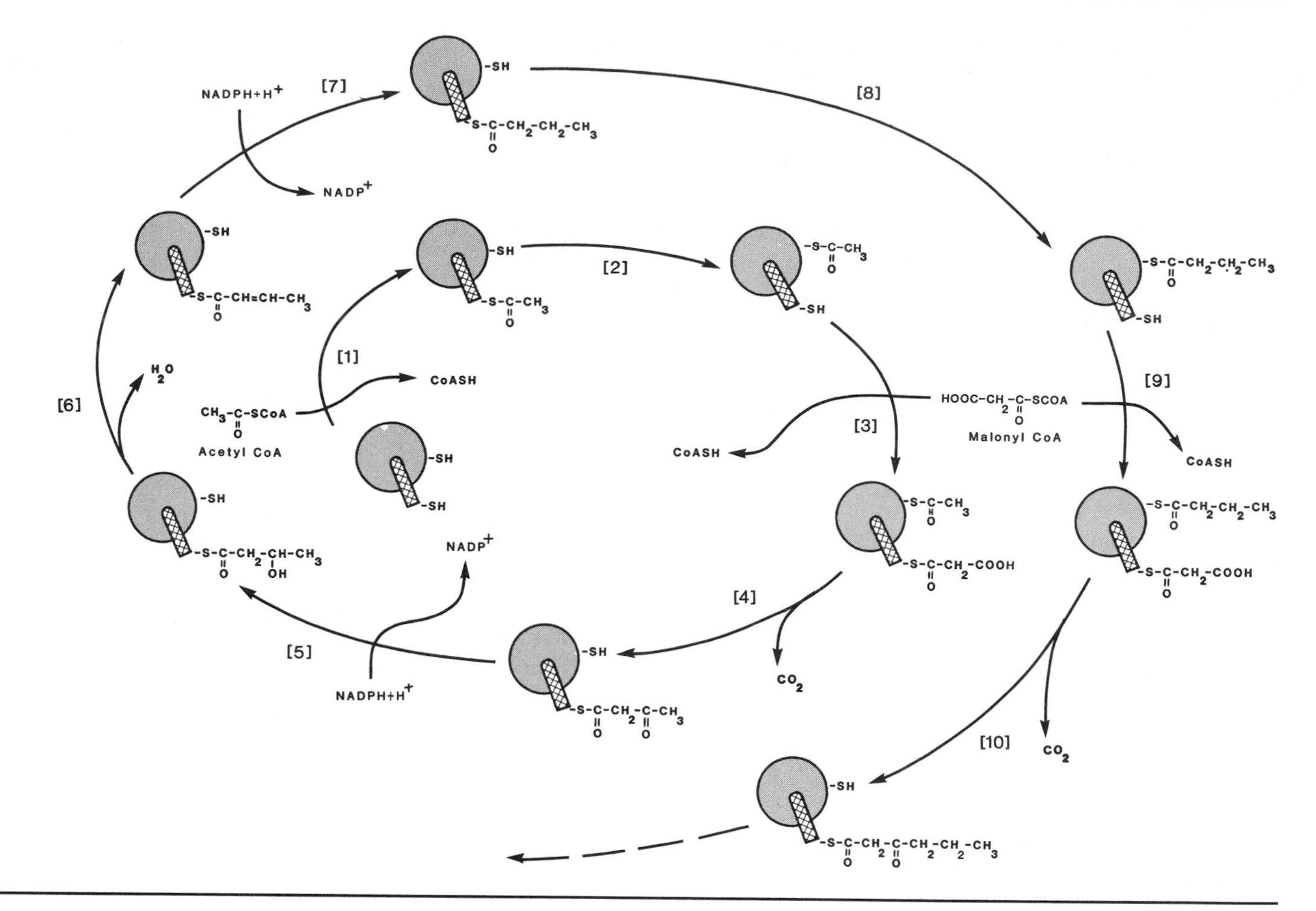

Figure 16.7
Synthesis of a fatty acid. The enzyme complex, *fatty acid synthase,* is represented as a gray circle, with the 4′-phosphopantetheine residue shaped like a textured cigar.

[7]: A second reduction step occurs:

Crotonyl-S-ACP + NADPH + $H^+ \rightarrow$

butyryl-S-ACP + $NADP^+$

Enzyme: *enoyl-ACP reductase*

4. The result of these seven steps is production of a four-carbon compound whose three-terminal carbons are fully saturated, and which remains attached to the ACP.
5. These seven steps are repeated, beginning with the transfer of the four-carbon chain from the ACP to the peripheral cysteine side group [8], the attachment of a molecule of malonate to the ACP [9], and the condensation of the two molecules liberating CO_2 [10]. The carbonyl group at the β-carbon (C3—the third carbon from the sulfur) is then reduced.
6. This cycle of reactions is repeated seven times, each time incorporating a two-carbon unit (derived from malonyl CoA) into

the growing fatty acid chain. Once the fatty acid reaches a length of 16 carbons, the synthetic process is terminated, producing a fully saturated molecule of palmitate.

Palmitoyl-S-ACP + H_2O → palmitate + ACP—SH
Enzyme: *palmitoyl thioesterase*

7. The overall reaction for palmitate synthesis is

   8 Acetyl CoA + 14 NADPH + 14 H^+ + 7 ATP →
   Palmitic acid + 8 CoA + 14 $NADP^+$ + 7 ADP + 7 P_i + 7 H_2O

   (Note: All the carbons in the palmitic acid have passed through malonyl CoA except the two donated by the original acetyl CoA, which are found at the methyl group end.)

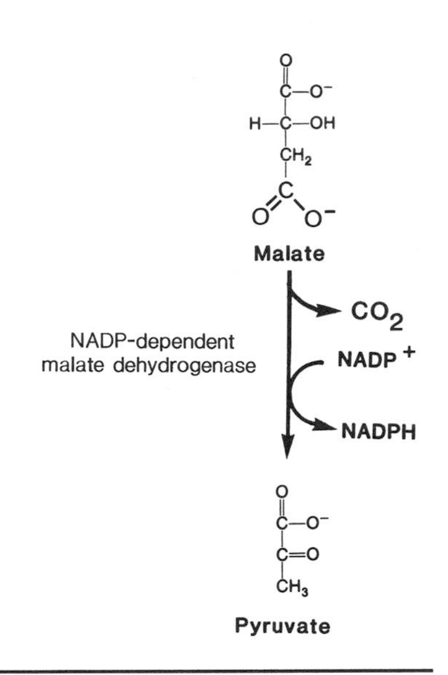

Figure 16.8
Cytoplasmic conversion of malate to pyruvate.

D. Major sources of the NADPH required for fatty acid synthesis

1. ***Hexose monophosphate pathway:*** This pathway is the major supplier of NADPH for fatty acid synthesis. Two NADPH are produced for each molecule of glucose that enters this pathway (see p. 143 for a discussion of this sequence of reactions.)

2. ***Cytoplasmic conversion of malate to pyruvate:*** Malate is oxidized and decarboxylated by a cytoplasmic *$NADP^+$-dependent malate dehydrogenase* (*malic enzyme*) to form pyruvate. Malate can arise from the reduction of oxaloacetate cytoplasmic *NAD^+-dependent malate dehydrogenase* (Figure 16.8). (The cytoplasmic NADH can be produced during glycolysis.) Oxaloacetate in turn can arise from citrate (recall from Figure 16.4 that citrate was shown to move from the mitochondria into the cytoplasm, where it is cleaved into acetyl CoA and oxaloacetate by the *citrate cleavage enzyme*).

E. A summary of the interrelationship between glucose metabolism and palmitate synthesis is shown in Figure 16.9.

1. The following points are illustrated in Figure 16.9. (The numbers in brackets below refer to the corresponding numbers on the figure.)

   [1]: The glycolytic pathway produces both pyruvate, which is the primary source of the mitochondrial acetyl CoA to be used for fatty acid synthesis, and the cytoplasmic reducing equivalents of NADH (see p. 114 for pathway details).

   [2]: Oxaloacetate (OAA) is produced by the first step in the gluconeogenic pathway (see p. 125) for pathway details).

   [3]: Acetyl CoA is produced in the mitochondria and condenses with OAA to form citrate, the first step in the tricarboxylic acid cycle (see p. 135 for pathway details).

   [4]: Citrate leaves the mitochondria and is cleaved in the cytoplasm to produce cytoplasmic acetyl CoA (see p. 161).

   [5]: Cytoplasmic reducing equivalents (NADH) produced during glycolysis contribute to the reduction of $NADP^+$ to NADPH needed for palmitoyl CoA synthesis (see p. 165).

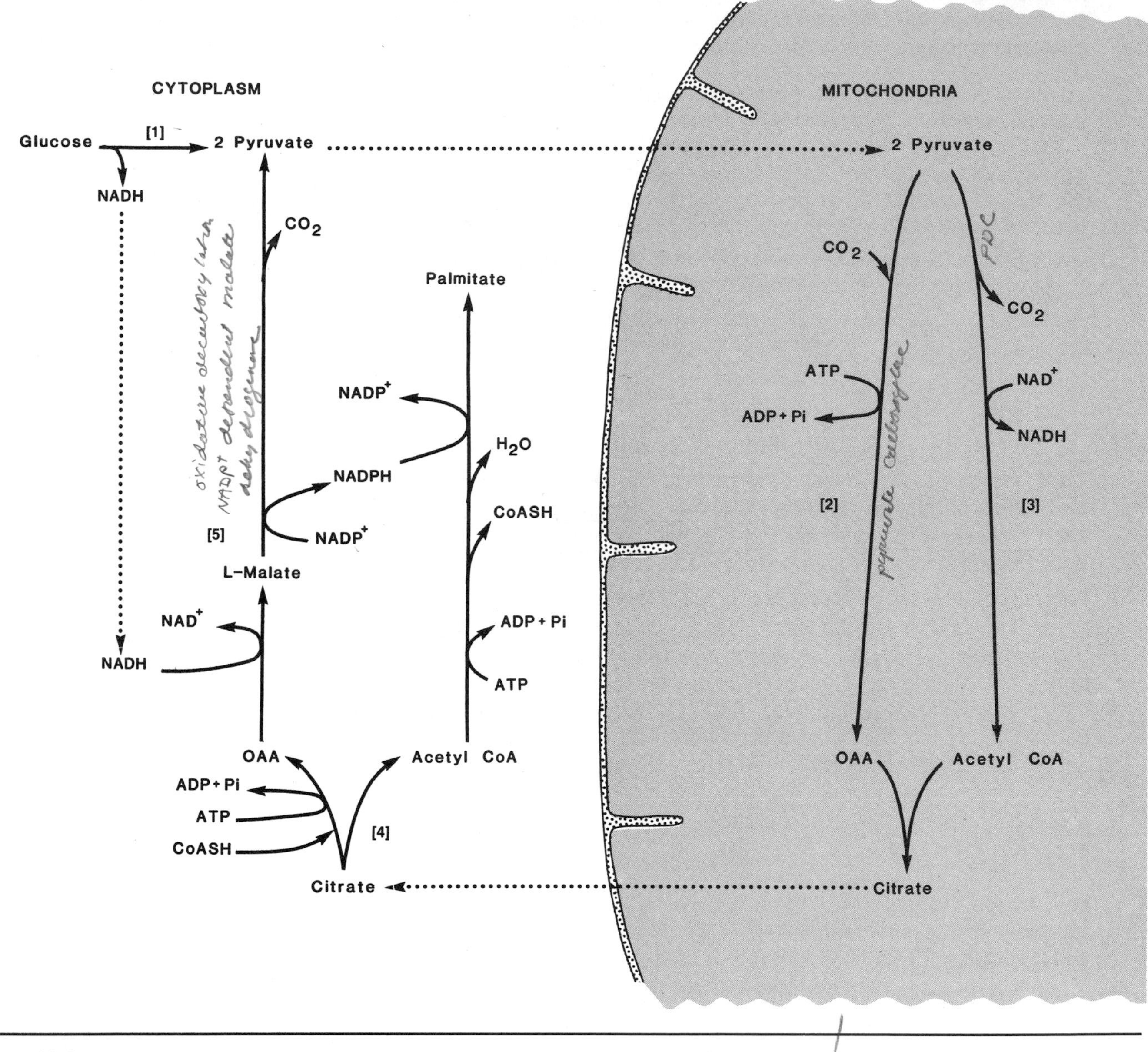

Figure 16.9
Interrelationship between glucose metabolism and palmitate synthesis. (The numbers in brackets on the figure refer to the corresponding numbers in the text.)

F. Regulation of fatty acid synthesis

1. ***Short-term control*** of fatty acid synthesis is accomplished by allosteric modifiers of synthetic enzymes. Two of the most important regulated synthetic enzymes are the following:
   a. *Acetyl CoA carboxylase*, which is activated by citrate and inhibited by malonyl CoA and palmitoyl CoA (see p. 162).
   b. *Fatty acid synthase*, which is also inhibited by palmitoyl CoA.
2. ***Long-term control*** of fatty acid synthesis is accomplished by regulating the synthesis of active enzymes: The synthesis of *acetyl CoA carboxylase*, *fatty acid synthase*, *citrate lyase*, *glucose 6-*

phosphate dehydrogenase, and the *malic enzyme* is decreased during fasting and increases dramatically when glucose is again available in the diet. Fat-free diets also lead to elevation of the levels of these enzymes, resulting in increased fatty acid synthesis.

G. Further elongation and desaturation of fatty acid chains

1. Although palmitate, a 16-carbon, fully saturated fatty acid, is the end product of the *fatty acid synthase* complex, the fatty acid chain itself can be further elongated and desaturated by separate enzymic processes. The enzymes involved are located in the mitochondria and endoplasmic reticulum and can use fatty acids of varying chain lengths and degrees of unsaturation as substrates. Humans lack the ability to introduce double bonds beyond that between carbons 9 and 10, and therefore must have the polyunsaturated fats linoleic and linolenic acid provided by the diet (see Table 16.1 for their structures).

H. Fatty acids are stored as components of triacylglycerol

1. ***Structure and storage of triacylglycerol:***

   a. Monoacylglycerols, diacylglycerols, and triacylglycerols (formerly called -glycerides, e.g., triglycerides) consist of one, two, or three molecules of fatty acid esterified to a molecule of glycerol. Fatty acids are esterified through their carboxyl groups, resulting in a loss of negative charge and formation of "neutral fat."

   b. The fatty acids on one glycerol molecule are usually not of the same type. The fatty acid on carbon #1 is usually saturated, the fatty acid on carbon #2 is usually unsaturated, and the fatty acid on carbon #3 can be either. The presence of the unsaturated fatty acid(s) decreases the melting temperature of the lipid. An example of a triacylglycerol molecule is shown in Figure 16.10.

   c. If a species of acylglycerol is solid at room temperature, it is called "fat"; if liquid, it is called "oil."

   d. Because triacylglycerols are only slightly soluble in water and cannot form stable micelles by themselves, they coalesce within adipocytes to form oily droplets that are nearly anhydrous. These lipid droplets are the major energy reserve of the body.

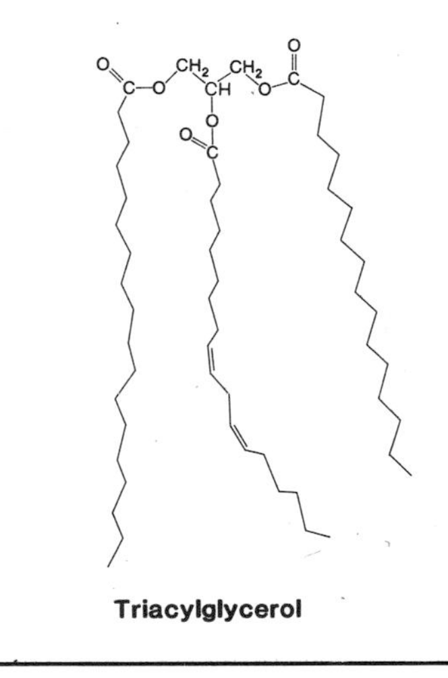

Figure 16.10
A triacylglycerol.

I. Synthesis of triacylglycerol

1. ***Synthesis of glycerol 3-phosphate:***

   a. There are two pathways for glycerol 3-phosphate production (Figure 16.11): First, in ***both adipose and liver cells*** (the primary sites of fatty acid synthesis), glycerol 3-phosphate can be produced from glucose, utilizing first the reactions of the glycolytic pathway to produce dihydroxyacetone phosphate (DHAP) (see p. 114). Next, the DHAP is reduced by *glycerol 3-phosphate dehydrogenase* to glycerol 3-phosphate (Figure 16.11).

   b. A second pathway found in the ***liver*** but NOT in the adipose converts free glycerol to glycerol 3-phosphate by *glycerol kinase* (Figure 16.11).

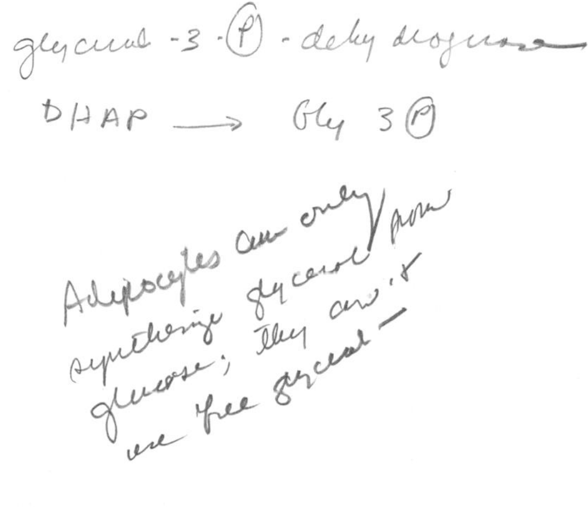

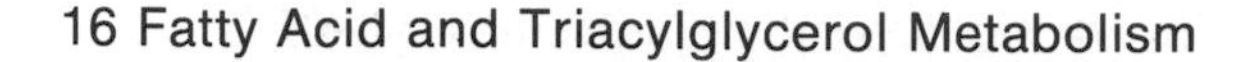

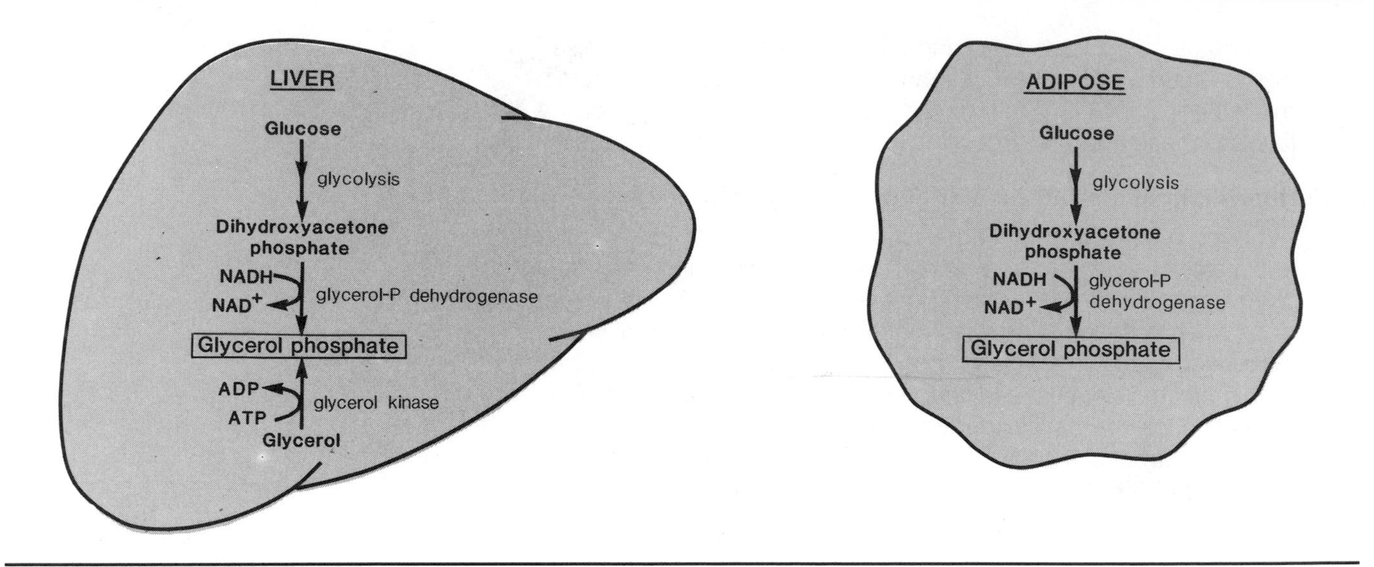

Figure 16.11
Pathways for production of glycerol 3-phosphate in liver and adipose.

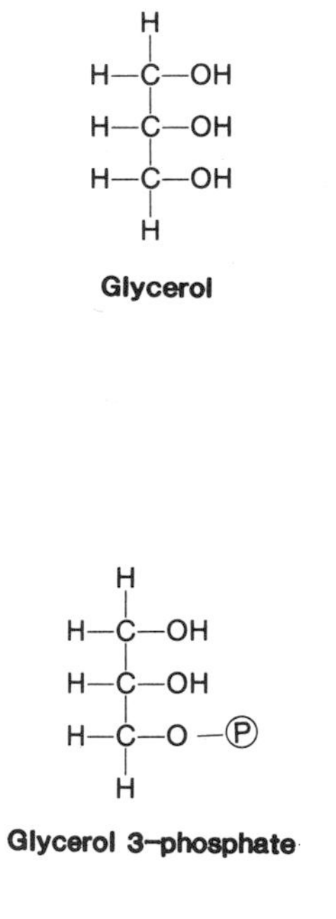

c. Adipocytes can take up glucose only in the presence of the hormone insulin (see p. 268). Thus when serum glucose—and therefore serum insulin—levels are low, adipocytes cannot synthesize glycerol 3-phosphate and cannot produce triacylglycerol.

2. ***Conversion of a free fatty acid to its activated form:***

   a. A free fatty acid must be converted to its activated form (attached to coenzyme A) before it can participate in triacylglycerol synthesis. This reaction is illustrated in Figure 15.9 and is catalyzed by *fatty acyl CoA synthetase (thiokinase)*.

3. ***Synthesis of a molecule of triacylglycerol from glycerol 3-phosphate and fatty acyl CoA:***

   a. This pathway involves four reactions, shown in Figure 16.12. These include the sequential addition of two fatty acids from fatty acyl CoA, the removal of phosphate, and the addition of the final fatty acid.

J. Different fates of triacylglycerol in the liver and adipose tissue

1. In the adipose, triacylglycerol is stored in the cytoplasm of the cells in a nearly anhydrous form. It serves as "depot fat," ready for mobilization when the body requires it for fuel.

2. In the liver, the triacylglycerol is combined with cholesterol and cholesterol esters, phospholipid, and protein to form lipoprotein particles called ***very low density lipoproteins (VLDL)***. These are secreted into the blood and deliver the newly synthesized lipids to the peripheral tissues (see discussion of serum lipoproteins on p. 210.)

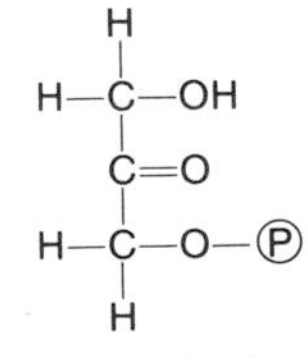

Study Questions

Choose the ONE best answer:

16.5 If radioactively labeled carbon dioxide ($^{14}CO_2$) is used to make malonyl

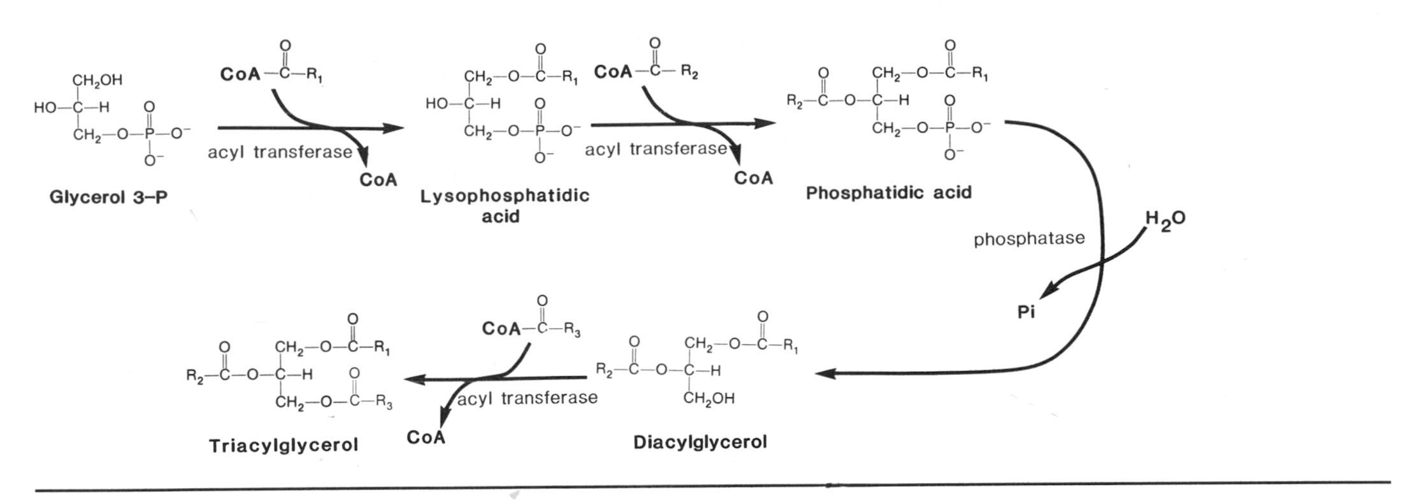

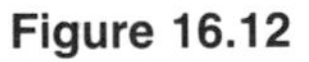

Figure 16.12
Synthesis of triacylglycerol.

CoA from acetyl CoA, and if the labeled malonyl CoA is then used in fatty acid biosynthesis, which positions in the fatty acid would be labeled?

A. Only the carbonyl carbon (carbon #1)
B. All odd-numbered carbons
C. All even-numbered carbons
D. Only the methyl terminal carbon
E. None of the carbons

16.6 The formation of fatty acids from malonyl CoA

A. is stimulated by citrate.
B. directly requires biotin as a cofactor.
C. uses NADPH as a reductant.
D. requires FAD as an oxidant.
E. requires ATP.

Answer A if 1, 2, and 3 are correct
B if 1 and 3 are correct
C if 2 and 4 are correct
D if only 4 is correct
E if all are correct

16.7 Characteristics of acetyl CoA carboxylase include which of the following?

1. Biotin is an essential cofactor.
2. Citrate catalyzes the polymerization of the enzyme into its active form.
3. It synthesizes malonyl CoA from acetyl CoA.
4. It is found in the tricarboxylic acid cycle.

16.8 Substances that play a direct role in the synthesis of palmitate by the fatty acid synthetase complex include

1. covalently bound phosphopantetheine.
2. covalently bound lipoic acid.
3. malonyl CoA.
4. thiamine pyrophosphate.

16.9 When glucose is converted to triacylglycerol in adipose tissue,

1. citrate serves to transport acetyl units across the mitochondrial membrane.
2. some reducing equivalents required for this synthesis are provided by the reactions in glycolysis.
3. CO_2 is a participant.
4. free glycerol is not an intermediate.

IV. MOBILIZATION OF STORED FATS AND OXIDATION OF FATTY ACIDS

Fatty acids stored in the adipose tissue in the form of neutral triacylglycerol serve as the body's major fuel storage depot. Triacylglycerols provide concentrated stores of metabolic energy because they are highly reduced and stored in an anhydrous state. The yield from the complete oxidation of fatty acids to CO_2 and H_2O is 9 kcal/g of fat (as compared to 4 kcal/g of protein or carbohydrate).

A. Release of fatty acids from triacylglycerol

1. The mobilization of stored fat is initiated by the release of free fatty acids from their triacylglycerol storage form. The three fatty acids are hydrolytically removed from triacylglycerol, releasing free glycerol. This process is initiated by *hormone-sensitive lipase*, which removes a fatty acid from either C1 or C3 of the triacylglycerol. Additional *lipases* specific for monoacylglycerol or diacylglycerol degradation remove the remaining fatty acids.
   a. *Hormone-sensitive lipase* is activated when phosphorylated by a *3′,5′-cyclic AMP-dependent protein kinase*. The process is similar to that of the activation of *glycogen phosphorylase* (see Figure 7.7 on p. 75).
   b. 3′,5′-Cyclic AMP is produced in the adipocyte when hormones, including epinephrine and glucagon, bind to receptors on the cell membrane and activate *adenyl cyclase* (Figure 16.13).

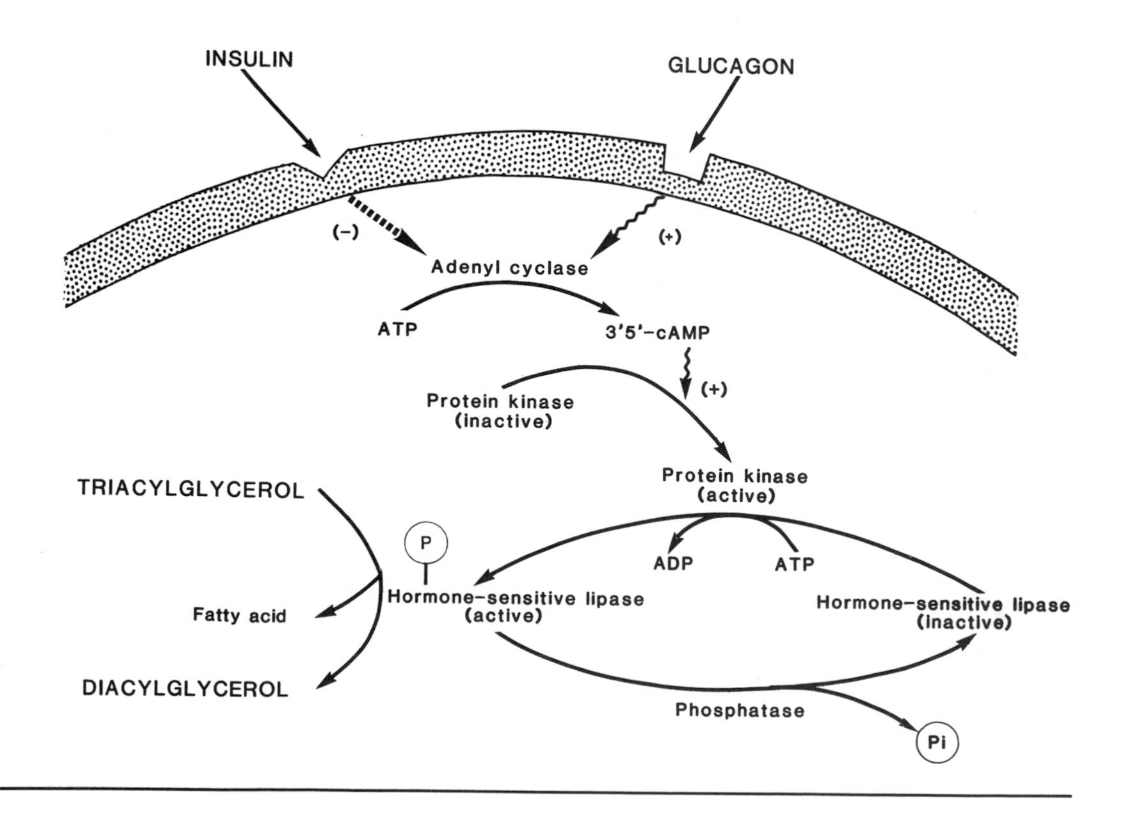

Figure 16.13
Hormonal regulation of triacylglycerol degradation in the adipocyte. Wavy lines (~~~) in figure indicate the process of activation; dashed lines (▪▪▪▪▪▪) indicate inactivation.

c. *Hormone-sensitive lipase* is not active in the presence of high serum levels of insulin and glucose.

d. A summary table of lipases is on p. 217.

2. The ***glycerol*** released by the action of the lipases cannot be metabolized by adipose cells which do not contain the enzyme *glycerol kinase*. Rather, glycerol is transported through the blood to the liver, which can phosphorylate glycerol. The resulting glycerol 3-phosphate can then be used to form triacylglycerol in the liver or can be converted to dihydroxyacetone phosphate (DHAP) by the reversal of the *glycerol dehydrogenase* reaction illustrated in Figure 16.11. DHAP can participate in either glycolysis or gluconeogenesis.

3. The ***free (unesterified) fatty acid*** moves through the cell membrane of the adipocyte and immediately binds to a molecule of albumin. The albumin carries the fatty acid through the blood to the tissues, where the fatty acid diffuses into the cells and is oxidized for energy; however, the brain and other nervous tissue, erythrocytes, and the adrenal medulla cannot use fatty acids for fuel regardless of the blood levels of fatty acid.

B. β-Oxidation of fatty acids

The major pathway for catabolism of saturated fatty acids is called β-oxidation, in which two-carbon fragments are successively removed from the carboxyl end of the fatty acid, producing acetyl CoA.

1. After the free fatty acid is taken up by a cell, the first step that occurs is its conversion to a CoA derivative. This reaction is catalyzed by *fatty acyl CoA synthetase (thiokinase)*, which was discussed on p. 152.

2. β-Oxidation occurs in the ***mitochondria;*** thus the fatty acid must be transported across the mitochondrial inner membrane. This membrane is generally impermeable to bulky, polar molecules such as coenzyme A. Therefore, a specialized carrier located in the inner membrane transports the acyl group from the cytoplasm into the mitochondrion. This carrier is ***carnitine,*** and the transport process is called the ***carnitine shuttle*** (Figure 16.14).

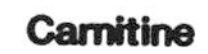

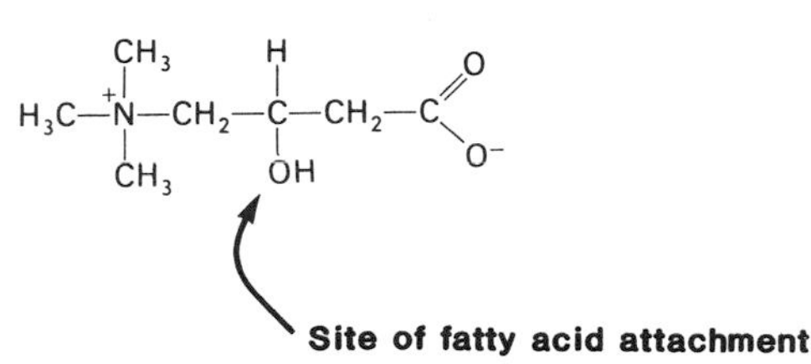

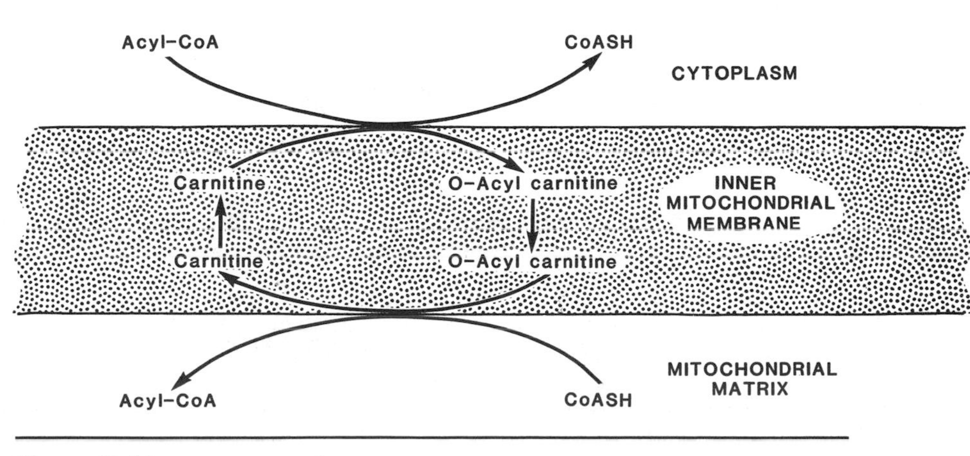

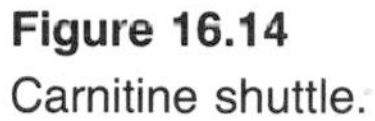

Figure 16.14
Carnitine shuttle.

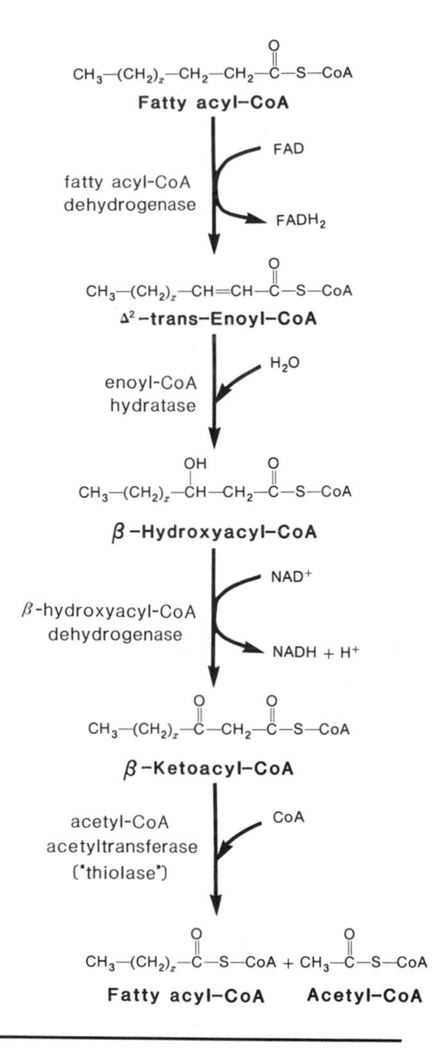

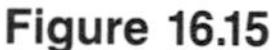

Figure 16.15
Initial steps in the β-oxidation of palmitic acid.

a. First an acyl group is transferred from the cytoplasmic coenzyme A to carnitine by *carnitine acyltransferase I*, forming O-acyl carnitine.

b. Second, the acyl group is then transported across the membrane to the mitochondrial matrix, where it is transferred to another molecule of coenzyme A by *carnitine acyl transferase II*.

c. Malonyl CoA inhibits *carnitine acyltransferase I*, thus inhibiting the entry of acyl groups into the mitochondria. Therefore, when fatty acid synthesis is occurring in the cytoplasm (as indicated by the presence of malonyl CoA, the building block of fatty acids), the newly made fatty acid chains cannot be transferred into the mitochondria and degraded.

d. The congenital absence of a *carnitine acyltransferase* in skeletal muscle or low concentrations of carnitine caused by defective synthesis result in an inability to use long-chain fatty acids as a metabolic fuel. This is an example whereby the impaired flow of a metabolite from one cell compartment to another results in a disease.

3. The steps in ***β-oxidation,*** the first cycle of which is shown in Figure 16.15, are a recurring sequence of four reactions that result in the shortening of the carbon chain by two carbons. The steps include an oxidation step that produces $FADH_2$, dehydration, a second oxidation step that produces NADH, and finally a thiolytic cleavage that releases a molecule of acetyl CoA. The last step is physiologically irreversible.

4. These four steps are repeated for saturated fatty acids of even-numbered carbon chains $(n/2) - 1$ times (where n is the number of carbons), each cycle producing an acetyl group plus one NADH and one $FADH_2$.

For example, the oxidation of a molecule of palmitoyl CoA to CO_2 and H_2O yields the following number of ATPs:

	ATP Yield
a. From palmitoyl CoA to 8 acetyl CoA:	
7 NADH which will each provide 3 ATP when oxidized by the electron transport chain (see p. 106):	21
7 $FADH_2$ which will each provide 2 ATP when oxidized by the electron transport chain (see p. 104):	14
b. The 8 acetyl CoA will each provide 12 ATP when converted to CO_2 and H_2O by the TCA cycle (see p. 140):	96
c. Total energy yield from one molecule of palmitoyl CoA:	131

(Note: When starting with the free fatty acid palmitate, the ATP required for the production of the palmitoyl CoA must be taken into consideration—two high-energy bonds are broken as a result of the thiokinase reaction—and therefore the total energy yield is only 129 ATP.)

5. The β-oxidation of a saturated fatty acid with an ***uneven*** number of carbon atoms proceeds by the same reaction steps as that of fatty acids with an even number of carbon atoms, until the final three carbons are reached. This compound, ***propionyl CoA,*** is metabolized by the following two-step pathway (Figure 16.16).
   a. First, propionyl CoA (3 carbons) is carboxylated, forming methylmalonyl CoA. The enzyme *propionyl CoA carboxylase* has an absolute requirement for the cofactor ***biotin,*** as do the other carboxylases (see pp. 127 and 317).
   b. Next, the carbons of methylmalonyl are rearranged, forming succinyl CoA, which can enter the tricarboxylic acid cycle (see p. 138). The enzyme *methylmalonyl CoA mutase* requires vitamin B_{12} for its action. (In patients with vitamin B_{12} deficiency, both propionate and methylmalonate are excreted in the urine; see p. 319 for a further discussion of vitamin B_{12}.)
   c. Two types of ***inheritable methylmalonic acidemia*** and ***aciduria*** have been described: one in which the *mutase* is missing, and the other in which the patient cannot convert the vitamin B_{12} into its coenzyme form.
6. The oxidation of unsaturated fatty acids provides less energy than that of the saturated fatty acids because they are less highly reduced, and therefore fewer reducing equivalents can be produced from these structures.

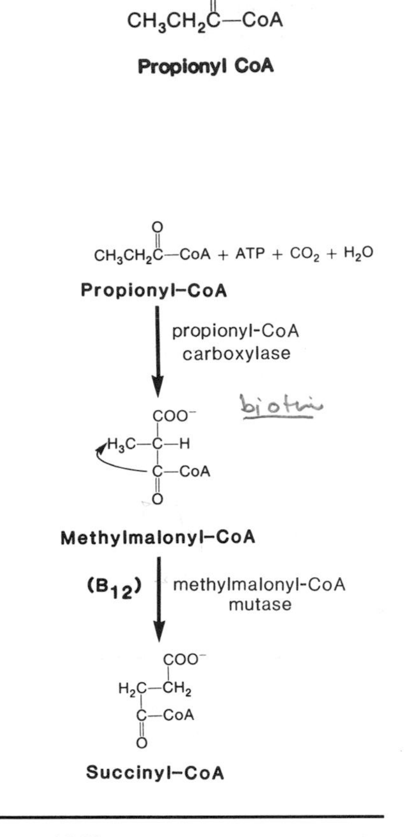

Figure 16.16
Metabolism of propionyl CoA.

C. A summary comparison of the processes of fatty acid synthesis and degradation is provided in Table 16.2.

Study Questions

Choose the ONE best answer

16.10 The lipolysis of triacylglycerol in adipose tissue leads to the formation of

A. glycerol 3-phosphate, which leaves the adipose cell and is metabolized by the liver.
B. glycerol, which is converted to glycerol 3-phosphate in the fat cell.
C. glycerol, which is converted to glucose in the liver.
D. glycerol, which is oxidized by muscle.
E. glycerol 3-phosphate, which is converted to glucose in the fat cell.

16.11 Which one of the following best describes the number of ATPs produced by the oxidation of palmitic acid to CO_2 and H_2O?

A. 40 ATP
B. 70 ATP
C. 100 ATP
D. 130 ATP
E. 160 ATP

Answer A if 1, 2, and 3 are correct
B if 1 and 3 are correct
C if 2 and 4 are correct
D if only 4 is correct
E if all are correct

16.12 Among the differences between fatty acid synthesis and fatty acid oxidation are the fact(s) that

1. synthesis uses NADPH and oxidation uses NAD^+ as a cofactor.
2. synthesis is accelerated and oxidation depressed in the presence of insulin.
3. malonyl CoA is an intermediate in synthesis but not in oxidation.
4. synthesis occurs in the mitochondria whereas oxidation occurs in the cytoplasm.

16.13 Propionyl CoA

1. arises from the oxidation of a fatty acid with an odd number of carbon atoms.
2. enters the tricarboxylic acid cycle after being converted to succinyl CoA.
3. metabolism is affected in patients with vitamin B_{12} deficiency.
4. is a direct precursor of acetyl CoA.

16.14 In humans, carnitine

1. stimulates the activity of acetyl CoA carboxylase.
2. is important for fatty acid oxidation.
3. inhibits the formation of triacylglycerol.
4. cannot serve its function in the presence of malonyl CoA.

TABLE 16.2

SUMMARY OF FATTY ACID SYNTHESIS AND DEGRADATION

	SYNTHESIS	DEGRADATION
Greatest flux through pathway	After carbohydrate-rich meal	In starvation
Hormonal state favoring pathway	High insulin/glucagon ratio	Low insulin/glucagon ratio
Major tissue site	Adipose, liver	Muscle, liver
Subcellular location	Primarily cytoplasm	Primarily mitochondria
Carriers of acyl/acetyl groups between mitochondria and cytoplasm	Citrate (mitochondria to cytoplasm)	Carnitine (cytoplasm to mitochondria)
Phosphopantetheine-containing active carriers	Acyl carrier protein, Coenzyme A	Coenzyme A
Oxidation/reduction cofactors	NADPH	NAD^+, FAD
Two-carbon donor/product	Malonyl CoA: donor	Acetyl CoA: product
Activator	Citrate	
Inhibitor	Fatty acyl CoA (inhibits acetyl CoA carboxylase)	Malonyl CoA (inhibits carnitine acyl transferase)
Product of pathway	Palmitate	Acetyl CoA

V. SPECIALIZED FATTY ACIDS: PROSTAGLANDINS AND RELATED COMPOUNDS

Prostaglandins, and the related compounds ***thromboxanes*** and ***leukotrienes,*** are extremely potent compounds that elicit a wide range of physiologic responses. These compounds have been very difficult to study because they have an extremely short half-life and are produced in extremely small amounts. Although they have been compared to hormones in terms of their actions, prostaglandins differ from the true hormones in that they are formed in almost all tissues rather than in specialized glands and they generally act locally rather than by circulating in the blood to distant sites of action. Prostaglandins are metabolized to inactive products at their site of synthesis and are not stored in any tissues to an appreciable extent. Examples of prostaglandin structures are shown in Figure 16.17.

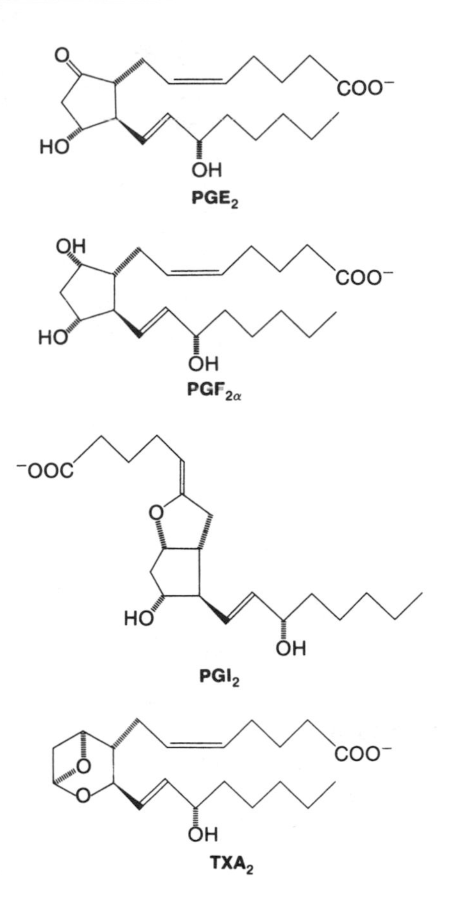

Figure 16.17
Examples of prostaglandin structures. Prostaglandins are named as follows: PG plus a third letter (e.g., A, E, D, F), which corresponds to the type and arrangement of functional groups in the molecule. The subscript number indicates the number of double bonds in the molecule. Thromboxanes are designated by TX and leukotrienes by LT.

A. Synthesis of prostaglandins

1. The dietary precursor of the prostaglandins is the essential fatty acid ***linoleic acid*** (18 carbons, 2 double bonds). It is converted to the immediate precursors of the prostaglandins—20-carbon, polyunsaturated fatty acids containing 3, 4, or 5 double bonds. ***Arachidonic acid*** (20:5, 8, 11, 14) (see Figure 16.3) is the precursor of the predominant classes of prostaglandins.
2. The first step in the synthesis of prostaglandins is the oxidation and cyclization of arachidonic acid to yield PGG_2 and PGH_2 (Figure 16.18). This is catalyzed by the *prostaglandin endoperoxide synthase complex*—a microsomal enzyme with two catalytic activities:
   a. *Fatty acid cyclooxygenase*, which requires two molecules of O_2.
   b. *Peroxidase*, which is dependent on reduced glutathione. (A further discussion of glutathione is presented on p. 146.)
3. PGH_2 is the precursor for a number of prostaglandins and thromboxanes, as shown in Figure 16.19.
4. The synthesis of prostaglandins can be inhibited by a number of unrelated compounds:
   a. ***Cortisol*** inhibits phospholipase A_2 activity, and thus the precursor of the prostaglandins, arachidonic acid, is not available.
   b. ***Aspirin, indomethacin,*** and ***phenylbutazone*** (all anti-inflammatory agents) inhibit *prostaglandin endoperoxide synthase*, and therefore prevent the synthesis of the parent prostaglandins, PGG_2 and PGH_2. These agents do not affect the synthesis of the leukotrienes.

B. Synthesis of leukotrienes

1. Arachidonic acid is converted to a variety of hydroperoxy acids by a separate pathway that involves a family of enzymes called *lipoxygenases*. For example, neutrophils contain *5-lipoxygenase*, which converts arachidonic acid to 5-hydroperoxy-6,8,11,14 eicosatetraenoic acid (5-HPETE, Figure 16.19).
2. 5-HPETE is converted to a series of leukotrienes, the nature of the final products varying according to the tissue.
3. In contrast to prostaglandin synthesis, no drugs are known that specifically inhibit the lipoxygenase pathway.

C. Biological actions of prostaglandins, thromboxanes, and leukotrienes

1. The biological actions of prostaglandins are different in each organ system (Figure 16.20). Excess production of prostaglandins

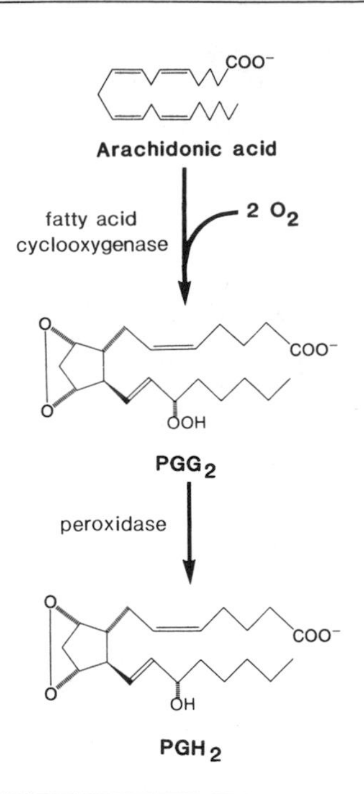

Figure 16.18
Oxidation and cyclization of arachidonic acid.

results in a diverse group of symptoms, including pain, inflammation, fever, nausea, and vomiting.

2. Two prostaglandins are particularly important in hemostasis. Prostacyclin (PGI_2), produced by the endothelial cells of the blood vessels, acts to inhibit platelet aggregation. In the healthy vascular system this action of PGI_2 prevents the formation of unwanted clots or thrombi. If the vascular endothelium is damaged, circulating platelets aggregate at the site of injury. This clumping of platelets is accompanied by the release of a number of compounds from the platelets, including thromboxane A_2 (TXA_2). TXA_2 promotes the further aggregation of platelets. Thus, the tendency of platelets to aggregate is determined by the balance between the opposing effect of TXA_2 produced by platelets and PGI_2 synthesized by the endothelial cells.

3. Leukotrienes appear to be mediators of allergic reactions and inflammation. Leukotrienes C_4, D_4, and E_4 are potent bronchoconstrictors, increase vascular permeability, and stimulate mucus secretion. LKB_4 causes chemotactic movement of leukocytes and stimulates aggregation, enzyme release, and the generation of superoxides in neutrophils.

Study Questions

Choose the ONE best answer

16.15 Which one of the following statements about prostaglandins is ***incorrect***?

A. Prostaglandins have a very short half-life.
B. Prostaglandins are synthesized only in the liver and the adrenal cortex.
C. Prostaglandins generally act locally on or near the tissue that produced them.
D. The common precursor of the prostaglandins is arachidonic acid.
E. Prostaglandin synthesis can be inhibited by a number of unrelated compounds, including cortisol and aspirin.

16.16 Which of the following has as one of its major effect the ability to inhibit platelet aggregation?

A. Leukotriene A_4
B. Prostacyclin
C. Thromboxane A_2
D. Prostaglandin H_2
E. Arachidonic acid

VI. KETONE BODIES: AN ALTERNATE FUEL FOR CELLS

A. Structure and physiologic role of ketone bodies

1. The liver has the enzymatic capacity to divert any excess acetyl CoA derived from fatty acid or pyruvate oxidation into ***ketone bodies***. They are transported by the blood to the peripheral tissues, where they can be reconverted to acetyl CoA, and oxidized by means of the TCA cycle (see p. 133).

2. The compounds categorized as ketone bodies are ***acetoacetate***, ***β-hydroxybutyrate***, and ***acetone*** (a nonmetabolizable side product).

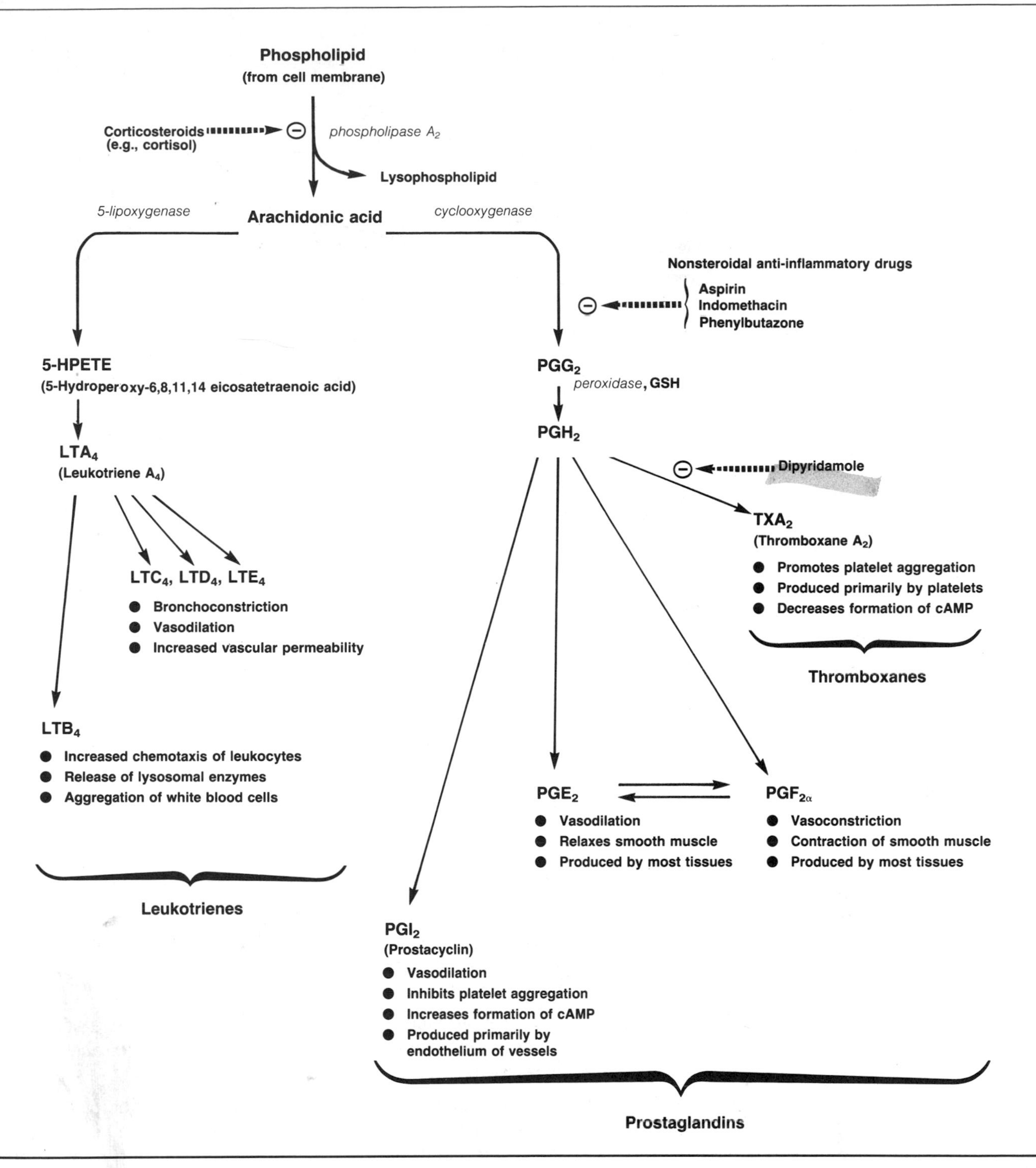

Figure 16.19
Biosynthesis of prostaglandins, thromboxanes, and leukotrienes from arachidonic acid.

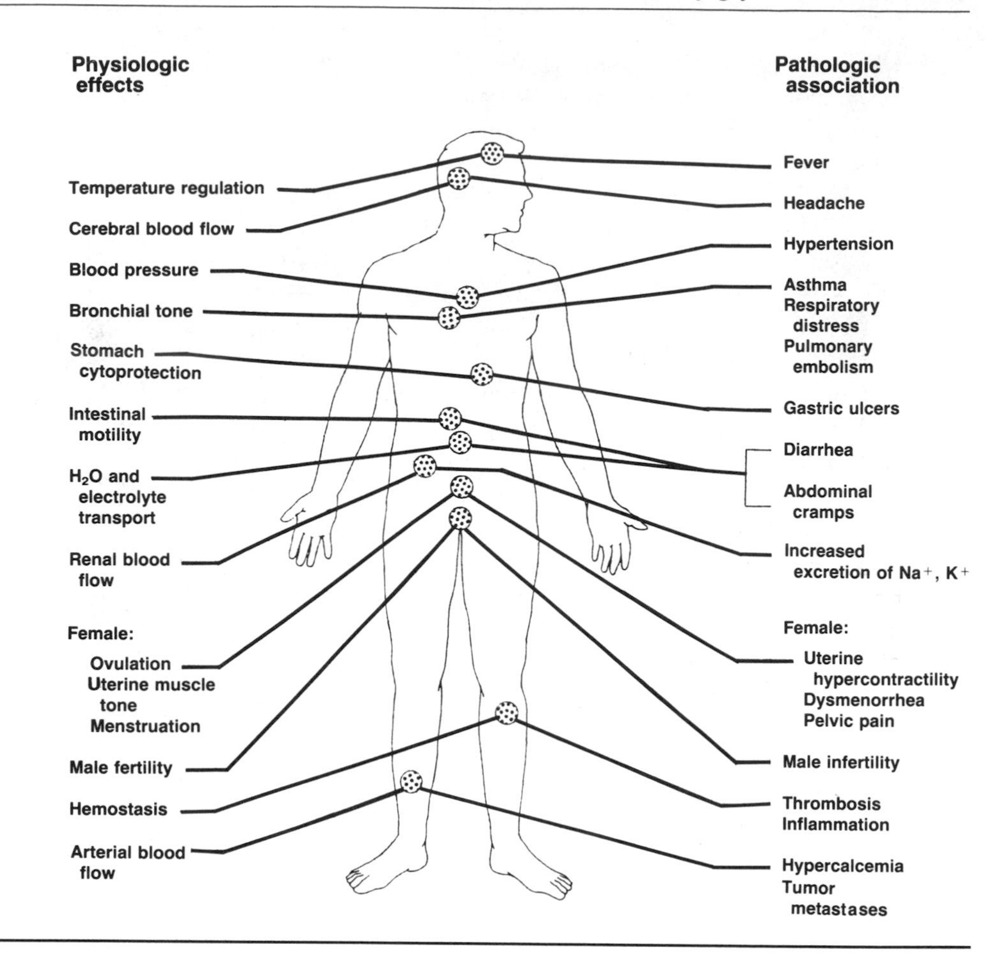

Figure 16.20
Summary of physiologic and pathologic effects of prostaglandins.

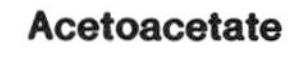

Acetoacetate

3. Ketone bodies are important sources of energy for the peripheral tissues for a number of reasons:
   a. They are soluble in aqueous solution, and therefore do not need to be incorporated in lipoproteins or carried by albumin as do the other lipids.
   b. They are produced in the liver in response to elevated levels of acetyl CoA during periods when the amount of acetyl CoA exceeds the oxidative capacity of the liver.
   c. They are used in extrahepatic tissues in proportion to their concentration in the blood. Even the ***brain*** can use ketone bodies for fuel if the level rises sufficiently. (This is important during prolonged periods of fasting—see p. 288).

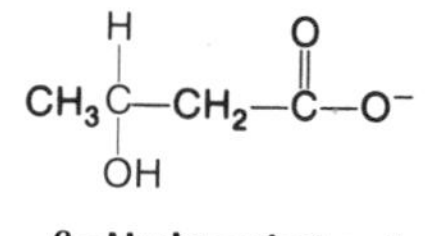

β-Hydroxybutyrate

B. Synthesis of ketone bodies by the liver

1. The first step, formation of acetoacetyl CoA, can occur by one of two processes:
   a. the incomplete breakdown of fatty acid.
   b. the reversal of the *thiolase* reaction of fatty acid oxidation (Figure 16.21).

2. Next, a third molecule of acetyl CoA can combine with the acetoacetyl CoA to produce ***3-hydroxy-3-methylglutaryl CoA*** (HMG CoA) (Figure 16.21). (Note: HMG-CoA is also a structural intermediate in the catabolism of the amino acid leucine [see Figure 21.12, p. 251], and a precursor of cholesterol [see Figure 19.3, p. 201]. This enzyme, *HMG-CoA synthase*, is the rate-limiting step in the synthesis of ketone bodies and is present in significant quantities only in the liver.
3. Finally, HMG CoA is cleaved to produce acetoacetate and acetyl CoA, as shown in Figure 16.21.
4. Acetoacetate can be converted into the other two ketone bodies as shown in Figure 16.21. It can be reduced to β-hydroxybutyrate with NADH as the hydrogen donor, or spontaneously decarboxylated to form acetone.
5. Release of ketone bodies by the liver is an ongoing process. These compounds are usually found in the blood at concentrations below 3 mg/dl because they are removed and used efficiently for fuel by skeletal and cardiac muscle, the renal cortex, and other peripheral tissues. Their production becomes much more significant in providing energy to the peripheral tissues during starvation.

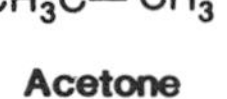

C. Use of ketone bodies by the peripheral tissues

1. Although the liver actively produces ketone bodies, it cannot reconvert acetoacetate to acetoacetyl CoA, and therefore cannot itself use them as fuels. Extrahepatic tissues, however, perform the following reactions:
   a. β-Hydroxybutyrate is reoxidized to acetoacetate by *β-hydroxybutyrate dehydrogenase*, producing NADH.
   b. Acetoacetate receives a coenzyme A molecule from succinyl CoA as shown in Figure 16.22. This reaction is reversible, but the product, acetoacetyl CoA, is actively removed by its conversion to two acetyl CoA. The liver lacks *succinyl-CoA-acetoacetate-CoA transferase* (*thiophorase*), and therefore cannot use acetoacetate as a fuel.
2. When the rate of formation of ketone bodies is greater than the rate of their use, their levels begin to rise in the blood ***(ketonemia)*** and eventually in the urine ***(ketonuria)***. These two conditions are seen most often in cases of starvation or severe diabetes mellitus.
   a. In diabetic individuals with severe ketosis, urinary excretion of ketone bodies may be as high as 5000 mg/24 hours and the blood concentration may reach 90 mg/dl (versus less than 3 mg/dl in normal individuals).

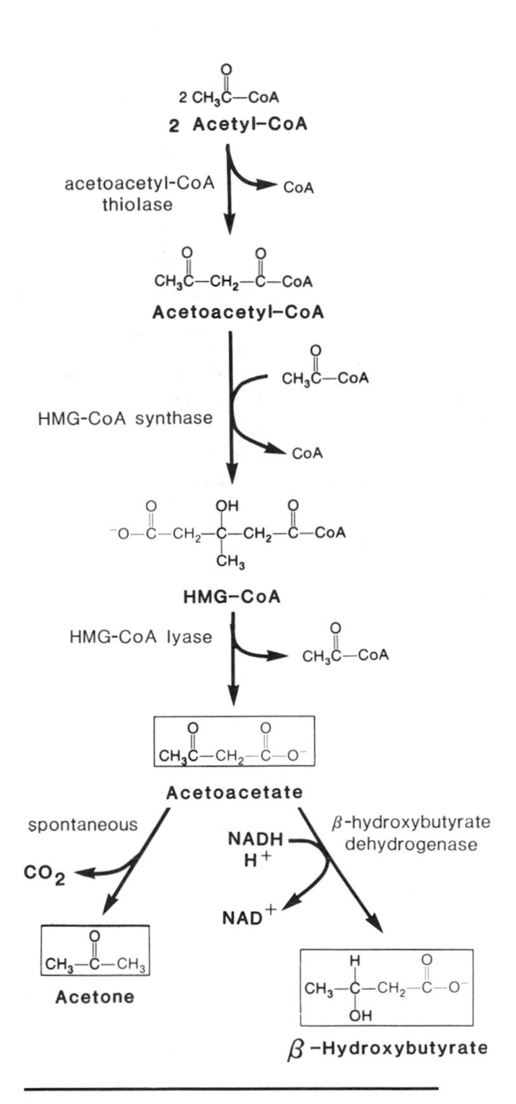

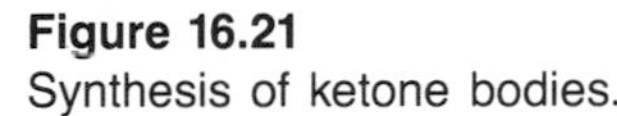

Figure 16.21
Synthesis of ketone bodies.

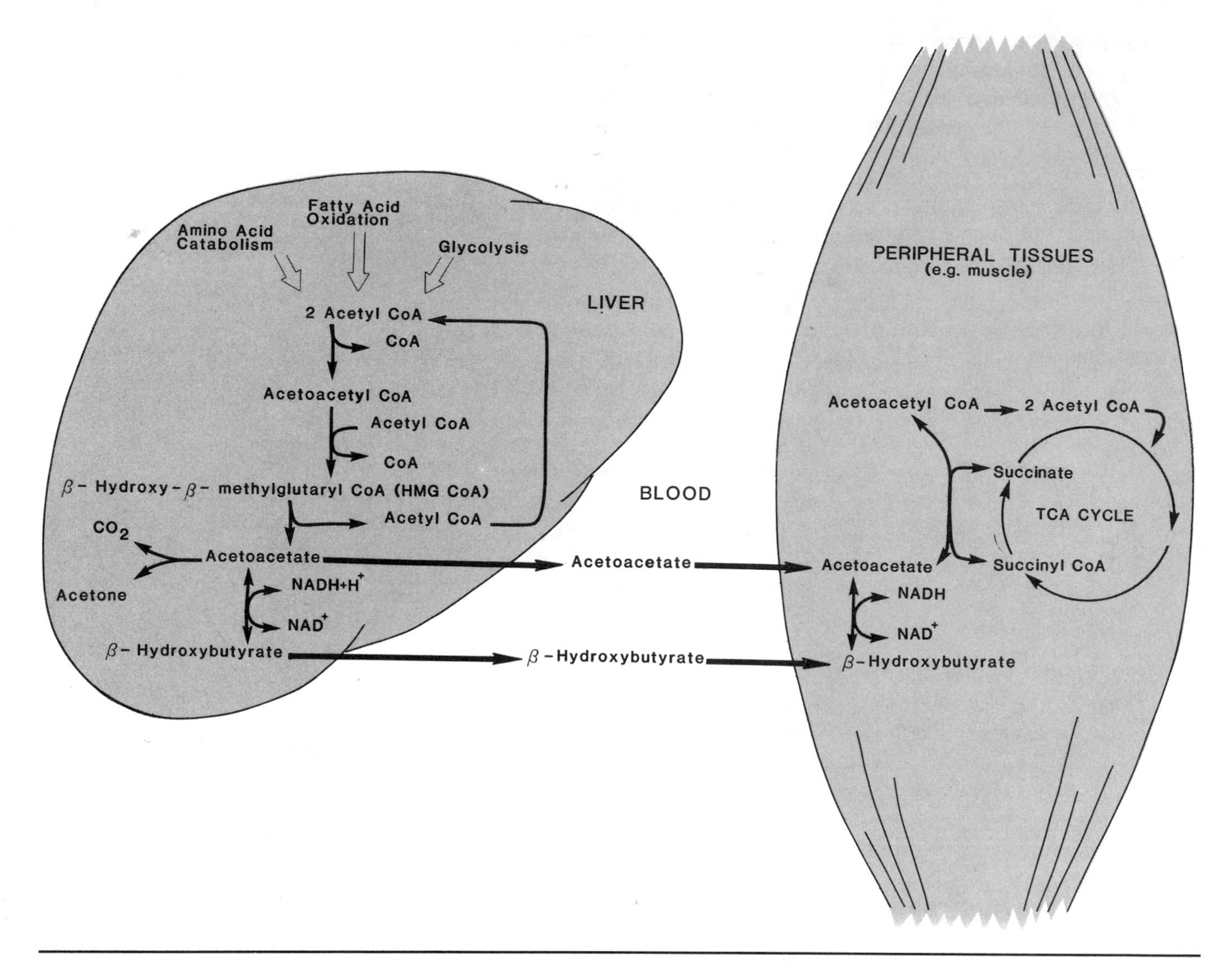

Figure 16.22
Use of ketone bodies.

b. An elevation of ketone bodies in the blood results in the following: The carboxyl group of a ketone body has a pK_a around 4. Therefore, each ketone will lose a proton (H^+) as it circulates in the blood, which will lower the pH of the body. Also, excretion of excess ketone bodies results in an increased dehydration of the body. (They are hydrophilic compounds that increase the rate of water loss when they are excreted in the urine). Therefore, the increased number of H^+, circulating in a decreased volume of plasma, can cause a severe acidosis ("ketoacidosis").

Study Questions

Choose the ONE best answer

16.17 In the major pathway by which liver produces ketone bodies, the immediate precursor of acetoacetate is

A. acetoacetyl CoA.
B. β-hydroxybutyrate.
C. 3-hydroxy-3-methylglutaryl CoA.
D. two molecules of acetyl CoA.
E. malonyl CoA.

16.18 Which one of the following statements about use of ketone bodies as a fuel by the body is ***incorrect***?

A. They are soluble in aqueous solution and therefore do not require carriers in the blood.
B. They are made in response to elevated levels of fatty acids in the liver, where the amount of acetyl CoA exceeds the oxidative capacity of the liver.
C. Acetone is not used by the body as a fuel.
D. Unlike fatty acids, they can be oxidized by the brain.
E. When plasma ketone body levels are elevated, the liver efficiently oxidizes them for energy.

Phospholipid Metabolism

17

I. OVERVIEW

Phospholipids are polar, ionic compounds composed of an alcohol that is attached by a phosphodiester bridge to either diacylglycerol or sphingosine. Like fatty acids, phospholipids are ***amphipathic*** in nature: Each has a hydrophilic head (the phosphate group plus whatever is attached to it—e.g., serine, ethanolamine, choline) and a long, hydrophobic tail (made of two fatty acid chains). The hydrophobic portions of the molecules are associated with other nonpolar compounds of membranes, including glycolipids, protein, and cholesterol. The hydrophilic head of the phospholipid extends out of the membrane (Figure 17.1). Phospholipids are also an essential component of the bile, where their detergent properties aid in the solubilization of cholesterol. A decrease of phospholipids in the bile can result in the formation of ***gallstones***.

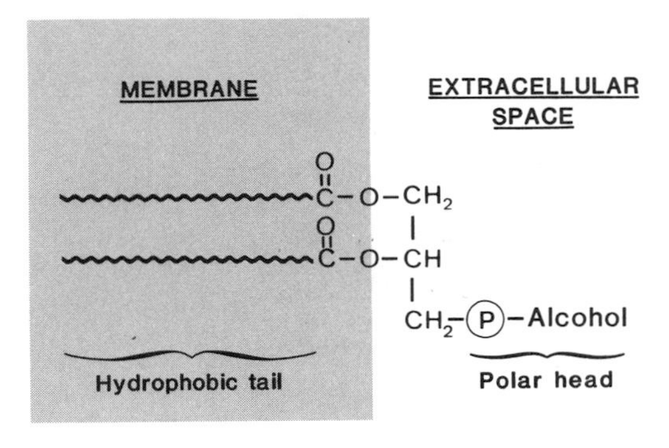

Figure 17.1
Structure of a phospholipid showing its orientation in a membrane.

II. STRUCTURE OF PHOSPHOLIPIDS

A. Phosphoglycerides

1. Phospholipids that contain glycerol are called phosphoglycerides. Phosphoglycerides compose the major class of phospholipids. All contain ***phosphatidic acid*** (diacylglycerol with a phosphate group on the third carbon). Phosphatidic acid is the simplest phosphoglyceride and is the precursor of the other members of this group (see p. 168 for a discussion of phosphatidic acid synthesis.)
2. The phosphate on the phosphatidic acid (PA) can itself be esterified to another compound containing an ***alcohol group*** (Figure 17.2). For example,

Serine	+ PA →	phosphatidylserine
Ethanolamine	+ PA →	phosphatidylethanolamine (cephalin)
Choline	+ PA →	phosphatidylcholine (lecithin)
Glycerol	+ PA →	phosphatidylglycerol
Inositol	+ PA →	phosphatidylinositol

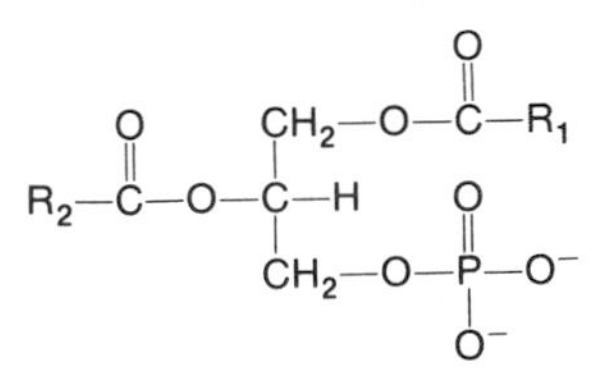
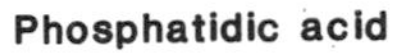

3. Two molecules of phosphatidic acid esterified through their phosphate groups to an additional molecule of glycerol are called

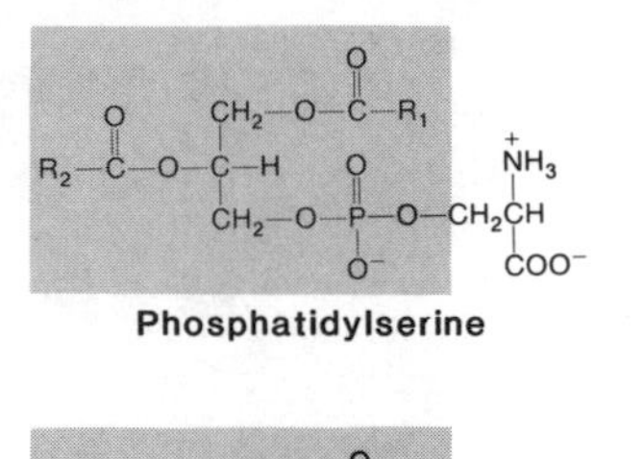
Phosphatidylserine

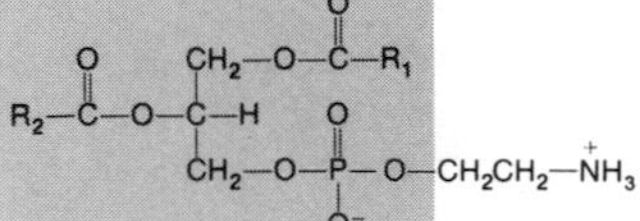
Phosphatidylethanolamine

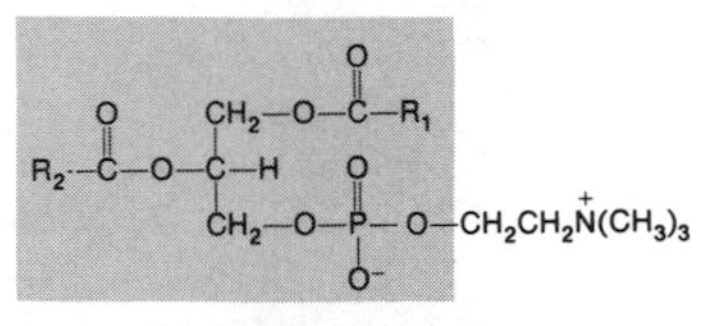
Phosphatidylcholine

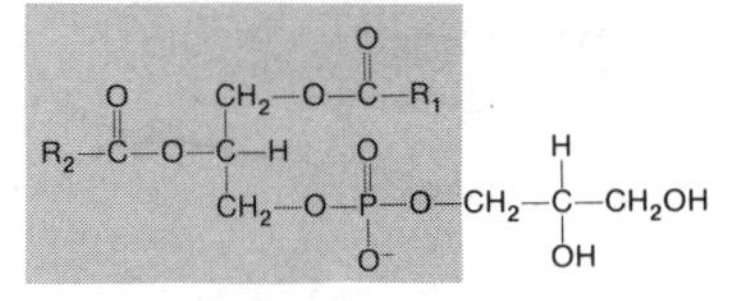
Phosphatidylglycerol

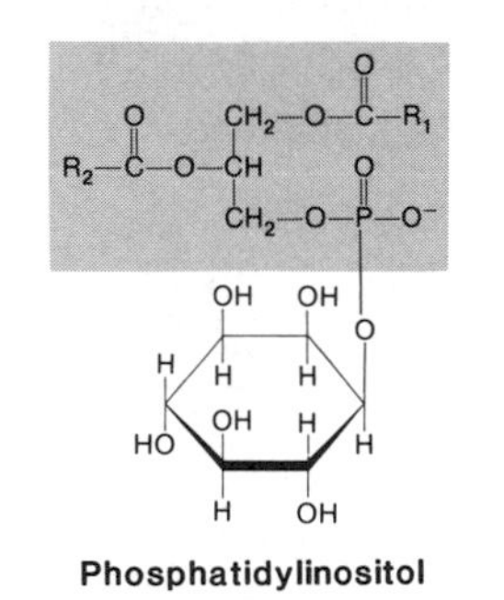
Phosphatidylinositol

Figure 17.2
Structures of some phosphoglycerides.

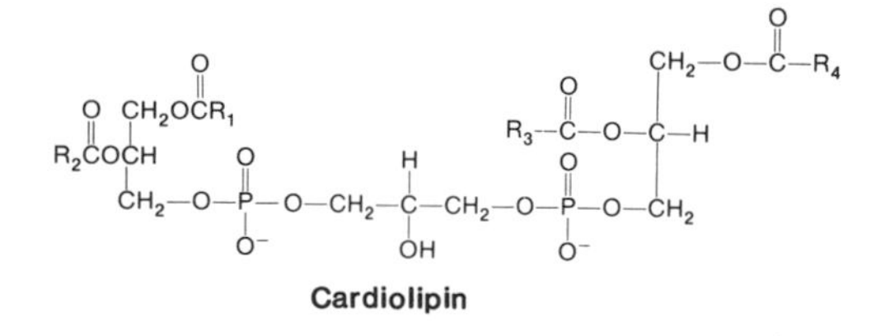
Cardiolipin

cardiolipin. This is the only human phosphoglyceride that is antigenic.

4. When a fatty acid is attached by an ***ether*** rather than by an ester linkage at carbon #1 of the core glycerol molecule, a ***plasmalogen*** is produced. For example, phosphatid***al***ethanolamine is the plasmalogen that is similar in structure to phosphatid***yl***ethanolamine.
5. If the fatty acid at either carbon #1 or #2 of a phosphoglyceride is removed, a ***lyso***phosphoglyceride results, for example, lysolecithin.

B. Sphingomyelin

1. The backbone of sphingomyelin is the amino alcohol ***sphingosine*** rather than glycerol (Figure 17.3).
2. A fatty acid is attached to the amino group of sphingosine by an amide linkage, producing a ***ceramide***. The fatty acids found most frequently in sphingomyelin are palmitic, stearic, lignoceric, and nervonic acid.
3. The alcohol group at carbon #1 of sphingosine is esterified to phosphorylcholine, producing ***sphingomyelin***.

III. SYNTHESIS OF PHOSPHOLIPIDS

Phosphoglyceride synthesis involves either the donation of phosphatidic acid from CDP-diacylglycerol to an alcohol, or the donation of the phosphomonoester of the alcohol from CDP-alcohol to 1,2-diacylglycerol. In both cases, CMP is released (see p. 334 for a discussion of the structures of CTP, CDP, and CMP). A key concept in phospholipid synthesis, therefore, is the activation of diacylglycerol OR the alcohol to be added by linkage with a nucleoside diphosphate (Figure 17.4).

A. Phosphatidic acid (PA)

1. The simplest of the phospholipids, PA is the precursor of many other phosphoglycerides. The steps in the synthesis of this compound were described on p. 168 and Figure 16.12, where it was shown as a precursor of triacylglycerol. (Note: Essentially all cells except mature erythrocytes can synthesize phospholipids, whereas triacylglycerol synthesis occurs only in liver, adipose, and intestine.)
2. The fatty acids attached to the glycerol phosphate can vary widely, contributing to the heterogeneity of this group of compounds.

B. Phosphatidylethanolamine (PE); common name: cephalin

1. The synthetic pathway for PE involves the phosphorylation of ethanolamine followed by its conversion to the activated form, CDP-ethanolamine. Finally, ethanolamine phosphate is transfered

from the nucleotide (leaving CMP) to a molecule of diacylglycerol (Figure 17.5).

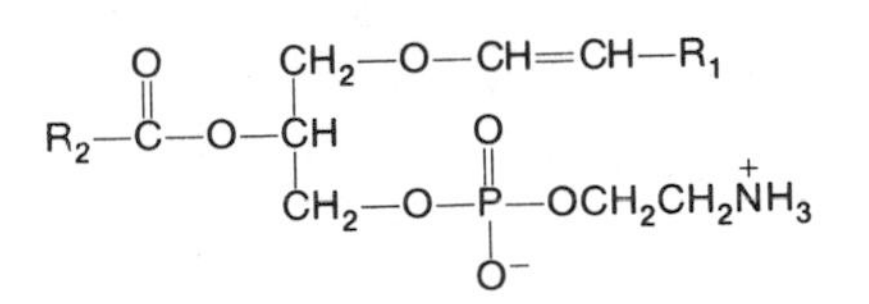

Phosphatidalethanolamine

C. Phosphatidylcholine (PC); common name: lecithin

1. There are two different pathways for the synthesis of PC from the choline that is obtained from the diet or from the catabolism of membrane phospholipids. If, however, there is insufficient choline provided by these routes for the body's needs, the liver can synthesize choline *de novo*.

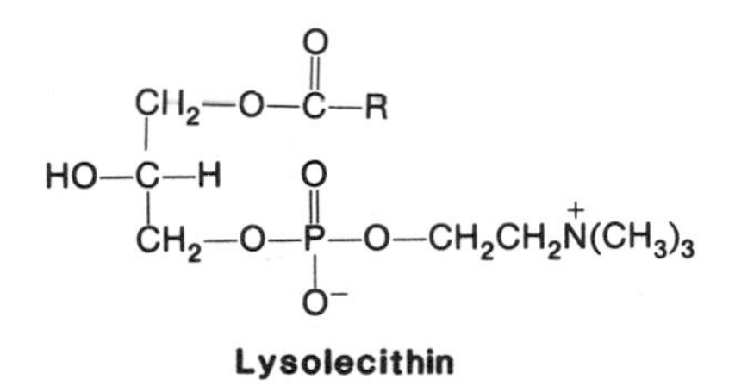

Lysolecithin

2. The first pathway using preexisting choline involves the production of CDP-choline as the ***activated intermediate*** (Figure 17.6). Here, once choline enters the cell, it is immediately phosphorylated. It is next converted to the activated-CDP choline form. Finally, choline phosphate is transferred to diacylglycerol, releasing CMP. (This pathway is essentially the same as that described for ethanolamine above.)
   a. This is the principal pathway for the synthesis of ***dipalmitoyl-lecithin*** in the lung. In this compound, both positions 1 and 2 on the glycerol are occupied by palmitate. This phospholipid is the major component of lung ***surfactant***—the extracellular fluid layer that lines the alveoli. Surfactant serves to decrease the surface tension of this fluid layer, thereby preventing alveolar collapse.
   b. ***Respiratory Distress Syndrome (Hyaline Membrane Disease)*** in infants is associated with insufficient surfactant production. Respiratory failure caused by an insufficient amount of surfactant can also occur in adults whose surfactant-producing pneumocytes have been destroyed as an adverse side-effect of the use of immunosuppressive medication or chemotherapeutic drugs.
3. The second pathway for the synthesis of PC from free choline involves the production of CDP-diacylglycerol as the activated intermediate. In this pathway, CTP is used to activate the ***diacylglycerol*** portion of phosphatidic acid, after which the PA can be transferred to a choline, releasing CMP.
4. *De novo* synthesis of phosphatidylcholine from phosphatidylserine in the membrane by a decarboxylation step followed by three methylation steps is illustrated in Figure 17.7:
   a. The *methyltransferases* that catalyze the methylation reactions shown in Figure 17.7 are stimulated by the binding of catecholamine neurotransmitters, lectins, immunoglobulins, or chemotactic peptides to receptors on the cell surface.
   b. The methylation of membrane phospholipids is coupled to an influx of calcium and to the release of arachidonic acid, lysophosphatidylcholine, and prostaglandins. These biochemical events facilitate the transmission of a number of signals through membranes, resulting in the production of 3′,5′-cyclic AMP in many cell types as well as the release of histamine from mast cells and basophils, cell division of lymphocytes, and enhanced chemotaxis in neutrophils.

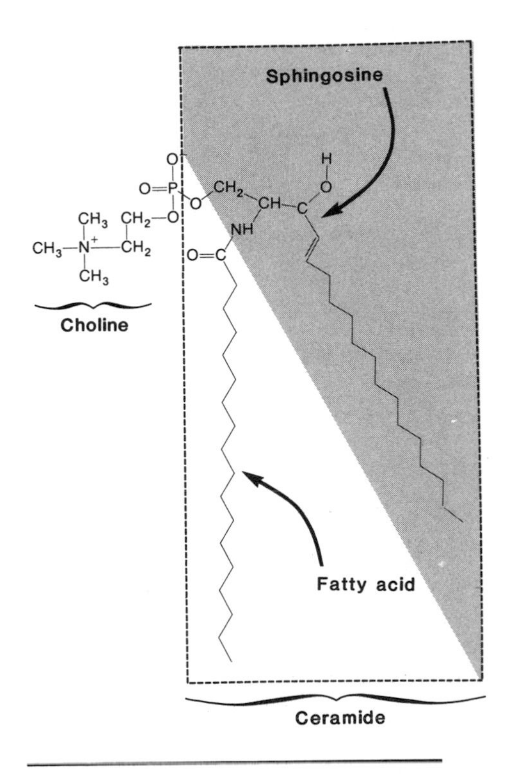

Figure 17.3
Structure of sphingomyelin showing the sphingosine and ceramide components.

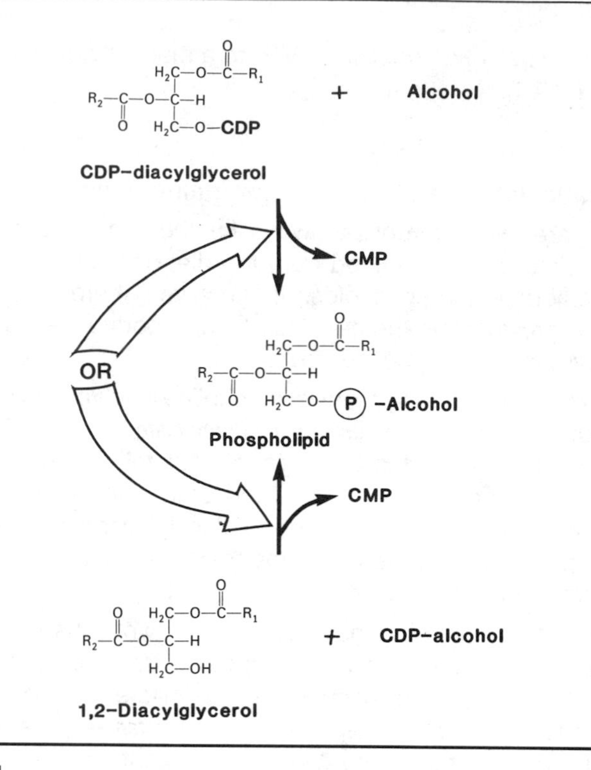

Figure 17.4
Activation of either diacylglycerol OR an alcohol by linkage to a nucleoside diphosphate promotes phospholipid synthesis.

D. Phosphatidylserine (PS)

1. The primary pathway for the synthesis of PS appears to be the exchange of the ethanolamine of PE for free serine (Figure 17.8). This reaction, although reversible, is used primarily to produce the PS required for membrane synthesis.

E. Phosphatidylinositol (PI)

1. PI is synthesized from free **myo**inositol and CDP diacylglycerol, as shown in Figure 17.9.
2. PI is an unusual phospholipid in that it often contains stearic acid on carbon #1 and arachidonic acid on carbon #2 of the glycerol. PI therefore serves as a reservoir of arachidonic acid in the membrane, and thus provides the substrate for prostaglandin synthesis when required (see p. 174 for a discussion of these compounds.)
3. The phosphorylation of membrane-bound phosphatidyl-inositol occurs in response to the binding of various neurotransmitters, hormones, and growth factors to receptors on the cell membrane. The degradation of these ***poly***phosphoinositides results in the mobilization of intracellular calcium and the activation of protein kinase C, both of which act synergistically to evoke specific

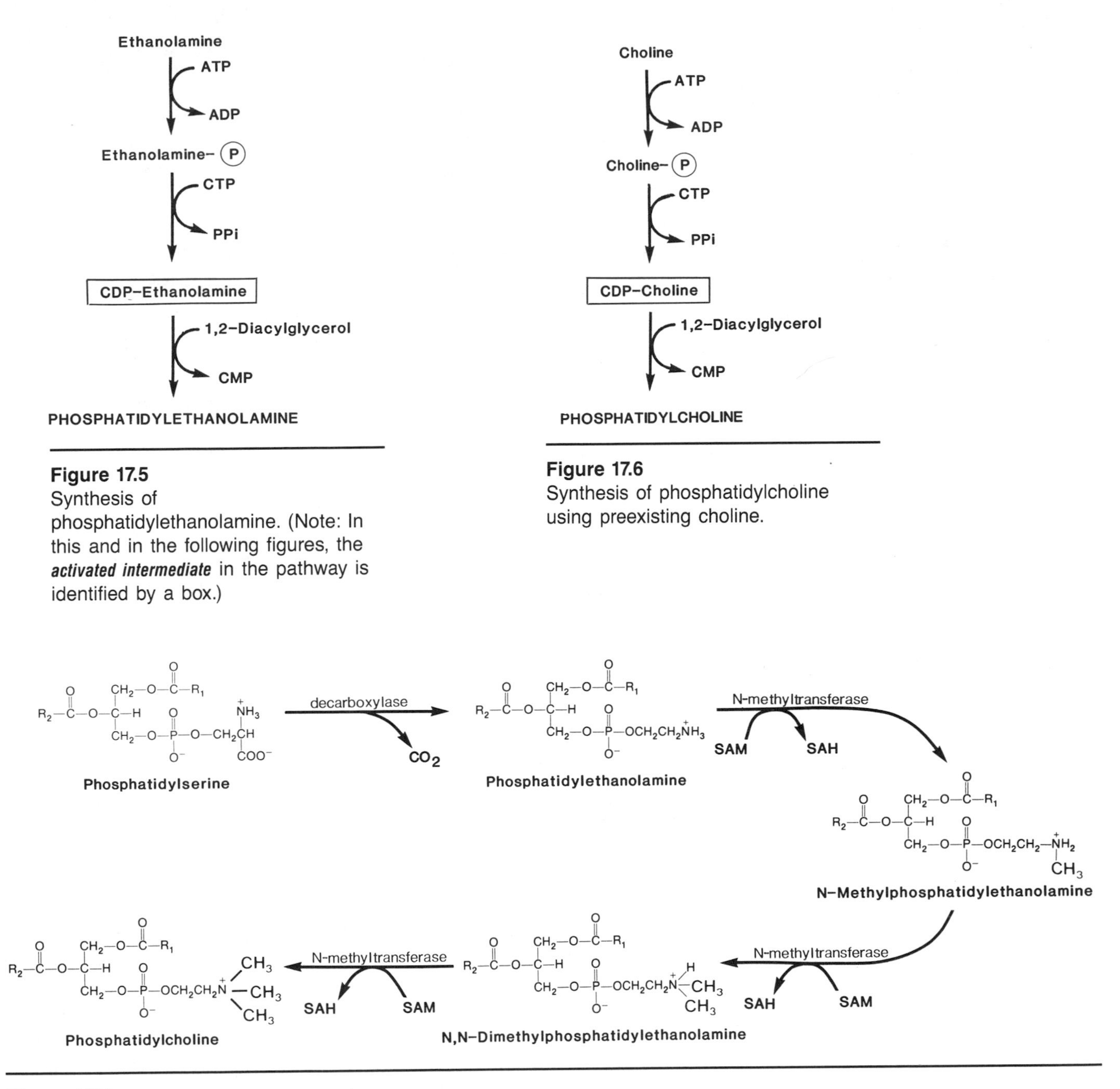

Figure 17.5
Synthesis of phosphatidylethanolamine. (Note: In this and in the following figures, the ***activated intermediate*** in the pathway is identified by a box.)

Figure 17.6
Synthesis of phosphatidylcholine using preexisting choline.

Figure 17.7
De novo synthesis of phosphatidylcholine in cell membranes.

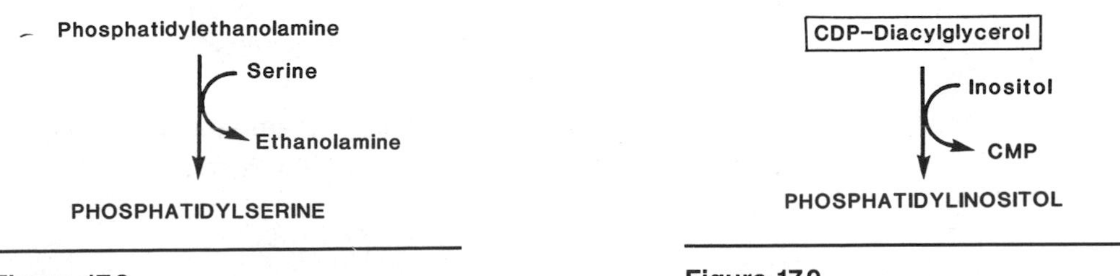

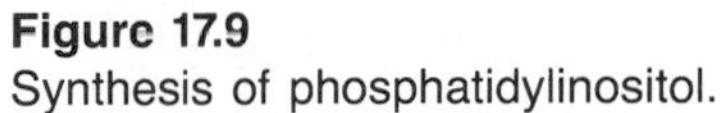

Figure 17.8
Synthesis of phosphatidylserine.

Figure 17.9
Synthesis of phosphatidylinositol.

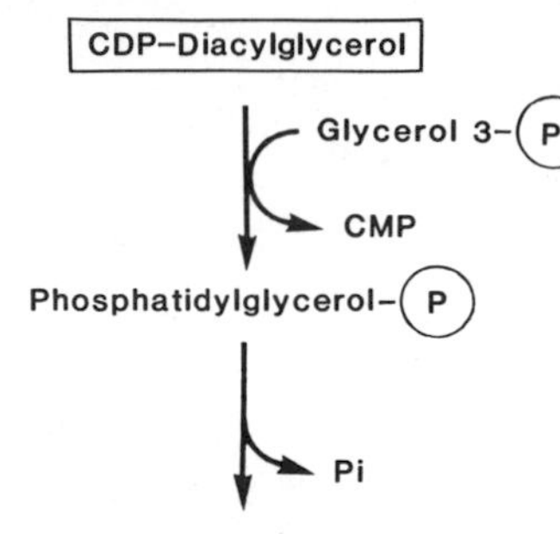

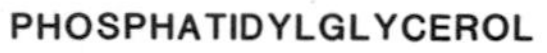

Figure 17.10
Synthesis of phosphatidylglycerol.

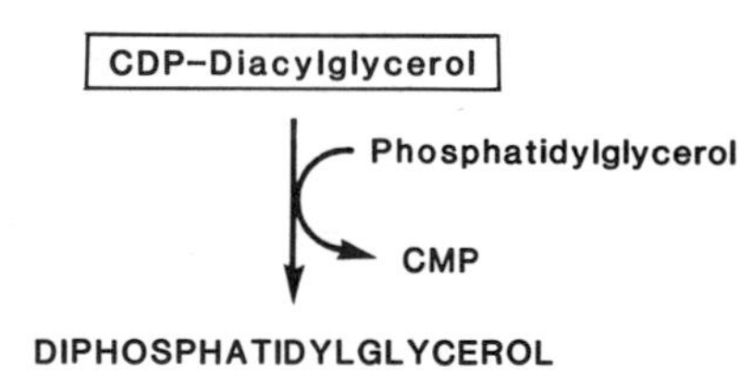

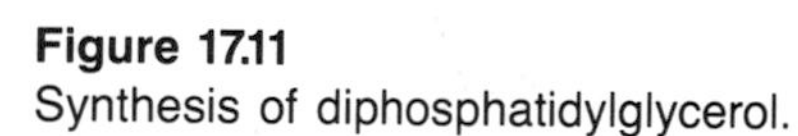

Figure 17.11
Synthesis of diphosphatidylglycerol.

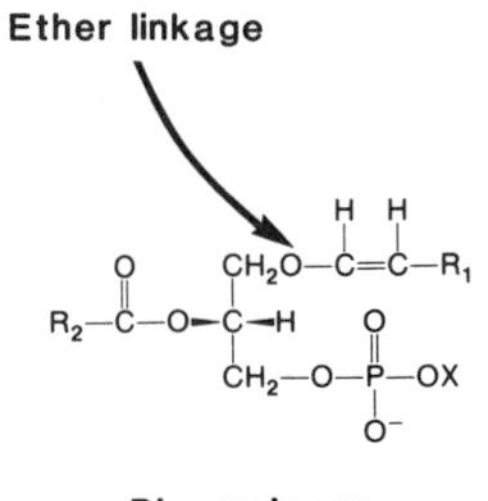

Figure 17.12
A plasmalogen illustrating the ether linkage.

cellular responses. Signal transmission across the membrane is thus accomplished.

F. Phosphatidylglycerol (PG)

1. PG is synthesized in a two-step reaction from CDP-diacylglycerol and glycerol 3-phosphate as shown in Figure 17.10.
2. PG is a precursor of ***diphosphatidylglycerol***.

G. Diphosphatidylglycerol

1. Diphosphatidylglycerol comprises two phosphatidic acids joined by a molecule of glycerol. It is synthesized as shown in Figure 17.11 by the transfer of diacylglycerolphosphate from CDP-diacylglycerol to a preexisting molecule of phosphatidylglycerol.
2. An important example of diphosphatidylglycerol is ***cardiolipin,*** which is found in significant amounts in the inner mitochondrial membrane. (It is named cardiolipin because it was originally isolated from heart tissue.)

H. Plasmalogens

1. There are three major classes of plasmalogens: phosphatidalcholines, phosphatidalethanolamines, and phosphatidalserines. They have in common a replacement of the fatty acid found at carbon #1 in the previously discussed phospholipids with an α, β-unsaturated fatty aldehyde. The linkage is an ***ether*** rather than an ester linkage (Figure 17.12).
2. One plasmalogen—1-alkyl-2-acetyl-phosphatidalcholine—is a very powerful chemical mediator. It has two potent physiologic actions: It reduces blood pressure and activates blood platelets, causing them to aggregate. It is therefore called ***platelet-activating factor*** (PAF) and has biological effects at concentrations as low as 10^{-10} M.

I. Sphingomyelin

1. The sphingomyelin class of phospholipid has ***sphingosine*** rather than glycerol as the alcohol portion of the molecule. The synthesis of sphingosine is shown in Figure 17.13. Briefly, palmitoyl CoA loses the coenzyme A portion of its structure and becomes attached to serine. (This reaction requires pyridoxal phosphate as a cofactor). This molecule is converted to sphingosine (newer name for this compound is ***sphingenine***),which can then be acylated to produce a ***ceramide***—an immediate precursor of ***sphingomyelin***.
2. There are several pathways for the synthesis of sphingomyelins. The one that accounts for most of the synthesis transfers a molecule of choline from CDP-choline to a ceramide as shown in Figure 17.13. Note that the phosphorylcholine is attached to a carbon that was the β-carbon of serine.
3. Sphingomyelin is found in significant amounts in brain and other nervous tissue but is present in membranes of other tissues as well.

J. A summary of the interrelated pathways of phospholipid synthesis is shown in Figure 17.14.

IV. DEGRADATION OF PHOSPHOLIPIDS

The degradation of phosphoglycerides is performed by ***phospholipases***. These enzymes are found in all tissues and are also present in pancreatic juice (see discussion of lipid digestion, p. 150). In addition, a number of toxins and venoms have phospholipase activity, and several pathogenic bacteria produce phospholipases that dissolve cell membranes and allow the spread of infection.

A. Types of phospholipases

1. *Phospholipases* hydrolyze the ester and phosphodiester bonds of phospholipids. Each enzyme cleaves a phospholipid at a specific site. The major enzymes responsible for degrading phosphoglycerides are shown in Figure 17.15.
2. Sphingomyelin is degraded by *sphingomyelinase*, which hydrolytically removes phosphorylcholine, leaving a ceramide. The ceramide is, in turn, cleaved by *ceramidase* into sphingosine and a free fatty acid (Figure 17.16).

B. Niemann-Pick Disease

1. Niemann-Pick disease is a genetic disease caused by the inability to degrade sphingomyelin. The deficient enzyme is *sphingomyelinase*. In the severe form (type A), the liver and spleen are the sites of lipid deposits and are therefore tremendously enlarged. The lipid consists primarily of sphingomyelin (which cannot be degraded) and also of phosphatidyl choline. Infants with this disease suffer severe mental retardation and death in early childhood. The type A form of the disease is detected predominantly in Ashkenazi Jews, with a carrier frequency of 1:100.
2. A number of less severe variants are known in which there is minimal damage to neural tissues, but kidney, spleen, liver, and bone marrow are affected, resulting in a chronic form of the disease and a life expectancy to early adulthood.

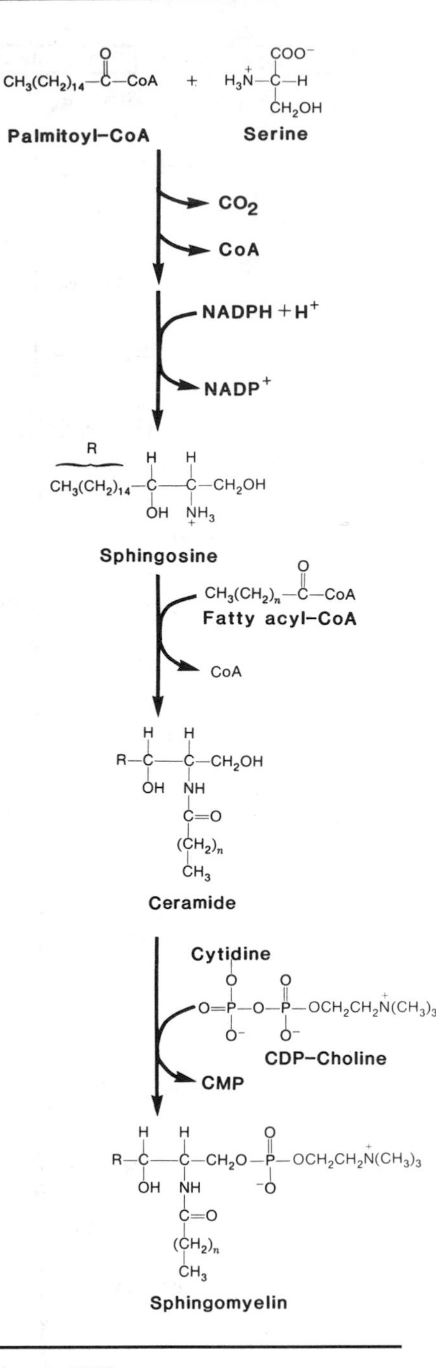

Figure 17.13
Synthesis of sphingosine and sphingomyelin.

Study Questions

Choose the ONE BEST answer

17.1 The neurologic disturbances seen in Niemann-Pick disease are associated with the accumulation in central nervous tissue of which one of the following:

A. Prostaglandins
B. Gangliosides
C. Cerebrosides
D. Sphingomyelin
E. Phosphatidylserine

Answer	
A if 1, 2, and 3 are correct	D if only 4 is correct
B if 1 and 3 are correct	E if all are correct
C if 2 and 4 are correct	

17.2 Phospholipid(s) that contain(s) glycerol is(are)

1. lecithin.
2. sphingomyelin.
3. cardiolipin.
4. cerebroside.

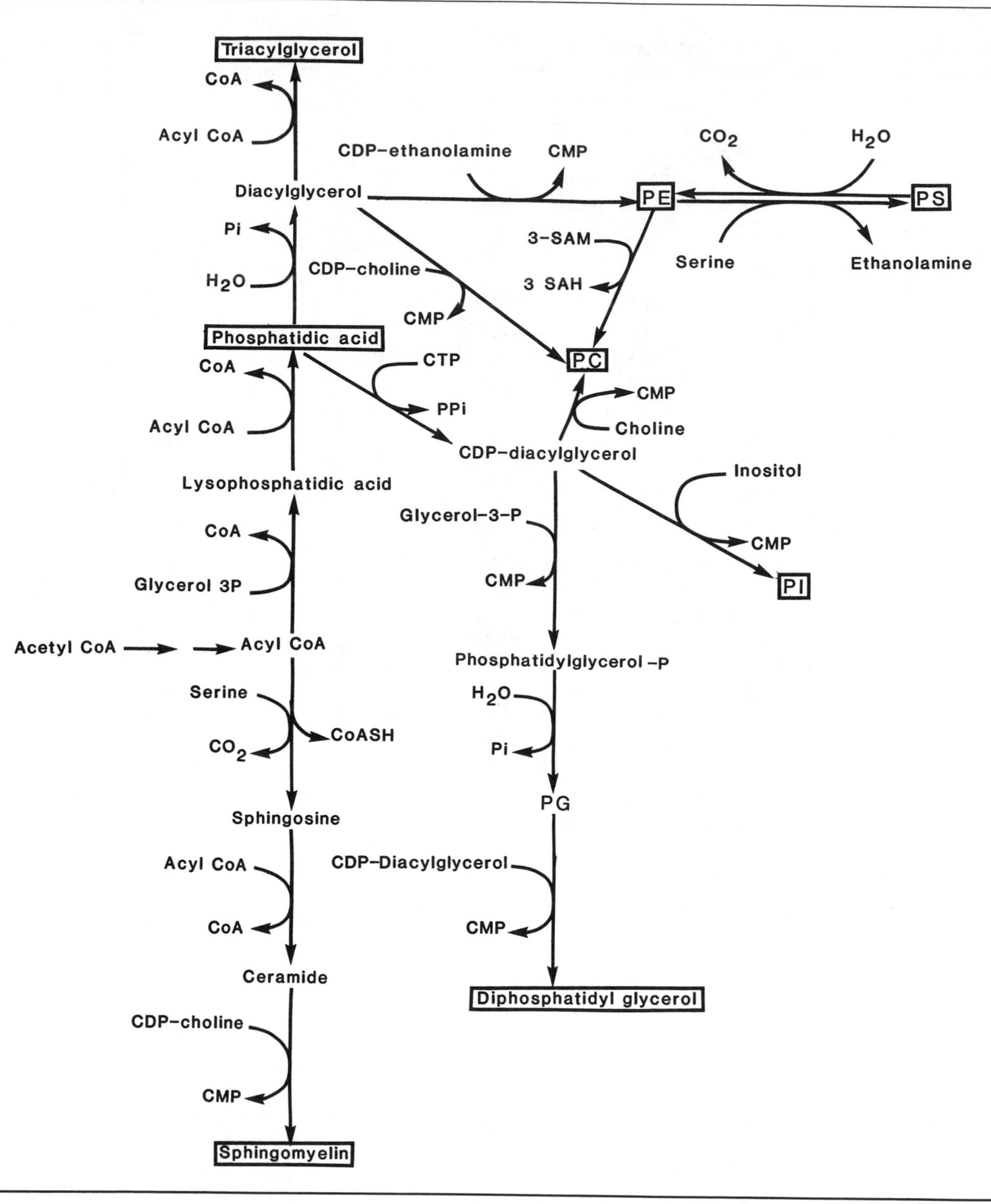

Figure 17.14
Summary pathways of phospholipid synthesis. Their relation to triacylglycerol synthesis is also shown. Major products of the pathway are in boxes. (PS, phosphatidylserine; PE, phosphatidylethanolamine; PC, phosphatidylcholine; PI, phosphatidylinositol; PG, phosphatidylglycerol)

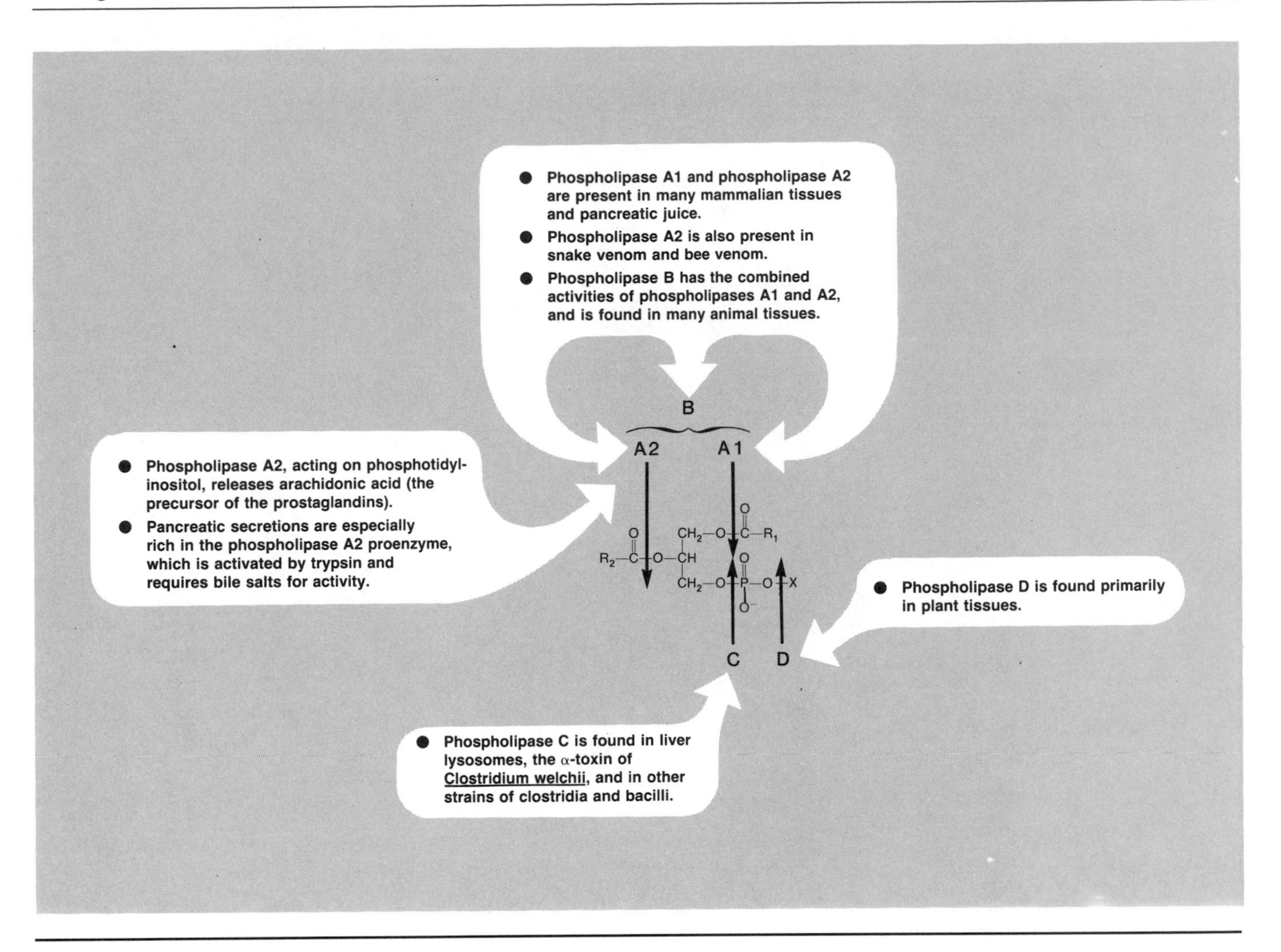

Figure 17.15
Degradation of phosphoglycerides by phospholipases.

17.3 Which of the following statements about phosphatidylcholine (PC) metabolism in humans is(are) correct?

1. PC can give rise to lysophosphatidylcholine by the action of phospholipase A.
2. PC can be synthesized from phosphatidylethanolamine by transmethylation.
3. Cytidine triphosphate (CTP) is required for PC synthesis from 1,2-diacylglycerol.
4. PC is derived exclusively from dietary choline.

17.4 Hydrolysis of a mixture of phosphoglycerides will yield which of the following compounds?

1. Choline
2. Glycerol
3. Phosphate
4. Serine

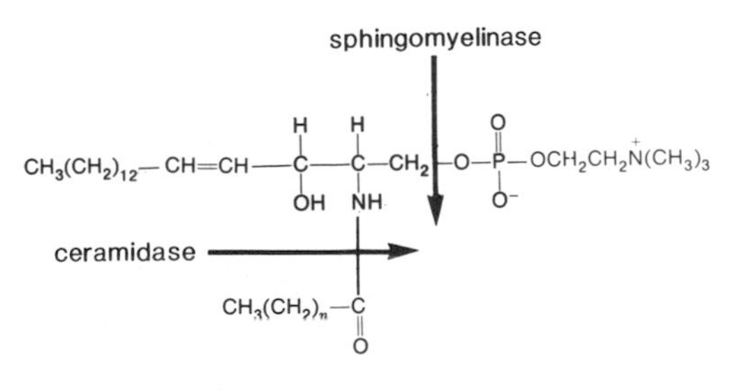

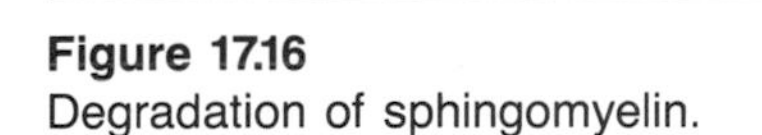

Figure 17.16
Degradation of sphingomyelin.

Glycolipid Metabolism

18

I. OVERVIEW

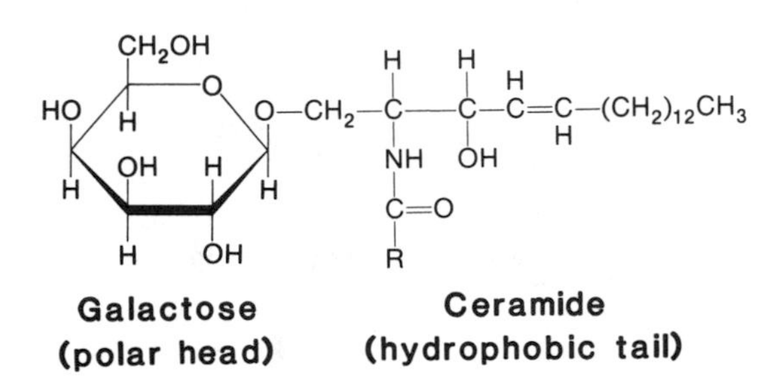

Figure 18.1
Structure of a neutral glycosphingolipid (galactocerebroside).

Like the phospholipid sphingomyelin, almost all glycolipids are derivatives of ceramides (in which a molecule of fatty acid is attached to the amino alcohol, sphingosine). They are therefore more precisely called glycosphingolipids. The glycosphingolipids differ from sphingomyelin in that (1) they contain no phosphate and (2) the polar head function is provided by a monosaccharide or oligosaccharide attached directly to the ceramide by an O-glycosidic bond (Figure 18.1). The number and type of carbohydrate moieties present help determine the type of glycosphingolipid.

Like the phospholipids, glycosphingolipids are essential components of all membranes in the body. When cells are transformed there is a dramatic change in the glycolipid composition of the membrane. This suggests that glycolipids may play a role in the regulation of cellular interactions, growth, and development. Glycolipids are very antigenic and have been identified as a source of blood group antigens, various embryonic antigens specific for particular stages of fetal development, and some tumor antigens. They also serve as cell surface receptors for cholera and diphtheria toxins and for certain viruses.

II. STRUCTURE OF GLYCOLIPIDS

A. Neutral glycosphingolipids

1. The simplest neutral (uncharged) glycosphingolipids are the ***cerebrosides***. These are ceramide monosaccharides that contain either a molecule of galactose (galactocerebroside, the most common cerebroside found in membranes; Figure 18.1) or glucose (glucocerebroside, serving primarily as an intermediate in the synthesis and degradation of the more complex glycosphingolipids).
2. Members of a group of galactocerebrosides (or glucocerebrosides) may differ from each other in the type of fatty acid attached to the sphingosine.
3. As their name implies, cerebrosides are found predominantly in the brain and peripheral nervous tissue, with high concentrations in the myelin sheath.

4. ***Ceramide oligosaccharides*** are produced by attaching additional monosaccharides to a glucocerebroside. Examples of these compounds include

Ceramide dihexoside:	Cer-Glc-Gal
Globoside:	Cer-Glc-Gal-Gal-GalNAc
Forssman antigen:	Cer-Glc-Gal-Gal-GalNac-GalNac

(Cer = ceramide, Glc = glucose, Gal = galatose, GalNac = N-acetylgalactosamine)

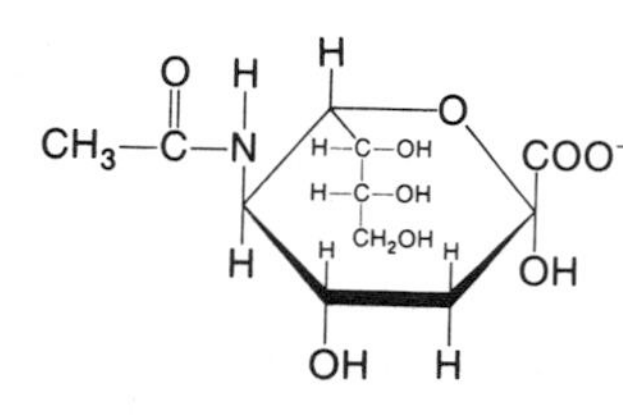

N-Acetylneuraminic acid

B. Acidic glycosphingolipids

1. Acidic glycosphingolipids are negatively charged at physiologic pH. The negative charge can be provided by N-acetylneuraminic acid (NANA) or by sulfate groups.
2. ***Gangliosides*** are the most complex glycosphingolipids. They are derivatives of the ceramide oligosaccharides and contain one or more molecules of NANA. The notation for these compounds is G (for ganglioside) plus a subscript M, D, or T to indicate whether there is one, two, or three molecules of NANA in the ganglioside. Additional numbers and letters in the subscript designate the sequence of the carbohydrate attached to the ceramide (see Figure 18.2 for the structure of G_{M2}, the ganglioside that accumulates in Tay-Sachs disease.)
3. Gangliosides are of medical interest because several lipid storage disorders involve the accumulation of NANA-containing glycosphingolipids in cells (Figure 18.3).

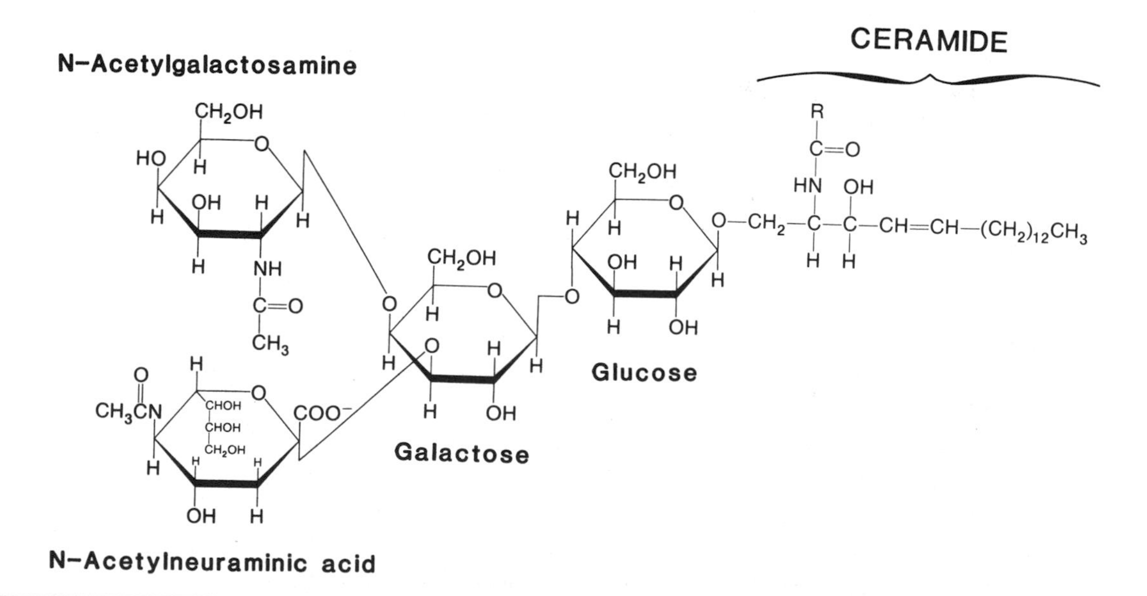

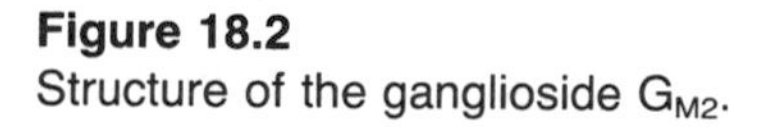

Figure 18.2
Structure of the ganglioside G_{M2}.

4. ***Sulfoglycosphingolipids (sulfatides)*** are cerebrosides that contain a galactosyl residue that has been sulfated and is therefore negatively charged at physiologic pH.

III. METABOLISM OF GLYCOLIPIDS

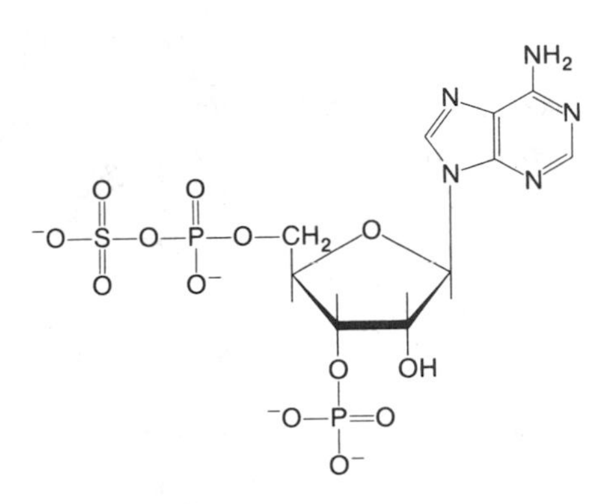

3′–Phosphoadenosine–5′–phosphosulfate

A. Synthesis of glycolipids

1. The synthesis of glycosphingolipids occurs by the sequential addition of glycosyl monomers that are transferred from sugar-nucleotide donors to the acceptor molecule. The mechanism is similar to that used in glycoprotein synthesis (see p. 92).
2. The enzymes that are involved in the synthesis are all *glycosyl transferases,* each specific for a particular sugar-nucleotide and acceptor. These enzymes may use both glycolipids and glycoproteins as substrates.
3. Sulfate groups are added to a galactocerebroside by the transfer of the sulfate from ***3′-phosphoadenosine-5′-phosphosulfate*** (PAPS) to the 3′-hydroxyl group of the galactose by the enzyme *sulfotransferase.*

B. Degradation of glycolipids

1. The degradation process involves lysosomal enzymes that hydrolytically cleave specific bonds in the glycolipid. These include *α- and β-galactosidases*, a *β-glucosidase*, a *neuraminidase* (also called *sialidase*), *hexosaminidase*, *sphingomyelinase*, a *sulfatase* (*sulfate esterase*), and a *ceramidase* (see Figure 18.3 for an outline of the degradative pathway).
4. Some major features of the degradative pathway follow.
   a. All the enzymes are present in the ***lysosomes,*** where degradation of these compounds occurs, and all are hydrolases.
   b. Most of the enzymes are relatively stable and may occur as isozymes. For example, *hexosaminidase* occurs in two isomeric forms: A and B.
   c. The enzymes degrade the sulfolipids by a stepwise removal of the components of the structure, such as sulfate and sugars.
   d. These hydrolytic reactions are irreversible.

C. Sphingolipidoses

1. In a normal individual, the synthesis and degradation of the sphingolipids are balanced so that the amount of these compounds present in membranes is constant. If one of the specific hydrolases required for the degradation process is partially or totally missing, sphingolipids will accumulate in the lysosomes. The diseases caused by these enzyme deficiencies are called ***sphingolipidoses.*** The result of a specific hydrolase deficiency may be seen dramatically in nervous tissue, in which neurologic deterioration occurs that can lead to early death.
2. The sphingolipidoses have in common the following properties.
   a. A specific lysosomal hydrolytic enzyme is deficient in each disorder.

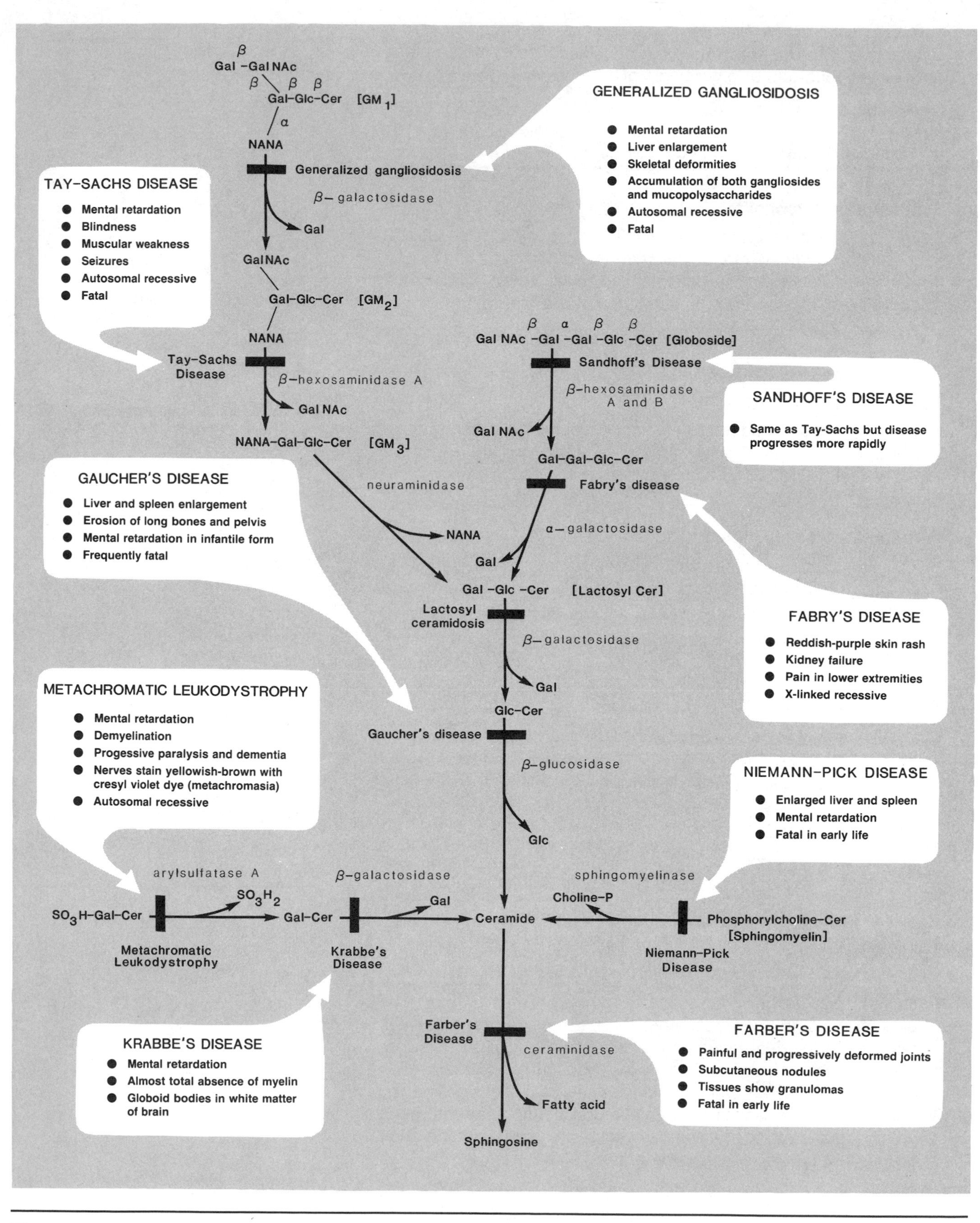

Figure 18.3
Degradation of glycolipids showing enzymes missing in related genetic diseases, the sphingolipidoses.

b. Usually only a single sphingolipid accumulates in the involved organs in each disease.

c. The rate of biosynthesis of the accumulating lipid is normal.

d. With the exception of the adult form of Gaucher's disease, and of Fabry's disease, the enzyme deficiencies cause death usually after the first months of life.

e. With the exception of Fabry's disease, which is linked to the X chromosome, the sphingolipidoses are all autosomal recessive diseases.

f. A specific sphingolipidosis can be diagnosed by analyzing tissue samples for the presence of enzyme activity and for accumulated lipid. Histologic examination of the affected tissue is also useful.

3. A summary of the sphingolipidoses is shown in Figure 18.3. From this figure you can learn the enzyme missing in a particular genetic disease and the main characteristics of the individual diseases. The sphingolipid that accumulates in the lysosomes in each disease is shown as the structure that cannot be further degraded owing to the specific enzyme deficiency.

Study Questions

Answer A if 1, 2, and 3 are correct
B if 1 and 3 are correct
C if 2 and 4 are correct
D if only 4 is correct
E if all are correct

18.1 Sphingolipidoses are a group of diseases caused by related enzyme deficiencies. Which of the following statements about sphingolipidoses is(are) correct?

1. A specific catabolic enzyme is missing in each disorder.
2. A specific sphingolipidosis can be diagnosed by analyzing tissue samples for the presence of enzyme activity and for accumulation of a particular lipid.
3. Usually only a single species of sphingolipid accumulates in the affected organs in each disease.
4. The rate of biosynthesis of the accumulating lipid is normal.

18.2 Which of the following compounds is(are) direct precursor(s) for the synthesis of the sphingosine found in glycolipids?

1. Asparagine
2. Serine
3. Malonyl CoA
4. Palmitoyl CoA

Choose the ONE BEST answer:

18.3 Which one of the following compounds would be found in a ***total*** hydrolysate of a typical mammalian tissue glycolipid?

A. Serine
B. Choline
C. Lecithin
D. Glucosylceramide
E. Fatty acid

18.4 To be defined as a ganglioside, a lipid substance isolated from nerve tissue must contain in its structure

A. N-acetylneuraminic acid (NANA), hexoses, sphingosine, long chain fatty acid.
B. NANA, a hexose, a fatty acid, sphingosine, phosphorylcholine.
C. NANA, sphingosine, ethanolamine.
D. an N-acyl fatty acid derivative of sphingosine, hexose.
E. NANA, hexoses, fatty acid, glycerol.

Cholesterol and Steroid Metabolism

19

I. CHOLESTEROL

Cholesterol is synthesized by virtually all tissues in humans, although liver, intestine, adrenal cortex, and reproductive tissues including ovaries, testes, and placenta make the largest contributions to the body's cholesterol pool. Cholesterol is the most abundant sterol in humans and performs a number of essential functions in the body. For example, cholesterol is a component of all ***cell membranes*** and functions as a precursor of ***bile acids, steroid hormones,*** and ***vitamin D.***

A. Cholesterol balance

1. Given the critical role of cholesterol in the structure and function of cells, it is important that the body be assured an adequate and continuous supply of this sterol. The ***liver*** plays a central role in the regulation of the body's cholesterol balance. Cholesterol ***enters*** the liver's cholesterol pool from a number of sources (Figure 19.1), including
   a. ***Dietary cholesterol: Chylomicron remnants*** contain dietary cholesterol or cholesterol synthesized in the intestinal mucosal cells. The processing of dietary cholesterol and cholesteryl esters in the small intestine and the uptake of cholesterol by the intestinal mucosal cells, with its subsequent packaging and export from the cell as a component of chylomicrons, have been previously described (see p. 152).
   b. ***Extrahepatic cholesterol:*** Cholesterol synthesized in other extrahepatic tissues that reaches the liver carried in ***high-density lipoproteins (HDL).***
   c. Cholesterol synthesized *de novo* in the liver itself.
2. Cholesterol ***leaves*** the liver (Figure 19.1):
   a. After synthesis and secretion of HDL and very low density lipoproteins (VLDL) that contain cholesterol.
   b. By being secreted into the bile as free cholesterol.
   c. After its conversion into bile salts which are secreted into the bile.

B. Structure of cholesterol

1. The structure of cholesterol includes four fused rings (identified by the first four letters of the alphabet), with the carbons numbered

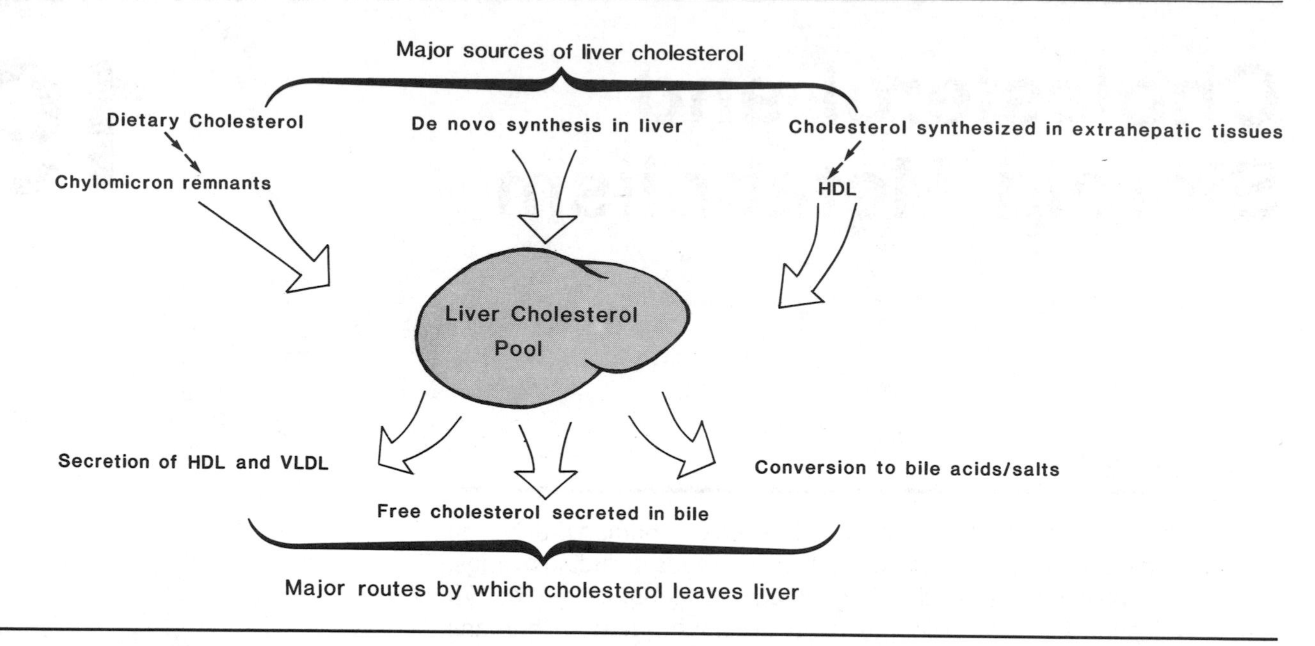

Figure 19.1
Sources of liver cholesterol and routes by which cholesterol leaves the liver.

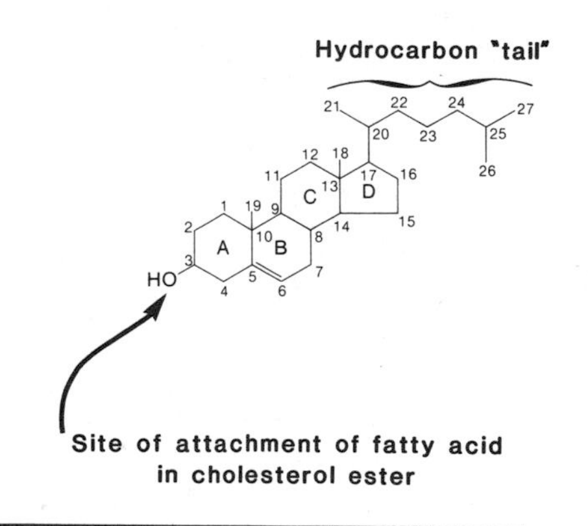

Figure 19.2
Structure of cholesterol showing site of attachment of fatty acid in cholesterol esters.

in sequence (Figure 19.2). Cholesterol also contains an eight-membered, branched hydrocarbon chain attached to the D ring. Cholesterol is therefore a very ***hydrophobic*** compound.

2. Steroids with 8 to 10 carbon atoms in the side chain at C-17 and an alcoholic hydroxyl group at C-2 are classified as ***sterols***. Cholesterol is the major sterol in animal tissues.
   a. Plant sterols such as β-sitosterol are poorly absorbed by humans. They can block the uptake of cholesterol, however, by interfering competitively with their binding to intestinal mucosal cell membranes before uptake.
3. Much of the serum cholesterol is in an esterified form (with a fatty acid attached at carbon #3; see Figure 19.2), which makes the structure even more hydrophobic.
4. Because of its hydrophobicity, cholesterol must be transported in the body either in association with protein as a lipoprotein (for a discussion of these compounds, see p. 208) or solubilized in the bile.

C. Synthesis of cholesterol

1. All the carbon atoms in cholesterol are provided by acetate. NADPH provides the reducing equivalents. Energetically, the pathway is driven by the hydrolysis of the high-energy thioester bond of acetyl CoA and the terminal phosphate bond of ATP. Synthesis occurs in the cytoplasm, with enzymes in both the cytosol and the endoplasmic reticulum.
2. The first two reactions in the cholesterol synthetic pathway are shared by the pathway that produces ketone bodies (see p. 176) and result in the production of ***3-hydroxy-3-methylglutaryl CoA*** (HMG CoA) (Figure 19.3).

a. Two acetyl CoA molecules condense to form acetoacetyl CoA.

b. Next, a third molecule of acetyl CoA is added, producing HMG CoA. (Note: Liver parenchymal cells contain two isozyme forms of *HMG CoA synthase*. The cytoplasmic enzyme participates in cholesterol synthesis, whereas the mitochondrial is in the pathway for ketone body synthesis.)

3. The next step, the synthesis of ***mevalonic acid,*** is catalyzed by *HMG CoA reductase* and is the ***rate-limiting step*** in cholesterol synthesis. It occurs in the endoplasmic reticulum, uses two molecules of NADPH as the reducing agent, and hydrolytically removes CoA, making the reaction irreversible (Figure 19.4).

4. The reactions and enzymes involved in the synthesis of cholesterol from mevalonate are illustrated in Figure 19.5. The numbers shown in brackets below correspond to reactions shown in this figure.

[1] Mevalonic acid is converted to ***5-pyrophosphomevalonate*** in two steps, each of which transfers a phosphate group from ATP.

[2] A five-carbon isoprene unit—***isopentenyl pyrophosphate*** (IPP)—is formed by the decarboxylation of 5-pyrophosphomevalonate. The reaction requires ATP.

[3] IPP can be isomerized to ***3,3-dimethylallyl pyrophosphate*** (DPP).

[4] These two compounds (IPP and DPP) condense to form ***geranyl pyrophosphate (GPP)***.

[5] A second molecule of IPP then condenses with GPP to form ***farnesyl pyrophosphate.***

[6] Two molecules of the 15-carbon farnesyl pyrophosphate combine to form ***presqualene pyrophosphate.***

[7] The atoms of presqualene are then rearranged and reduced with NADPH, producing the 30-carbon hydrocarbon compound ***squalene.*** In each of these two steps, a pyrophosphate molecule is released.

[8] Squalene is converted to ***lanosterol*** by two reactions that use molecular oxygen and NADPH. The hydroxylation of squalene triggers the cyclization of the structure to lanosterol.

[9] The conversion of lanosterol to ***cholesterol*** is a multistep process, resulting in the shortening of the carbon chain from 30 to 27. All of the enzymes catalyzing this conversion are located in the endoplasmic reticulum.

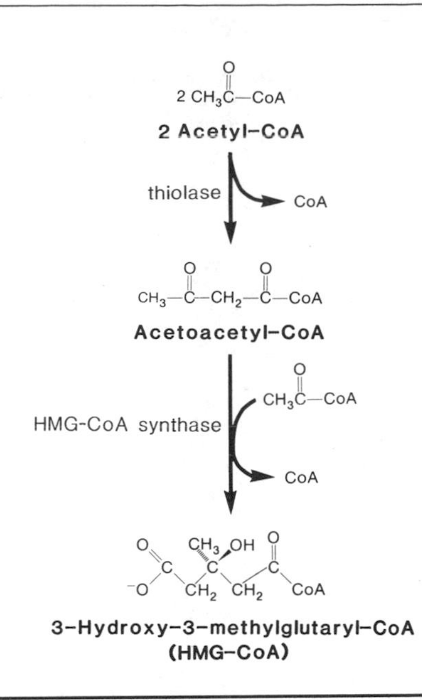

Figure 19.3
Synthesis of 3-hydroxy-3-methylglutaryl CoA (HMG CoA).

HMG–CoA
HMG-CoA reductase
2 NADPH + 2 H^+
CoA
2 $NADP^+$
Mevalonic acid

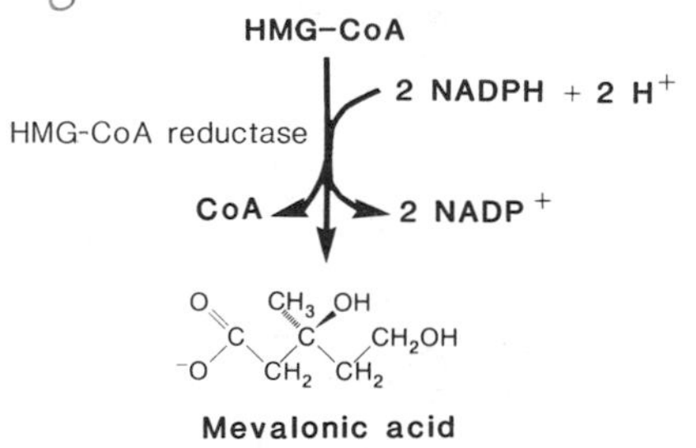

Figure 19.4
Synthesis of mevalonic acid.

D. Regulation of cholesterol synthesis

1. *HMG CoA reductase* is the ***rate-limiting enzyme*** in cholesterol synthesis and is subject to a number of different kinds of metabolic controls.

a. *HMG CoA reductase* activity is controlled hormonally through a complex cascade of enzyme activations and inhibitions shown in Figure 19.6. The net effect is that glucagon favors the formation of the inactive form of *HMG CoA reductase* and, hence, the rate of cholesterol synthesis is decreased. In contrast, insulin favors the formation of the active form of *HMG CoA reductase,* resulting in an increase in the rate of cholesterol synthesis.

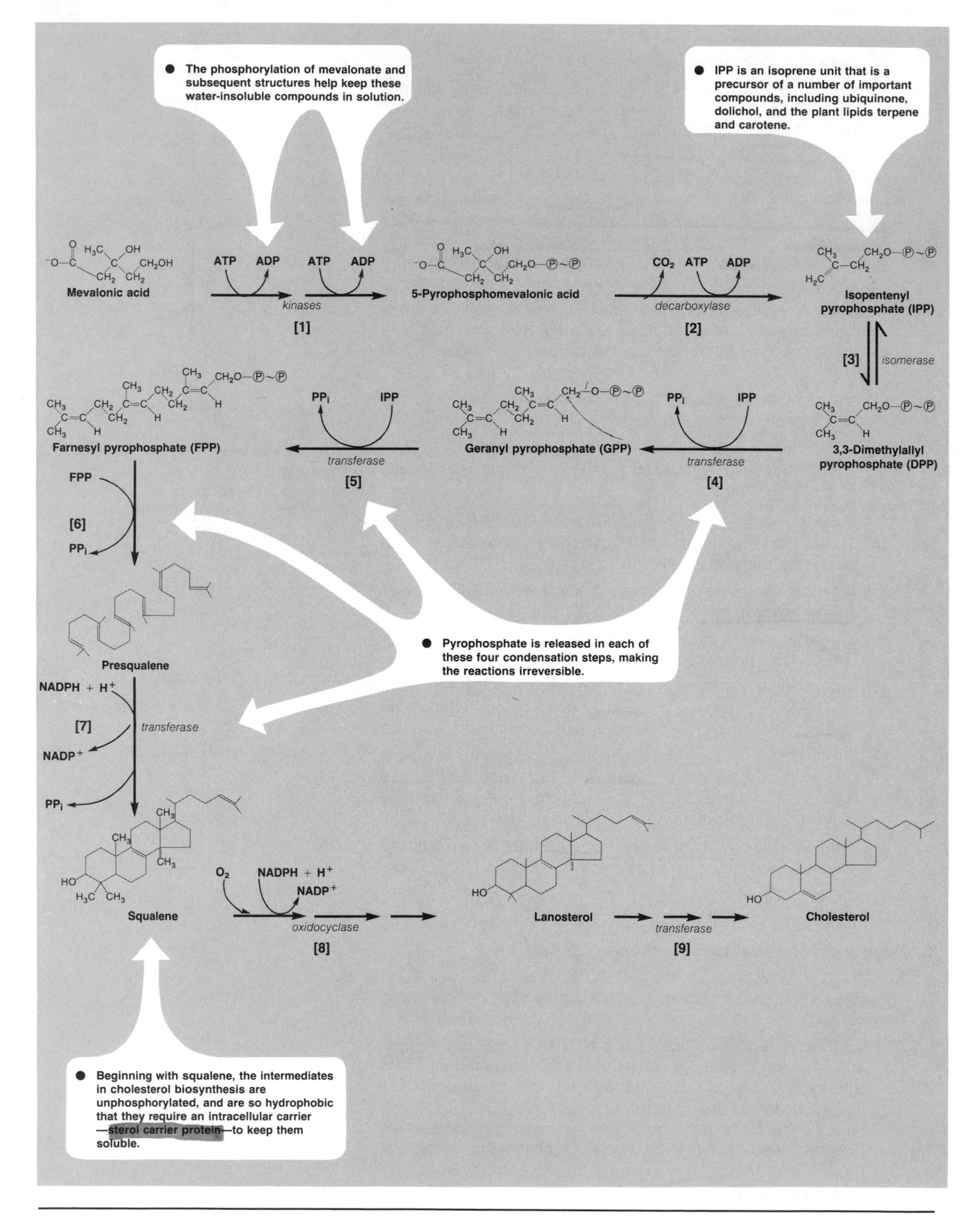

Figure 19.5
Synthesis of cholesterol from mevalonic acid.

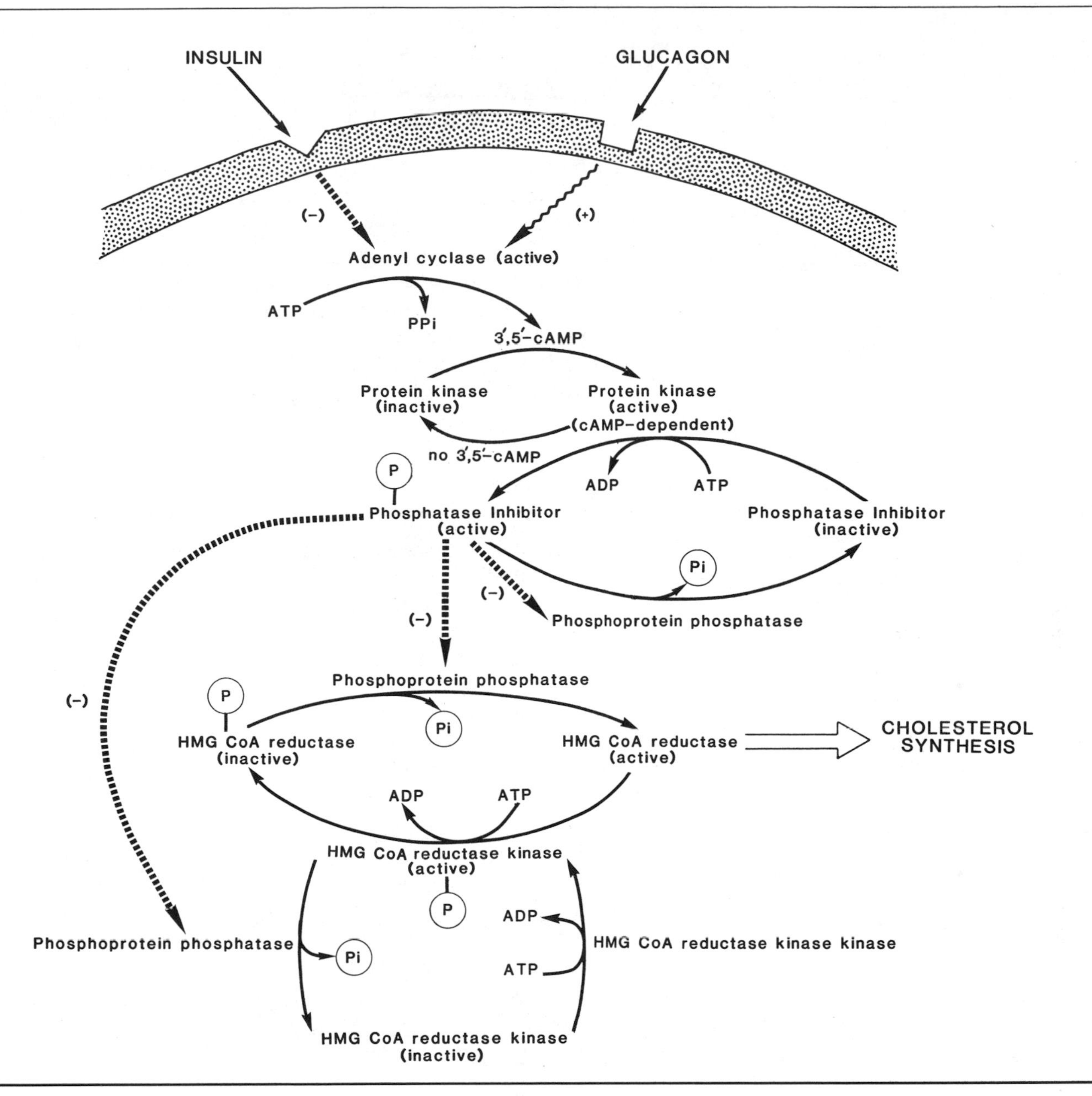

Figure 19.6
Hormonal regulation of HMG CoA reductase activity. Wavy lines (~~~~) in figure indicate the process of activation; dashed lines (▮▮▮▮▮▮) indicate deactivation.

b. The synthesis of cholesterol is also regulated by the amount of cholesterol taken up by the cells during lipoprotein metabolism. Chylomicron remnants internalized by liver cells, and LDL internalized by cells of the liver and peripheral tissues, provide cholesterol, which causes a decrease in *de novo* cholesterol synthesis. This process is described in section III of this chapter.

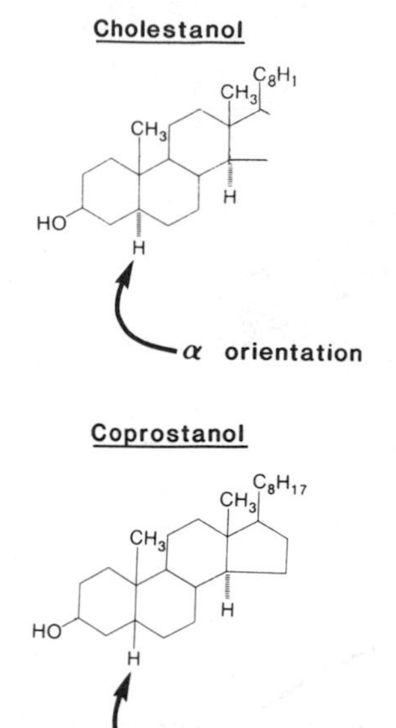

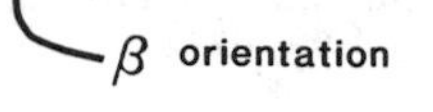

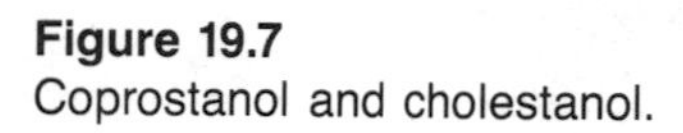

Figure 19.7
Coprostanol and cholestanol.

E. Degradation of cholesterol

1. The ring structure of cholesterol cannot be metabolized to CO_2 and H_2O in humans. Rather, the intact sterol ring is eliminated from the body by two routes: (1) conversion to bile acids, which can be excreted in the feces, and (2) solubilization of cholesterol in the bile, which transports it to the intestine for elimination.
2. Some of the cholesterol in the intestine is modified by bacteria before excretion. The primary compounds made, ***coprostanol*** and ***cholestanol,*** are reduced derivatives of cholesterol, and together these three compounds compose the bulk of neutral fecal sterols. (Note: Coprostanol and cholestanol are isomers, the only difference between them being the orientation of the hydrogen atom between the A and B rings; Figure 19.7.)

II. BILE ACIDS

Bile is composed of a watery mixture of organic and inorganic compounds. Phosphatidylcholine (lecithin, p. 185) and the bile salts are quantitatively the most important components of bile. Bile can either pass directly from the liver into the duodenum through the common bile duct or be stored in the gallbladder when not needed immediately for digestion. The most common are cholic acid and chenodeoxycholic acid. Their structure contains 24 carbons, with two or three hydroxyl groups and a side chain that terminates in a carboxyl group. The carboxyl group has a pK_a of about 6, and therefore is not fully ionized at physiologic pH.

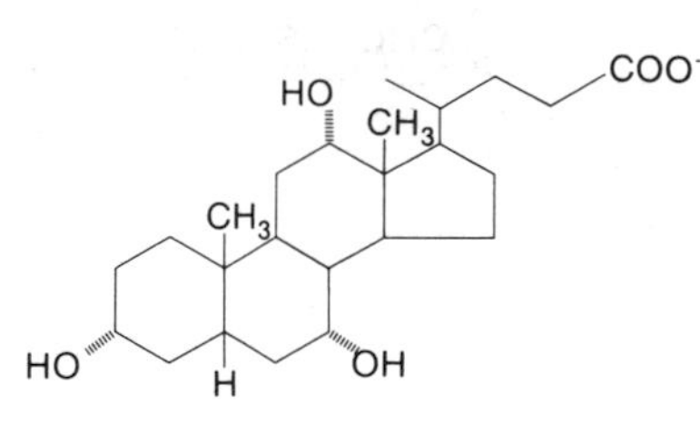

The bile acids are amphipathic in that all the hydroxyl groups are alpha in orientation (lie "above" the plane of the rings) and the methyl groups are beta (lie "below" the plane of the rings). Therefore the molecules have both a polar and a nonpolar face and can act as emulsifying agents in the intestine, helping to prepare dietary triacylglycerol and other lipids (including the fat-soluble vitamins) for degradation by pancreatic enzymes. Bile salts provide the only significant route for cholesterol excretion—both as a metabolic product of cholesterol and as an essential aid to cholesterol excretion through the bile.

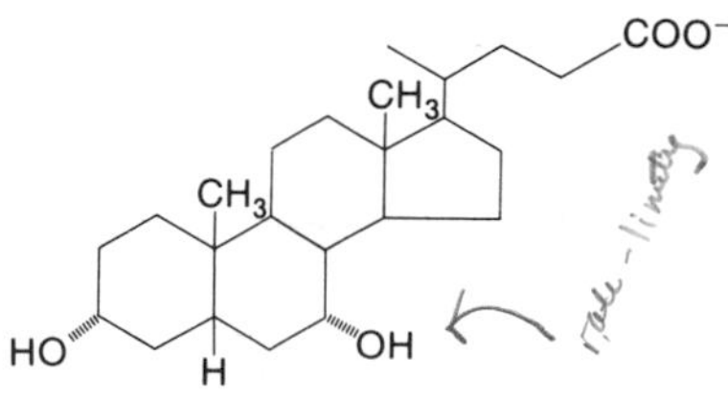

A. Synthesis of bile acids

1. Bile acids are synthesized in the liver by a multistep pathway in which hydroxyl groups are inserted at specific positions on the steroid structure, the double bond of the cholesterol B ring is reduced, and the hydrocarbon chain is shortened by three carbons, introducing a carboxyl group at the end of the chain. The resulting compounds, ***cholic*** and ***chenodeoxycholic acids,*** are called the ***"primary" bile acids.***
   a. The rate-limiting step in bile acid synthesis is the introduction of a hydroxyl group at carbon #7 of the steroid ring. The enzyme is *7-α-hydroxylase* and is inhibited by cholic acid (Figure 19.8).
2. Before the bile acids leave the liver, they are conjugated to a molecule of either glycine or taurine by a peptide bond between the carboxyl group of the bile acid and an amino group on the added compound. These new compounds are called ***bile salts***

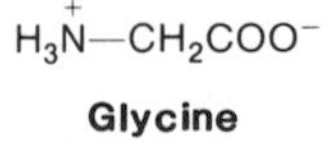

and include glycocholic and glycochenodeoxycholic acids and taurocholic and taurochenodeoxycholic acids.

a. The addition of glycine or taurine results in the presence of either a carboxyl group with a lower pK_a (from glycine) or a sulfate group (from taurine), both of which are negatively charged at physiologic pH. The ratio of the glycine to taurine forms in the bile is about 3:1.

b. The bile salts are more effective detergents than bile acids because of their enhanced amphipathic nature (having both a polar and a nonpolar end). Only the conjugated forms—that is, the bile ***salts***—are found in the bile.

3. Bacteria in the intestine remove some of the glycine and taurine from the bile salts. They then convert some of the primary bile acids into ***secondary bile acids*** by removing a hydroxyl group, producing ***deoxycholic*** from cholic acid and ***lithocholic*** from chenodeoxycholic acid.

4. The bile salts secreted into the intestine are efficiently reabsorbed and reused. Between 15 and 30 g of bile salts is secreted from the liver into the duodenum each day, yet only about 0.5 g is lost daily in the feces. Approximately 0.5 g is synthesized per day in the liver to replace the lost bile acids (Figure 19.9).

a. The mixture of primary and secondary bile salts and acids is absorbed primarily in the ileum. They move from the intestinal mucosal cells into the portal blood and are efficiently removed by the liver parenchymal cells.

b. The liver converts both primary and secondary bile acids into bile salts by conjugation with glycine or taurine, and they are then ready to be secreted in the bile.

c. The continuous process of secretion of the bile salts into the bile, their passage through the duodenum where some are converted to bile acids, and their subsequent return to the liver as a mixture of bile acids and salts are termed the ***enterohepatic circulation*** (Figure 19.9).

d. The bile acids are so hydrophobic that they require a carrier in the portal blood. Albumin carries them in a noncovalent complex, similar to the way it transports free fatty acids in blood.

C. Bile salt deficiency: cholelithiasis

1. The movement of cholesterol from the liver into the bile must be accompanied by the simultaneous secretion of phospholipid and bile salts. If this coupled process is disrupted and more cholesterol enters the bile than can be solubilized by the bile salts and lecithin present, the cholesterol can precipitate in the gallbladder, initiating the pathogenesis of cholesterol gallstone disease—***cholelithiasis.***

2. Bile salt deficiency can result from a number of different causes, including the following:

a. Gross malabsorption of bile acids from the intestine, as seen in patients with severe ileal disease.

b. Obstruction of the biliary tract, interrupting the enterohepatic circulation.

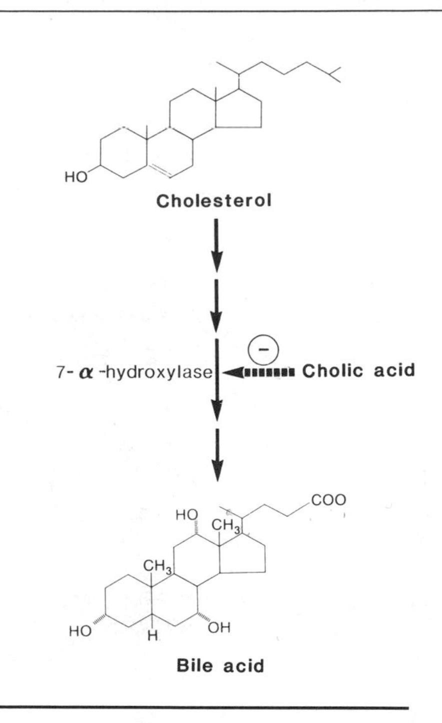

Figure 19.8
Rate-limiting step in bile acid synthesis.

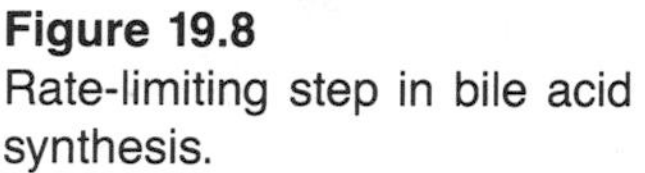

Taurine

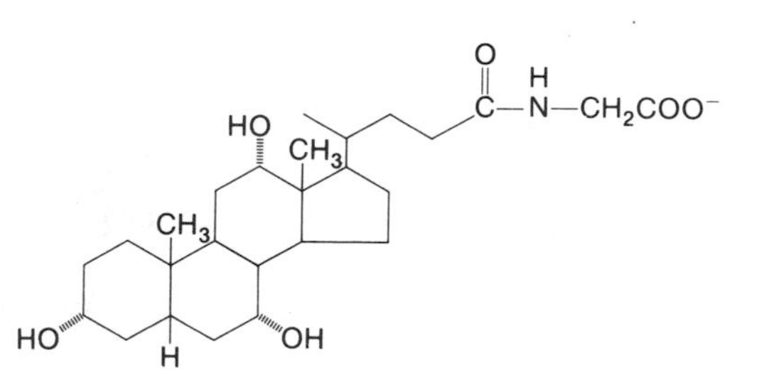

Glycocholic acid

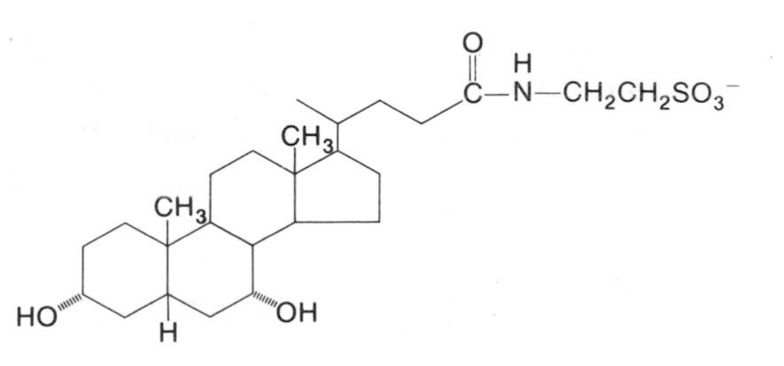

Taurochenodeoxycholic acid

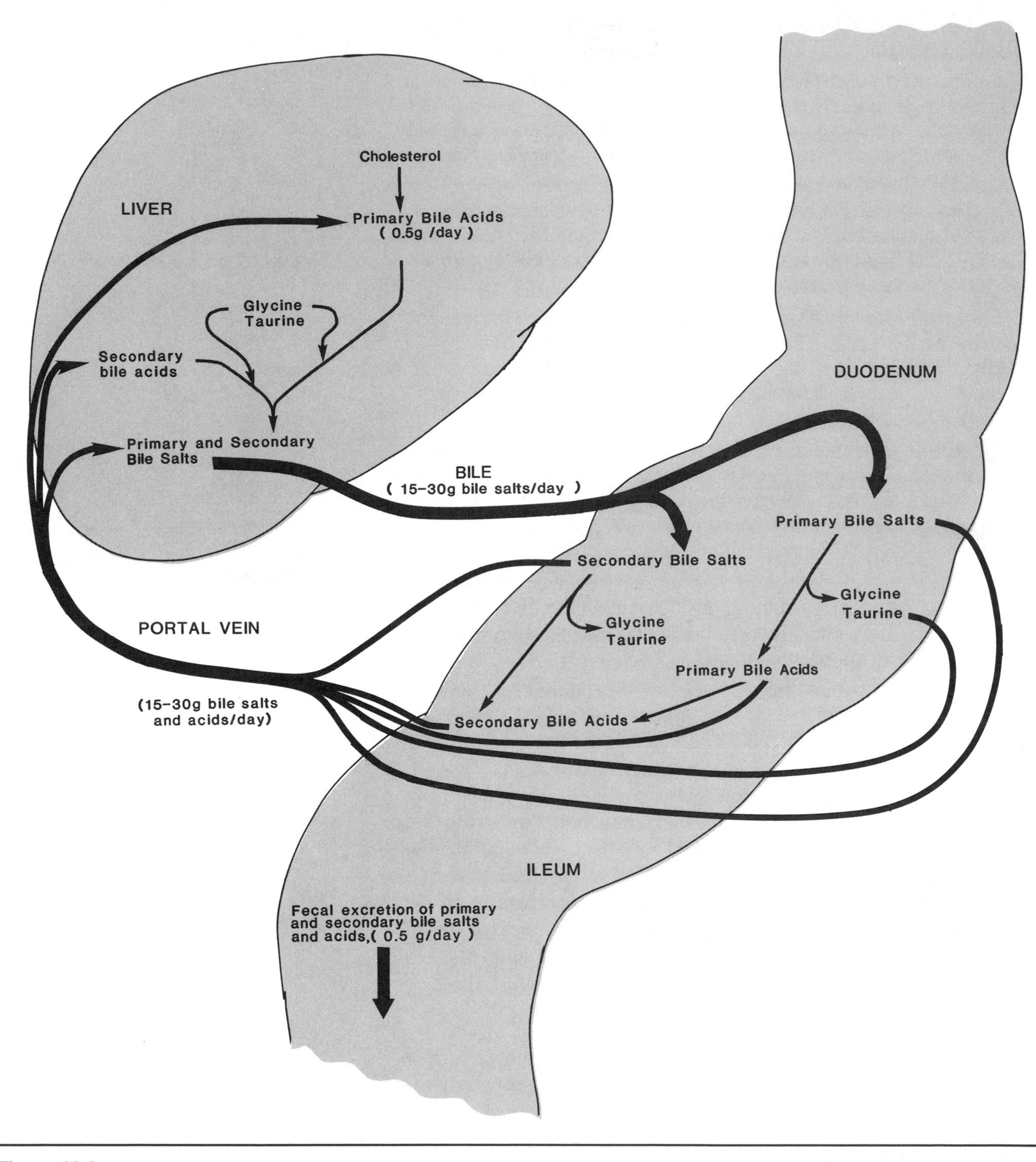

Figure 19.9
Enterohepatic circulation of bile salts and acids.

c. Severe hepatic dysfunction that leads to a decreased synthesis of bile salts or other abnormalities in bile production.

d. Excessive feedback suppression of bile acid synthesis as a result of an accelerated rate of recycling of bile acids.

3. Until recently the only treatment for severe cases of cholelithiasis was surgical removal of the gallbladder. However, some patients with gallstones primarily composed of precipitated cholesterol (about 80% of the total cholelithiasis population) respond to administration of chenodeoxycholic acid, commonly called chenodiol. Chenodiol supplements the body's supply of bile acids, resulting in a gradual (months to years) dissolution of gallstones.

Study Questions

Choose the ONE BEST answer:

19.1 The immediate precursor of mevalonic acid is

A. mevalonyl CoA.
B. mevalonyl pyrophosphate.
C. acetoacetyl CoA.
D. 3-hydroxy-3-methylglutaryl CoA.
E. isopentenyl pyrophosphate.

19.2 Which one of the following statements about sterols found in nature is INCORRECT?

A. Cholesterol is the most abundant sterol found in animal tissue.
B. All the carbon atoms of cholesterol are derived from acetyl CoA.
C. β-Sitosterol is the most abundant plant sterol.
D. Dietary β-sitosterol and cholesterol are absorbed to about the same extent in the intestine of normal humans.
E. The cholesterol ring structure cannot be broken down enzymatically by humans into smaller molecules for excretion.

19.3 Which one of the following compounds is a precursor in the biosynthesis of cholesterol?

A. Cholestanol
B. Progesterone
C. Lanosterol
D. Cholic acid
E. Pregnenolone

19.4 Which one of the following compounds is NOT a precursor for the biosynthesis of cholesterol?

A. Mevalonic acid
B. Squalene
C. Isopentenyl pyrophosphate
D. Aldosterone
E. Farnesyl pyrophosphate

19.5 Animals fed a high cholesterol diet exhibit decreased cholesterol synthesis by liver because of the inhibition of which one of the following enzymes?

A. 3-Hydroxy-3-methyl glutaryl CoA (HMG CoA) synthetase
B. HMG CoA reductase
C. Mevalonate kinase
D. HMG CoA lyase
E. Squalene synthetase

19.6 Which one of the following is NOT a bile ***acid***?

A. Glycocholate
B. Deoxycholate
C. Lithocholate
D. Cholate
E. Chenodeoxycholate

III. SERUM LIPOPROTEINS

The serum lipoproteins are complexes of lipids and specific proteins called ***apoproteins***. These particles are in a constant state of synthesis, degradation, and removal from the plasma. These particles include the ***chylomicrons*** (CM), ***very low density lipoproteins*** (VLDL), ***low density lipoproteins*** (LDL), and ***high density lipoproteins*** (HDL). Lipoproteins function both to keep lipids soluble as they transport them in the serum and to provide an efficient mechanism for delivering their lipid contents to the tissues. In humans, the delivery system is less perfect than in other animals, and, as a result, humans experience a gradual deposition of lipid—especially cholesterol—in tissues. This is a potentially life-threatening occurrence when the lipid deposition causes the occlusion of blood vessels—a condition known as ***atherosclerosis*** (see p. 304).

A. Composition of serum lipoproteins

1. The principal lipids carried by lipoprotein particles are triacylglycerol and cholesterol, obtained either from the diet or *de novo* synthesis.
2. Lipoproteins are composed of a neutral lipid core surrounded by a shell of apoproteins, phospholipid, and nonesterified cholesterol, all oriented so that their polar portions are exposed on the surface of the lipoprotein, thus making the particle soluble in aqueous solution.
3. The chylomicrons are the lowest of the lipoproteins in density and the largest in size and contain the most lipid and the smallest percentage of protein. The VLDLs and LDLs are successively more dense, having a higher content of protein and a lower content of lipid. The HDL particles are the most dense of the serum lipoproteins (see Figure 19.10 for a comparison of their relative compositions.) The serum lipoproteins can also be separated on the basis of their electrophoretic mobility, as shown in Figure 19.11.
4. The apoproteins associated with the lipoprotein particles have a number of diverse functions: They serve as structural components of the particles, provide recognition sites for cell-surface receptors, and serve as co-factors for enzymes involved in lipoprotein metabolism.

B. Metabolism of chylomicrons

1. Chylomicrons are produced in intestinal mucosal cells and carry dietary triacylglycerol and cholesterol esters (plus lipids made in these cells) to the peripheral tissues. Their production was discussed on p. 152.

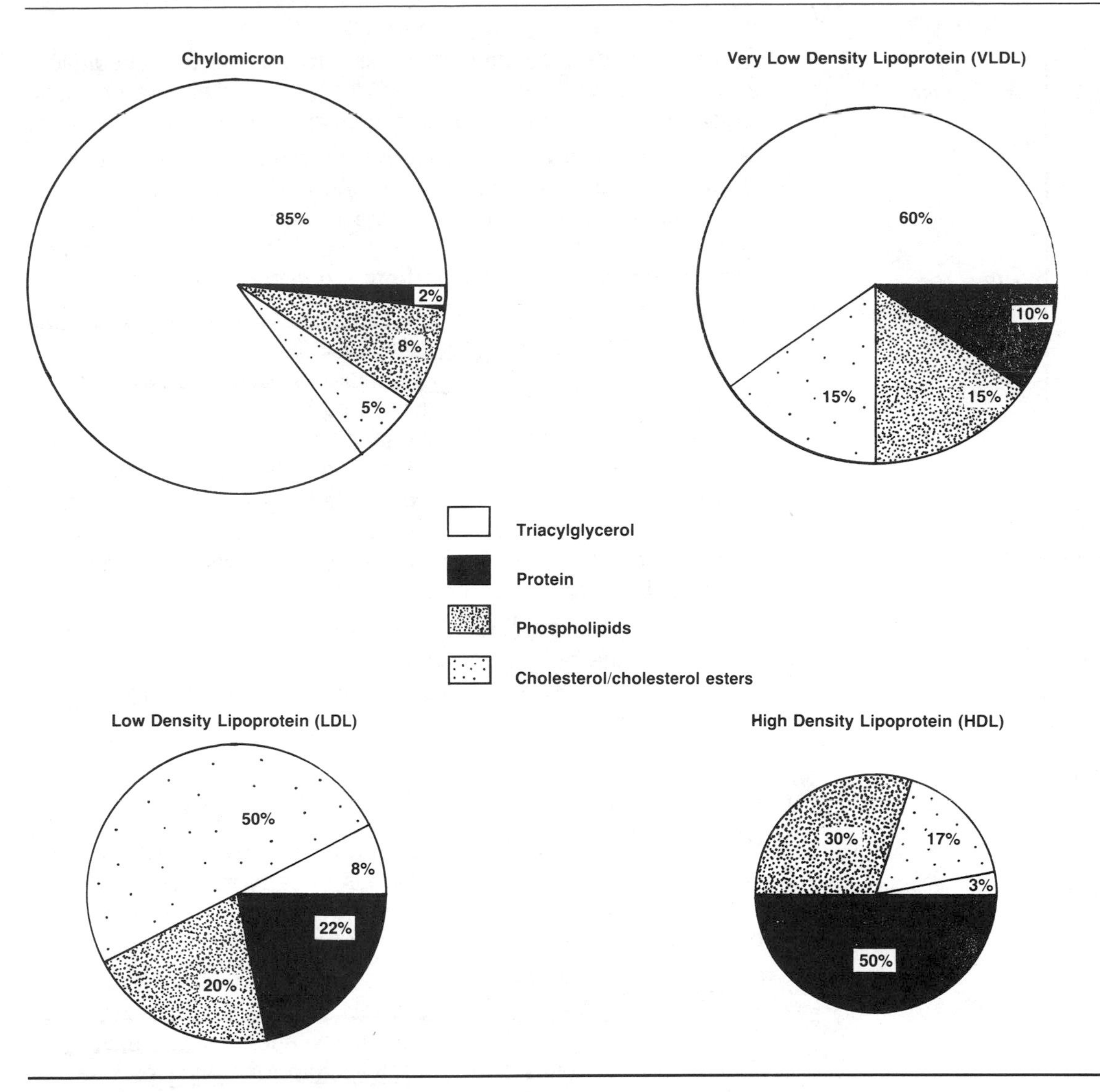

Figure 19.10
Compositions of the serum lipoproteins.

2. The particle released by the intestinal mucosal cell is called a "nascent" chylomicron and contains predominantly apoprotein B (apoB). When it reaches the plasma, it is rapidly modified, receiving apoprotein E (which, along with apoB, is recognized by hepatic receptors) and the C apoproteins (including apoC-II, necessary for the activation of *lipoprotein lipase*, the enzyme that degrades the triacylglycerol contained in the chylomicron). The source of these apoproteins is circulating HDL (Figure 19.12).
    a. *Lipoprotein lipase* is a negatively charged extracellular enzyme attached by ionic bonds to the surface of capillary cells. It is found predominantly in the capillaries of the adipose, cardiac, and skeletal muscle and tissues. *Lipoprotein lipase* catalyzes the hydrolysis of triacylglycerol contained in circulating lipoprotein particles to yield fatty acids and glycerol.
    b. *Lipoprotein lipase* is essential for the degradation of the

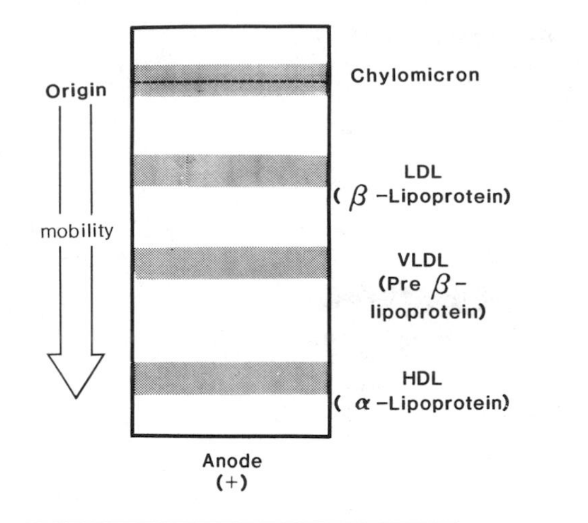

Figure 19.11
Electrophoretic mobility of serum lipoproteins.

triacylglycerol component of lipoproteins in the circulation. Patients with a deficiency of *lipoprotein lipase* show a dramatic accumulation of triacylglycerol-rich lipoproteins in the plasma.

3. As the chylomicron circulates and the triacylglycerol in its core is degraded by *lipoprotein lipase,* the particle begins to shrink. In addition, the C apoproteins are returned to the HDLs. The remaining particle is called a "remnant." In humans, these ***chylomicron remnants*** are removed from the circulation by the liver:
   a. ***Hepatocyte membranes*** contain ***lipoprotein receptors*** that recognize the combination of ***apoproteins B and E*** on the same particle. Chylomicron remnants, containing apoB and apoE, bind to these receptors and are taken into the cells by endocytosis. The endocytosed vesicle then fuses with a lysosome, and the apoproteins, cholesteryl esters, and other components of the remnant are hydrolytically degraded, releasing amino acids, free cholesterol, and fatty acids. (A more detailed discussion of the mechanism of ***receptor-mediated endocytosis*** is illustrated for LDL in Figure 19.15.)
   b. The cholesterol released from the chylomicron appears to regulate the rate of *de novo* cholesterol synthesis in the liver by causing a decrease in cell content of HMG CoA reductase, rather than by allosterically inhibiting the enzyme directly.

C. Metabolism of very low density lipoproteins (VLDL)

1. VLDL are produced in the ***liver.*** They are composed predominantly of triacylglycerol, and their function is to carry this lipid from the liver to the peripheral tissues. There, the triacylglycerol is degraded by *lipoprotein lipase,* as discussed for chylomicron degradation.
   a. "Fatty liver" occurs in clinical conditions in which there is an imbalance between hepatic triacylglycerol synthesis and the secretion of VLDL. Human diseases such as hepatitis, uncontrolled diabetes, and excessive ethanol ingestion can cause fatty liver.
2. When VLDL are released from the liver, they are nascent particles and must obtain apoprotein C-II from circulating HDL before their triacylglycerol can be degraded (Figure 19.13). (As with chylomicrons, apoC-II is required for *lipoprotein lipase* to function.) The primary apoprotein of circulating VLDL is apoB. VLDL also receive apoE from the HDL.
3. As the VLDL pass through the circulation their structure is altered by the following mechanisms:
   a. Triacylglycerol is removed by *lipoprotein lipase,* causing the VLDL to shrink and become more dense.
   b. Surface components, including phospholipid, cholesterol, and the C and E apoproteins (that originally had been donated to the VLDL from HDL), are transferred to HDL.
   c. Cholesteryl esters are transferred from HDL to VLDL in an ***exchange reaction*** that concomitantly transfers triacylglycerol or phospholipid from VLDL to the HDL. This exchange is accomplished by cholesteryl ester transfer protein—a component of HDL (see Figure 19.14 for a summary of these processes).

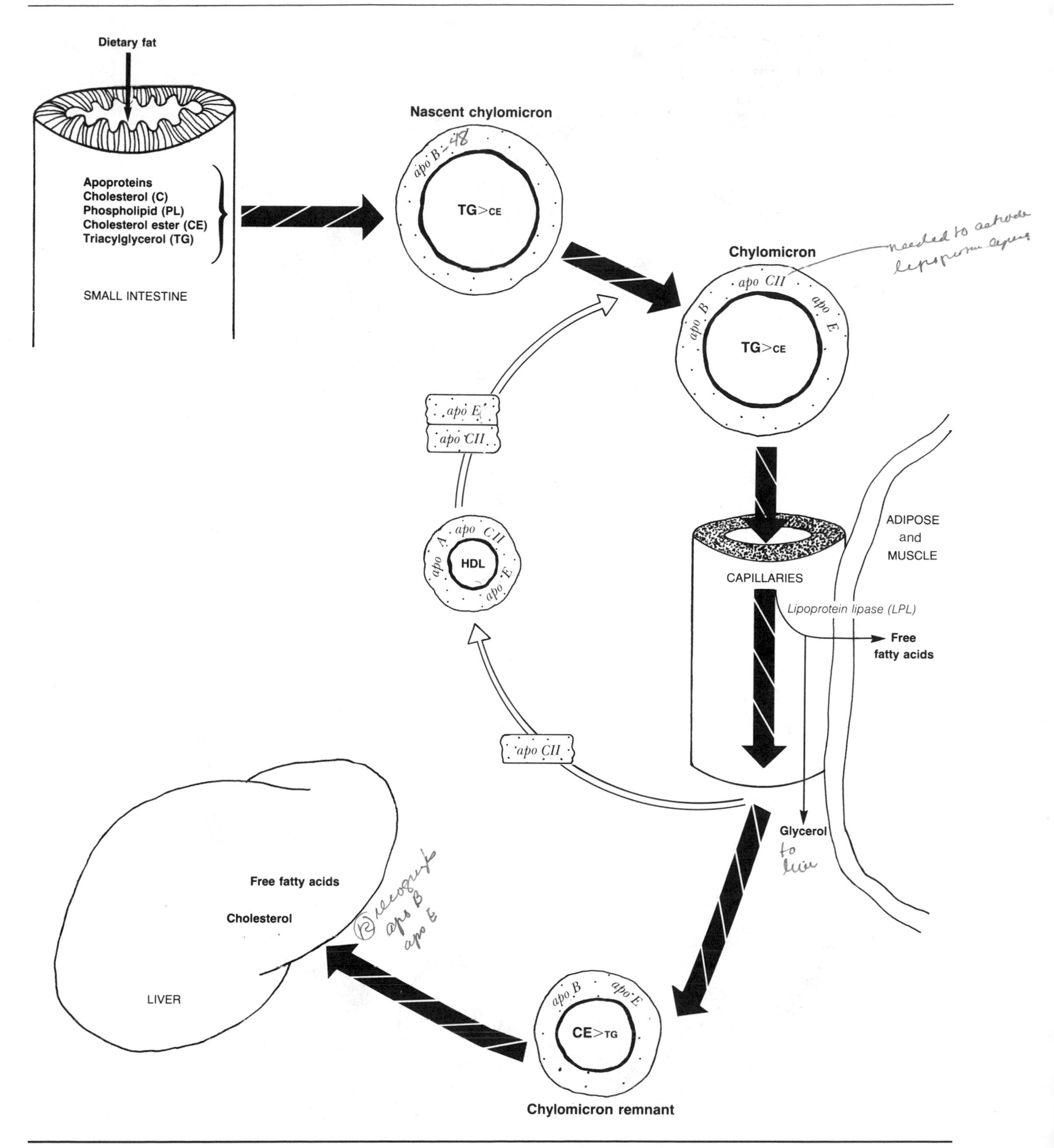

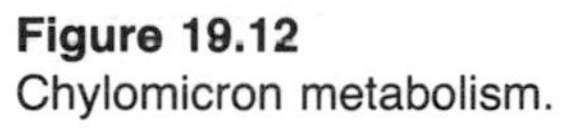

Figure 19.12
Chylomicron metabolism.

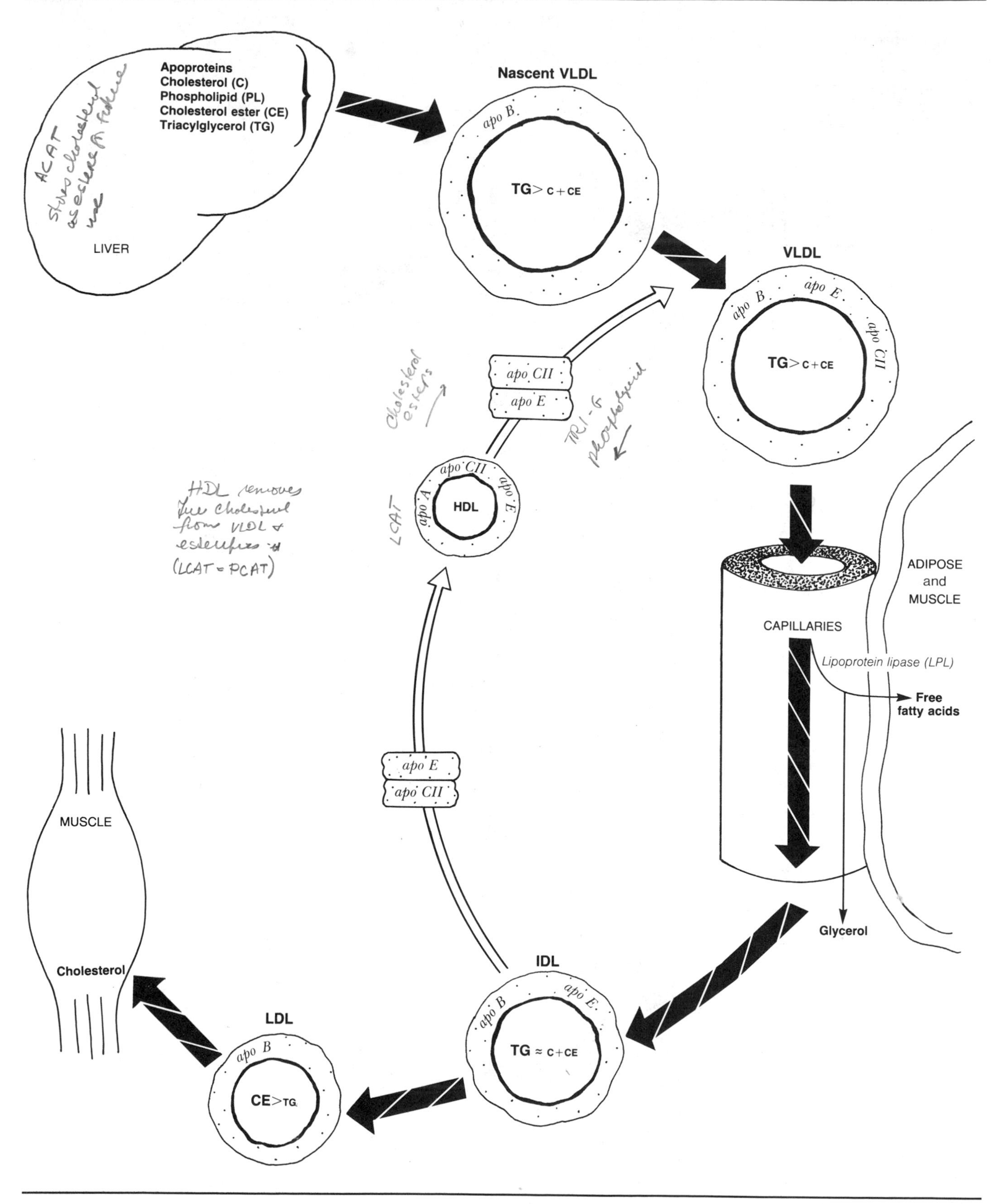

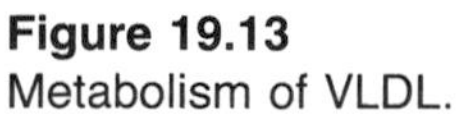
Figure 19.13
Metabolism of VLDL.

4. After these modifications, the VLDL has been converted in the plasma to LDL. (Note: An intermediate-sized particle, the intermediate density lipoprotein, IDL, is observed during the transition from VLDL to LDL in the serum.)

D. Metabolism of LDL

1. The LDL particles retain apoprotein B but have lost their other apoproteins to HDL. They have also lost most of the triacylglycerol contained in their VLDL predecessors and have a high concentration of cholesterol and cholesteryl esters. LDL particles are small enough to leave the blood vessels and enter the extracellular matrix, where they can move between cells.

2. The primary function of LDL particles is to provide cholesterol to the peripheral tissues. They do so both by depositing free cholesterol on the membranes of cells as they bump against the cell surface and by binding to receptors on cell-surface membranes that recognize apoprotein B. A summary of the uptake and degradation of LDL particles is presented in Figure 19.15. A similar mechanism is presumably used for the cellular uptake and degradation of chylomicron remnants and HDLs. (The numbers in brackets refer to corresponding numbers on the figure.)

   [1] The LDL receptors are negatively charged glycoprotein molecules that are clustered in pits on cell membranes. The intracellular side of the pit is coated with the protein ***clathrin***.

   [2] After binding, the LDL are internalized as intact particles by ***endocytosis***.

   [3] The vesicle containing the LDL rapidly loses its clathrin coat and fuses with other similar vesicles, forming larger vesicles called ***endosomes***.

   [4] The pH of the contents of the endosome falls, allowing separation of the LDL from its receptor. The receptors then migrate to one side of the endosome while the LDL stay free within the lumen of the vesicle. (This structure is called CURL—the Compartment of Uncoupling of Receptor and Ligand.

   [5] The receptors can be recycled, whereas the lipoprotein remnants are degraded by lysosomal (hydrolytic) enzymes, releasing cholesterol, amino acids, fatty acids, and phospholipid skeletons. These compounds can be recycled by the cell.

3. The number of receptors for lipoproteins varies according to the availability of these lipoprotein particles and according to the needs of the cell. For example, if there is a large amount of circulating serum lipoprotein, the number of cell-surface receptors will decrease. If cells are starved for cholesterol, however, they will increase the number of cell-surface receptors.

4. The chylomicron remnant-, HDL-, and LDL-derived cholesterol affects cellular cholesterol content in several ways:

   a. *HMG CoA reductase* activity is decreased so that *de novo* cholesterol synthesis decreases.

   b. If the cholesterol is not required immediately for some structural or synthetic purpose, it can be esterified by the enzyme *acyl*

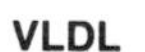

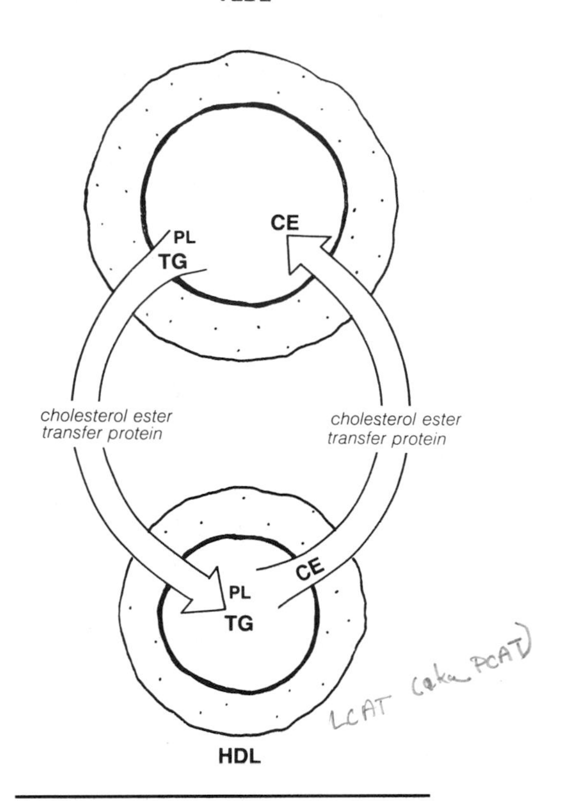

Figure 19.14
Transfer of cholesteryl esters from HDL to VLDL in exchange for triacylglycerol or phospholipid.

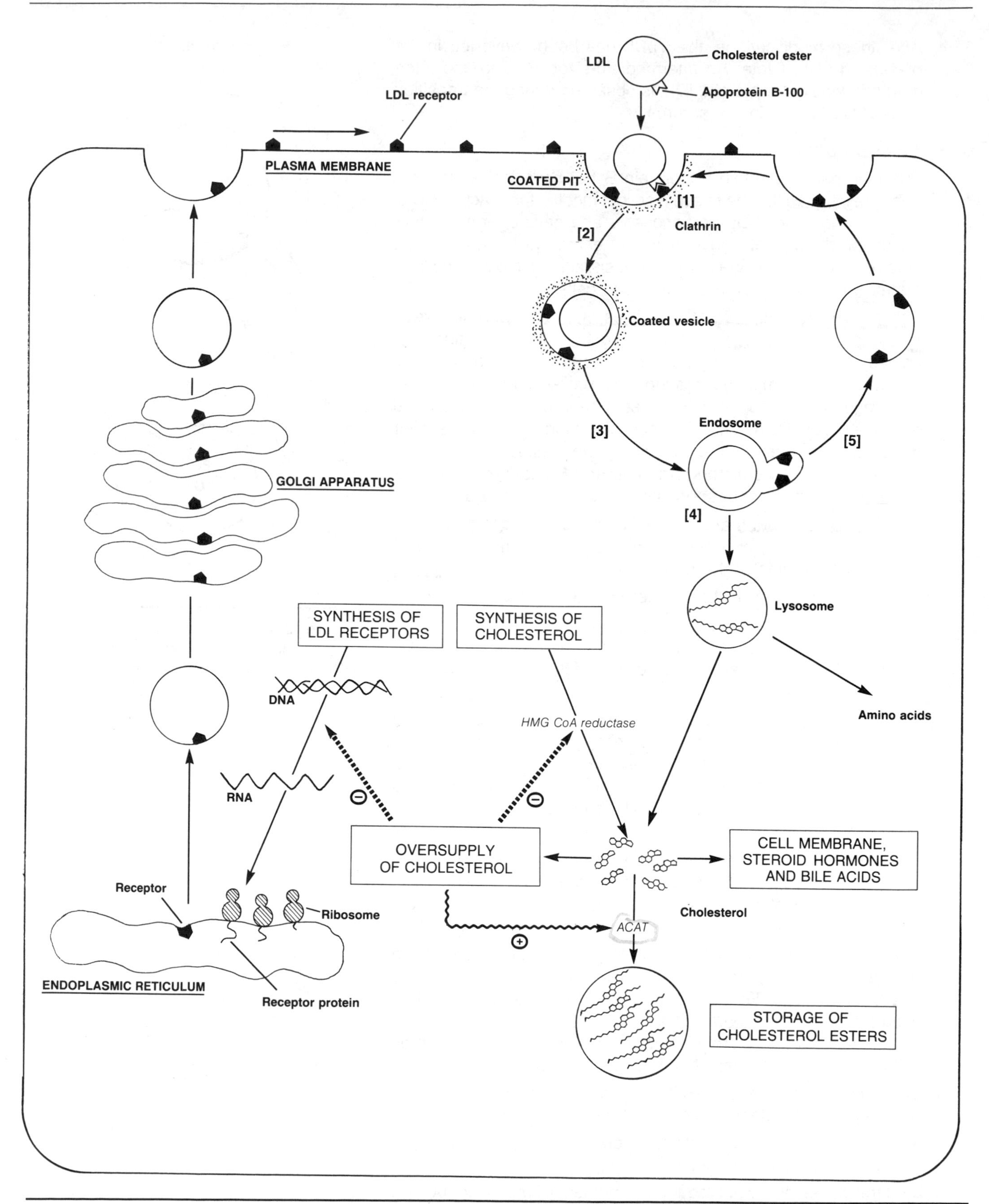

Figure 19.15
Cellular uptake and degradation of LDL.

CoA:cholesterol acyltransferase (*ACAT*) and stored in the cell for future use. The activity of this enzyme is enhanced in the presence of increased intracellular cholesterol. *ACAT* transfers a fatty acid from a fatty acyl CoA derivative to cholesterol, producing a cholesteryl ester that can be stored in the cell (Figure 19.16).

c. Synthesis of new LDL receptor protein is decreased, so that further entry of LDL cholesterol into the cell is limited.

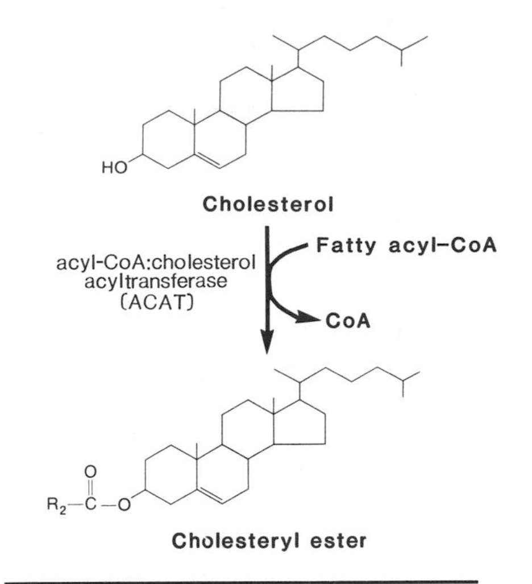

Figure 19.16
Synthesis of intracellular cholesteryl ester.

E. Metabolism of HDL

1. HDL particles are synthesized in the liver and released into the bloodstream by ***exocytosis***. They perform a number of important functions, including the following.

   a. Serving as a circulating reservoir of apoC-II, the apoprotein that is transferred to VLDL and chylomicrons and used as an activator of *lipoprotein lipase*.

   b. Removing free (unesterified) cholesterol from extrahepatic tissues and esterifying it, using the plasma enzyme *phosphatidylcholine:cholesterol acyl transferase* (*PCAT*—also known as *LCAT*, where "L" stands for lecithin).

   c. Transferring cholesteryl esters to VLDL and LDL in exchange for triacylglycerol.

   d. Carrying cholesteryl esters to the liver, where the HDL is degraded and cholesterol released.

2. Newly secreted HDL are disk-shaped particles containing predominantly unesterified cholesterol, phospholipid (largely phosphatidyl choline), and a number of apoproteins, including apoA-I, apoE, and the C apoproteins. They are rapidly converted to spherical particles through their accumulation of cholesterol (Figure 19.17).

   a. HDL particles are excellent acceptors of unesterified cholesterol, both from the surface of cell membranes and also from other circulating lipoproteins.

   b. Once the free cholesterol is taken up, it is immediately esterified by *PCAT*, a plasma enzyme, which is activated by apoA-I of the HDL. The fatty acid from carbon #2 of phosphatidyl choline is transferred directly to the cholesterol, leaving lysophosphatidyl choline.

   c. The resulting cholesteryl ester is so hydrophobic that it is effectively "trapped" in the HDL and can no longer be transferred to a membrane. The only mechanism for removing it from HDL in the plasma is through transfer to VLDL (see Figure 19.14) or LDL by the cholesteryl ester transfer protein, and it will remain in the LDL until the particle is taken up by a cell. About two thirds of the cholesterol in the plasma is esterified with fatty acid.

   d. In liver disease, a decreased concentration of plasma cholesteryl esters is observed. This may be due either to a deficiency in phosphatidyl choline production or a lack of *PCAT*.

3. HDL particles not only serve as the source of apoproteins required for the proper metabolism of other serum lipoproteins, but also

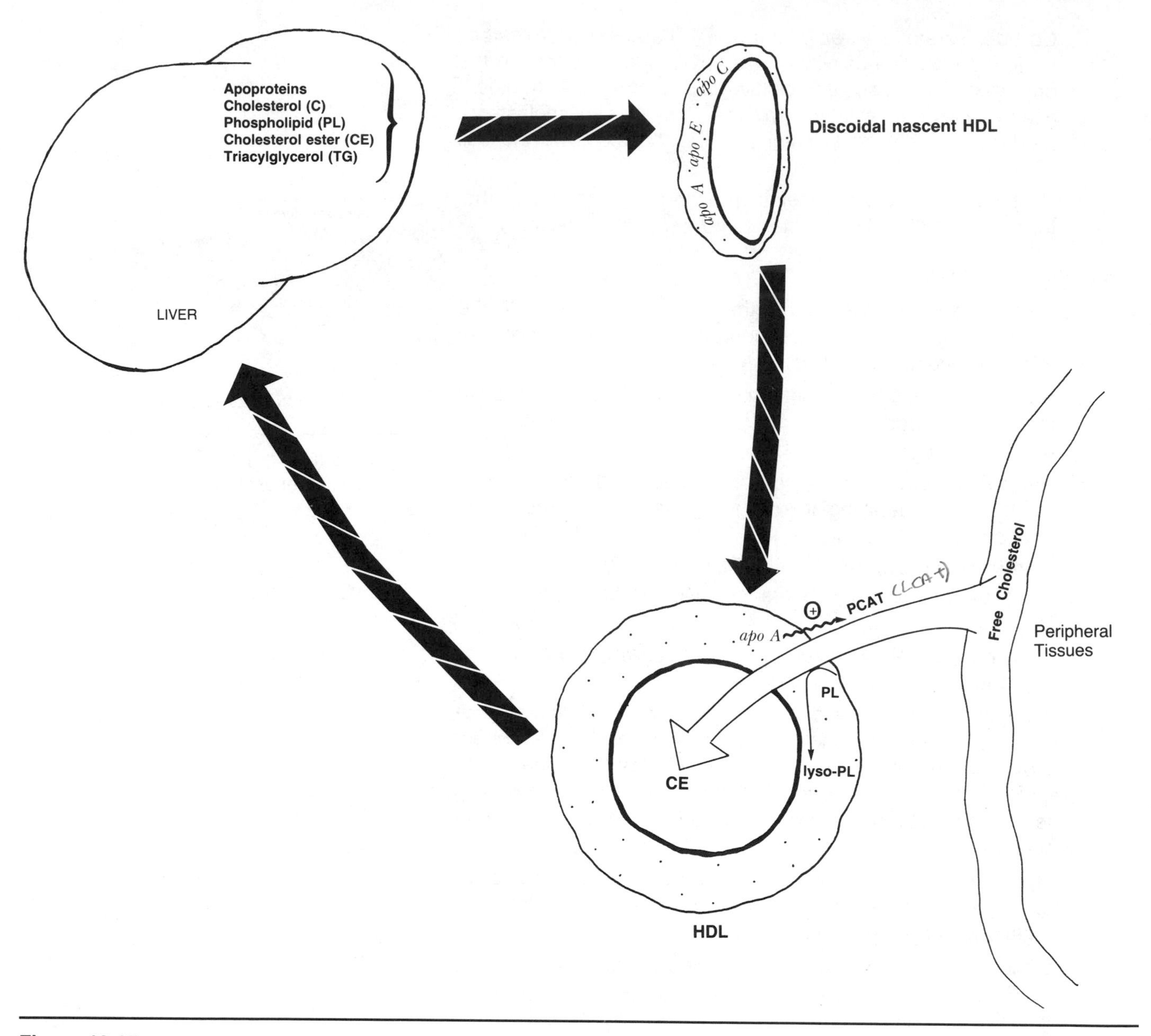

Figure 19.17
Metabolism of HDL.

TABLE 19.1: SUMMARY OF LIPASES

Enzyme	Origin	Site of Action	Function	Special Properties
Gastric lipase	Stomach	Stomach	Degrade dietary triacylglycerol (removes short-chain fatty acids)	Acid-stable
Pancreatic lipase	Pancreas	Small intestine (lumen)	Degrade dietary triacylglycerol (removes fatty acid from carbon #1 and #3, leaving 2-monoacylglycerol)	Requires co-lipase for stabilization
Lipoprotein lipase	Extrahepatic tissues	Surface of endothelial cells lining the capillaries	Degrade triacylglycerol circulating in chylomicrons or VLDL, releasing non-esterified fatty acid and glycerol	Can be released into plasma by heparin. Activated by apoprotein C-II
Hormone-sensitive lipase	Adipocytes	Adipocytes (cytoplasm)	Degradation of stored triacylglycerol	Activated by cyclic AMP-dependent protein kinase
Acid lipase	Most tissues	Lysosomes	Remove fatty acids from lipids taken into cells during phagocytosis	Acid pH optimum

take back most of these proteins before the chylomicron remnants and LDL bind to their cell-surface receptors and are endocytosed.

4. Spherical HDL particles are taken up by the liver and the cholesteryl esters degraded. The cholesterol thus released can be either repackaged in lipoproteins, converted into bile acids, or secreted into the bile for removal from the body.

F. A summary of the properties and functions of some important lipases is presented in Table 19.1.

Study Questions

Choose the ONE BEST answer:

19.7 Which of the following functions is NOT performed by high density lipoproteins (HDL)?

A. HDL contains apoprotein apoA-I, which activates phosphatidylcholine:cholesterol acyl transferase.
B. HDL contains apoA-III, which transfers cholesterol esters from the HDL to other circulating lipoproteins in exchange for triacylglycerol.
C. HDL carries cholesterol from the peripheral tissues to the liver.
D. HDL is an important source of cholesterol esters for the extrahepatic tissues.
E. HDL donates apoprotein E to chylomicra. This apoprotein, together with apoprotein B, is recognized by the chylomicron receptor on hepatocytes.

19.8 Which one of the following statements about serum lipoproteins is CORRECT?

A. Chylomicrons are synthesized primarily in adipose tissue and transport triacylglycerol to the liver.
B. HDL are produced from LDL particles in the circulation by the action of lipoprotein lipase.
C. VLDL are the precursors of LDL in the circulation.
D. HDL competes with LDL for binding to receptors on the surface of cells in extrahepatic tissues.
E. Cholesterol ester transfer protein in HDL is important for the efficient uptake of cellular cholesterol esters by HDL in extrahepatic tissues.

19.9 Which one of the following statements about familial hypercholesterolemia is INCORRECT?

A. This is a group of disorders characterized by elevations of total serum and especially LDL cholesterol.
B. The disease is manifested clinically by xanthomas and accelerated atherosclerosis.
C. Heterozygotes for this disease may have plasma cholesterol levels that are approximately twice normal.
D. The primary metabolic defect is a lack of binding of LDL to cell surface receptors caused by a lack of LDL apoprotein B.
E. Homozygotes for this disease are able to metabolize chylomicrons normally.

19.10 Which one of the following changes would you expect in a patient with decreased activity of lipoprotein lipase?

A. Elevation of serum chylomicrons only.
B. Elevation of both serum chylomicrons and VLDL.
C. Elevation of serum HDL only.
D. Elevation of serum LDL only.
E. Elevation of both serum HDL and LDL.

19.11 The lipoprotein particles that have the highest percent concentration of cholesterol are

A. the chylomicrons.
B. the VLDL.
C. the LDL.
D. the HDL.
E. serum albumin-associated lipid.

19.12 The lipoprotein particles that have the highest percent concentration of triacylglycerol are

A. the chylomicrons.
B. the VLDL.
C. the LDL.
D. the HDL.
E. serum albumin-associated lipid.

19.13 A patient has a genetic defect that results in a deficiency of lipoprotein lipase. After eating a meal containing a large amount of fat, one would expect to see a plasma elevation of

A. the chylomicrons.
B. the VLDL.
C. the LDL.
D. the HDL.
E. serum albumin-associated lipid.

VI. STEROID HORMONES

Cholesterol is the precursor of the five classes of steroid hormones: glucocorticoids (e.g., cortisol and corticosterone), mineralocorticoids (e.g., aldosterone), and the sex hormones—the androgens, estrogens, and progestagens. Synthesis occurs in the adrenal cortex, ovaries, testes, and ovarian corpus luteum. Steroid hormones are transported by the blood from their sites of synthesis to their target organs. Because of their hydrophobicity, they must be complexed with a serum protein: ***serum albumin*** can act as a nonspecific carrier for the steroid hormones. However, specific plasma steroid-carrier proteins can bind the steroid hormones more tightly than does albumin. ***Transcortin*** is responsible for transporting cortisol and corticosterone. ***Sex hormone-binding protein*** transports the sex steroids. A large number of genetic diseases have been identified that are associated with specific steps in the metabolism of steroid hormones. Some representative diseases are described in Figure 19.18.

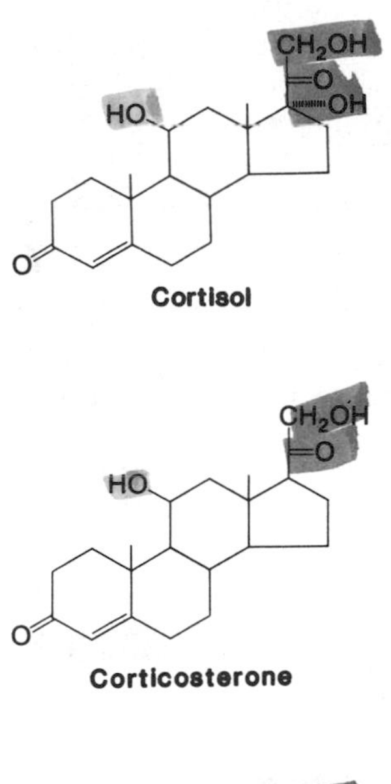

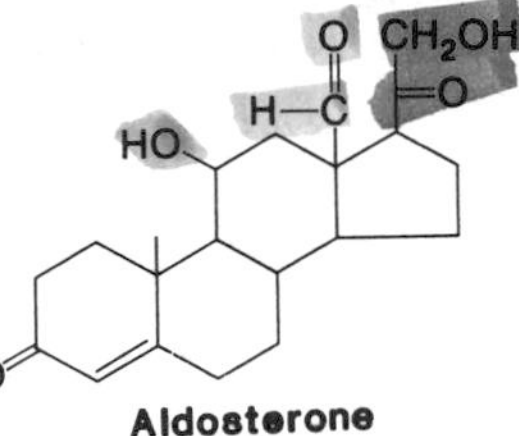

Aldosterone

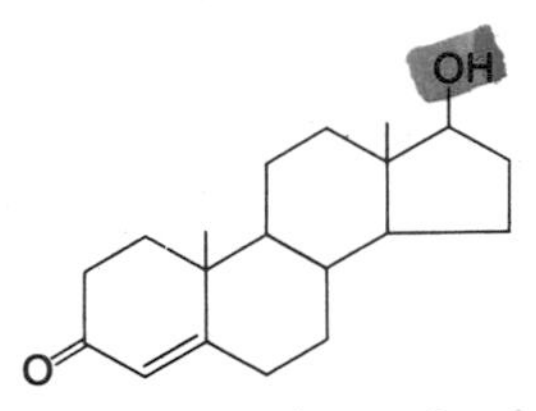

Testosterone (an androgen)

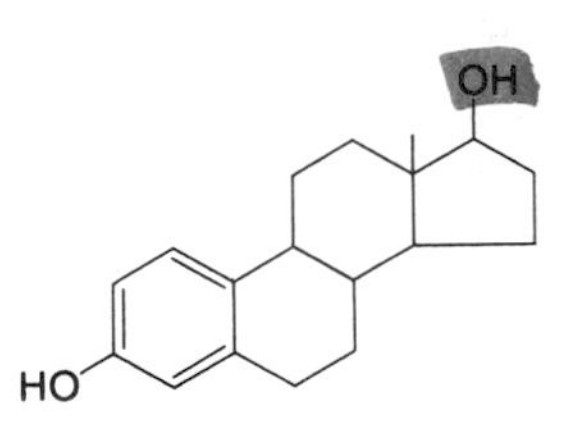

Estradiol (an estrogen)

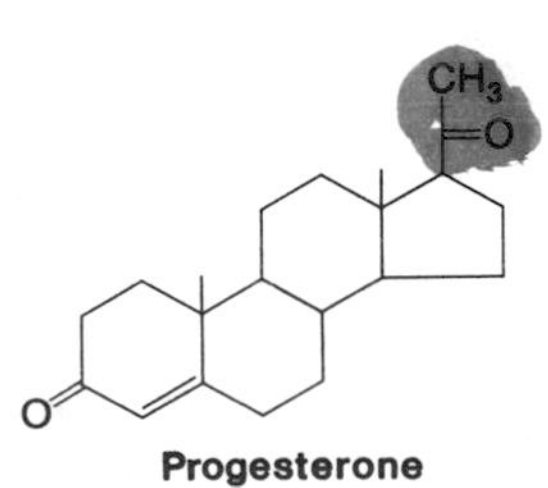

Progesterone

A. Synthesis of steroid hormones

1. Synthesis involves the shortening of the hydrocarbon chain of cholesterol and hydroxylation of the steroid nucleus. The initial reaction, catalyzed by the enzyme complex *desmolase*, converts cholesterol to pregnenolone. This is the ***rate-limiting step*** in steroid hormone biosynthesis. It requires NADPH and molecular oxygen. All the steroid hormones are derived from pregnenolone.
2. Pregnenolone is next oxidized and then isomerized to progesterone.
3. Progesterone is further modified by a series of hydroxylation reactions to other steroid hormones (see Figure 19.18 for a summary of these reactions). These enzymes are *mixed-function oxidases* requiring NADPH and molecular oxygen.
4. A defect in the activity or amount of an enzyme in this pathway can lead to both a deficiency in the synthesis of hormones beyond the affected step and to an excess in the hormones or metabolites before that step. Since all members of the pathway have potent biological activity, serious metabolic imbalances may occur if enzyme deficiencies are present.

B. Further metabolism of steroid hormones

1. Steroid hormones are generally converted into metabolic excretion products in the liver. Reactions include reductions of unsaturated bonds and the introduction of additional hydroxyl groups.
2. The resulting structures are made more soluble by conjugation with either glucuronic acid or sulfate. About 20% to 30% of these metabolites are secreted into the bile and then excreted in the feces, whereas the remainder are released into the blood and are filtered from the plasma in the kidney, passing into the urine. These conjugated metabolites are soluble in blood or bile and do not need protein carriers.

C. Secretion of adrenal steroid hormones

1. Adrenal cortical hormone secretion is controlled by the ***hypothalamus***, to which the pituitary gland is attached (Figure 19.19).

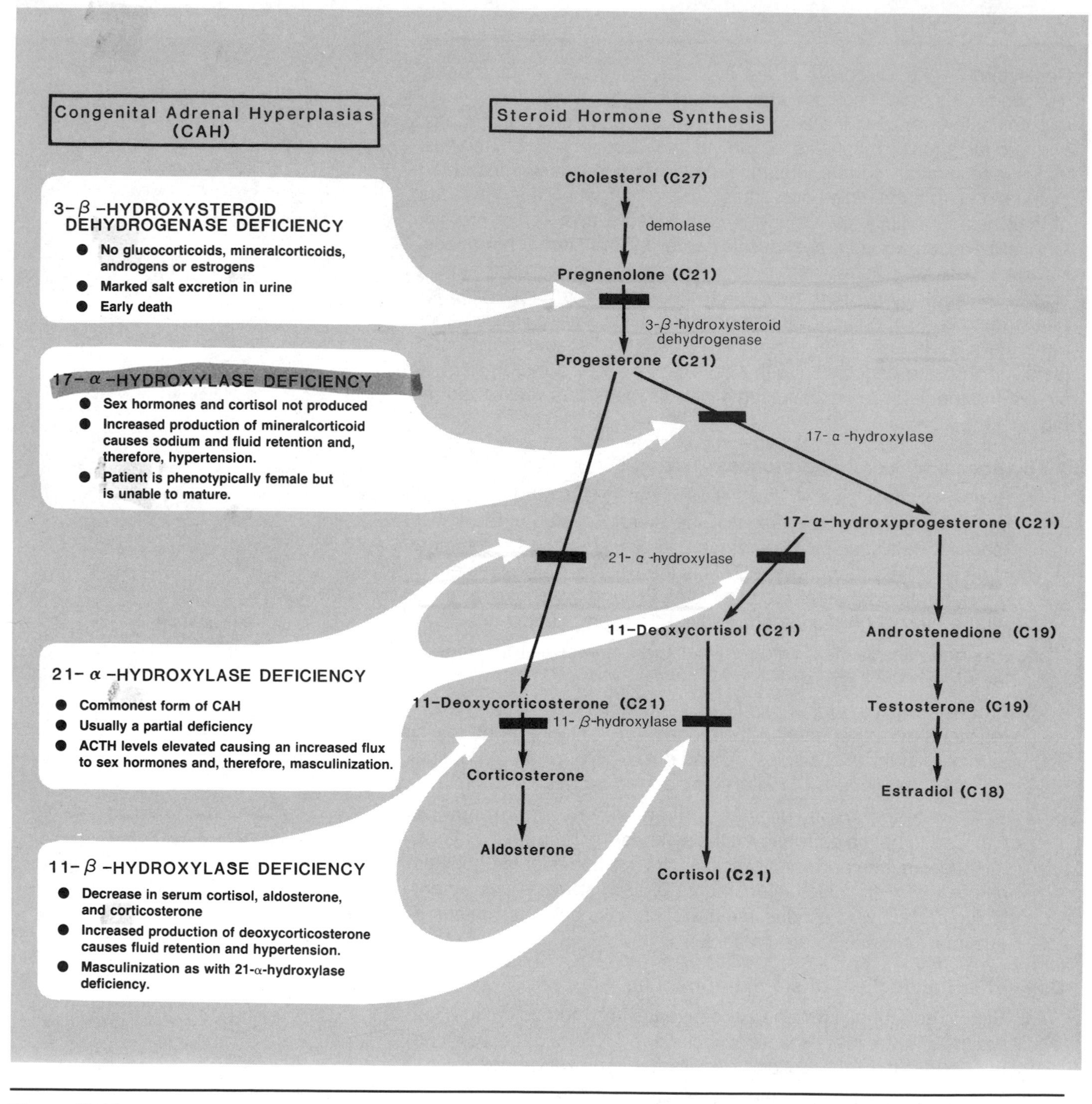

Figure 19.18
Steroid hormone synthesis.

When the body is stressed, release factors produced by the hypothalamus travel through a network of capillaries to the ***anterior lobe*** of the ***pituitary***, where they induce the production and secretion of the anterior pituitary hormone ***adrenocorticotropin*** (ACTH).

2. ACTH, often called the "stress hormone," stimulates the adrenal cortex to synthesize and secrete the ***mineralocorticoid aldos-***

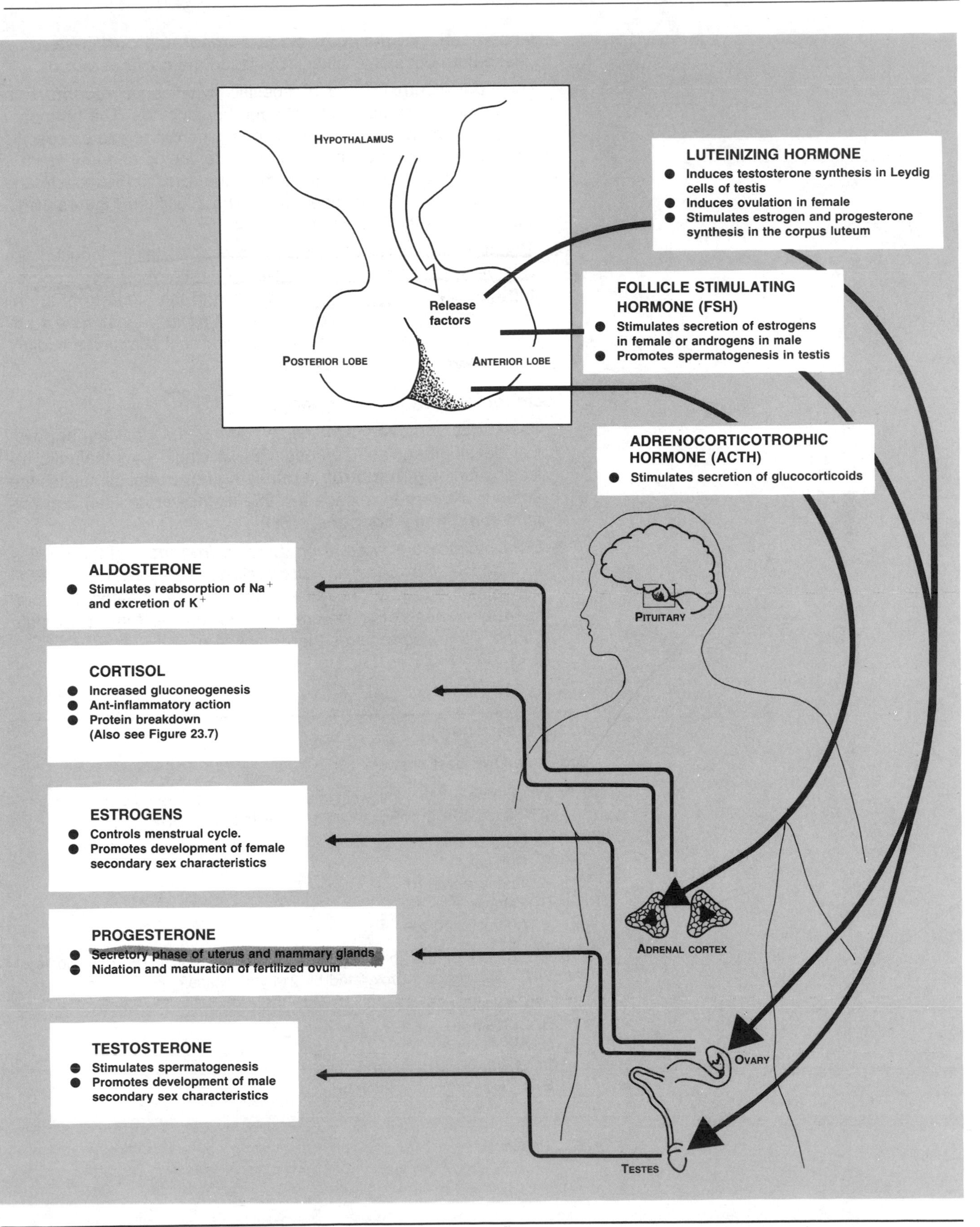

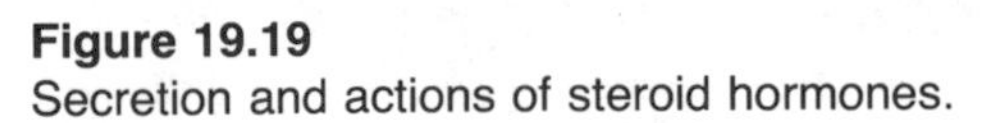

Figure 19.19
Secretion and actions of steroid hormones.

terone and the ***glucocorticoids cortisol*** and ***corticosterone***. These hormones are collectively called the **corticosteroids**.

3. The corticosteroids bind to specific cytoplasmic ***receptors*** in target cells, such as fibroblasts and hepatocytes. The hormone/receptor complex enters the nucleus, where it regulates specific gene expression. For example, glucocorticoids generally stimulate the degradation of proteins to amino acids in the muscle and the initiation of gluconeogenesis in the liver (see Figures 19.19 and 23.7 for other actions of cortisol).
4. ***Aldosterone*** secretion from the adrenal cortex is induced not only by ACTH, but also by the Na^+/K^+ ratio of the body and by **angiotensin**, an octapeptide produced in the blood from an inactive precursor by the kidney enzyme *renin*. Aldosterone's primary effect is on the kidney tubules, where it stimulates sodium retention and potassium excretion.

D. Secretion of steroid from gonads

1. The ***testes*** and ***ovary*** synthesize hormones necessary for physical development and reproduction. A single hypothalamic releasing factor, **gonadotropin releasing hormone**, stimulates the anterior pituitary to release ***luteinizing hormone*** (LH) and ***follicle-stimulating hormone*** (FSH).
2. LH stimulates the testis to produce ***androgens*** and the ovaries to produce ***estrogens*** and ***progesterone*** (Figure 19.19). FSH regulates the growth of ovarian follicles and stimulates testicular spermatogenesis. For maximum effect on the male or female gonad, FSH also requires the presence of LH.

Study Questions

Choose the ONE best answer

19.14 Which one of the following steroids is synthesized from cholesterol WITHOUT being hydroxylated by 17 α-hydroxylase?

A. Corticosterone
B. Cortisol
C. Testosterone
D. Estradiol
E. Androstenedione

19.15 Which one of the following steroids is synthesized from cholesterol WITHOUT being hydroxylated by 21-hydroxylase?

A. Corticosterone
B. Cortisol
C. Aldosterone
D. 11-Deoxycorticosterone
E. 17 α-Hydroxyprogesterone

Disposal of Nitrogen

20

I. OVERVIEW

After the digestion and absorption of dietary amino acids (see p. 224), the catabolism of most amino acids involves two sequential processes. The first phase of catabolism described in this chapter involves the removal of the α-amino groups, which occurs by transamination and oxidative deamination, forming ammonia and the corresponding α-ketoacids. A portion of the free ammonia is excreted in the urine, but most is used in the synthesis of urea, which is quantitatively the most important route for disposing of nitrogen from the body. In the second phase of catabolism, described in Chapter 21, the carbon skeletons of the α-ketoacids are converted to common intermediates of energy metabolism. These compounds can be metabolized to CO_2 and water, glucose, fatty acids, or ketone bodies by the central pathways of metabolism described in Chapters 11 through 16. Chapter 22 concludes this unit with a discussion of some specialized products that are derived from amino acids.

II. OVERALL NITROGEN ECONOMY

A. Protein turnover

1. Most proteins in the body are constantly being repetitively synthesized and then degraded. In healthy adults, the total amount of protein in the body remains constant, since the rate of protein synthesis is just sufficient to replace the protein that is degraded. This process, called ***protein turnover,*** leads to the hydrolysis and resynthesis of 125 to 220 g of body protein each day.
2. The ***rate*** of protein turnover varies widely for individual proteins. For example, the plasma proteins and most intracellular proteins are rapidly degraded, having half-lives of hours or days. However, some proteins, such as the extracellular structural protein collagen, are metabolically stable and have half-lives of years.

B. Amino acid pool

1. Amino acids released as a result of protein hydrolysis join other free amino acids distributed throughout the body and collectively constitute the ***amino acid pool*** (Figure 20.1). The amino acid pool, containing about 100 g of amino acids, is small in comparison to the amount of protein in the body (about 12 kg in a 70-kg

1/6

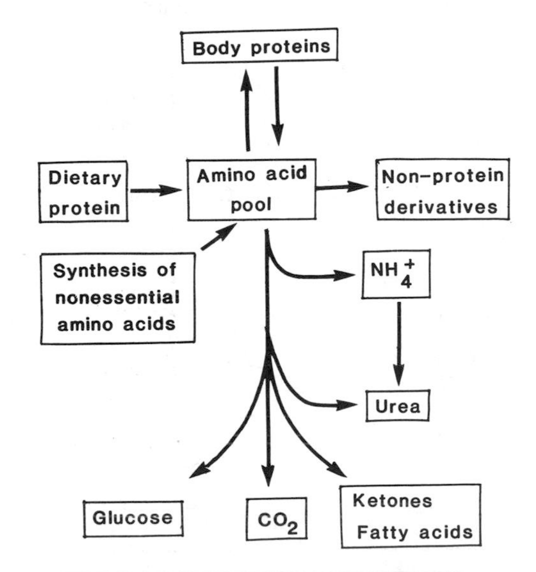

Figure 20.1
Sources and fates of amino acids.

man). Of this 100 g of amino acids, about 50% is in the form of glutamate plus glutamine.

2. If the only fate of the amino acids contributed to the pool by the degradation of the body's proteins was to reform those proteins, adults would not have a significant need for additional dietary protein. However, only about 75% of the amino acids obtained through hydrolysis of body protein are recaptured through the biosynthesis of new tissue protein. The remainder serve as precursors for a variety of compounds shown in Figure 20.1, some of which are described in detail in Chapter 22.

C. The role of dietary protein

1. In contrast to carbohydrates and triacylglycerols whose major function is to provide energy, the primary role of amino acids is to serve as building blocks in biosynthetic reactions, particularly the synthesis of tissue protein. Protein is used secondarily as a fuel and in a typical American diet provides only about one fifth of the daily energy requirement.

2. The catabolism of amino acids leads to a net loss of nitrogen from the body, corresponding to approximately 30 to 55 g of protein each day in healthy adults. This loss must be compensated by the diet to maintain a constant amount of body protein. The ***Recommended Dietary Allowance*** (RDA) of 56 g of protein per day for a 70-kg man (see p. 302) provides a safe margin for replenishing the amino acids lost through anabolic and catabolic pathways.

D. Consequences of high and low intakes of dietary protein

1. ***Diets low in protein:*** If the diet does not provide adequate amounts of protein, there will be a deficiency of essential amino acids required for the synthesis of important body proteins. This will result in the net breakdown of tissue protein, which can lead to clinical symptoms of protein deficiency, such as those described for ***kwashiorkor*** (see p. 303 for a discussion of nitrogen balance).

2. ***Diets high in protein:*** There is no storage form for amino acids analogous to that for lipid (triacylglycerol) or carbohydrate (glycogen). Therefore, if the diet contains excess protein, providing more amino acids than can be rapidly incorporated into protein or other nitrogen-containing molecules, the excess amino acids are metabolized, with their carbon skeletons converted to glucose or to fat.

III. DIGESTION OF DIETARY PROTEINS

Most of the nitrogen in the diet is consumed in the form of protein (Figure 20.1), typically amounting to 70 to 100 g/day in the American diet. Proteins are too large to be absorbed by the intestine and therefore must be hydrolyzed to yield their constituent amino acids, which can be absorbed. The proteolytic enzymes responsible for degrading proteins are produced by three different organs: the stomach, the pancreas, and the small intestine (Figure 20.2).

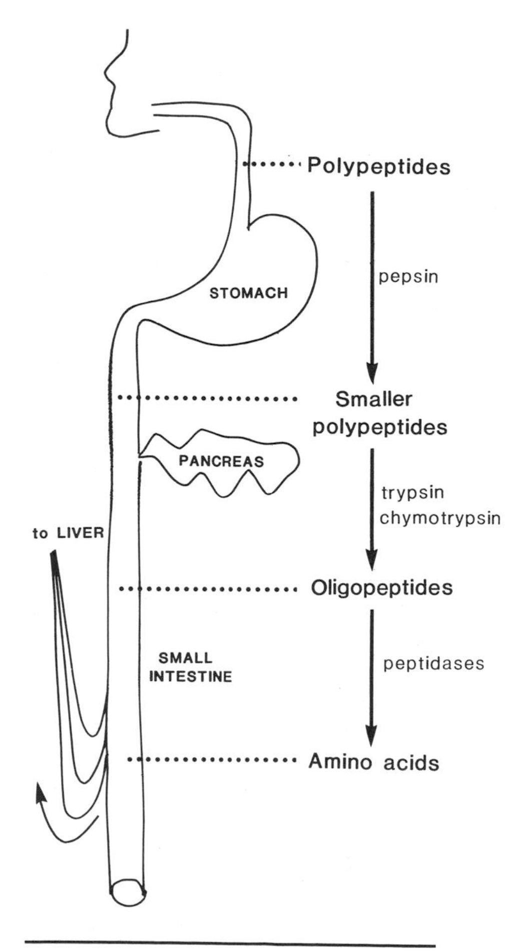

Figure 20.2
Digestion of dietary proteins by the proteolytic enzymes of the gastrointestinal tract.

A. Digestion of proteins by gastric secretions

The digestion of proteins begins in the stomach, which secretes ***gastric juice,*** a unique solution containing hydrochloric acid and the enzyme *pepsin*:

1. ***Hydrochloric acid*** in the stomach (pH 2–3) is too dilute to hydrolyze proteins; however, the acid functions to kill some bacteria and to denature proteins, making them more susceptible to subsequent hydrolysis by proteases.
2. *Pepsin,* an acid-stable endopeptidase, is secreted by the serous cells of the stomach as an inactive ***zymogen*** (or proenzyme), ***pepsinogen***. In general, zymogens contain one or more extra amino acid sequences, which prevent the protein from being a catalytically active enzyme. Removal of these amino acid sequences permits the proper folding of the enzyme, thus forming an active structure. Pepsinogen is activated to *pepsin* either by HCl or autocatalytically by other *pepsin* molecules that have already been activated. *Pepsin* releases large peptides and a few free amino acids from dietary proteins.

B. Digestion of proteins by pancreatic enzymes

On entering the small intestine, large polypeptides produced in the stomach by the action of *pepsin* are further cleaved to oligopeptides and amino acids by a group of pancreatic proteases.

1. Each of these enzymes has a different specificity for the amino acids adjacent to the susceptible peptide bond (Figure 20.3). For example, *trypsin* cleaves only when the carbonyl group of the peptide bond is contributed by arginine or lysine. These enzymes, like *pepsin* described above, are synthesized and secreted as inactive zymogens. They are activated in the lumen of the intestine by *trypsin* which cleaves a limited number of specific peptide bonds in the zymogen.
2. The release and activation of the pancreatic zymogens is mediated by the secretion of ***cholecystokinin*** and ***secretin,*** two polypeptide hormones of the digestive tract (see p. 150).
3. *Enteropeptidase* (also called *enterokinase*), an enzyme synthesized by and present on the luminal surface of intestinal mucosal cells of the brush border membrane, converts the pancreatic zymogen ***trypsinogen*** to *trypsin* by removal of a hexapeptide from the NH_2-terminus of trypsinogen. Active *trypsin* can subsequently convert other trypsinogen molecules to *trypsin*. *Enterokinase* thus unleashes a cascade of proteolytic activity, since *trypsin* is the common activator of all the pancreatic zymogens (Figure 20.3).
4. In individuals with a deficiency in pancreatic secretion (e.g., due to chronic pancreatitis or surgical removal of the pancreas), the digestion and the absorption of fat and protein are incomplete, resulting in the abnormal appearance of lipids and protein in the feces (see p. 152).

C. Digestion by enzymes of the small intestine

1. The luminal surface of the intestine contains *aminopeptidase* activity , which cleaves oligopeptides to dipeptides and tripeptides and free amino acids.

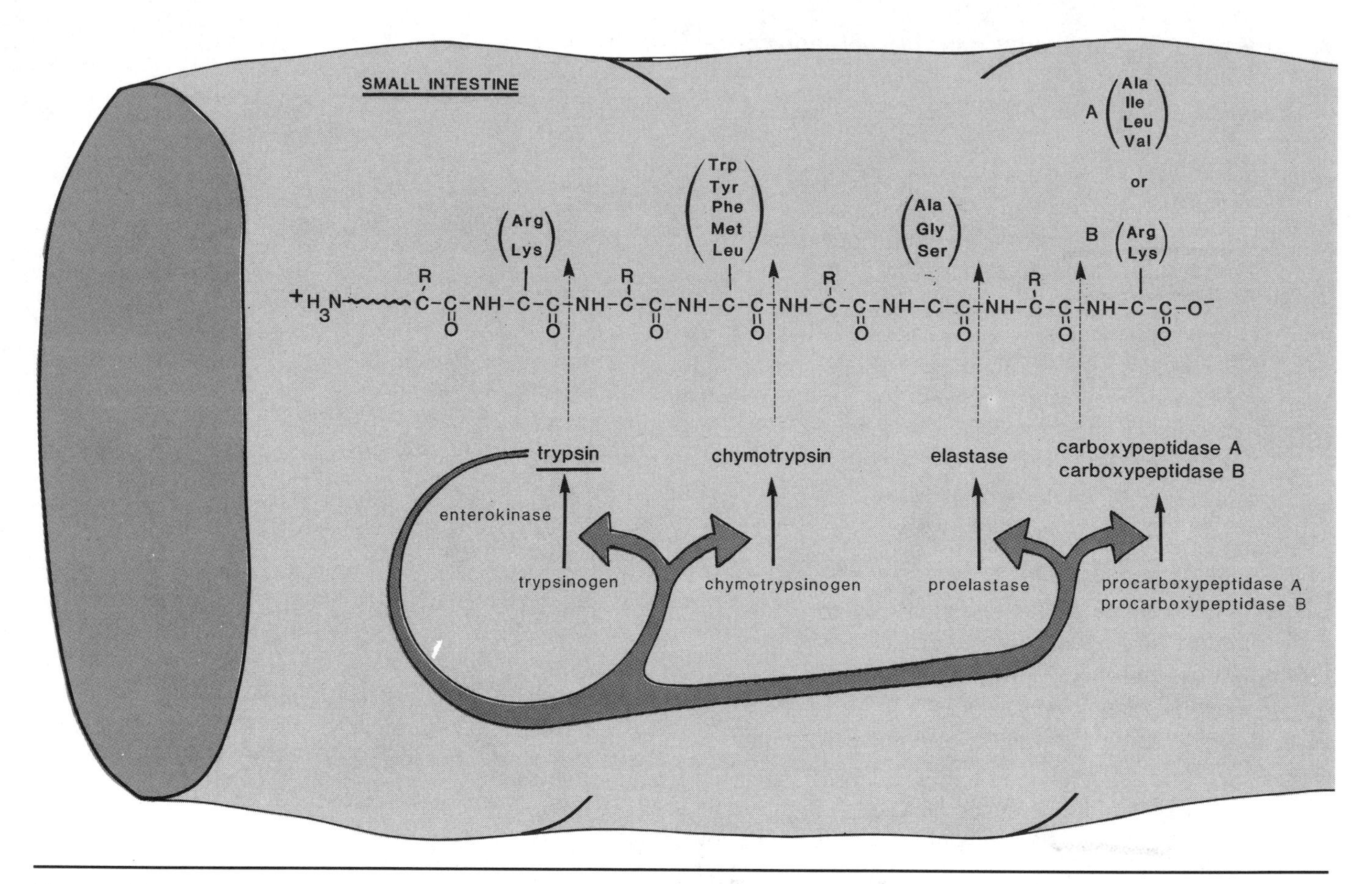

Figure 20.3
Cleavage of dietary protein by proteases from the pancreas. The peptide bonds susceptible to hydrolysis are shown for each of the five major pancreatic proteases.

Cystinuria:
defect in basic a.a. transporter
Cysteine
Ornithine
arginine
lysine

Oxoprolinuria
↓ in glutathione synthetase
accum of γ-glutamyl cysteine

trypsin = arg
lys

chymotrypsin = phe
met
try
tyr
leu

2. Free amino acids and dipeptides are absorbed by the intestinal epithelial cells in which the peptides are hydrolyzed to amino acids in the cytoplasm before they enter the portal system. Thus, only free amino acids are found in the portal vein after a meal containing protein. These amino acids are either metabolized by the liver or released into the general circulation.

IV. TRANSPORT OF AMINO ACIDS INTO CELLS

A. Specific transport systems

1. The concentration of free amino acids in the extracellular fluids is significantly lower than that within the cells of the body. This concentration gradient is maintained because active transport systems, driven by the hydrolysis of ATP, are required for movement of amino acids from the extracellular space into the cell. At least seven different transport systems are known, which have overlapping specificity for different amino acids.

2. One transport system is responsible for reabsorption of the basic amino acids cysteine, ornithine, arginine, and lysine. In the inherited disorder ***cystinuria***, this carrier system is defective, resulting in the appearance of all four amino acids in the urine. Cystinuria is the most common genetic error of amino acid transport.

B. General amino acid transport system: the γ-glutamyl cycle

1. The ***γ-glutamyl cycle*** occurs in brain, intestine, and kidney. Although it is most active in the transport of neutral amino acids, such as methionine and glutamine, it can transport a broad spectrum of amino acids across the cell membrane into the cytoplasm.

2. The γ-glutamyl cycle is the only transport system for amino acids whose mechanism is known in any detail (Figure 20.4). The amino acid to be transported reacts with ***glutathione*** (γ-glutamylcysteinylglycine) at the surface of the cell to form a dipeptide that is transported across the membrane into the cytoplasm of the cell (reaction 1, Figure 20.4). The subsequent reactions of the cycle serve to regenerate glutathione (reactions 2–5, Figure 20.4). Thus the cycle serves two functions:

   a. transportation of amino acids from the extracellular space into the cytoplasm; and

   b. synthesis of glutathione, which, in addition to functioning in the transport of amino acids, is an important reductant in the cell (see p. 146).

3. In the γ-glutamyl cycle, transport of amino acids across the membrane is driven by the hydrolysis of three molecules of ATP for each molecule of amino acid that enters the cell. This allows the efficient extraction of amino acids from the extracellular fluid despite the presence of high concentrations of amino acids within the cell. *Oxoprolinase*, which converts 5-oxoproline to glutamate (reaction 3, Figure 20.4), is the rate-limiting reaction of the cycle.

4. ***Oxoprolinuria*** is an inherited disease in which elevated levels of 5-oxoproline occur in blood and urine, resulting in acidosis and

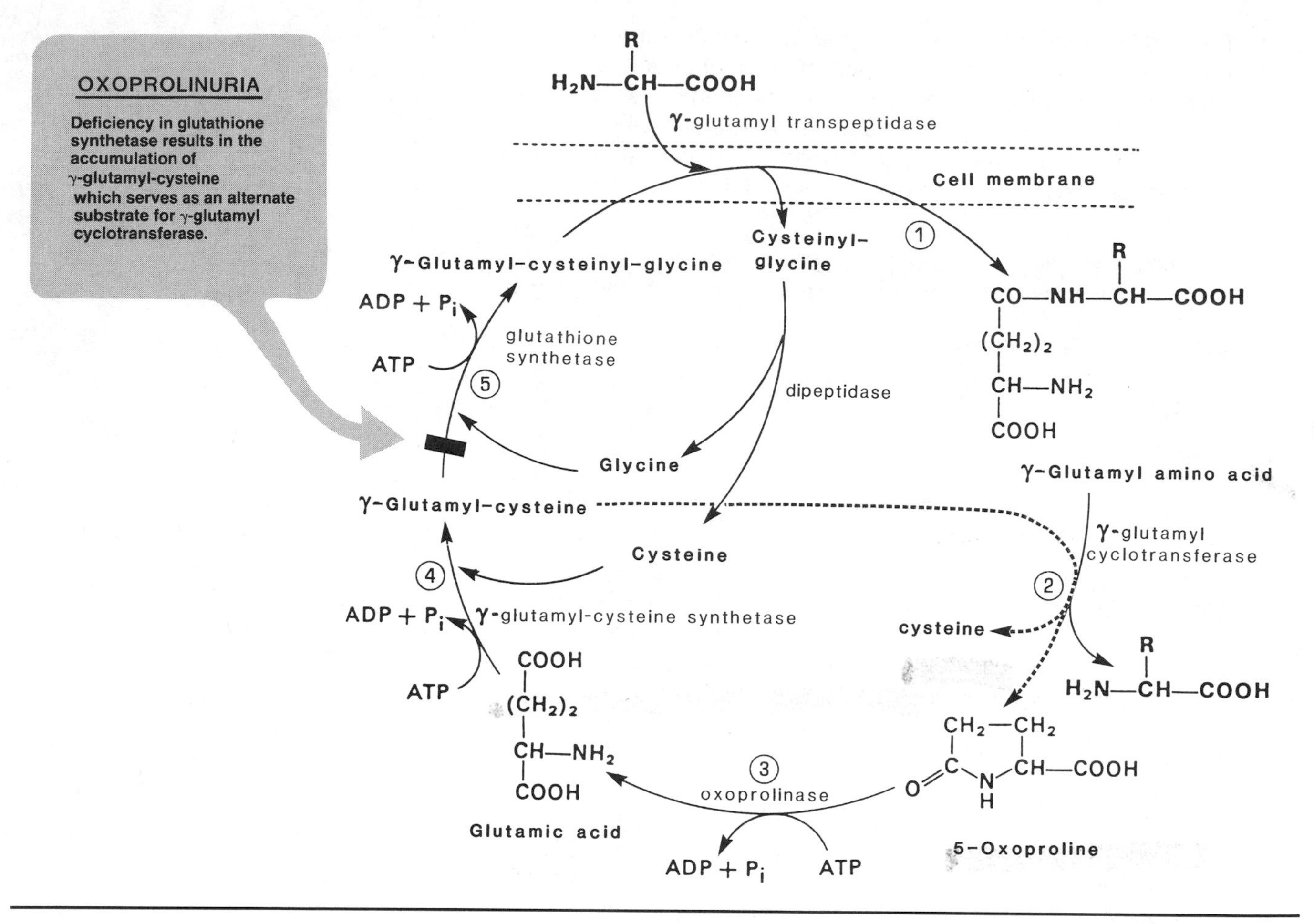

Figure 20.4
Reactions of γ-glutamyl cycle. The dashed lines show the alteration of the cycle in individuals with oxoprolinuria

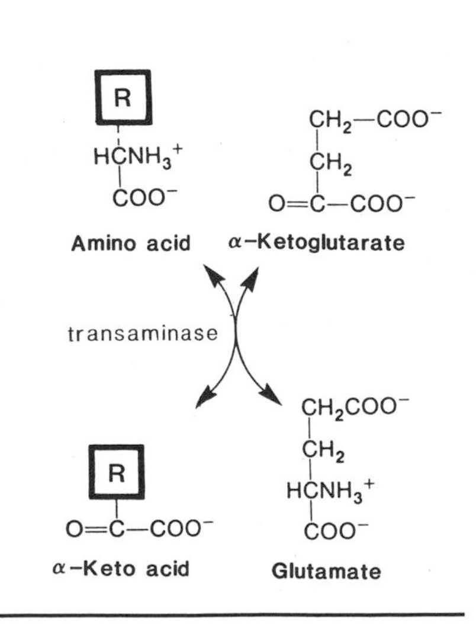

Figure 20.5
Transaminase reactions using α-ketoglutarate as amino-acceptor.

neurologic damage. The disease is due to a deficiency in the enzyme *glutathione synthetase* (reaction 5 in Figure 20.4.) This enzyme deficiency causes the accumulation of γ-glutamylcysteine, the substrate of the defective enzyme. At high concentrations this dipeptide can act as a substrate for *γ-glutamyl cyclotransferase* (reaction 2 in Figure 20.4). Cysteine and 5-oxoproline are the products; cysteine is readily metabolized, but 5-oxoproline accumulates.

V. REMOVAL OF NITROGEN FROM AMINO ACIDS

The first step in amino acid catabolism generally involves the removal of the α-amino group. Once released, this nitrogen can be incorporated into other compounds or excreted. This section describes ***transamination*** and ***oxidative deamination,*** two important reactions that ultimately provide ammonia and aspartate, the two sources of urea nitrogen (see p. 231).

A. Transamination: the funneling of amino groups to glutamate

The first step in the catabolism of most amino acids is the transfer of their α-amino group to α-ketoglutarate (Figure 20.5). The products are an α-keto acid (derived from the original amino acid) and glutamate. α-Ketoglutarate plays a unique role in amino acid metabolism by accepting the amino groups from other amino acids, thus becoming ***glutamate***. This transfer of amino groups from one carbon skeleton to another is catalyzed by a family of *transaminases* (also called *aminotransferases*). Most amino acids, with the exception of lysine and threonine, participate in transamination at some point in their catabolism.

1. ***Substrate specificity of transaminases:*** Each *transaminase* is specific for one or at most a few amino acid nitrogen donors. *Transaminases* are named after the specific amino acid nitrogen donor, since the acceptor of the amino group is almost always α-ketoglutarate. The two most important *transaminase* reactions are catalyzed by *alanine transaminase* and *aspartate transaminase*.

   a. *Alanine transaminase,* also called *glutamate:pyruvate transaminase* (GPT), is present in many tissues. The enzyme catalyzes the transfer of the amino group of alanine to α-ketoglutarate, resulting in the formation of pyruvate and glutamate (Figure 20.6). The reaction is readily reversible; however, during amino acid catabolism, this enzyme (like most transaminases) functions in the direction of glutamate synthesis. Thus glutamate, in effect, acts as a "collector" of nitrogen from alanine.

   b. *Aspartate transaminase,* also called *glutamate: oxaloacetate transaminase* (GOT), is an exception to the general rule that *transaminases* funnel amino groups to form glutamate. During amino acid catabolism, *aspartate transaminase* transfers amino groups ***from*** glutamate to oxaloacetate, forming aspartate, which is itself used as a source of nitrogen in the urea cycle (see Figure 20.7 and p. 231).

2. ***Mechanism of action of transaminases:*** All transaminases require the cofactor ***pyridoxal phosphate*** (a derivative of vitamin B_6, see p. 316), which is covalently linked to the ε-amino group of a specific lysine residue at the active site of the enzyme. Transaminases act by transferring the amino group of an amino acid to the pyridoxal cofactor to generate pyridoxamine. The ***pyridoxamine*** form of the cofactor then reacts with an α-ketoacid to form an amino acid and regenerates the original aldehyde form of the cofactor. Figure 20.8 shows these two component reactions for the transformation catalyzed by *aspartate transaminase*.

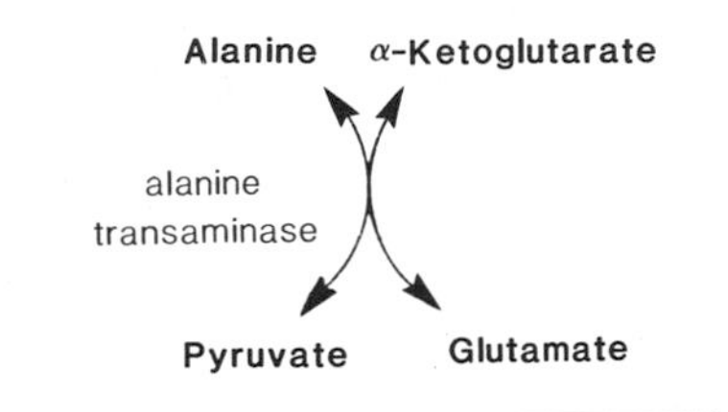

Figure 20.6
Reaction catalyzed by *alanine transaminase*

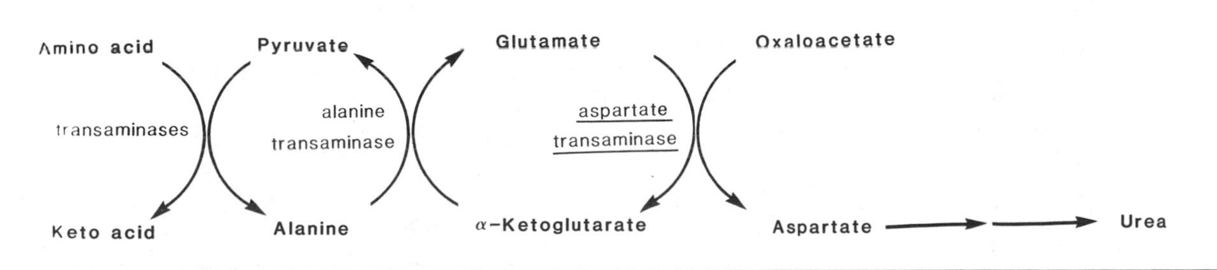

Figure 20.7
Role of transaminases in the flow of amino nitrogen from amino acids to urea.

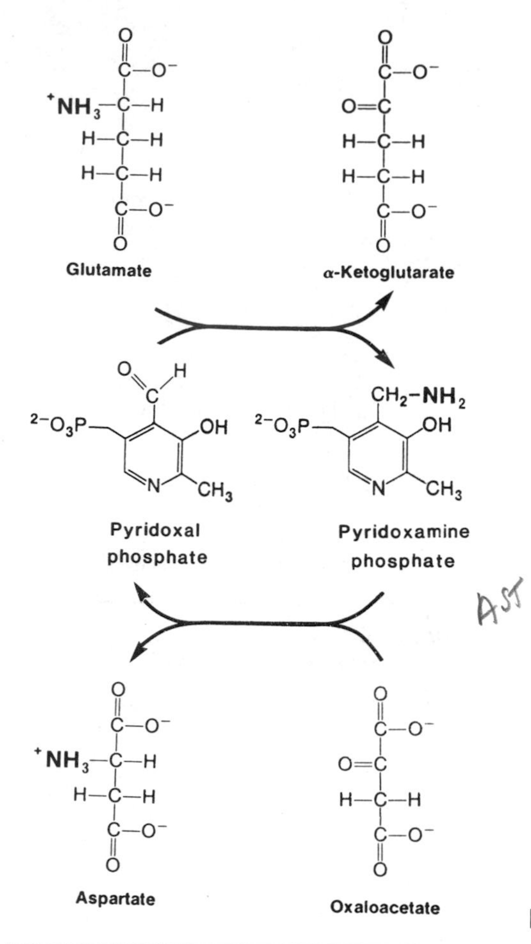

Figure 20.8
Cyclic interconversion of pyridoxal phosphate and pyridoxamine phosphate during the *aspartate transaminase* reaction.

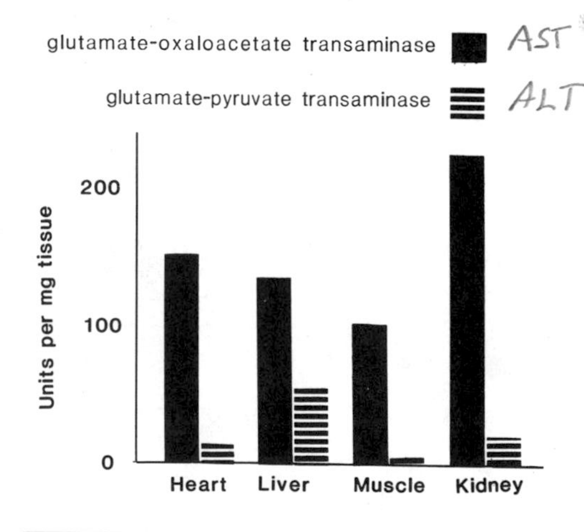

Figure 20.9
Glutamate:oxaloacetate transaminase (GOT) and *glutamate:pyruvate transaminase (GPT)* in human tissues.

3. ***Equilibrium of transaminase reactions:*** For most transaminase reactions the equilibrium is near one, allowing the reaction to function in both amino acid degradation through removal of α-amino groups (e.g., after consumption of a protein-rich meal) and biosynthesis through addition of amino groups to the carbon skeletons of α-ketoacids (e.g., when the supply from the diet is not adequate to meet the synthetic needs of the cell).

4. ***Diagnostic value of transaminases:*** Transaminases are normally ***intracellular*** enzymes. Thus, the presence of elevated levels of transaminases in the ***serum*** indicates damage to cells rich in the enzyme. For example, physical trauma or a disease process can cause cell lysis, resulting in release of intracellular enzymes into the blood. Two transaminases are of particular diagnostic value when found in the serum: *serum glutamate:oxaloacetate transaminase (SGOT)* and *serum glutamate:pyruvate transaminase (SGPT)*. Figure 20.9 shows that these two enzymes are present in differing amounts in each tissue.

   a. An elevated level of both *SGOT* and *SGPT* indicates possible damage to the liver (which results in hepatic enzymes escaping into the blood), however, a rise in *SGOT* accompanied by only a moderate rise in *SGPT* suggests damage to heart muscle, skeletal muscle, or kidney.

   b. Damage to heart and skeletal muscle can be diagnosed with greater specificity and predictive accuracy by measuring the serum levels of *lactate dehydrogenase* and *creatine phosphokinase* isoenzymes, described on p. 42.

B. Oxidative deamination results in the release of free ammonia

1. ***Glutamate dehydrogenase:*** As described above, the amino groups of most amino acids are ultimately funneled to glutamate by means of transamination with α-ketoglutarate. Glutamate is unique in that it is the only amino acid that undergoes rapid ***oxidative deamination,*** a reaction catalyzed by *glutamate dehydrogenase* (Figure 20.10). Therefore the sequential action of transamination (resulting in the collection of amino groups from other amino acids onto α-ketoglutarate to produce glutamate) and the subsequent oxidative deamination of that glutamate (reproducing α-ketoglutarate) provide a pathway whereby the amino groups of most amino acids can be released as ammonia.

   a. In contrast to transamination reactions that transfer amino groups, oxidative deamination results in the liberation of the amino group as ***free ammonia***.

   b. *Glutamate dehydrogenase* is unusual in that it can use either NAD^+ or $NADP^+$ as a cofactor.

   c. The direction of the reaction depends on the relative concentrations of glutamate, α-ketoglutarate, and ammonia and the ratio of oxidized to reduced cofactors. For example, after ingestion of a meal containing protein, glutamate levels in the liver are elevated, and the reaction proceeds in the direction of amino acid degradation and the formation of ammonia.

2. ***D-amino acid oxidase:*** D-Amino acids are found in plants and in the cell walls of microorganisms but are not used in the synthesis

of mammalian proteins. D-Amino acids are, however, present in the diet and are efficiently metabolized by the liver. *D-Amino acid oxidase* is an FAD-dependent enzyme that catalyzes the oxidative deamination of these ***unnatural*** isomers of amino acids. The resulting α-ketoacids can then enter the general pathways of amino acid metabolism, being reaminated to an L-isomer or catabolized for energy (Figure 20.11).

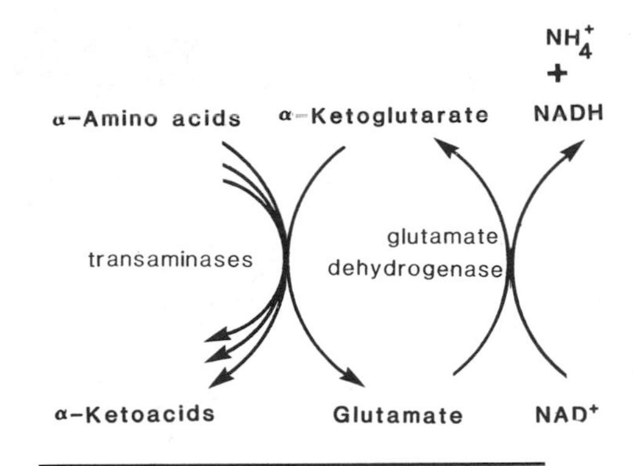

Figure 20.10
Combined actions of *transaminase* and *glutamate dehydrogenase*.

VI. UREA CYCLE: THE MAJOR PATHWAY FOR DISPOSAL OF NITROGEN

Urea is the major disposal form of amino groups derived from amino acids and accounts for about 90% of the nitrogen-containing components of urine. The nitrogens of urea are derived from ammonia and aspartate by the five enzyme-catalyzed reactions of the urea cycle. Urea is produced by the liver and then is transported in the blood to the kidney for ultimate excretion in the urine.

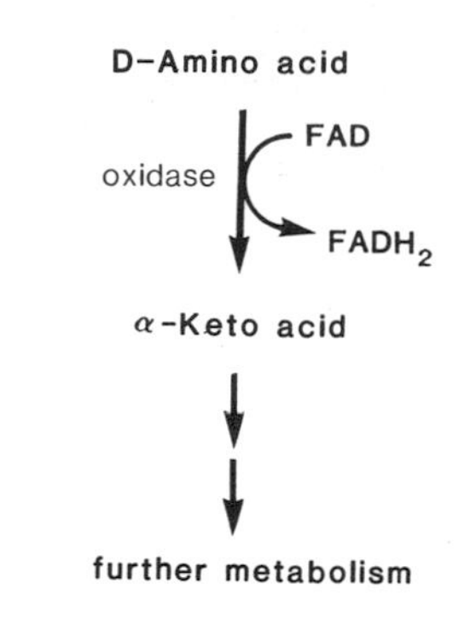

Figure 20.11
The deamination of D-amino acids followed by reamination to form L-amino acids.

A. Reactions of the cycle

The first two reactions leading to the synthesis of urea occur in the mitochondria, whereas the remaining cycle enzymes are located in the cytoplasm (see Figure 20.12). *Glutamate dehydrogenase* also occurs in the mitochondria, providing ammonia for incorporation into carbamoyl phosphate.

1. ***Formation of carbamoyl phosphate***
   a. Formation of carbamoyl phosphate is driven by cleavage of two molecules of ATP.
   b. Ammonia incorporated into carbamoyl phosphate is provided primarily by the oxidative deamination of glutamate (see p. 230). Ultimately, the nitrogen atom derived from this ammonia becomes one of the nitrogens of the urea molecule. Carbon dioxide (CO_2) used in this reaction is a product primarily of the citric acid cycle.
   c. *Carbamoyl phosphate synthetase I* requires N-acetylglutamate for activity (Figure 20.12).
2. ***Formation of citrulline***
   a. Both ornithine and citrulline are basic amino acids that participate in the urea cycle but are not incorporated into cellular proteins. Ornithine is regenerated with each turn of the urea cycle, much in the same way that oxaloacetate is regenerated by the reactions of the citric acid cycle.
   b. The release of the high-energy phosphate of carbamoyl phosphate as P_i drives the reaction to the right.
   c. The reaction product, citrulline, is transported to the cytoplasm.
3. ***Synthesis of argininosuccinate***
   a. The α-amino group of aspartate provides the second nitrogen that is ultimately incorporated into urea.
   b. The formation of argininosuccinate is driven by the cleavage of ATP to AMP and PP_i. This is the third and final molecule of ATP consumed in the formation of urea.

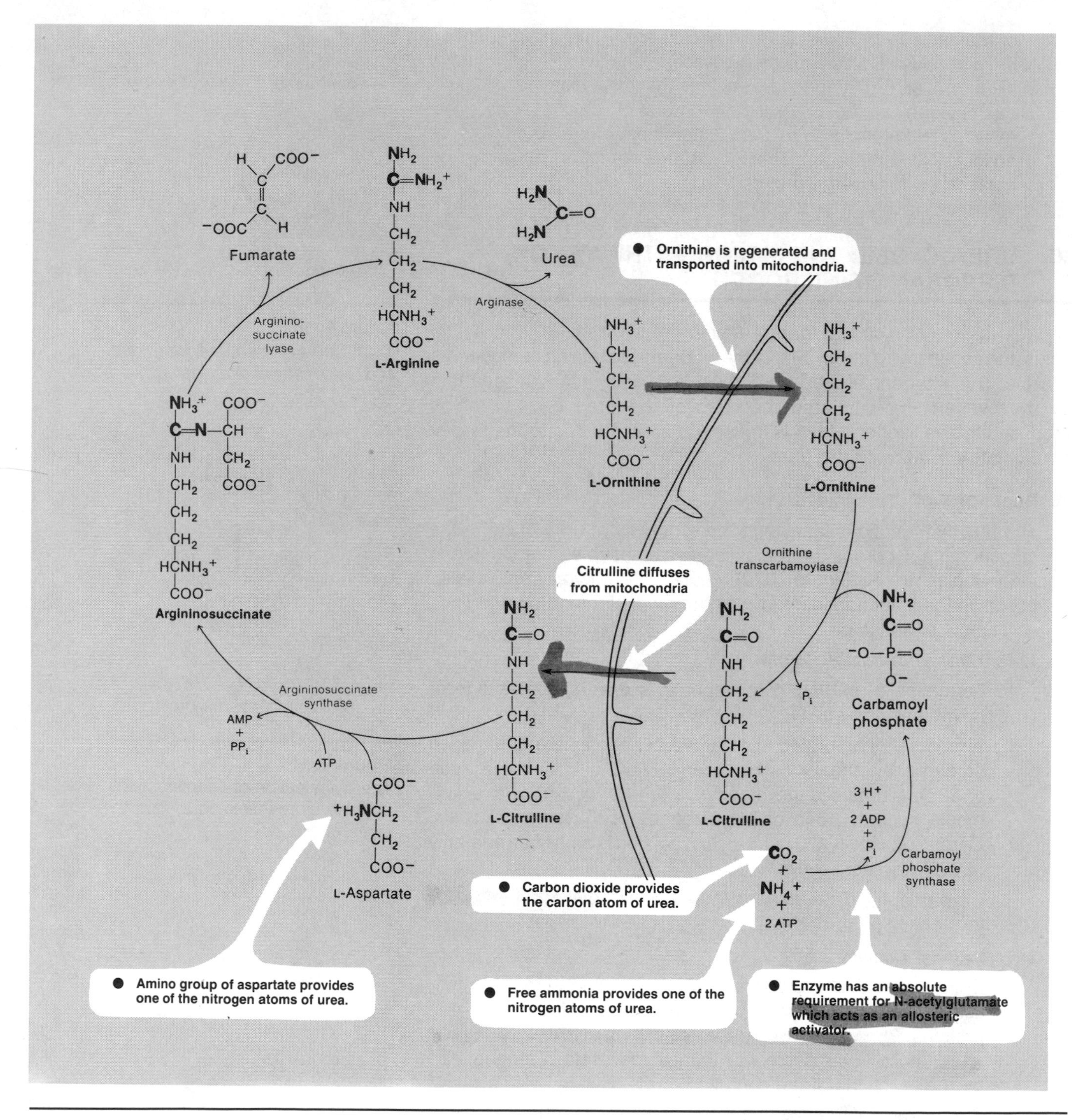

Figure 20.12
Reactions of the urea cycle.

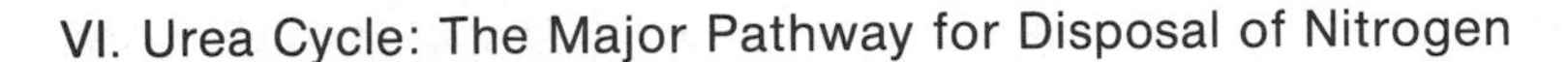

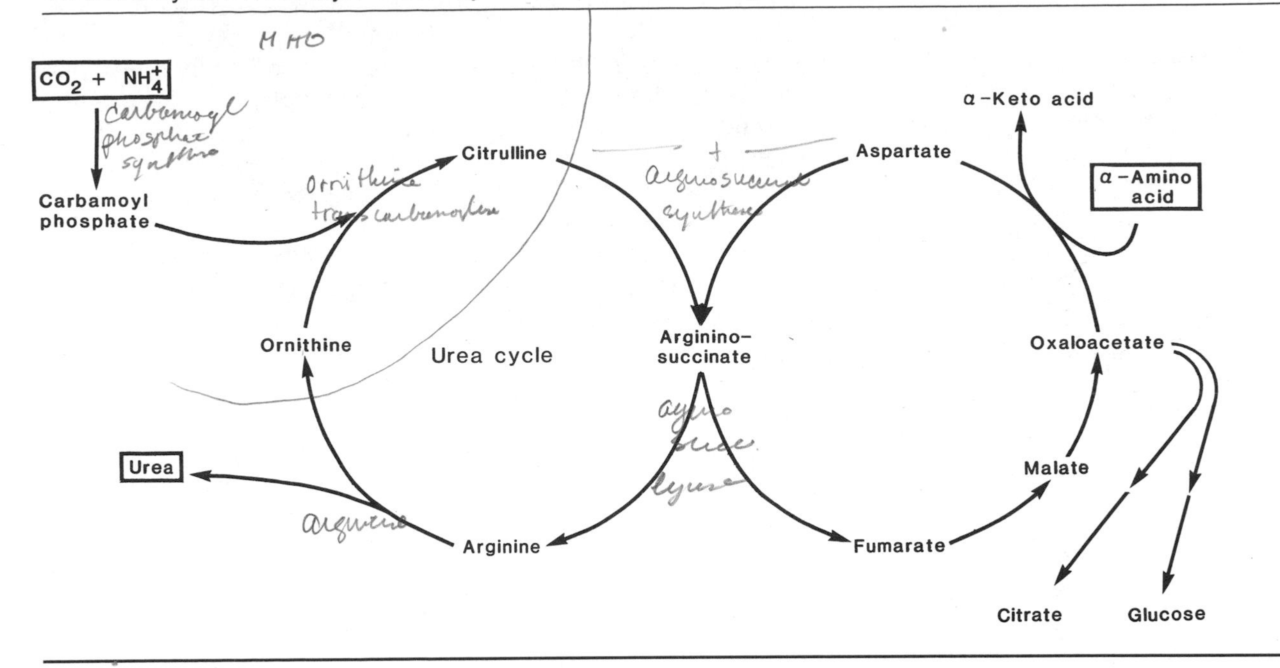

Figure 20.13
Fate of fumarate produced by the urea cycle.

c. Citrulline is transported from the mitochondria to the cytoplasm, where it condenses with aspartate to form argininosuccinate.

4. ***Cleavage of argininosuccinate***

a. The arginine formed by this reaction serves as the immediate precursor of urea.

b. Fumarate produced in the urea cycle provides a link with several metabolic pathways: Fumarate is hydrated to malate, which is transported into the matrix of the mitochondria. There, malate is oxidized to oxaloacetate, which can subsequently be converted to aspartate or glucose or enter the TCA cyle (Figure 20.13).

5. ***Cleavage of arginine to ornithine and urea***

a. The regeneration of ornithine and its subsequent transport into the mitochondria enables the cycle to continue with no net consumption of intermediates.

b. *Arginase* occurs almost exclusively in the liver. Thus whereas other tissues can synthesize arginine, only the liver can cleave arginine and thereby synthesize urea.

c. Urea diffuses from the liver and is transported in the blood to the kidneys, where it is filtered and excreted into the urine.

B. Overall stoichiometry of the urea cycle

$$\text{Aspartate} + NH_3 + CO_2 + 3ATP \rightarrow 3H_2O + \text{urea} + \text{fumarate} + 2ADP + AMP + 2P_i + PP_i$$

1. Four high-energy phosphates are consumed in the synthesis of each molecule of urea: Two ATP are needed to restore 2ADP to 2ATP, plus two to restore AMP to ATP.

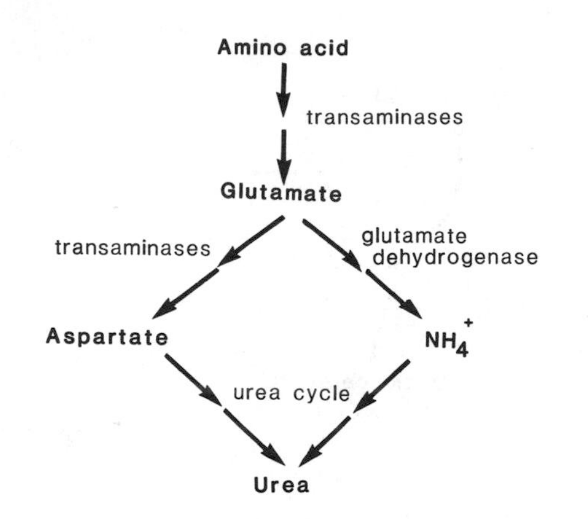

Figure 20.14
Flow of nitrogen from amino acids to urea.

2. One nitrogen of the urea molecule is supplied by free NH_3, and the other nitrogen is obtained from aspartate. Glutamate is the immediate precursor of both ammonia (through oxidative deamination by *glutamate dehydrogenase*) and aspartate nitrogen (through transamination of oxaloacetate by *aspartate transaminase*). In effect, both nitrogen atoms of urea arise from glutamate, which in turn gathers nitrogen from other amino acids. Figure 20.14 shows this convergent flow of nitrogen from amino acids to glutamate and ultimately to urea.
3. The carbon and oxygen of urea are derived from CO_2.

C. Regulation of the urea cycle

1. ***N-Acetylglutamate*** is an essential activator for *carbamoylphosphate synthetase I*, the rate-limiting step in the urea cycle (see Figure 20.12). N-Acetylglutamate is synthesized from acetyl CoA and glutamate. The intracellular concentration of this compound increases after ingestion of a protein-rich meal, leading to an increased rate of the urea synthesis.

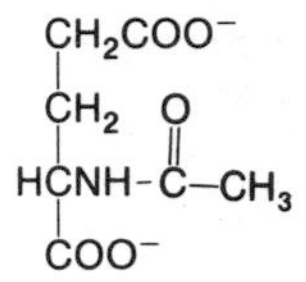

N-Acetylglutamate

VII. METABOLISM OF AMMONIA

Although free ammonia is involved in the formation of urea in the liver, the level of ammonia in the blood must be kept low because even slightly elevated concentrations (hyperammonemia) are ***toxic*** to the ***central nervous system***. There must, therefore, be a metabolic mechanism by which nitrogen is moved from the peripheral tissues to the liver for ultimate disposal as urea, at the same time maintaining low levels of circulating ammonia.

A. Sources of ammonia

1. Many tissues, particularly liver, form ammonia from amino acids by the *transaminase* and *glutamate dehydrogenase* reactions previously described (see p. 230).
2. Ammonia is formed in the intestinal mucosa by several reactions, including the hydrolysis of glutamine by intestinal *glutaminase* (Figure 20.15). The intestinal cells obtain glutamine either from the blood or from the digestion of dietary protein. Ammonia is also formed by the bacterial degradation of urea in the lumen of the intestine. Ammonia from either source is absorbed from the intestine by way of the portal vein and is almost quantitatively removed by the liver.
3. The kidneys form ammonia from glutamine by the action of renal *glutaminase* (Figure 20.15). Most of this ammonia is excreted into the urine as NH_4^+, which is an important mechanism for maintaining the body's acid–base balance.
4. Amines obtained from the diet and monoamines that serve as hormones or neurotransmitters give rise to ammonia by the action of *amine oxidase* (see p. 261 for the metabolism of epinephrine, serotonin, and histamine).
5. In both purine and pyrimidine metabolism, the amino groups attached to the rings are released as ammonia.

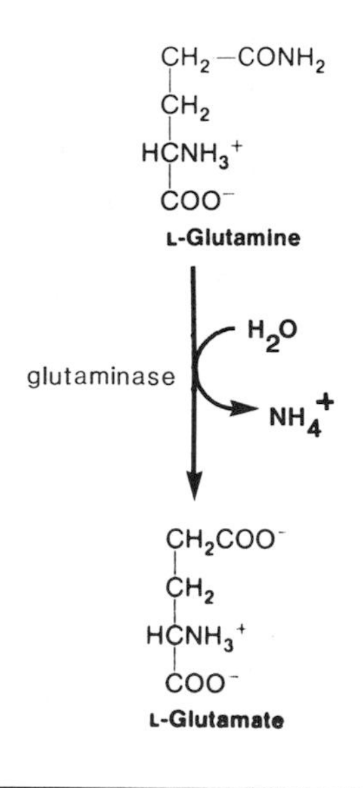

Figure 20.15
Hydrolysis of glutamine to form ammonia.

B. Transport of ammonia in the circulation

1. Although ammonia is constantly produced in the tissues, it is present at very low levels in blood. This is due to both the rapid removal of ammonia from the blood by the liver and the fact that many tissues, particularly muscle, release amino acid nitrogen in the form of glutamine or alanine, rather than as free ammonia. (The metabolism of ammonia is summarized in Figure 20.17.)

   a. Formation of urea in the liver is quantitatively the most important disposal route for ammonia.

   b. Glutamine provides a nontoxic storage and transport form of ammonia (Figure 20.16). The formation of glutamine occurs primarily in the muscle and liver but also is important in the nervous system, where it is the major mechanism for the removal of ammonia in the brain. Glutamine is found in plasma at concentrations higher than other amino acids, a finding consistent with its transport function. Circulating glutamine is removed by the kidney and deaminated by *glutaminase*, as described on p. 234.

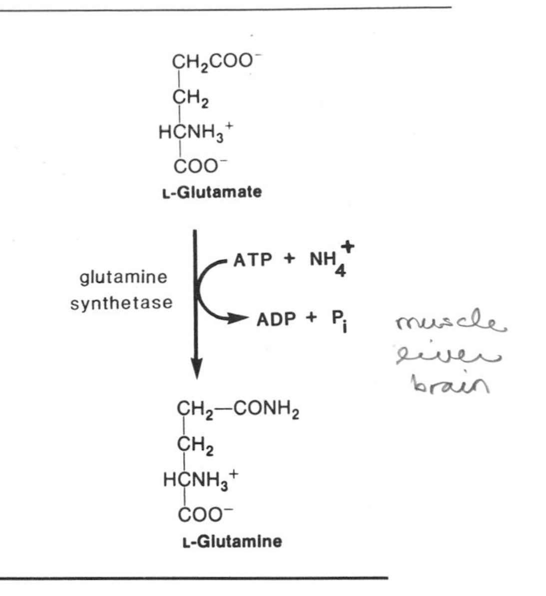

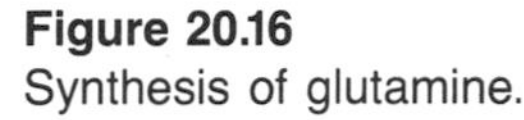

Figure 20.16
Synthesis of glutamine.

C. Hyperammonemia

1. Elevated concentrations of ammonia in the blood cause the symptoms of ***ammonia intoxication,*** which include tremors, slurring of speech, and blurring of vision. At high concentrations ammonia

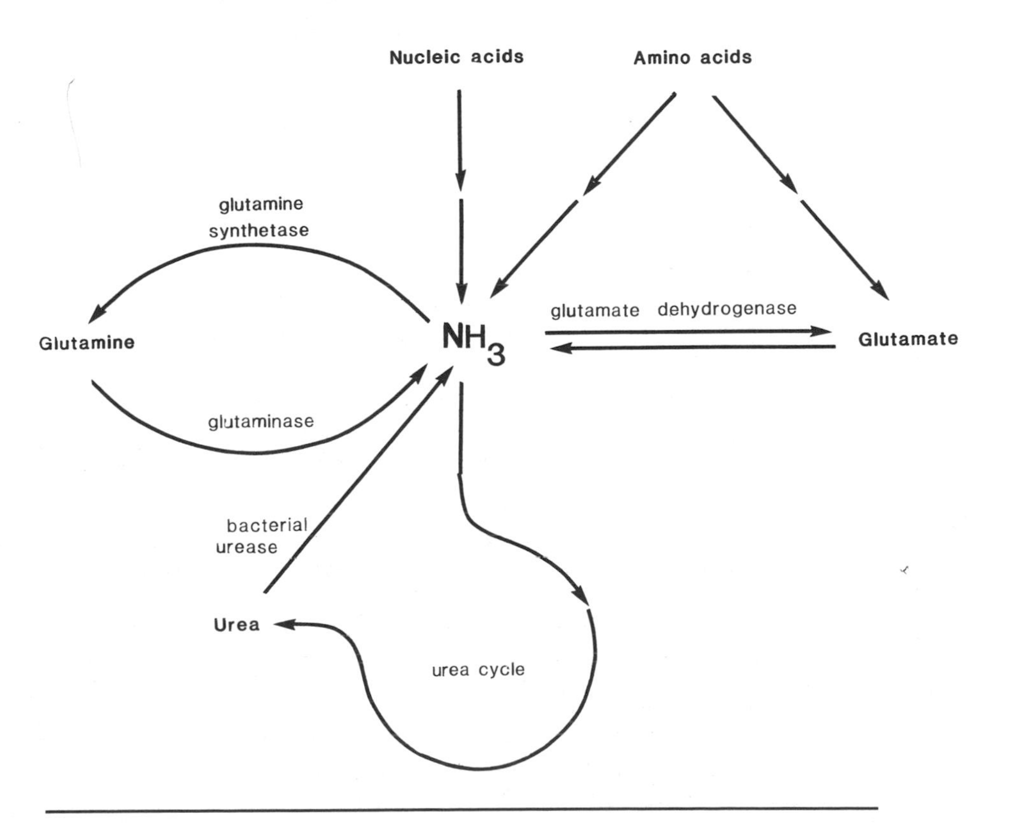

Figure 20.17
Metabolism of ammonia.

can cause coma and death. The two major types of hyperammonemia are as follows:

a. ***Acquired hyperammonemia:*** Cirrhosis of the liver caused by alcoholism, hepatitis, or biliary obstruction may result in formation of collateral circulation around the liver. As a result, portal blood is shunted directly into the systemic circulation and does not have access to the liver. The detoxification of ammonia is therefore severely impaired, leading to elevated levels of circulating ammonia.

b. ***Inherited hyperammonemia:*** Genetic deficiencies of each of the five enzymes of the urea cycle have been described, with an overall prevalence estimated to be 1 in 30,000 live births. In each case the failure to synthesize urea leads to hyperammonemia during the first week after birth. All inherited deficiencies of the urea cycle enzymes result in mental retardation.

2. The toxicity of high levels of ammonia is thought to result, in part, from a shift in the equilibrium of the reaction catalyzed by *glutamate dehydrogenase* toward the direction of glutamate formation:

$$\alpha\text{-ketoglutarate} + \text{NADH} + \text{H}^+ + \text{NH}_3 \rightarrow \text{glutamate} + \text{NAD}^+$$

This depletes α-ketoglutarate, an essential intermediate in the citric acid cycle, resulting in a decrease in cellular oxidation and ATP production. The brain is particularly vulnerable to hyperammonemia, presumably because it depends on the citric acid cycle to maintain its high rate of energy consumption.

Study Questions

Answer A if 1, 2, and 3 are correct
B if 1 and 3 are correct
C if 2 and 4 are correct
D if only 4 is correct
E if all are correct

20.1 In humans, amino acids can be used

1. as building blocks for the biosynthesis of proteins and other nitrogen-containing molecules.
2. for the synthesis of tissue proteins.
3. as sources of energy.
4. as carriers for other small molecules in body fluids.

20.2 Chymotrypsin acts

1. in the stomach on peptide bonds formed by the amino acid glycine.
2. in the intestinal mucosa on carboxy-terminal amino acids in proteins and peptides.
3. in the intestine on peptide bonds formed by the amino acids arginine or aspartate.
4. in the intestine on peptide bonds formed by amino acids with aromatic side-chains.

20.3 Which of the following statements about glutamine is(are) correct?:

1. Glutamine is responsible for the transport and excretion of ammonium ions in a nontoxic form.
2. The high level of activity of glutamine synthetase in the liver effectively traps ammonium ions as glutamine.
3. ATP is required for the reaction leading to the synthesis of glutamine from glutamate and ammonia.
4. The kidneys can hydrolyze glutamine to glutamate and ammonia.

20.4 Given the following reactions, numbered I to IV,

I.

$$^{-}OOC{-}\underset{NH_3^+}{\underset{|}{C}}H{-}CH_2{-}CH_2{-}COO^- + NAD^+ \rightarrow$$

$$^{-}OOC{-}\underset{O}{\underset{\|}{C}}{-}CH_2{-}CH_2{-}COO^- + NADH + NH_3$$

II.

$$^{-}OOC{-}\underset{NH_3^+}{\underset{|}{C}}H{-}CH_2{-}COO^- + {}^{-}OOC{-}\underset{O}{\underset{\|}{C}}{-}CH_2{-}CH_2{-}COO^- \rightleftarrows$$

$$^{-}OOC{-}\underset{O}{\underset{\|}{C}}{-}CH_2{-}COO^- + {}^{-}OOC{-}\underset{NH_3^+}{\underset{|}{C}}H{-}CH_2{-}CH_2{-}COO^-$$

III.

$$^{-}OOC{-}\underset{NH_3^+}{\underset{|}{C}}H{-}CH_2{-}CH_2{-}COO^- + NH_3 \rightarrow$$

$$^{-}OOC{-}\underset{NH_3^+}{\underset{|}{C}}H{-}CH_2{-}CH_2{-}CONH_2$$

IV.

$$NH_3 + CO_2 + 2ATP \rightarrow NH_2{-}\overset{O}{\overset{\|}{C}}{-}O{-}\underset{OH}{\underset{|}{\overset{O}{\overset{\|}{P}}}}{-}OH + 2ADP + P_i$$

Which of the following statements about these amino acids is(are) correct?

1. Reaction IV is activated by N-acetyl glutamate.
2. Reaction II is catalyzed by aspartate aminotransferase.
3. Reaction III requires ATP.
4. Reaction I is catalyzed by glutaminase.

20.5 Which of the following statements about the urea cycle is(are) correct?

1. The two nitrogen atoms that are incorporated into urea enter the cycle as ammonia and aspartate.
2. Urea is produced directly by the hydrolysis of ornithine.
3. ATP is required for the reaction in which argininosuccinate is formed.
4. The urea cycle occurs primarily in the kidney.

Choose the ONE best answer

20.6 In humans, the major route of nitrogen metabolism from amino acids to urea is catalyzed by which of the following enzymatic activities?

A. Amino acid oxidases and decarboxylases.
B. Amino acid decarboxylases and amino acid oxidases.
C. Transaminases and glutaminase.
D. Glutamate dehydrogenase and transaminases.
E. Glutaminase and amino oxidase.

20.7 Which of the following statements about the synthesis of carbamoyl phosphate by carbamoyl phosphate synthetase I is NOT true?

A. The enzyme catalyzes the rate-limiting reaction in the urea cycle.
B. The reaction occurs in the mitochondria.
C. The reaction requires two high-energy phosphates for each carbamoyl phosphate molecule synthesized.
D. The enzyme requires biotin.
E. The reaction is irreversible.

Amino Acids: Metabolism of Carbon Atoms

21

I. CATABOLISM OF THE CARBON SKELETONS OF AMINO ACIDS

The catabolism of the 20 amino acids found in proteins involves the removal of α-amino groups followed by the breakdown of the resulting carbon skeletons. The catabolism of the carbon skeletons converges to form seven products: pyruvate, acetyl CoA, acetoacetyl CoA, α-ketoglutarate, succinyl CoA, fumarate, and oxaloacetate. These products enter the pathways of intermediary metabolism, resulting either in the synthesis of glucose or lipid or in the production of energy through their oxidation to CO_2 and water by the citric acid cycle. The catabolism of the amino acid carbon skeletons is described below and summarized in Figure 21.1.

A. Glycogenic and ketogenic amino acids

Amino acids can be classified as (1) ***ketogenic*** or ***glycogenic*** according to the nature of their metabolic end products (Figure 21.2), and (2) ***essential*** or ***nonessential*** depending on whether they can be synthesized in man (see p. 245).

1. ***Ketogenic:*** Amino acids whose catabolism yields either ***acetoacetate*** or one of its precursors, ***acetyl CoA*** or ***acetoacetyl CoA,*** are termed ketogenic (see Figure 21.1). Acetoacetate is one of the triad of "ketone bodies," which also include β-hydroxybutyrate and acetone (see p. 176 for a discussion of the metabolism of ketone bodies). Leucine is the only exclusively ketogenic amino acid found in proteins.
2. ***Glycogenic:*** Amino acids whose catabolism yields ***pyruvate*** or one of the intermediates of the ***citric acid cycle*** are termed glucogenic or glycogenic (see Figure 21.1). These intermediates are substrates for gluconeogenesis and therefore can give rise to the ***net*** formation of glycogen in liver and muscle.

B. Amino acids forming oxaloacetate

1. ***Asparagine*** is hydrolyzed by the enzyme *asparaginase*, liberating ammonia and aspartate. ***Aspartate*** loses its amino group by transamination to form oxaloacetate (Figure 21.3).

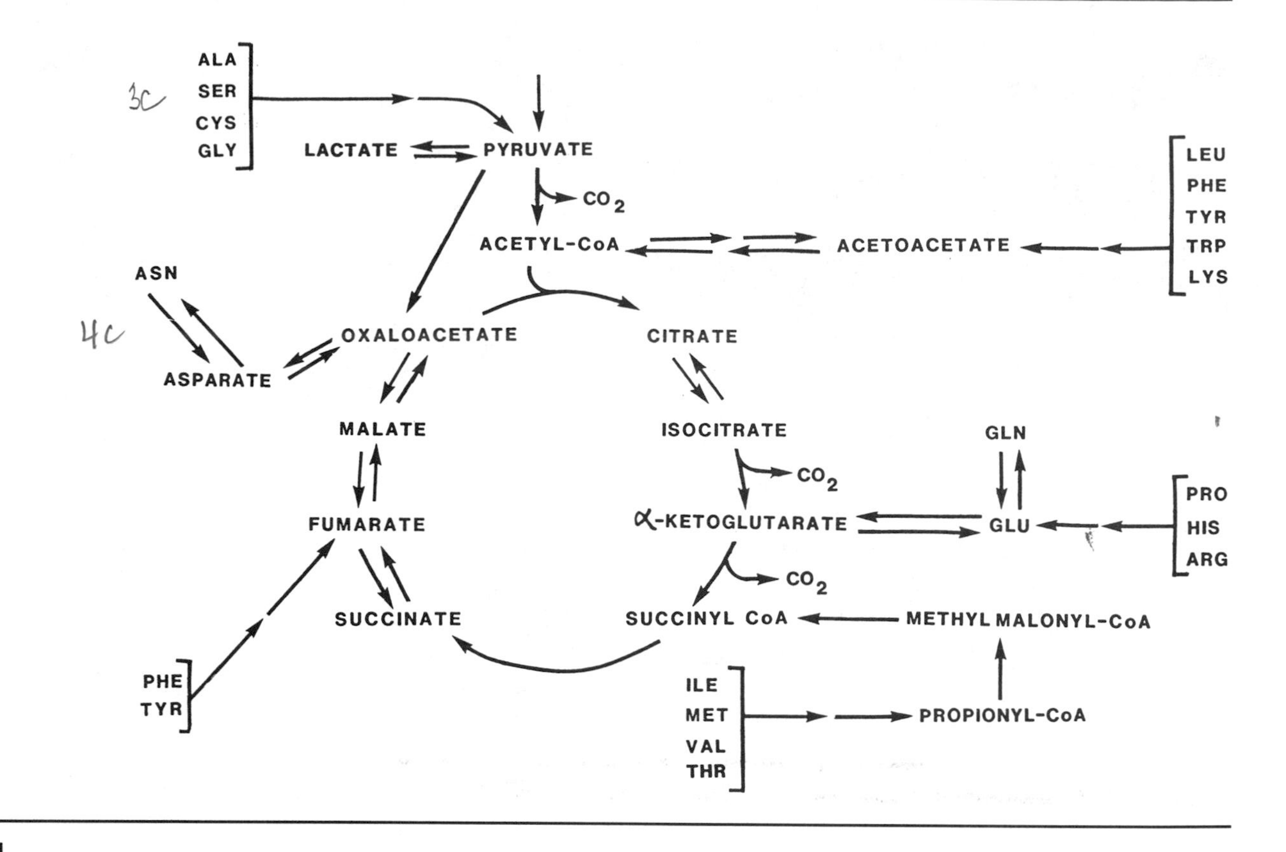

Figure 21.1
Conversion of carbon skeletons of amino acids into the intermediates of energy metabolism.

C. Amino acids forming α-ketoglutarate

1. ***Glutamine*** is converted to glutamate and ammonia by the enzyme *glutaminase* (see p. 234). ***Glutamate*** is converted to α-ketoglutarate by transamination or through oxidative deamination by *glutamate dehydrogenase* (see p. 230).
2. ***Proline*** is oxidized to Δ^1-pyrroline semialdehyde, which is hydrated and oxidized to glutamate (Figure 21.4). Glutamate is transaminated or oxidatively deaminated to form α-ketoglutarate.
3. ***Arginine*** is cleaved by *arginase* to produce ornithine; this reaction occurs primarily in the liver as part of the urea cycle (see p. 233). Ornithine subsequently undergoes transamination to yield glutamate-γ-semialdehyde, which is converted to α-ketoglutarate, as described for proline.
4. ***Histidine*** is deaminated to urocanate, which is converted to 4-imidazolone 5-propionate (Figure 21.5). Hydrolysis of the latter yields ***N-formiminoglutamate*** (FIGlu), which donates its formimino group to tetrahydrofolate, leaving glutamate, which is degraded as described above. Individuals deficient in folic acid excrete increased amounts of FIGlu in the urine, particularly after ingestion of a large dose of histidine. The ***FIGlu excretion test*** is therefore useful in diagnosing a deficiency of folic acid (see p. 245 for a discussion of folic acid and one-carbon metabolism).

D. Amino acids forming pyruvate

1. ***Alanine*** loses its amino group by transamination to form pyruvate (see Figure 21.6).

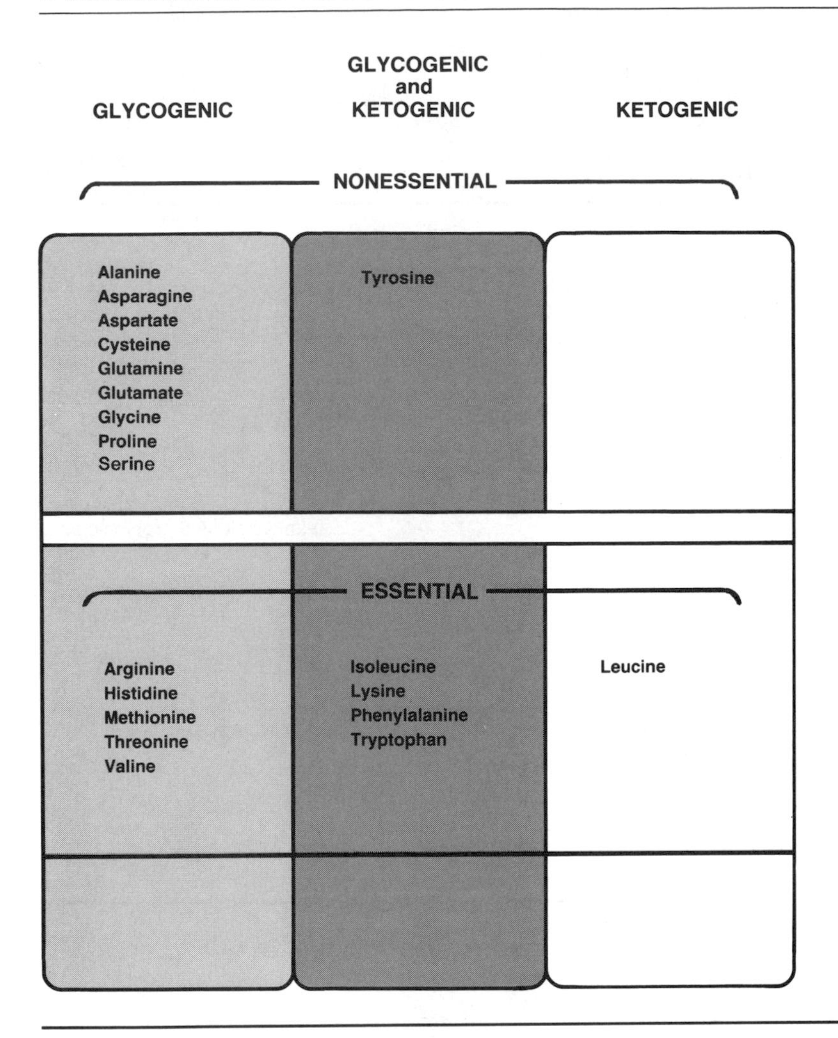

Figure 21.2
Classification of amino acids found in proteins as (1) essential or nonessential and as (2) glycogenic or ketogenic, or both.

2. ***Serine*** can be degraded to pyruvate by the action of *serine dehydratase* (Figure 21.7A). Serine can also be converted to glycine and N^5,N^{10}-methylenetetrahydrofolic acid (Figure 21.7B). The role of tetrahydrofolic acid in the transfer of one-carbon units is presented on p. 245.
3. ***Glycine*** can either be converted to serine by addition of a methylene group from N^5,N^{10}-methylenetetrahydrofolic acid (Fig 21.7B) or oxidized to CO_2 and NH_4^+.
4. ***Cystine*** is reduced to cysteine using NADH as a reductant. ***Cysteine*** undergoes desulfuration to yield pyruvate (Figure 21.8).

E. Amino acids forming fumarate

1. The hydroxylation of ***phenylalanine*** leads to the formation of ***tyrosine*** (see Figure 21.9). This reaction, catalyzed by the enzyme *phenylalanine hydroxylase,* is also the first reaction in the catabolism of phenylalanine. Thus the metabolism of phenylalanine and tyrosine merge, as shown in Figure 21.9, leading ultimately to the formation of fumarate and acetoacetate. Phenylalanine and tyrosine are therefore both glycogenic and ketogenic.

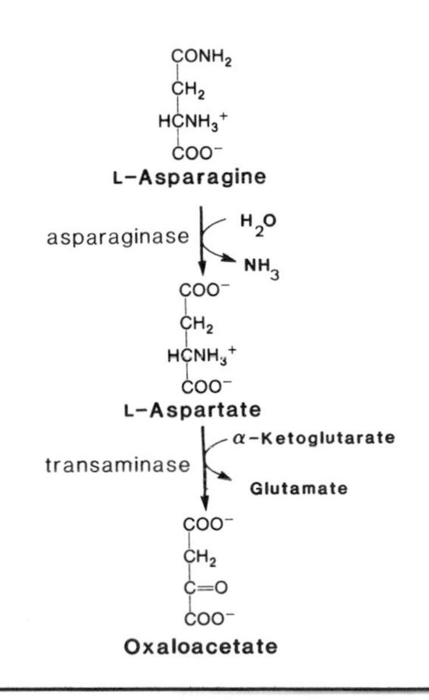

Figure 21.3
Metabolism of asparagine and aspartate.

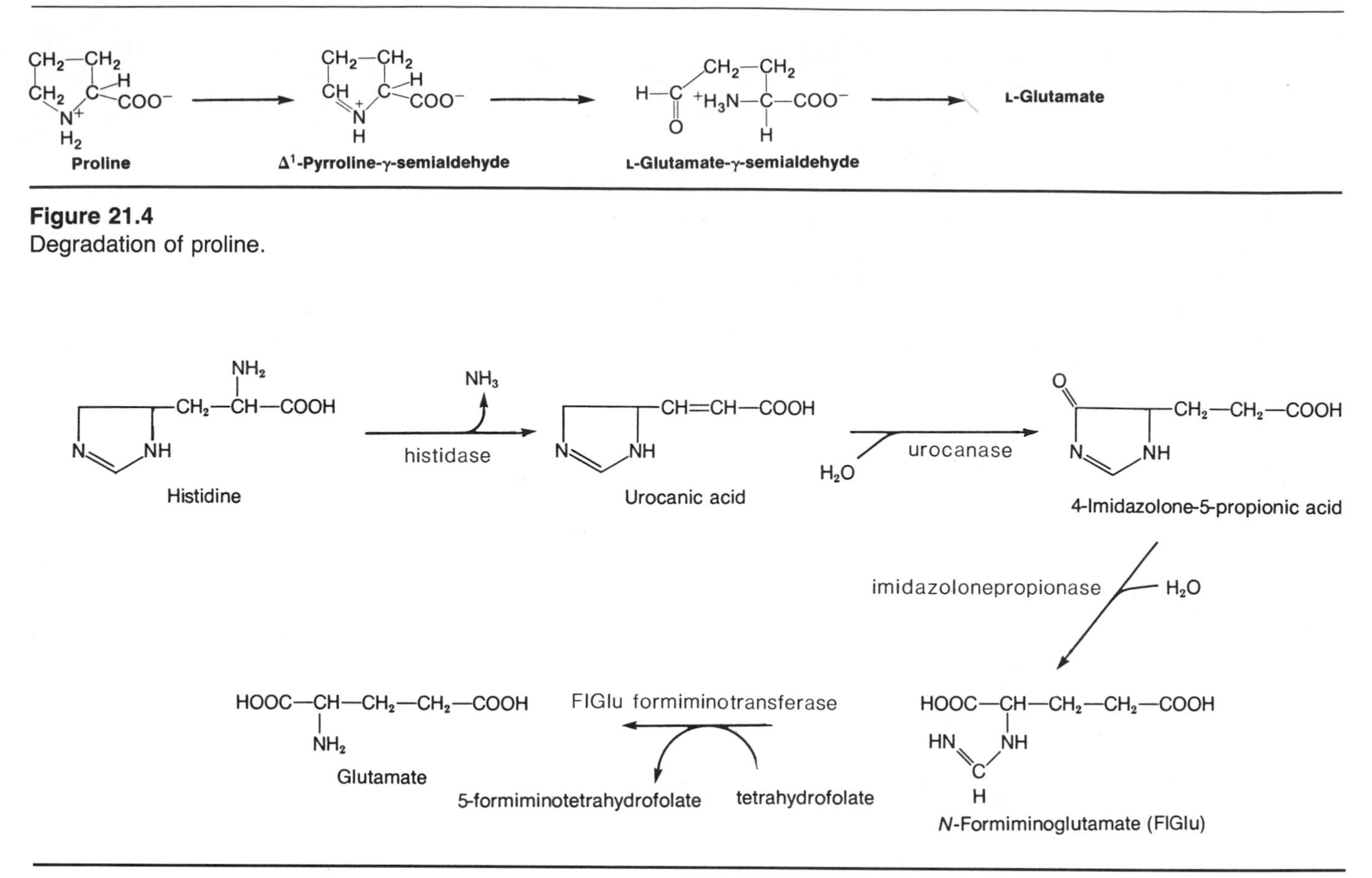

Figure 21.4
Degradation of proline.

Figure 21.5
Degradation of histidine.

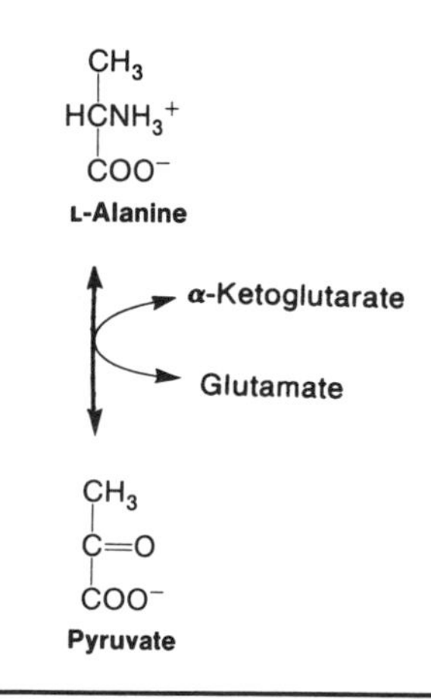

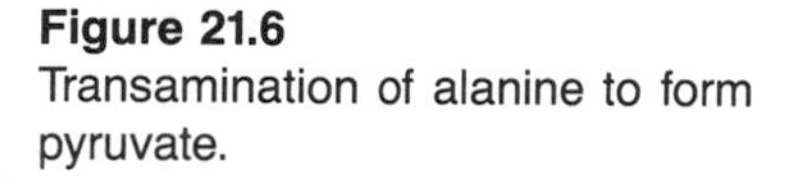

Figure 21.6
Transamination of alanine to form pyruvate.

2. Inherited deficiencies in the enzymes of phenylalanine and tyrosine metabolism, shown in Figure 21.20, lead to the diseases ***phenylketonuria*** and ***alkaptonuria***. Diseases of amino acid metabolism are discussed in more detail on p. 249.

F. Amino acids forming acetyl CoA or acetoacetyl CoA

The following five amino acids form acetyl CoA or acetoacetyl CoA directly, without pyruvate serving as an intermediate (through the pyruvate dehydrogenase reaction, p. 133). As mentioned previously, phenylalanine and tyrosine also give rise to acetoacetate during their catabolism (see Figure 21.9). Therefore, there are a total of seven ketogenic amino acids.

1. ***Leucine,*** the only amino acid that is exclusively ketogenic in its catabolism, forms acetyl CoA and acetoacetate. The initial steps in the catabolism of leucine are similar to those of the other branched-chain amino acids, isoleucine and valine, which are discussed on p. 244 (see Figure 21.12).
2. ***Isoleucine*** is both ketogenic and glycogenic, since its metabolism yields acetyl CoA and propionyl CoA. The first three steps in the metabolism of isoleucine are virtually identical to the initial steps in the degradation of the other branched-chain amino acids, valine and leucine, which are discussed on p. 244 (see Figure 21.12).

3. ***Threonine*** may be degraded by several routes. A major pathway in humans is the cleavage of threonine to glycine and acetaldehyde. Acetaldehyde is oxidized to acetate, which is converted to acetyl CoA (see Figure 21.20). An alternate pathway, the conversion of threonine to succinyl CoA, is described on p. 244.
4. ***Lysine*** is unusual in that neither of its amino groups undergoes transamination as the first step in catabolism. Rather, lysine forms α-aminoadipate-δ-semialdehyde, which is ultimately converted to acetoacetyl CoA (see Figure 21.20).
5. ***Tryptophan*** is converted to acetoacetyl CoA by the reactions shown in Figure 21.20.

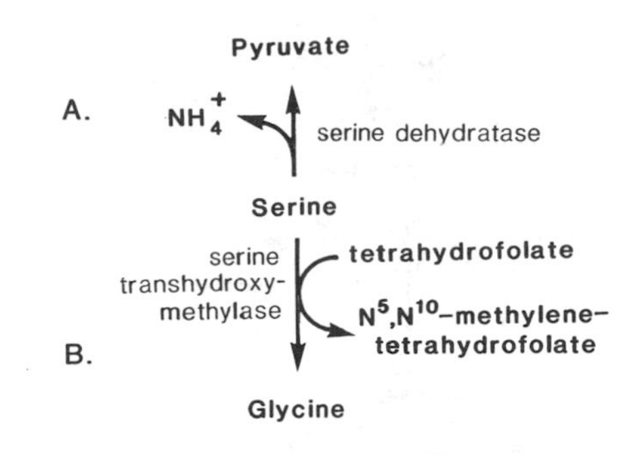

Figure 21.7
A. Dehydration of serine to form pyruvate. B. Interconversion of serine and glycine.

G. Amino acids forming succinyl-CoA

1. ***Methionine*** is metabolized to ***S-adenosylmethionine*** (SAM), the major methyl-group donor in one-carbon metabolism (Figure 21.10):
   a. Methionine condenses with ATP, forming S-adenosylmethionine (SAM), an unusual high-energy compound in that it contains no phosphate. The formation of SAM is driven, in effect, by the hydrolysis of all the phosphate bonds in ATP (Figure 21.10).
   b. The methyl group attached to the tertiary sulfur in SAM is "activated" and can be transferred to a variety of acceptor molecules, usually by attachment to oxygen or nitrogen atoms but sometimes to carbon atoms. The reaction product, S-adenosylhomocysteine, is a simple thioether, analogous to methionine, and the resulting loss of free energy makes methyl transfer essentially irreversible.
   c. After donation of the methyl group, S-adenosylhomocysteine is hydrolyzed to L-homocysteine and adenosine. Homocysteine has two fates:
      1) ***Synthesis of cysteine:*** Homocysteine can combine with serine, forming ***cystathionine,*** which is hydrolyzed to L-homoserine and cysteine (see Figure 21.18). This sequence has the net effect of converting serine to cysteine and homocysteine to homoserine. Homoserine is converted to α-ketobutyrate, which is oxidatively decarboxylated to form propionyl CoA. Propionyl CoA is converted to succinyl CoA (see Figures 16.16 and 21.20).
      2) ***Resynthesis of methionine:*** Homocysteine can accept a methyl group from N^5-methyltetrahydrofolate (N^5-methyl-THF) in a reaction requiring methylcobalamin (B_{12}) as cofactor (see p. 319 and Figure 21.11). The methyl group is transferred from the B_{12} derivative to homocysteine, and cobalamin is recharged from N^5-methyl-THF. In vitamin B_{12} deficiency, the rate of methyl group transfer in the above reaction is

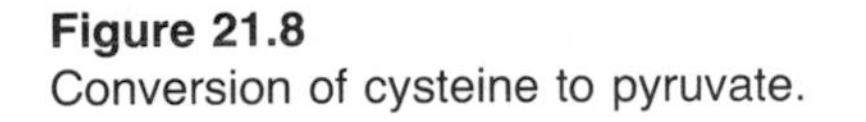

Figure 21.8
Conversion of cysteine to pyruvate.

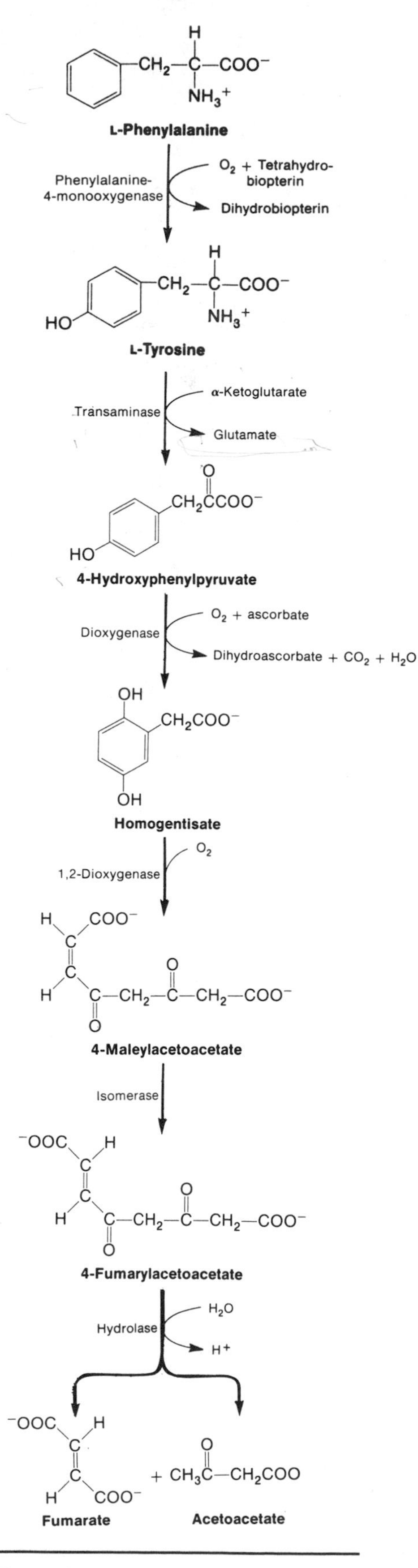

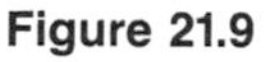

Figure 21.9
Degradation of phenylalanine and tyrosine to fumarate and acetoacetate.

decreased, resulting in an increase in N^5-methyl-THF that cannot be converted to other folic acid derivatives, and thus "traps" a portion of the folic acid pool in an unusable form. Therefore the effect of vitamin B_{12} deficiency includes an accompanying deficiency of the other essential forms of folate, in addition to an impairment of methionine synthesis. This imposed secondary folate "deficiency" results in the characteristic megaloblastic anemia seen with true folate deficiency (see p. 319 for a discussion of folic acid deficiency on the synthesis of purines and pyrimidines.)

3) Note: Administration of large quantities of folate can mask some of the early signs of B_{12} deficiency, since folate can ease the anemia, but it does not reverse the neurologic damage done by B_{12} deficiency (see p. 320).

2. ***Valine*** and ***isoleucine*** are branched-chain amino acids that yield succinyl CoA, and hence are included in this section. However, the details of their metabolism will be considered on p. 246, which describes the catabolism of the branched-chain amino acids (Figure 21.12).

3. ***Threonine*** has already been mentioned as a ketogenic amino acid because its degradation yields acetate (see p. 243). Alternatively, threonine is dehydrated to α-ketobutyrate, which is converted to propionyl CoA, the precursor of succinyl CoA (see Figures 16.16 and 21.20).

H. Catabolism of the branched-chain amino acids: isoleucine, leucine, and valine

1. The branched-chain amino acids isoleucine, leucine, and valine are all ***essential*** amino acids. In contrast to other amino acids, they are metabolized primarily by the peripheral tissues (particularly muscle) rather than by liver (see pp. 277 and 280). Since these three amino acids have a similar route of catabolism, it is convenient to describe them as a group (Figure 21.12):

   a. ***Transamination*** of all three amino acids appears to be catalyzed by a single enzyme, *branched-chain amino acid transaminase*.

   b. ***Oxidative decarboxylation*** of the α-keto acids derived from leucine, valine, and isoleucine is also catalyzed by a single enzyme, *α-keto acid dehydrogenase*, which uses thiamine pyrophosphate as a cofactor (see p. 311). This reaction is analogous to the conversion of pyruvate to acetyl CoA (see p. 133) and the oxidation of α-ketoglutarate to succinyl CoA (see p. 137). An inherited deficiency of *α-keto acid dehydrogenase* results in the accumulation of the keto acid substrates in the urine. Their sweet odor prompted the name ***maple-syrup urine disease***.

   c. Dehydrogenation of the acyl-CoA products formed in the above reaction yields α-β-unsaturated acyl-CoA derivatives. This reaction is reminiscent of the dehydrogenation described in the β-oxidation scheme of fatty acid degradation (see p. 171).

   d. The catabolism of isoleucine ultimately yields acetyl CoA and succinyl CoA, rendering it both ketogenic and glycogenic. Valine yields succinyl CoA and is glycogenic; leucine is ketogenic, being metabolized to acetoacetate and acetyl CoA.

II. ROLE OF FOLIC ACID IN AMINO ACID METABOLISM

A. Overview

1. Single carbon atoms can exist in a variety of oxidation states, including methane, methanol, formaldehyde, formate, and carbonic acid. It is possible to incorporate carbon units at each of these oxidation states, except methane, into other organic compounds.
2. These single carbon units can be transferred from carrier compounds such as ***folic acid*** and ***S-adenosyl methionine*** to specific structures that are being synthesized or modified (Figure 21.13). The ***"one-carbon pool"*** refers to this group of carriers. (Note: Carbonic acid, the hydrated form of CO_2, is carried by the vitamin biotin, which participates in carboxylation reactions but is not considered a member of the "one-carbon pool.")
3. Formaldehyde (HCHO) is a toxic substance that reacts spontaneously with amino groups of proteins and nucleic acids, hydroxymethylating them and forming methylene-bridged cross-links between them. Formic acid (HCOOH) is a nonreactive compound and must be activated before it can serve as an efficient formylating agent. Therefore, a major function of the one-carbon pool is to maintain formaldehyde and formic acid in a nontoxic but active state, available for essential synthetic processes when required by specific enzymes.

B. Folic acid: a carrier of one-carbon units

1. The chemistry and the metabolism of folic acid is presented on p. 317. Briefly, folic acid is composed of three components: a bicyclic, nitrogenous compound called ***pteridine***, a molecule of ***p-aminobenzoic acid*** (PABA), and one or more ***glutamic acid*** residues (Figure 21.13).
2. The ***active*** form of folic acid, ***tetrahydrofolic acid*** (THF), is produced by the enzyme *dihydrofolate reductase* (Figure 21.13) in a two-step reaction requiring NADPH.
3. The carbon unit carried by THF is bound to nitrogen N^5 or N^{10}, or to both N^5 and N^{10}.
4. Figure 21.13 shows the structures of the various members of the THF family, indicating the sources of the one-carbon units and the reactions in which the specific members participate.

III. BIOSYNTHESIS OF NONESSENTIAL AMINO ACIDS

The nutritional requirements of humans include certain of the amino acids commonly found in proteins (see Figure 21.2). These ***essential amino acids*** cannot be synthesized (or cannot be produced in sufficient amounts) by the body, and therefore must be obtained in the diet in order for normal protein synthesis to occur. In contrast, ***nonessential amino acids*** (shown in Figure 21.2) can be synthesized in sufficient amounts in the body from the intermediates of metabolism or, as in the case of

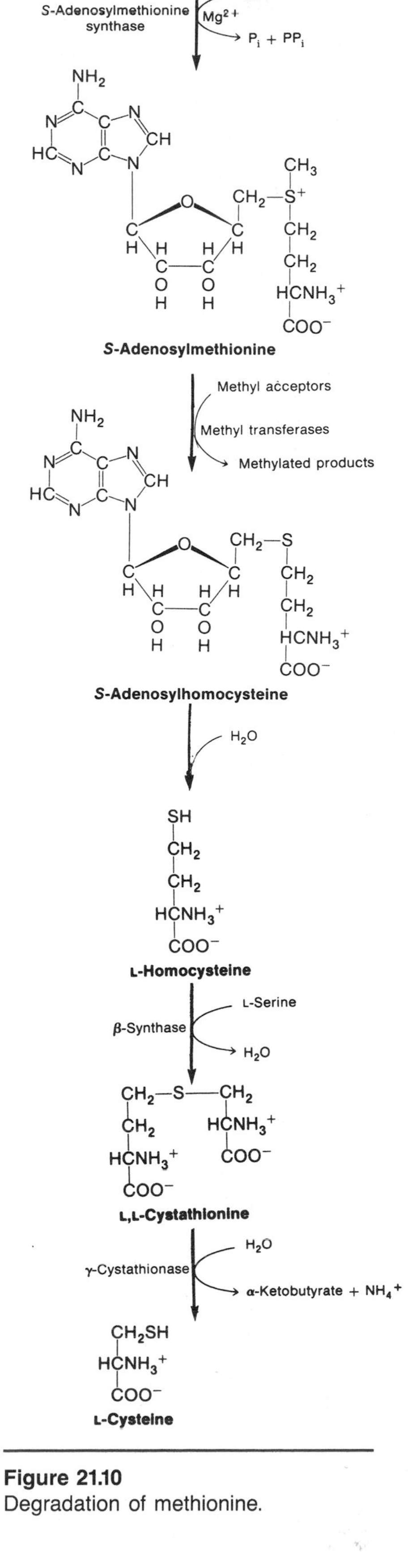

Figure 21.10
Degradation of methionine.

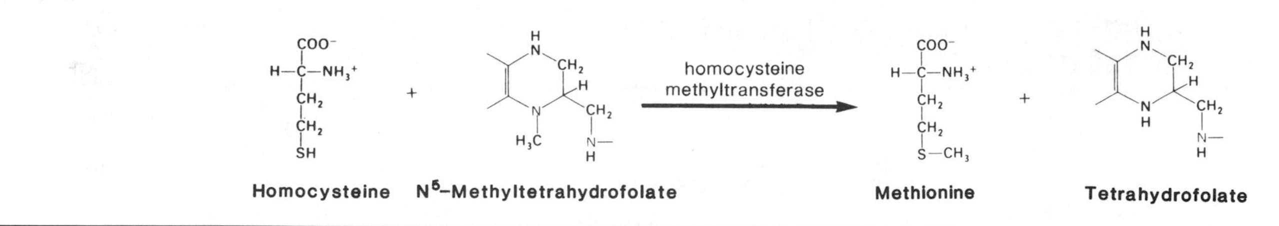

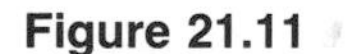

Figure 21.11
Resynthesis of methionine from homocysteine.

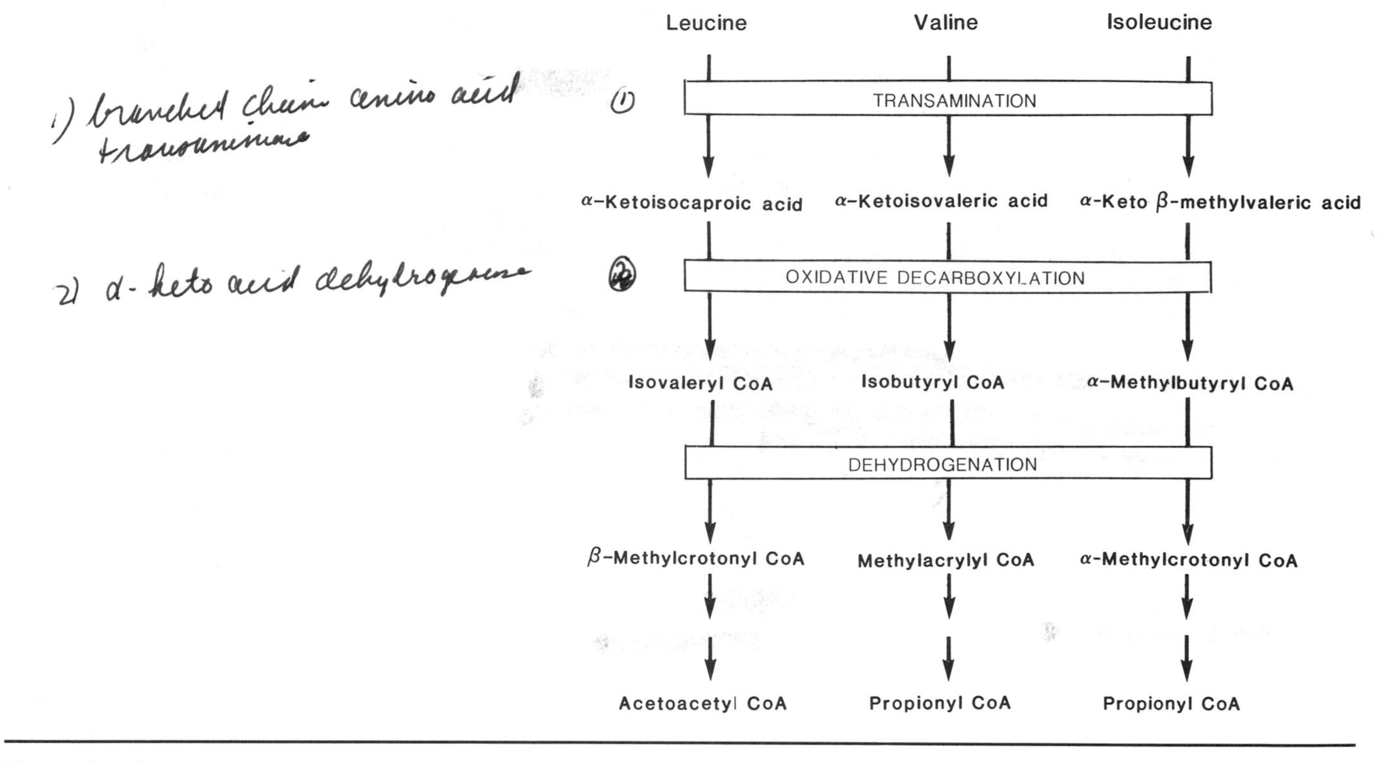

Figure 21.12
Degradation of leucine, valine, and isoleucine.

cysteine and tyrosine, from essential amino acids. These synthetic reactions are described below and summarized in Figure 21.20.

A. Synthesis from α-keto acids

1. ***Alanine, aspartate,*** and ***glutamate*** are synthesized by transfer of an amino group to the α-keto acids pyruvate, oxaloacetate, and α-ketoglutarate, respectively. These transamination reactions, shown in Figure 21.14, are the most direct of the biosynthetic pathways. (The role of transamination reactions in the maintenance of nitrogen balance is covered more thoroughly on p. 228.)
2. Glutamate is unusual in that it can also be synthesized by the reverse of oxidative deamination, catalyzed by *glutamate dehydrogenase* (see p. 230).

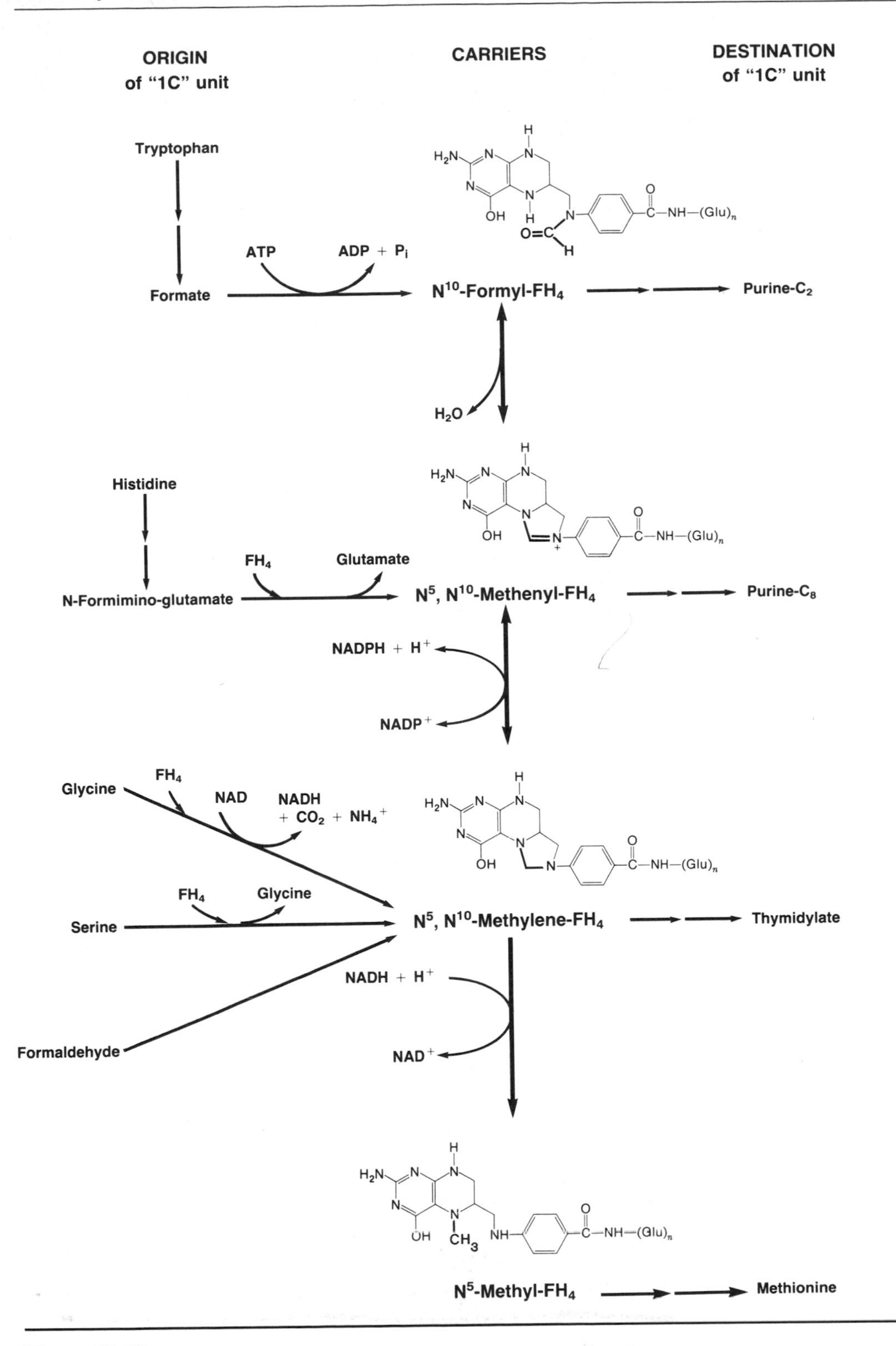

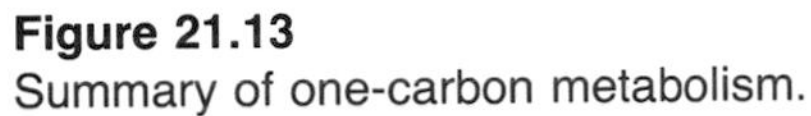

Figure 21.13
Summary of one-carbon metabolism.

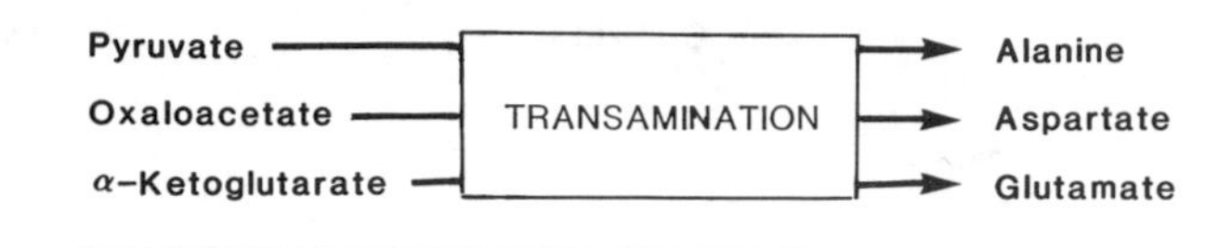

Figure 21.14
Formation of alanine aspartate and glutamate from the corresponding α-keto acids.

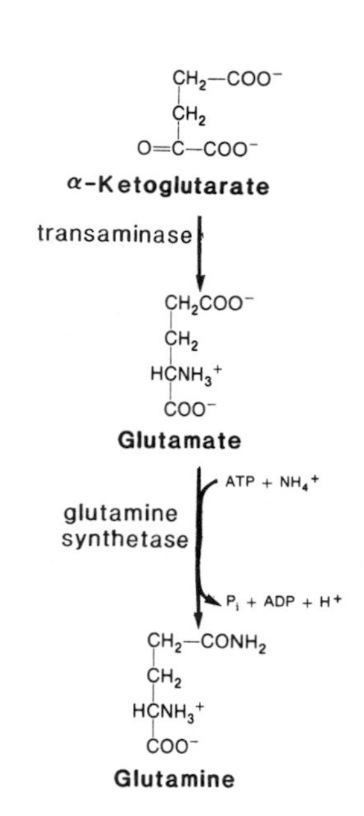

Figure 21.15
Biosynthesis of glutamine.

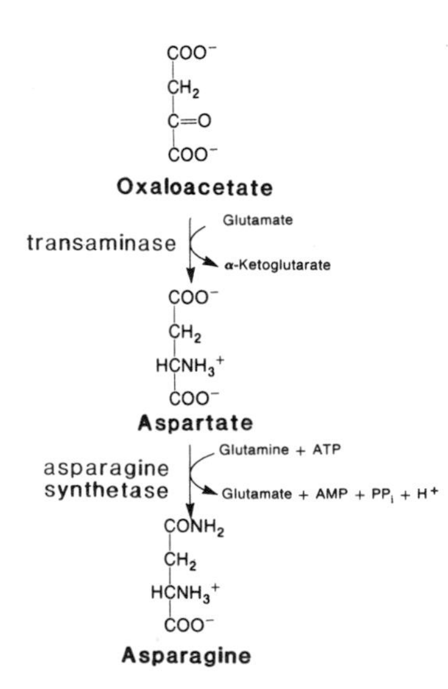

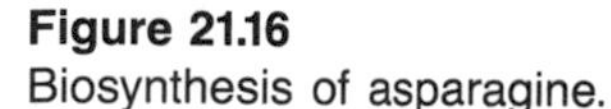

Figure 21.16
Biosynthesis of asparagine.

B. Synthesis by amidation

1. ***Glutamine,*** which contains an amide linkage with ammonia at the γ-carbon, is formed from glutamate in a reaction catalyzed by *glutamine synthetase*. The reaction is driven by the hydrolysis of ATP (see Figure 21.15). In addition to producing glutamine for protein synthesis, the reaction also serves as a major mechanism for the detoxification of ammonia in brain and liver (see p. 234 for a discussion of ammonia metabolism).
2. ***Asparagine*** is formed from aspartate in a reaction catalyzed by *asparagine synthetase,* using glutamine as amino donor (see Figure 21.16). The reaction requires ATP and, like the synthesis of glutamine, has an equilibrium far in the direction of asparagine synthesis.

C. Proline

Glutamate is converted to proline by the intermediate glutamate semialdehyde, which spontaneously cyclizes to form Δ^1-pyrroline semialdehyde (see Figure 21.4 for structures). Reduction of Δ^1-pyrroline semialdehyde yields proline.

D. Serine, glycine, and cysteine

1. ***Serine*** arises from 3-phosphoglyceric acid (an intermediate in glycolysis, p. 115), which is first oxidized to 3-phosphopyruvate and then transaminated to yield 3-phosphoserine. Serine is formed by hydrolysis of the phosphate ester (see Figure 21.17). Serine can also be formed from glycine by transfer of a methylene group (see Figure 21.7).
2. ***Glycine*** can be synthesized from serine by removal of a methylene group (see Figure 21.7B).
3. ***Cysteine*** is synthesized by two consecutive reactions in which homocysteine combines with serine, forming cystathionine, which in turn is hydrolyzed to homoserine and cysteine (Figure 21.18). Homocysteine is derived from methionine, as described on p. 243. Because methionine is an essential amino acid, cysteine synthesis can be sustained only if the dietary intake of methionine is adequate.

E. Tyrosine

1. ***Tyrosine*** is formed from phenylalanine in a reaction catalyzed by *phenylalanine hydroxylase*. The reaction requires molecular oxygen and the cofactor ***tetrahydrobiopterin*** (Figure 21.19). One atom of molecular oxygen becomes the hydroxyl group of tyrosine, and the other is reduced to water. During the reaction, tetrahy-

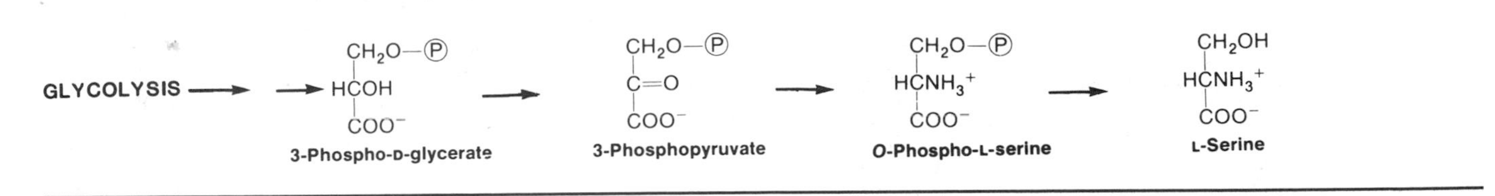

Figure 21.17
Biosynthesis of serine from 3-phosphoglycerate.

drobiopterin is oxidized to dihydrobiopterin. Tetrahydrobiopterin is regenerated from dihydrobiopterin in a separate reaction requiring NADPH.

2. Tyrosine, like cysteine, is formed from an essential amino acid; tyrosine is therefore nonessential only in the presence of adequate dietary phenylalanine.
3. A genetic deficiency of *phenylalanine hydroxylase* results in the disease phenylketonuria, described below. The biosynthesis and the degradation of amino acids are summarized in Figure 21.20.

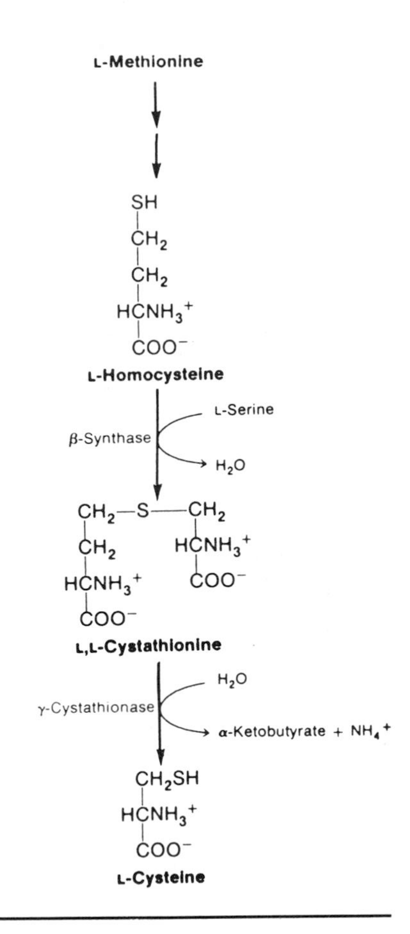

Figure 21.18
Biosynthesis of cysteine.

IV. METABOLIC DEFECTS IN AMINO ACID METABOLISM

Inborn errors of amino acid metabolism almost invariably result in mental retardation or other developmental abnormalities. The inherited defects may be expressed as a total loss of enzyme activity or, more frequently, as a partial deficiency in catalytic activity. Although more than 50 of these disorders have been described, most are rare, occurring less than 1 per 500,000 in most populations. Nevertheless, these deficiency diseases provide information about the intermediary metabolism of amino acids. Figure 21.20 summarizes some of the more commonly encountered diseases of amino acid metabolism. Phenylketonuria is discussed in some detail below because screening tests and prenatal diagnosis are available.

A. Phenylketonuria

1. ***Hyperphenylalaninemias:*** Phenylketonuria, caused by a deficiency of *phenylalanine hydroxylase* (see p. 241), is the most commonly encountered type of hyperphenylalaninemia (prevalence 1:11,000), accounting for about half of the patients with elevated levels of serum phenylalanine. Hyperphenylalaninemia may also be caused by other inborn errors of metabolism that result in the impaired ability to convert phenylalanine to tyrosine. For example, a partial deficiency in the enzymes that synthesize or reduce the cofactor biopterin can also lead to elevated concentration of phenylalanine in the serum. It is frequently important to distinguish among these various forms of hyperphenylalaninemia because their clinical management is different.
2. ***Diagnosis of PKU:*** The patient with untreated PKU will typically show symptoms of mental retardation by the age of 1 year. PKU is detected by neonatal screening for elevated blood levels of phenylalanine using the Guthrie Test. However, the infant with PKU frequently has normal blood levels of phenylalanine at birth

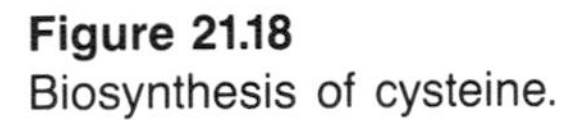

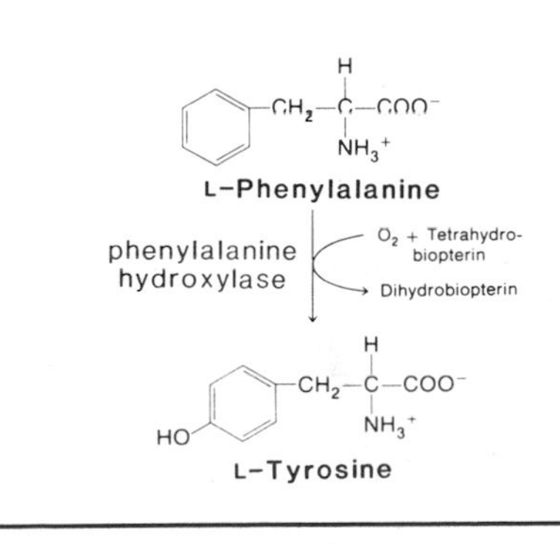

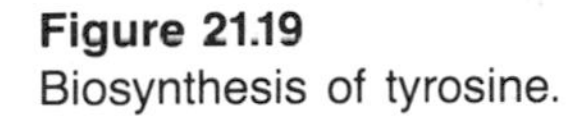

Figure 21.19
Biosynthesis of tyrosine.

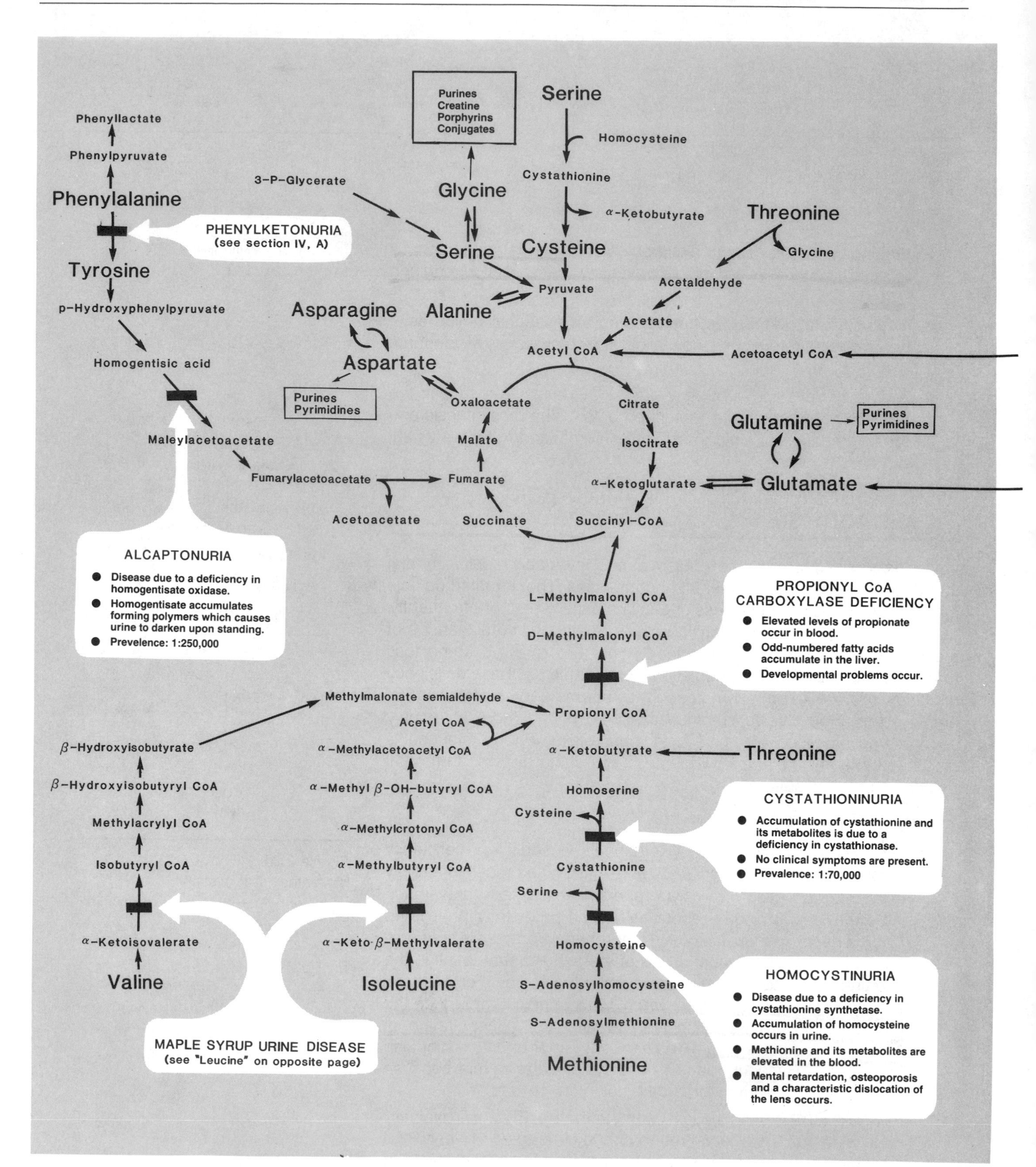

Purines
Creatine
Porphyrins
Conjugates
Serine
Homocysteine
Cystathionine
α-Ketobutyrate
Threonine
Glycine
Phenyllactate
Phenylpyruvate
Phenylalanine
3-P-Glycerate
Glycine
Serine
Cysteine
PHENYLKETONURIA
(see section IV, A)
Tyrosine
Pyruvate
Acetaldehyde
p-Hydroxyphenylpyruvate
Asparagine
Alanine
Acetate
Homogentisic acid
Aspartate
Acetyl CoA
Acetoacetyl CoA
Purines
Pyrimidines
Oxaloacetate
Citrate
Glutamine
Purines
Pyrimidines
Maleylacetoacetate
Malate
Isocitrate
Fumarylacetoacetate
Fumarate
α-Ketoglutarate
Glutamate
Acetoacetate
Succinate
Succinyl-CoA
ALCAPTONURIA
Disease due to a deficiency in homogentisate oxidase.
Homogentisate accumulates forming polymers which causes urine to darken upon standing.
Prevelence: 1:250,000
L-Methylmalonyl CoA
D-Methylmalonyl CoA
PROPIONYL CoA CARBOXYLASE DEFICIENCY
Elevated levels of propionate occur in blood.
Odd-numbered fatty acids accumulate in the liver.
Developmental problems occur.
Methylmalonate semialdehyde
Propionyl CoA
Acetyl CoA
β-Hydroxyisobutyrate
α-Methylacetoacetyl CoA
α-Ketobutyrate
Threonine
β-Hydroxyisobutyryl CoA
α-Methyl β-OH-butyryl CoA
Homoserine
Cysteine
CYSTATHIONINURIA
Methylacrylyl CoA
α-Methylcrotonyl CoA
Accumulation of cystathionine and its metabolites is due to a deficiency in cystathionase.
Isobutyryl CoA
α-Methylbutyryl CoA
Cystathionine
No clinical symptoms are present.
Prevalence: 1:70,000
Serine
α-Ketoisovalerate
α-Keto-β-Methylvalerate
Homocysteine
Valine
Isoleucine
S-Adenosylhomocysteine
HOMOCYSTINURIA
Disease due to a deficiency in cystathionine synthetase.
Accumulation of homocysteine occurs in urine.
Methionine and its metabolites are elevated in the blood.
Mental retardation, osteoporosis and a characteristic dislocation of the lens occurs.
S-Adenosylmethionine
MAPLE SYRUP URINE DISEASE
(see "Leucine" on opposite page)
Methionine

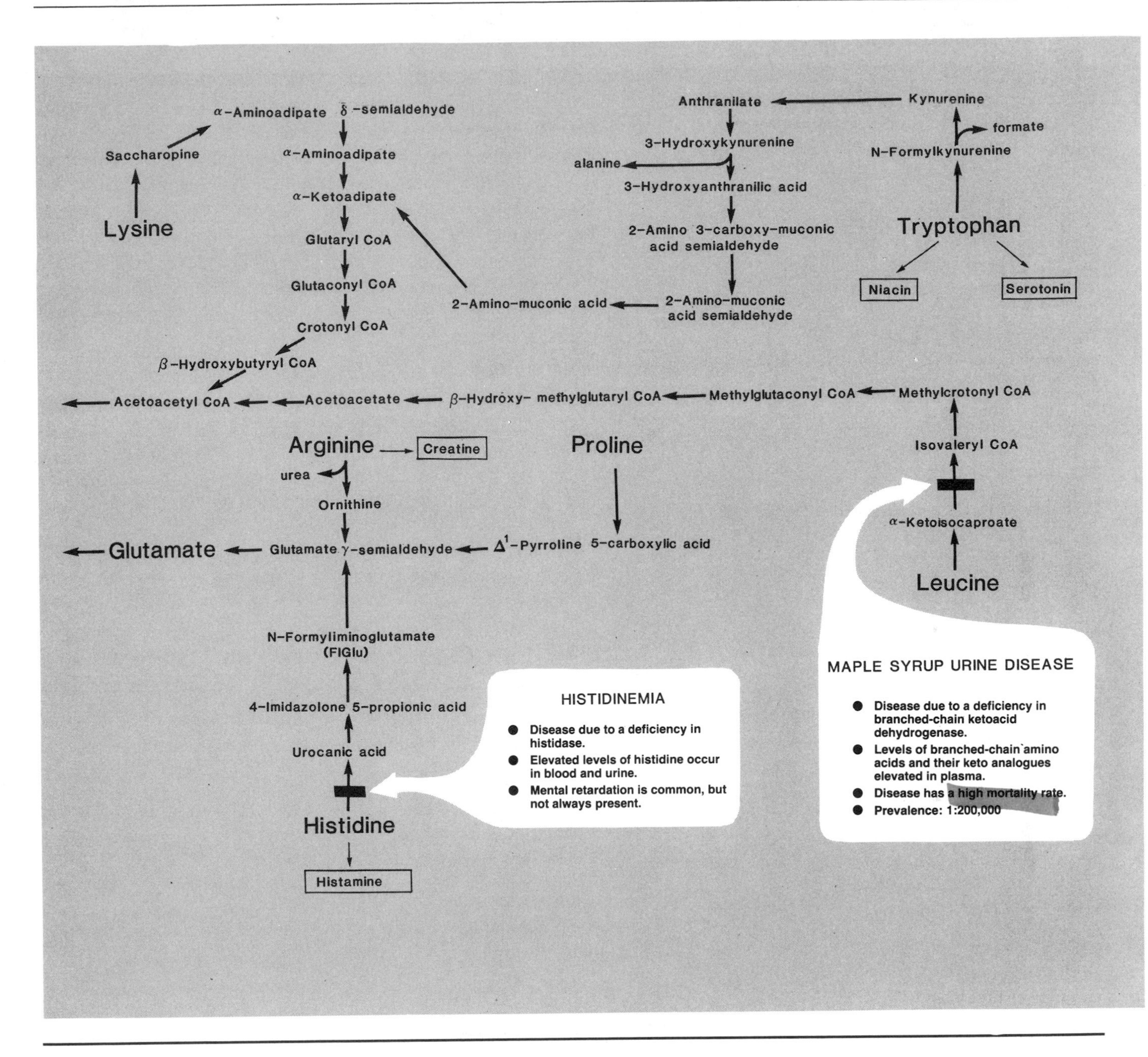

Figure 21.20
Summary of the metabolism of amino acids in humans. Genetically determined enzyme deficiencies are summarized in white boxes. Nitrogen-containing compounds derived from amino acids are shown in boxes.

and will have normal levels until exposed to at least 24 hours of protein feeding. Thus tests performed at birth may show false-negative results.

3. ***Characteristics of PKU***:

   a. Phenylalanine is present in elevated concentrations in tissues, serum, and urine. Phenyllactate, phenylacetate, and phenylpyruvate, which are not normally produced in significant amounts in the presence of a functional *phenylalanine hy-*

droxylase, are also elevated in PKU. The disease acquired its name from the high levels of the phenylketones present in the urine.

b. Mental retardation, failure to walk or talk, seizures, hyperactivity, tremor, microencephaly, and failure to grow are characteristic findings in PKU. Virtually all untreated patients show IQs below 50.

c. Patients with PKU show a deficiency of pigmentation (fair hair, light skin color, and blue eyes). The hydroxylation of tyrosine, which is the first step in the formation of the pigment melanin, is competitively inhibited by the high levels of phenylalanine present in PKU.

4. *Treatment of PKU:*

a. Blood phenylalanine is maintained in the normal range by feeding the patient low phenylalanine protein preparations. The amount is adjusted according to the tolerance of the individual as measured by blood phenylalanine levels. The earlier treatment is started, the more completely neurologic damage can be prevented. However, overzealous treatment that results in blood phenylalanine levels below normal should be avoided because it can lead to poor growth and neurologic symptoms.

b. In patients with PKU, tyrosine cannot be synthesized from phenylalanine and hence must be supplied in the diet.

Study Questions

Answer A if 1, 2, and 3 are correct
B if 1 and 3 are correct
C if 2 and 4 are correct
D if only 4 is correct
E if all are correct

21.1 In the degradation of amino acids,

1. arginine, proline, histidine, and glutamine all lead to the production of α-ketoglutarate by glutamate.
2. valine, isoleucine, and methionine all lead to the production of succinyl CoA by way of propionyl CoA and methylmalonyl CoA.
3. phenylalanine leads to the production of fumarate and acetoacetyl CoA by way of tyrosine and homogentisic acid.
4. asparagine and aspartic acid lead to the production of oxaloacetate.

21.2 The structures of four amino acids are listed below:

I.

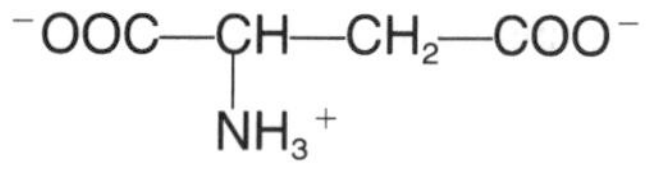

$$^{-}OOC{-}\underset{\displaystyle NH_3^{+}}{CH}{-}CH_2{-}COO^{-}$$

II.

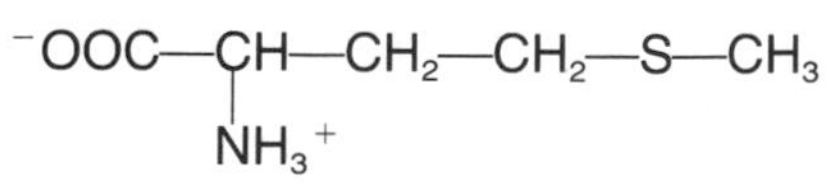

$$^{-}OOC{-}\underset{\displaystyle NH_3^{+}}{CH}{-}CH_2{-}CH_2{-}S{-}CH_3$$

III.

$$^{-}OOC{-}\underset{\displaystyle NH_3^{+}}{CH}{-}CH_2{-}CH_2{-}COO^{-}$$

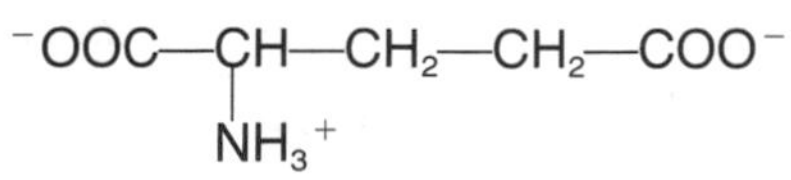

IV. $^{-}OOC—CH(NH_3^+)—CH_2—CH(CH_3^+)—CH_3$

Which of the following statements about these amino acids is(are) correct?

1. Amino acids I and II are glucogenic.
2. Amino acids II, III, and IV are essential amino acids.
3. Amino acid IV is ketogenic.
4. Amino acid III is degraded to pyruvate after transamination.

21.3 Which of the following are synthesized from essential amino acids?

1. Alanine
2. Cysteine
3. Proline
4. Tyrosine

21.4 From which of the following amino acids can the α-amino group be removed by a dehydration reaction?

1. Serine
2. Phenylalanine
3. Threonine
4. Arginine

Choose the ONE best answer:

21.5 In humans, essential amino acids (with two exceptions) may be replaced in the diet by which one of the following?

A. Reducing caloric requirements
B. Increasing tricarboxylic acid cycle activity
C. Adding an excess of all other essential amino acids
D. Adding the keto acids that correspond to the essential amino acids
E. None of the above

21.6 A normal adult is placed on a diet deficient only in phenylalanine. Which of the following statements is CORRECT?

A. Synthesis of proteins by the liver continues normally.
B. Tyrosine in the diet will be used to compensate for the missing phenylalanine.
C. Phenylalanine will be formed from alanine and benzoic acid, and therefore no metabolic changes will be observed.
D. Tyrosine becomes an essential amino acid because it is synthesized from phenylalanine by hydroxylation.
E. An increased dietary intake of both vitamin B_{12} and biotin will be required to remain in nitrogen balance.

21.7 Which one of the following statements about amino acid metabolism in a growing child is INCORRECT?

A. The basic (positively charged) amino acids are all essential, whereas the acidic (negatively charged) amino acids are nonessential.
B. The basic amino acids and acidic amino acids are all glycogenic and not ketogenic.
C. The aromatic amino acids are ketogenic and glycogenic.
D. Proline is degraded to glutamic acid by way of glutamic acid semi-aldehyde, and glutamic acid is converted to α-ketoglutarate by trans-amination.
E. The dietary requirement for the essential amino acid methionine is lowered if cysteine is included in the diet.

Conversion of Amino Acids to Specialized Products

22

I. OVERVIEW

In addition to serving as building blocks for proteins, amino acids are precursors of many nitrogen-containing compounds that have important physiologic functions. These compounds include heme, neurotransmitters, hormones, purines, and pyrimidines.

II. PORPHYRINS AND BILE PIGMENTS

Porphyrins readily bind metal ions, usually Fe^{+2} or Fe^{+3}. The most prevalent metalloporphyrin in humans is ***heme,*** which is the prosthetic group for hemoglobin, myoglobin, cytochromes, *catalase,* and *tryptophan pyrrolase*. Like most proteins, these hemeproteins have a short lifetime and are constantly being synthesized and degraded. Concomitant with the turnover of hemeproteins is the simultaneous synthesis and degradation of the associated porphyrins and recycling of the bound iron ions. The formation and the degradation of the porphyrin component of hemoglobin are of quantitative importance in the nitrogen balance of the body.

N
H
Pyrrole

A. Structure of porphyrins

1. Porphyrins are cyclic compounds formed by the linkage of four pyrrole rings through methenyl bridges (Figure 22.1).
2. Different porphyrins vary in the nature of the side chains that are attached to each of the four pyrrole rings. For example, uroporphyrin contains acetate ($—CH_2—COO^-$) and propionate ($—CH_2—CH_2—COO^-$) side chains (Figure 22.1A), whereas coproporphyrin is substituted with methyl ($—CH_3$) and propionate groups .
3. The side chains of porphyrins can be ordered around the tetrapyrrole nucleus in four different ways, designated by Roman numerals I to IV. Only ***type III*** porphyrins (which contain an ***asymmetric*** substitution on ring D) are physiologically important in

A.

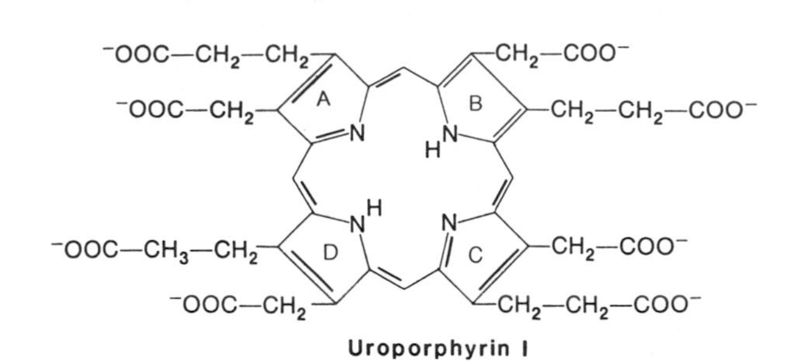

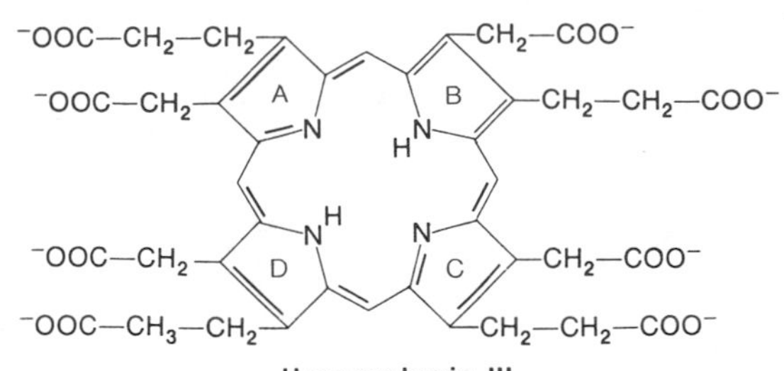

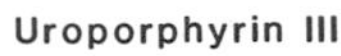

B.

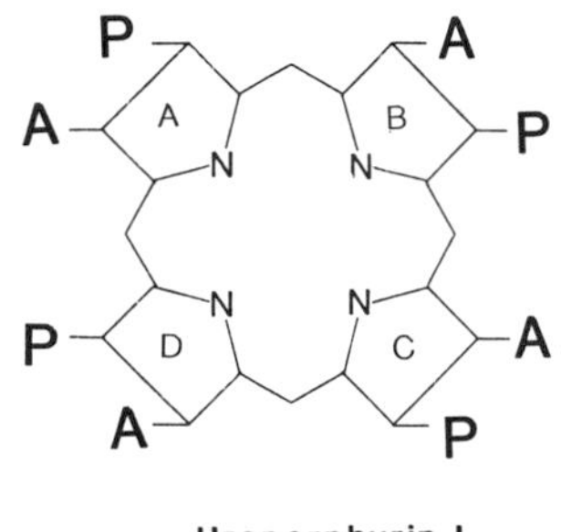

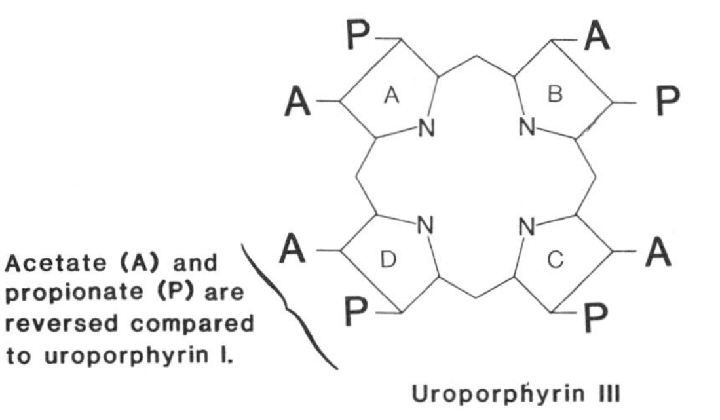

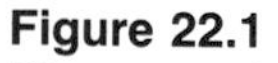

Figure 22.1
Structure of uroporphyrin I and uroporphyrin III.

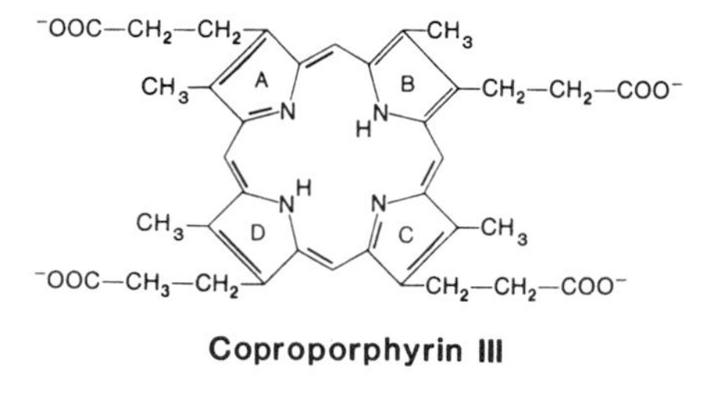

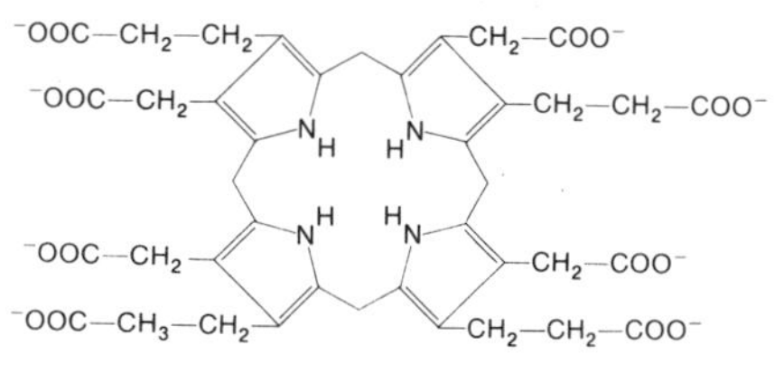

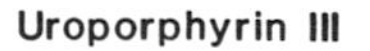

humans (Figure 22.1). In certain diseases (see p. 257) ***type I*** porphyrins (which contain a ***symmetric*** arrangement of substituents) may also be synthesized in appreciable quantities (Figure 22.1).

4. Porphyrins can exist in a chemically reduced form called ***porphyrinogens***. In contrast to the porphyrins, which are colored, the porphyrinogens, such as uroporphyrinogen, are colorless. As is described in the next section, porphyrinogens serve as intermediates in the biosynthesis of porphyrins.

5. ***Heme*** is the final product of the porphyrin synthetic pathway. Heme consists of one ferrous (Fe^{+2}) iron atom coordinated in the center of the tetrapyrrole ring of protoporphyrin IX. Heme is quantitatively the most important porphyrin in humans (see p. 21).

B. Biosynthesis of porphyrins

1. ***Tissues involved:*** Heme synthesis occurs in most mammalian tissues but is particularly active in the liver, which synthesizes a number of hepatic heme proteins, and in the blood-producing cells of the bone marrow, which are active in hemoglobin synthesis. (Note: Mature red blood cells lack mitochondria and cannot synthesize heme.) The initial reaction and the last three steps in the formation

of porphyrins occur in the mitochondria; the intermediate steps of the biosynthetic pathway occur in the cytosol (Figure 22.4).

2. ***Formation of δ-aminolevulinic acid (ALA)***

a. All the carbon atoms of the porphyrin molecule are provided by ***glycine*** (a nonessential amino acid) and ***succinyl CoA*** (an intermediate in the citric acid cycle). Glycine and succinyl CoA condense to form ALA in a reaction catalyzed by *ALA synthase* (Figure 22.2). This reaction, which requires ***pyridoxal phosphate*** as a cofactor, is the rate-controlling step in porphyrin biosynthesis.

b. The activity of *ALA synthase* is decreased by elevated concentrations of ***hemin,*** which is derived from heme by the oxidation of Fe^{+2} to Fe^{+3}. When porphyrin production exceeds the availability of globin, heme accumulates and is oxidized to hemin. This end-product inhibition causes the decreased synthesis of the enzyme *ALA synthase*.

c. Administration of any of a large number of drugs, such as ***phenobarbital,*** results in a marked increase in hepatic *ALA synthase* activity. These drugs are metabolized by cytochrome P_{450}, a *hemeprotein oxidase* system found in the liver (see p. 146). In response to these drugs the amount of cytochrome P_{450} increases, leading to an enhanced consumption of heme, a component of cytochrome P_{450}. This, in turn, causes a decrease in the concentration of heme in the liver cell. The lower intracellular heme concentration leads to an increase in the synthesis of *ALA synthase* (derepression) and prompts a corresponding increase in ALA synthesis.

3. ***Formation of porphobilinogen:*** The dehydration of two molecules of δ-aminolevulinic acid to form porphobilinogen, catalyzed by *δ-aminolevulinic acid dehydrase,* is extremely sensitive to ***inhibition by heavy metal ions.*** This inhibition is, in part, responsible for both the elevation in ALA and the anemia seen in ***lead poisoning*** (see Figures 22.2 and 22.4).

4. ***Formation of uroporphyrinogen:*** The condensation of four molecules of porphobilinogen results in the formation of uroporphyrinogen III. The reaction requires the participation of two enzymes:

a. *Uroporphyrinogen I synthetase,* which catalyzes the symmetric condensation of four porphobilinogen molecules to form uroporphyrinogen I.

b. A separate protein, *uroporphyrinogen II cosynthetase,* which alters the specificity of *uroporphyrinogen I synthetase* so that the asymmetrical uroporphyrinogen ***III*** is produced (Figure 22.3).

5. ***Formation of heme:*** Uroporphyrinogen III is converted to heme by a series of decarboxylations and oxidations summarized in Figure 22.3. The introduction of Fe^{+2} into protoporphyrin occurs spontaneously, but the rate is enhanced by the enzyme *ferrochelatase.*

C. Porphyrias

1. Porphyrias are a group of inherited or acquired diseases characterized by increased excretion of porphyrins or porphyrin precursors (Figure 22.4).

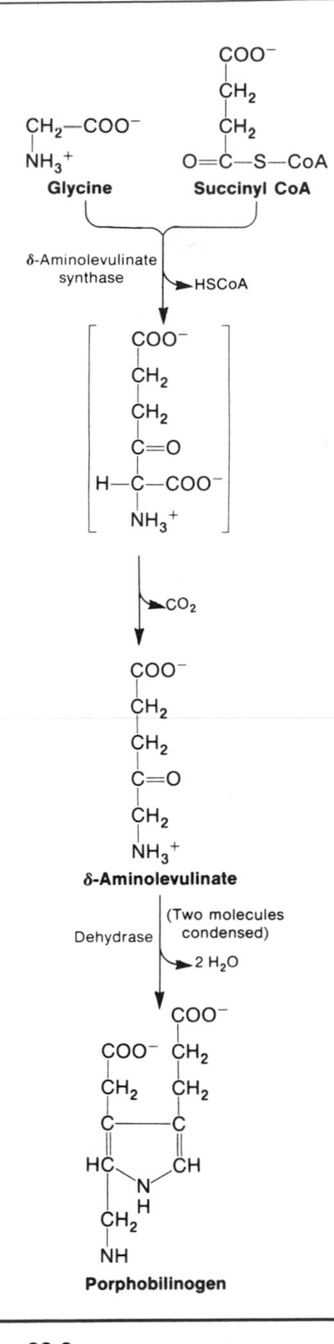

Figure 22.2
Pathway of porphyrin synthesis: formation of porphobilinogen.

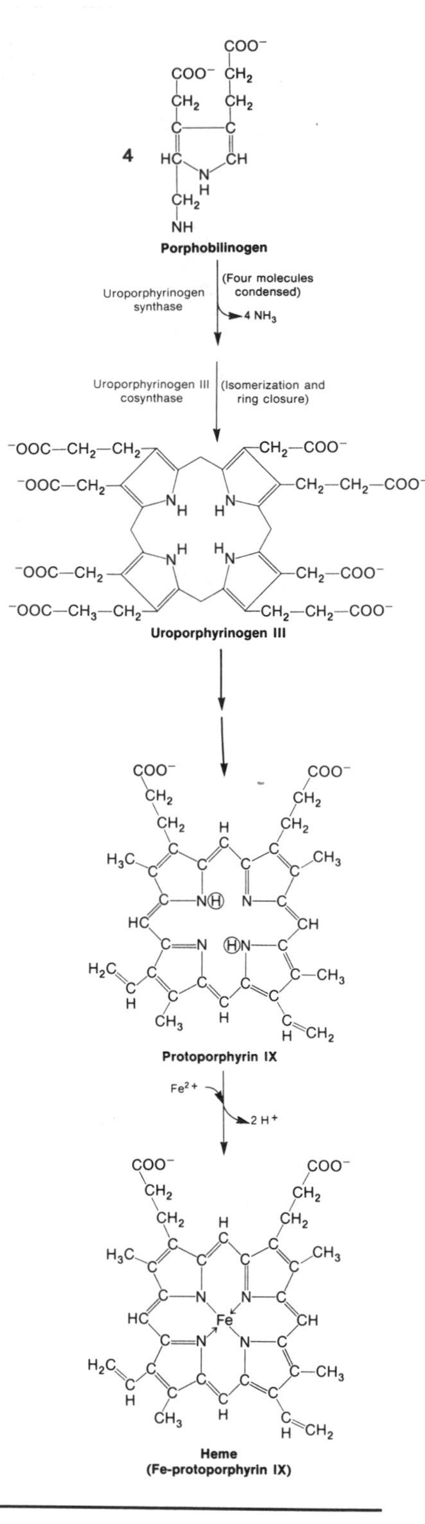

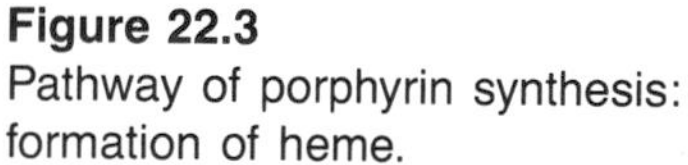
Figure 22.3
Pathway of porphyrin synthesis: formation of heme.

2. ***Cutaneous photosensitivity*** is seen in some porphyrias as a result of the accumulation of porphyrins in the tissues. Exposure of the skin to sunlight results in itching and burning, followed by skin lesions.
3. One of the common features of the porphyrias is a decreased synthesis of heme. Because heme normally functions as an inhibitor of *ALA synthase,* the absence of this end-product causes an increase in *ALA synthase* activity (derepression), which in turn causes an increased synthesis of intermediates that occurs before the genetic block.
4. The severity of symptoms of porphyrias can be diminished by intravenous injection of hemin, which acts to decrease the synthesis of *ALA synthase.*

D. Degradation of heme

1. ***Formation of bilirubin***
   a. Degradation of heme takes place in the reticuloendothelial cells (RE), particularly in the liver and spleen (Figure 22.5).
   b. The first step in the degradation of heme is catalyzed by the microsomal *heme oxygenase* system of the RE cells. In the presence of NADPH, the enzyme adds a hydroxyl group to the methenyl bridge between two pyrrole rings with a concomitant oxidation of ferrous iron (Fe^{+2}) to ferric iron (Fe^{+3}).
   c. A second oxidation by the same enzyme system results in cleavage of the porphyrin ring. Ferric iron and carbon monoxide are released, resulting in the production of the green pigment ***biliverdin*** (Figure 22.6).
   d. Biliverdin is reduced, forming ***bilirubin***. Bilirubin and its derivatives are collectively termed ***bile pigments***.
2. ***Uptake of bilrubin by the liver:*** Bilirubin is sparingly soluble in plasma and therefore is transported to the liver by binding noncovalently to albumin. Bilirubin dissociates from the carrier albumin molecule and enters a hepatocyte.
3. ***Formation of bilirubin diglucuronide:*** The solubility of bilirubin in aqueous solution is increased by the addition of two molecules of ***glucuronic acid,*** using UDP-glucuronic acid as the glucuronide donor.

(text continues on p. 260)

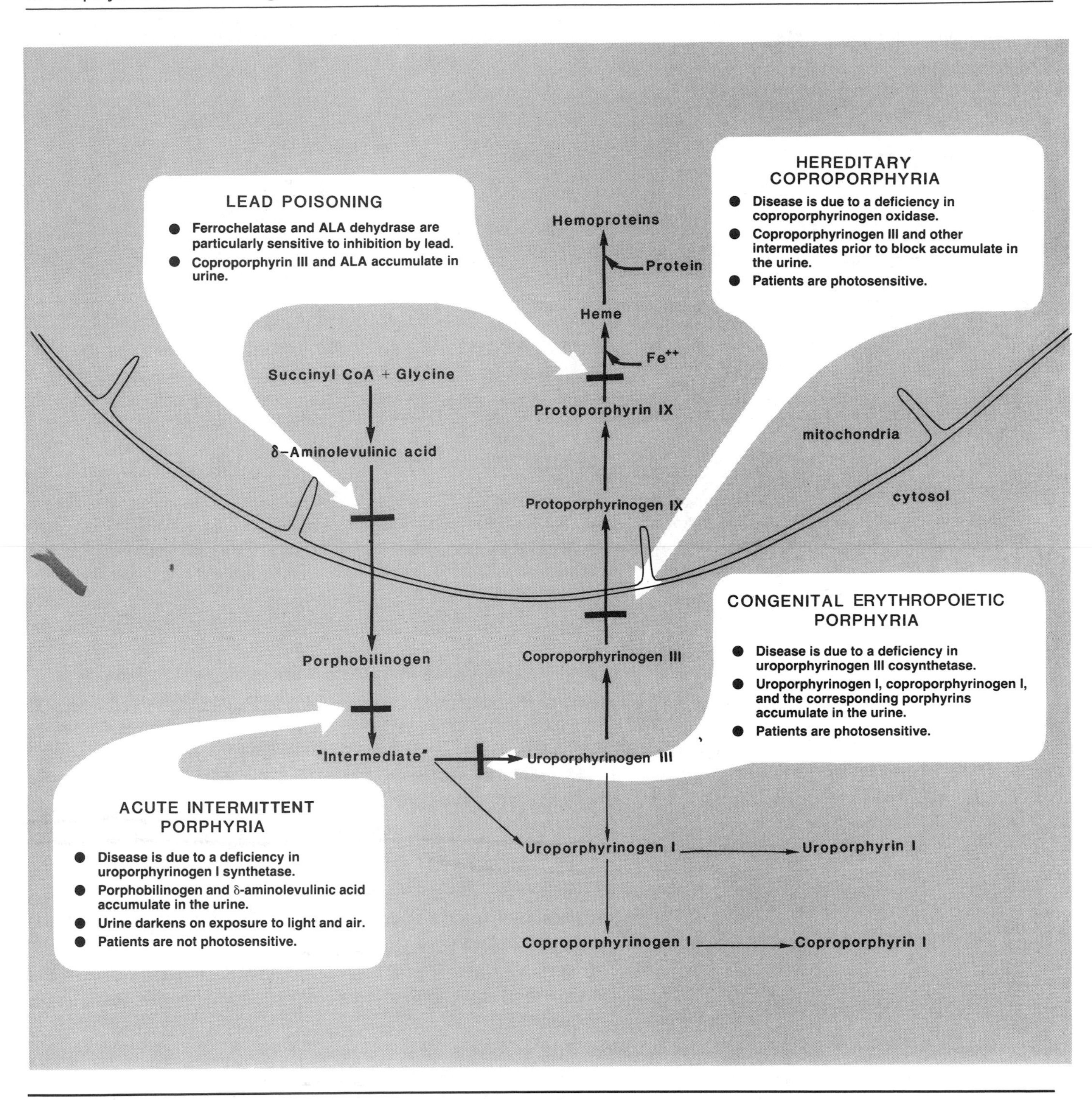

Figure 22.4
Summary of heme synthesis.

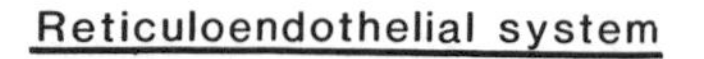

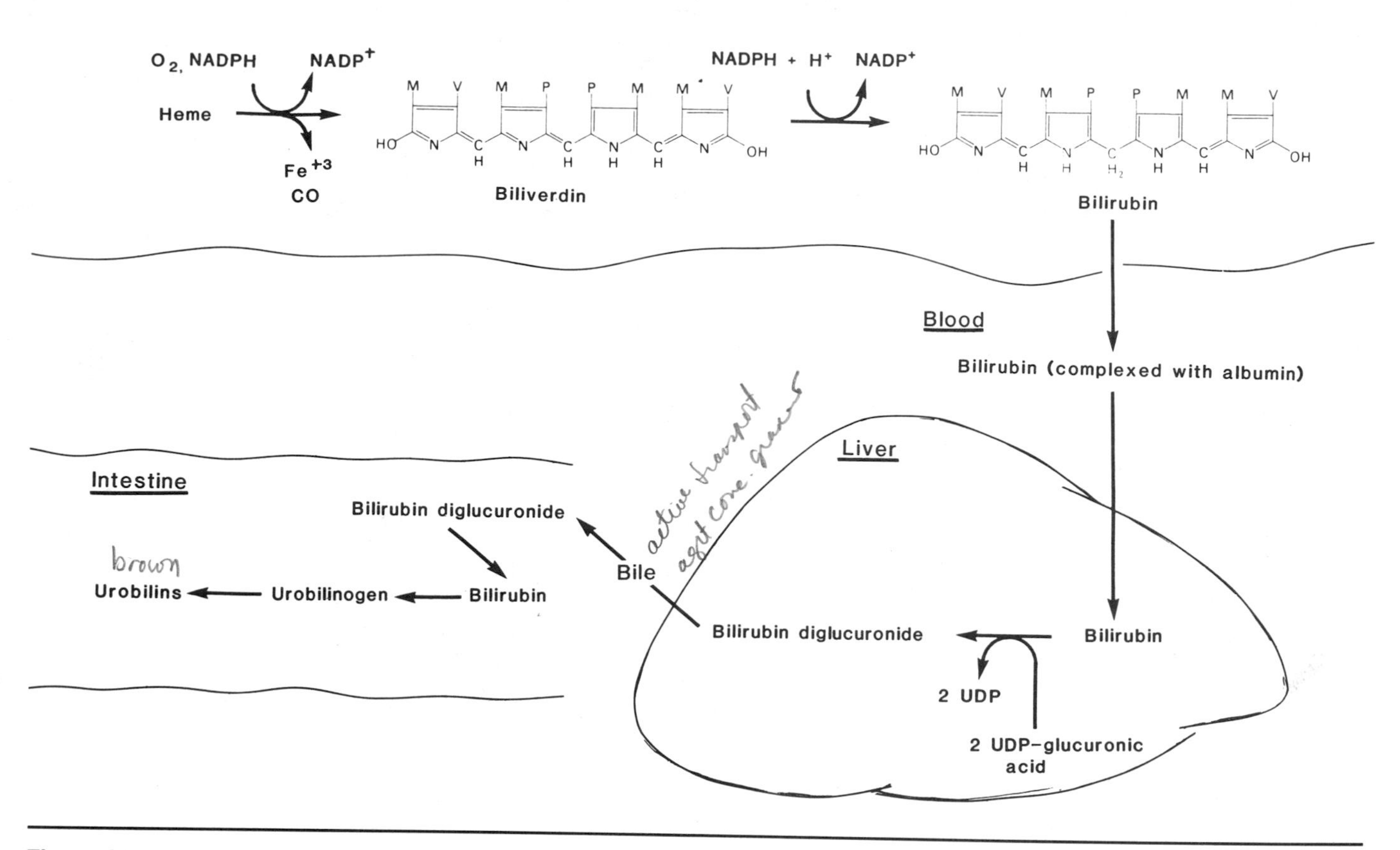

Figure 22.5
Catabolism of heme.

4. ***Secretion of bilirubin into bile:*** Bilirubin diglucuronide is actively transported against a concentration gradient into the bile canaliculi and then into the bile.
5. ***Formation of urobilins in the intestine***
   a. Bilirubin diglucuronide is hydrolyzed and reduced by bacteria in the gut to yield ***urobilinogens.***
   b. A small fraction of the urobilinogens is reabsorbed from the gut and subsequently re-excreted, forming the ***enterohepatic urobilinogen cycle***.
   c. The colorless urobilinogens of the feces are oxidized by intestinal bacteria to the ***urobilins***, the pigments that give stools their characteristic brown color. The metabolism of bilirubin is summarized in Figure 22.5.

III. CREATINE

A. Functions of creatine

1. ***Creatine phosphate,*** the phosphorylated derivative of creatine found in muscle, is a high-energy compound that can reversibly donate a phosphate group to ADP to form ATP (Figure 22.6).

2. The reaction, catalyzed by *creatine phosphokinase*, provides a small but rapidly mobilized reserve of high-energy phosphates that can be used to maintain the intracellular level of ATP during the first few minutes of intense muscular contraction.

B. Synthesis of creatine

1. Creatine is synthesized with carbon and nitrogen from glycine and arginine, plus a methyl group from S-adenosylmethionine (Figure 22.6).
2. Creatine is reversibly phosphorylated to ***phosphocreatine*** by *creatine kinase* using ATP as phosphate donor. Phosphocreatine functions as a store of high-energy phosphate in muscle.

C. Degradation of creatine

1. Creatine and phosphocreatine spontaneously cyclize at a slow but ***constant*** rate to form ***creatinine***, which is excreted in the urine.
2. The amount of creatinine excreted from the body is proportional to the total phosphocreatine content of the body, and thus can be used to estimate muscle mass. When muscle mass decreases for any reason (e.g., from paralysis or muscular dystrophy), the creatinine content of the urine falls. In addition, any rise in blood creatinine is a sensitive indicator of kidney malfunction, since creatinine is normally rapidly removed from the blood and excreted.
3. A typical adult man excretes about 15 mM of creatinine per day. The constancy of this excretion is sometimes used to test the reliability of collected 24-hour urine samples—too little creatinine in the total urine may indicate an incomplete sample.

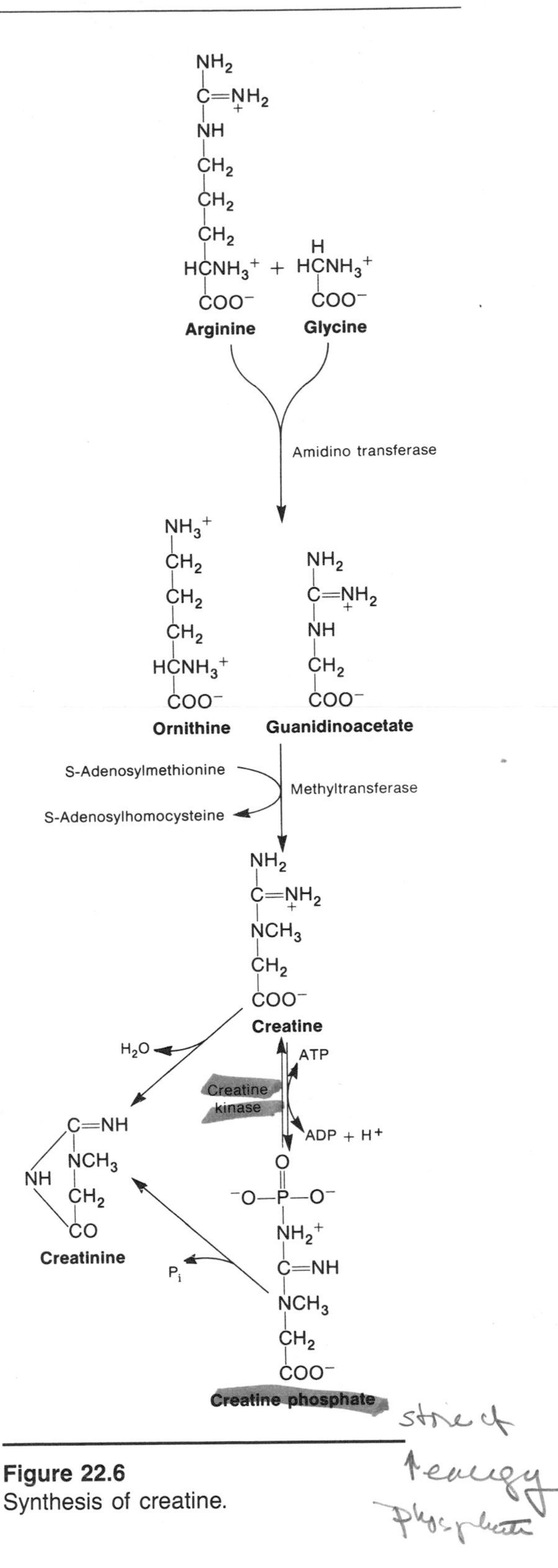

Figure 22.6
Synthesis of creatine.

IV. SYNTHESIS OF HISTAMINE

A. Histamine, a powerful ***vasodilator***, is formed by decarboxylation of histidine. Histamine is secreted by mast cells as a result of allergic reactions or trauma (Figure 22.7).

V. SEROTONIN

A. Functions of serotonin

1. ***Serotonin***, also called ***5-hydroxytryptamine***, is synthesized and stored at several sites in the body. By far the largest amount of serotonin is found in the cells of the intestinal mucosa. Smaller amounts of serotonin occur in platelets and in the central nervous system. Serotonin has multiple physiologic roles, including regulation of blood pressure and respiration. Serotonin also functions as a neurotransmitter in certain parts of the brain.

B. Synthesis of serotonin

1. Tryptophan is hydroxylated in a reaction analogous to that catalyzed by *phenylalanine hydroxylase* (Figure 22.8). The product, 5-hydroxytryptophan, is decarboxylated to serotonin.

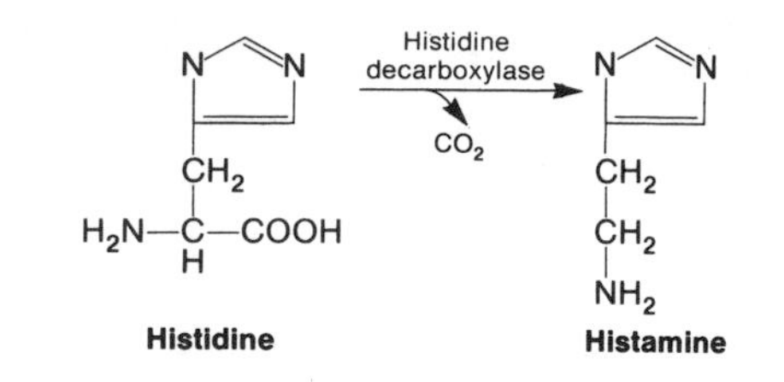

Figure 22.7
Synthesis of histamine.

VI. CATECHOLAMINES

A. Functions of catecholamines

1. ***Dopamine, norepinephrine,*** and ***epinephrine (adrenalin)*** are biologically active amines that collectively are termed ***catecholamines.*** Dopamine and norepinephrine function as a neurotransmitters in the brain. Norepinephrine is also synthesized in the adrenal medulla.
2. Outside the nervous system, norepinephrine and its methylated derivative epinephrine act as regulators of metabolism. Norepinephrine and epinephrine are released from storage vessels in the adrenal gland in response to fright, exercise, cold, and low levels of blood glucose. As outlined on p. 269, norepinephrine and epinephrine increase the degradation of triacylglycerol and glycogen as well as increase the output of the heart and blood pressure. These effects of the catecholamines are part of a coordinated response to prepare the individual for emergencies and are often called the "fight or flight" reactions.

B. Synthesis of catecholamines

1. The catecholamines are synthesized from tyrosine by the reactions shown in Figure 22.9. Tyrosine is first hydroxylated to form 3,4-dihydroxyphenylalanine ***(dopa)*** in a reaction analogous to that described for the hydroxylation of phenylalanine. This reaction is the rate-limiting step of the pathway; the enzyme is abundant in the central nervous system, the sympathetic ganglia, and the adrenal gland.
2. Dopa is decarboxylated to form ***dopamine,*** which is hydroxylated by a copper-containing *hydroxylase* to yield norepinephrine. Epinephrine is formed from norepinephrine by an N-methylation reaction using S-adenosylmethionine as methyl donor.

C. Degradation of catecholamines

1. The catecholamines are inactivated by oxidative deamination, catalyzed by *monoamine oxidase* (MAO) and by O-methylation carried out by *catechol-O-methyltransferase* (COMT). The two reactions can occur in either order. The aldehyde products of the MAO reaction are oxidized to the corresponding acids.

VII. MELANIN

A. Functions of melanin

1. Melanin is a ***pigment*** that occurs in a number of tissues in the

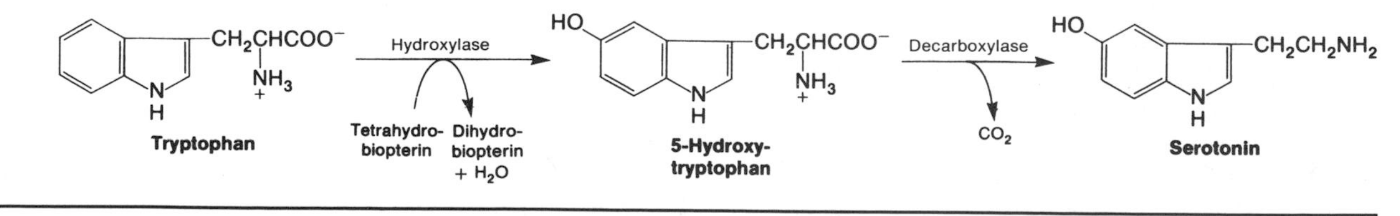

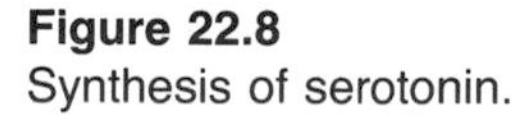

Figure 22.8
Synthesis of serotonin.

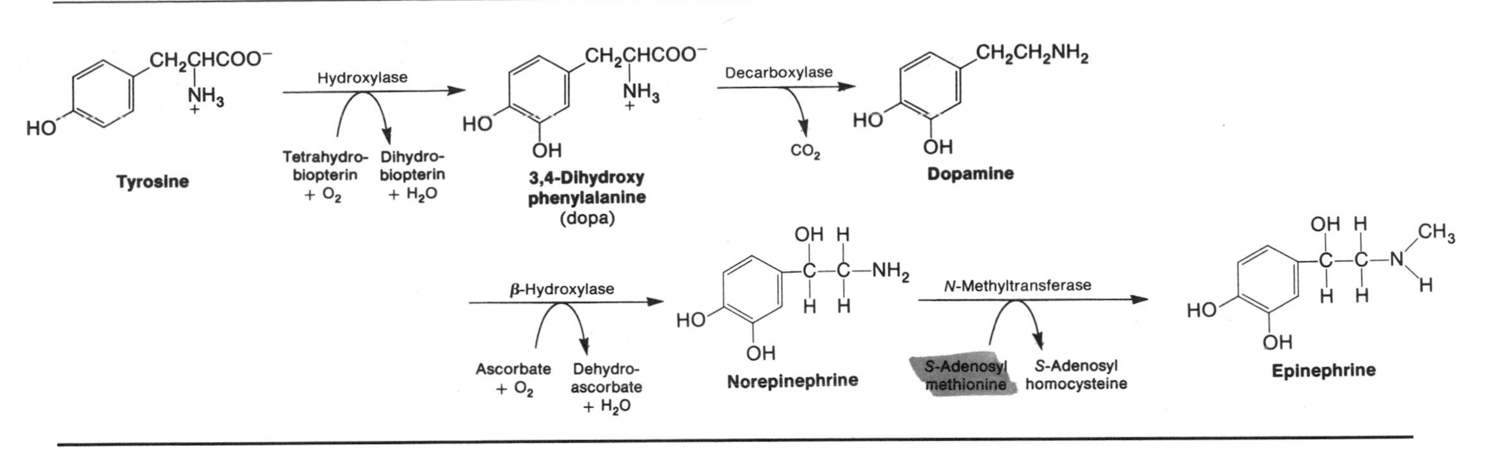

Figure 22.9
Synthesis of catecholamines.

body, particularly in the eye, hair, and skin. In the epidermis, the pigment-forming cells are called ***melanocytes***. Here melanin is synthesized to protect underlying cells from the harmful effects of sunlight.

B. Synthesis of melanin

1. The first step in melanin formation from tyrosine is a hydroxylation to form dopa, catalyzed by the copper-containing enzyme, *tyrosinase*. Subsequent reactions leading to the formation of brown and black pigments are thought to be catalyzed by *tyrosinase* or to be nonenzymic.

VIII. THYROID HORMONES

A. Functions of thyroid hormones

1. ***Thyroxine*** (T_4) and ***triiodothyronine*** (T_3), the two major hormones produced by the thyroid gland, increase heat production and oxygen consumption in most tissues, with the exception of brain, testis, and spleen. In addition, the thyroid hormones produce a variety of metabolic changes. Thyroid hormones, although not essential for life, act in conjunction with growth hormone as the major anabolic agents during growth; a thyroid deficiency during the prenatal period results in abnormal physical and mental development, a syndrome called ***cretinism***.
2. The synthesis and release of T_3 and T_4 are stimulated by **thyroid stimulating hormone** (TSH), released from the pituitary gland (see Figure 23.8, p. 272).

B. Synthesis of thyroid hormones

1. The thyroid contains many follicles, each composed of a single-layered shell of cells surrounding a central space filled with a glycoprotein, called ***thyroglobulin*** (TG).
2. Unlike other tissues, the thyroid cells can trap and oxidize iodide ions, I^-, forming iodine that is incorporated into the tyrosine residues of TG. The resulting monoiodo-tyrosine and diiodoty-

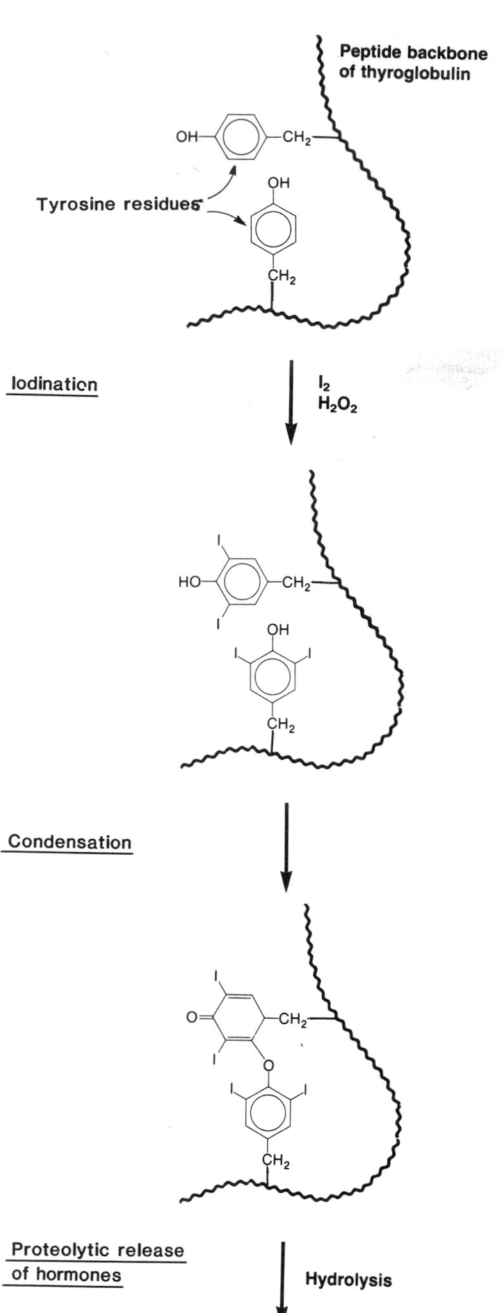

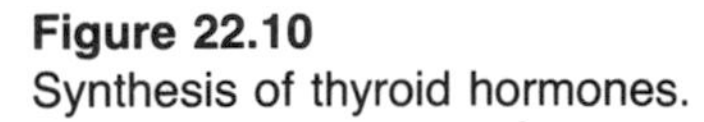

Figure 22.10
Synthesis of thyroid hormones.

rosine residues are coupled to yield either T_3 or T_4 residues, both of which are still part of the TG molecule (Figure 22.10).

3. Enzymic hydrolysis of thyroglobulin releases T_3 and T_4.

Study Questions

Answer A if 1, 2, and 3 are correct
B if 1 and 3 are correct
C if 2 and 4 are correct
D if only 4 is correct
E if all are correct

22.1 Which of the following is(are) heme proteins?

1. Catalase
2. Hemoglobin
3. Cytochrome oxidase
4. Myoglobin

22.2 δ-Aminolevulinic acid synthase activity

1. is frequently increased in individuals treated with drugs, such as the barbiturate phenobarbital.
2. catalyzes a rate-limiting reaction in porphyrin biosynthesis.
3. requires the cofactor pyridoxal phosphate.
4. is strongly inhibited by heavy metal ions such as lead.

22.3 The catabolism of heme

1. occurs in the cells of the reticuloendothelial system.
2. involves the oxidative cleavage of the porphyrin ring.
3. results in the liberation of carbon monoxide.
4. results in the formation of protoporphrinogen.

22.4 In intermittent acute porphyria,

1. the severity of the symptoms can be diminished by intravenous injection of hemin.
2. the disease is associated with decreased activity of ALA synthetase.
3. skin photosensitivity does not occur.
4. protoporphyrin accumulates in the liver and in the blood.

Choose the ONE best answer:

22.5 The normal brown-red color of feces results from the presence of

A. stercobilinogen.
B. urobilin.
C. bilirubin diglucuronide.
D. coproporphyrin III.
E. biliverdin.

22.6 Which one of the following is a direct precursor for the carbon atoms of the heme portion of hemoglobin?

A. Alanine
B. ALA
C. Aspartate
D. Succinyl CoA
E. Carbon monoxide

Metabolic Effects of Insulin and Glucagon

23

I. OVERVIEW

Individual tissues do not function in isolation, but rather are part of a community in which one tissue may provide substrates to another, or process compounds produced by other organs. Communication between tissues is mediated by the nervous system, by the availability of circulating substrates, and by variation in the levels of plasma hormones (Figure 23.1). Hormones act as chemical messengers that can trigger a response in the target tissue(s). Some hormones have very focused actions, affecting only one tissue. Other hormones may have a wide range of effects on many organs. For example, the steroid hormone aldosterone almost exclusively affects ion exchange in the kidney. In contrast, insulin and glucagon, which are hormones secreted by the pancreas, are pivotal in the integration of energy metabolism. Changes in the circulating levels of these hormones allow the body to store energy when food is available in abundance or to make stored energy available, for example, during "survival crises," such as famine, severe injury, and "fight or flight" situations. This chapter describes the structure, secretion, and metabolic effects of the major hormones secreted in humans.

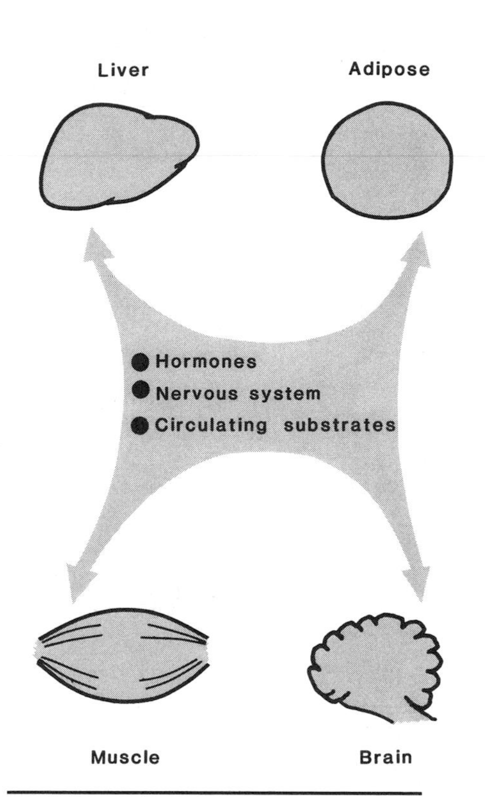

Figure 23.1
Mechanism of communication between four major tissues.

II. INSULIN

Insulin is a polypeptide hormone produced by the β-cells of the islets of Langerhans, clusters of cells that comprise about 1% of the pancreas. Insulin is one of the most important hormones coordinating the use of fuels by tissues. Its metabolic effects are ***anabolic,*** favoring, for example, synthesis of glycogen, triacylglycerol, and protein.

A. Structure of insulin

1. Insulin is composed of 51 amino acids arranged in two polypeptide chains, designated A and B, which are linked together by two disulfide bridges (Figure 23.2). The insulin molecule also contains an ***intra***molecular disulfide bridge between amino acid residues 6 and 11 of the A chain.
2. Human insulin, prepared by recombinant DNA techniques, is now commercially available. Human insulin has the same potency as pig insulin, which is similar in structure to the human hormone and has been used for treatment of diabetics (see p. 294). It is hoped that human insulin will show less long-term tendency to induce the unwanted immune response that can be caused by the use of nonhuman insulin.

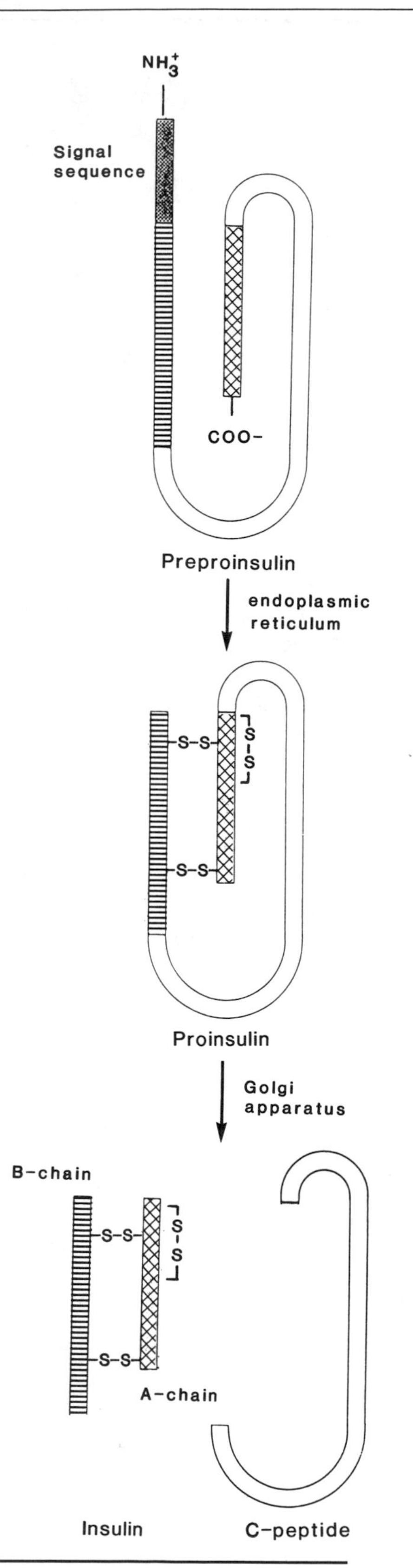

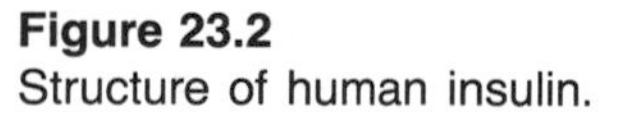

Figure 23.2
Structure of human insulin.

B. Biosynthesis of insulin

The processing and the movement of intermediates that occur during the synthesis of insulin is shown in Figure 23.3. Note that the biosynthesis involves two inactive precursors, ***preproinsulin*** and ***proinsulin,*** which are sequentially cleaved to form the active hormone. Insulin is stored in the cytoplasm in granules that, given the proper stimulus (see below), are released by exocytosis (see p. 383 for a discussion of the synthesis of proteins destined for secretion).

C. Regulation of insulin secretion

1. ***Stimulation of insulin secretion:*** Insulin secretion by the β-cells of the islets of Langerhans of the pancreas is closely coordinated with the release of glucagon by the pancreatic α-cells (see p. 269). The relative amounts of insulin and glucagon released by the pancreas are regulated so that the rate of hepatic glucose production is kept equal to the use of glucose by the peripheral tissues. In view of its coordinating role, it is not surprising that the β-cell responds to a variety of stimuli. In particular, insulin secretion is ***increased*** by

   a. ***Glucose:*** The β-cells are the most important glucose-sensing cells in the body. Ingestion of glucose or a carbohydrate-rich meal leads to a rise in blood glucose, which is a signal for increased insulin secretion (as well as decreased glucagon release; Figure 23.4).

   b. ***Amino acids:*** Ingestion of protein causes a transient rise in plasma amino acids levels, which in turn induces the immediate secretion of insulin.

   c. ***Gastrointestinal hormones:*** The gastric peptide ***secretin,*** as well as other gastrointestinal hormones, stimulates insulin secretion. These hormones are released after the ingestion of food. They cause an anticipatory rise in insulin levels in the portal vein before there is an actual rise in blood glucose. This may account for the fact that the same amount of glucose given orally induces a much greater secretion of insulin than if given intravenously.

2. ***Inhibition of insulin secretion:*** The synthesis and the release of insulin are ***decreased*** when there is a scarcity of dietary fuels and also during periods of trauma. These effects are mediated primarily by

   a. ***Epinephrine:*** This hormone is secreted in response to stress, trauma, or extreme exercise. Under these conditions, the release of epinephrine is controlled largely by the nervous system. Epinephrine has a direct effect on energy metabolism, causing a rapid mobilization of energy-yielding fuels, including glucose from the liver (see p. 74) and fatty acids from adipose tissue (see p. 170). In addition, epinephrine can override the normal glucose-stimulated release of insulin. Thus, in emergency situations, the sympathetic nervous system largely replaces plasma glucose concentration as the controlling influence over β-cell secretion. The regulation of insulin secretion is summarized in Figure 23.5.

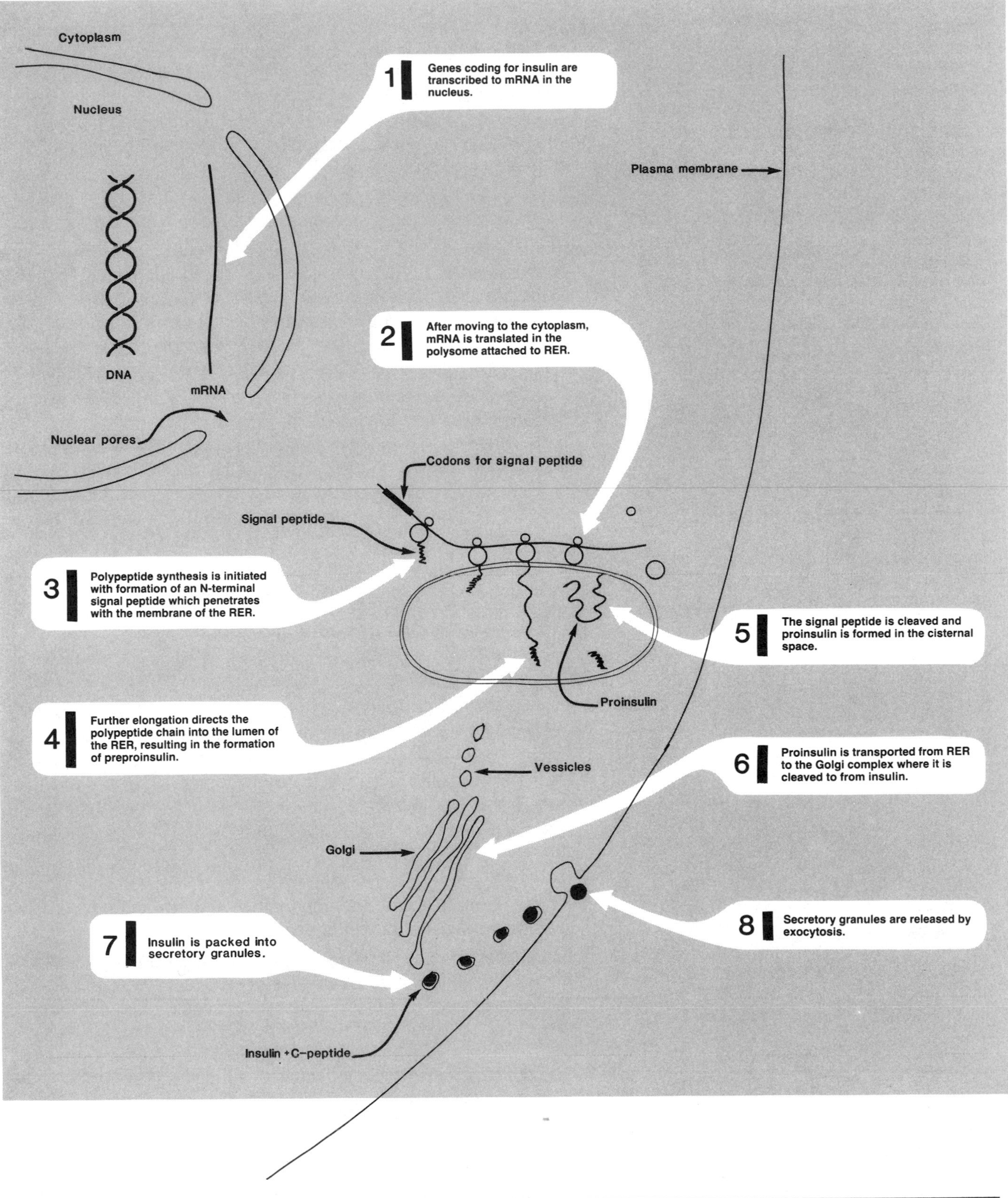

Figure 23.3
Intracellular movements of insulin and its precursors.

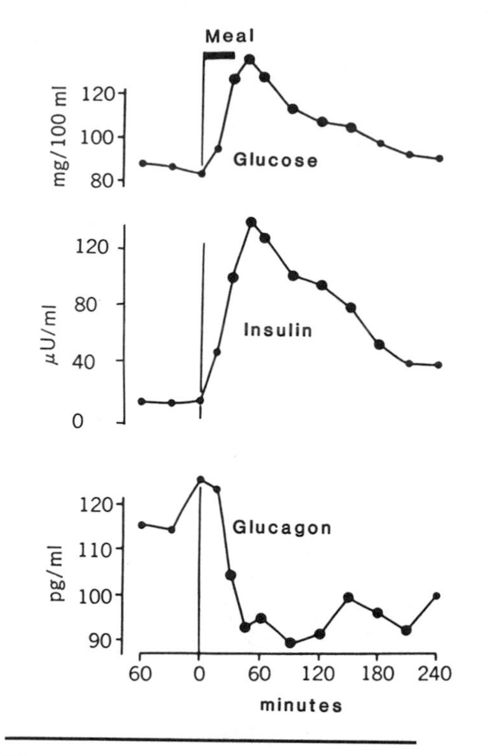

Figure 23.4
Changes in blood levels of glucose, insulin, and glucagon after ingestion of a carbohydrate-rich meal.

D. Metabolic effects of insulin

1. ***Effects on carbohydrate metabolism:*** The intravenous administration of insulin causes an immediate decrease in the concentration of blood glucose. This decrease is caused by increased glucose transport into cells (except for liver, brain, lens, intestinal mucosa, renal tubes, and the red blood cell in which glucose transport is ***not*** sensitive to insulin), increased glycogen synthesis, and decreased gluconeogenesis.
2. ***Effects on lipid metabolism:*** Adipose tissue responds within minutes to the administration of insulin, which causes a marked reduction in the release of fatty acids by the following processes:
   a. ***Decrease in triacylglycerol degradation:*** Insulin decreases the level of circulating fatty acids by inhibiting the activity of *hormone-sensitive lipase* in adipose tissue. Insulin acts primarily by countering the stimulation of *adenyl cyclase* by epinephrine and glucagon. This action reduces the intracellular levels of cAMP and leads to a diminished production of active *protein kinase* (see p. 170).
   b. ***Increased triacylglycerol synthesis:*** Insulin increases the transport and metabolism of glucose, providing the substrates (acetyl CoA, glycerol 3-phosphate) and the NADPH needed for fatty acid synthesis. These actions result in the increased availability of fatty acids for triacylglycerol synthesis (see p. 167).
3. ***Effects on protein synthesis:*** Insulin stimulates the entry of amino acids into cells and protein synthesis in most tissues.

E. Mechanism of insulin action

1. ***Insulin receptors:*** Like other peptide hormones, insulin binds to specific, high-affinity receptors in the cell membrane of most tissues, including liver, muscle, and adipose. This is the first step in a cascade of reactions, ultimately leading to a diverse array of biological actions. After binding to the cell surface, the insulin receptor complex enters the cell by pinocytosis, producing a membrane-bound vesicle. The insulin is ultimately degraded in the lysosomes and the receptor is recycled back to the membrane.
2. ***Membrane effects of insulin:*** Insulin, once bound to the receptor, causes an increase in the transport of glucose and amino acids across the plasma membrane.
3. ***Intracellular effects of insulin:*** The binding of insulin to its receptor triggers a series of reactions that lead to the activation or inhibition of key enzymes in the cell. These intracellular effects of insulin are probably mediated by a compound or compounds that act as a signal within the cell. The chemical nature of this molecule (sometimes called the "second messenger") is currently under active investigation.

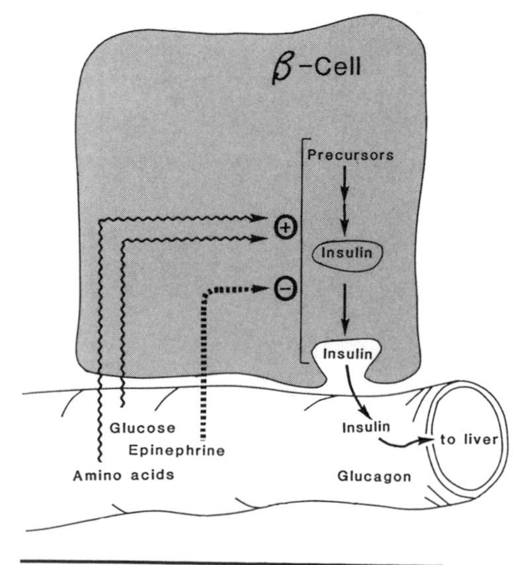

Figure 23.5
Regulation of insulin and glucagon release from pancreatic cells.

III. GLUCAGON

Glucagon is a polypeptide hormone secreted primarily by the α-cells of the pancreatic islets. Glucagon, along with epinephrine, cortisol, and growth hormone (the "counterregulatory hormones"), opposes many of the actions of insulin (see p. 268). Most importantly, glucagon acts to maintain blood glucose levels by activation of hepatic glycogenolysis and gluconeogenesis.

A. Structure of glucagon

1. Glucagon is composed of 29 amino acids arranged in a single polypeptide chain. Unlike insulin, the amino acid sequence of glucagon is the same in all mammalian species examined to date.

B. Biosynthesis of glucagon

1. Glucagon is synthesized as a larger precursor molecule that is converted to glucagon through a series of selective proteolytic cleavages, similar to those described for insulin biosynthesis (see Figure 23.3).

C. Regulation of glucagon secretion

1. ***Stimulation of glucagon secretion:*** The α-cell is responsive to a variety of stimuli that signal actual or potential hypoglycemia (Figure 23.6). Specifically, glucagon secretion is increased by
   a. ***Low blood glucose:*** A decrease in plasma glucose concentration is the primary stimulus for glucagon release. During an overnight or prolonged fast, elevated glucagon levels prevent hypoglycemia.
   b. ***Amino acids:*** Amino acids derived from a protein-containing meal stimulate the release of both glucagon and insulin. The glucagon effectively prevents hypoglycemia that would otherwise occur as a result of increased insulin secretion that occurs after a protein meal.
   c. ***Epinephrine:*** Elevated levels of circulating epinephrine produced by the adrenal medulla, or epinephrine produced by direct innervation of the pancreas, or both, stimulate the release of glucagon. Thus during periods of stress, trauma, or severe exercise, the elevated epinephrine levels can override the effect on the α-cell of circulating substrates. In these situations—regardless of the concentration of blood glucose—glucagon levels are elevated in anticipation of increased glucose use. In contrast, insulin levels are depressed.
2. ***Inhibition of glucagon secretion:*** Glucagon secretion is markedly decreased by elevated blood sugar. This occurs after ingestion of glucose or a carbohydrate-rich meal (see Figures 23.4 and 23.6).

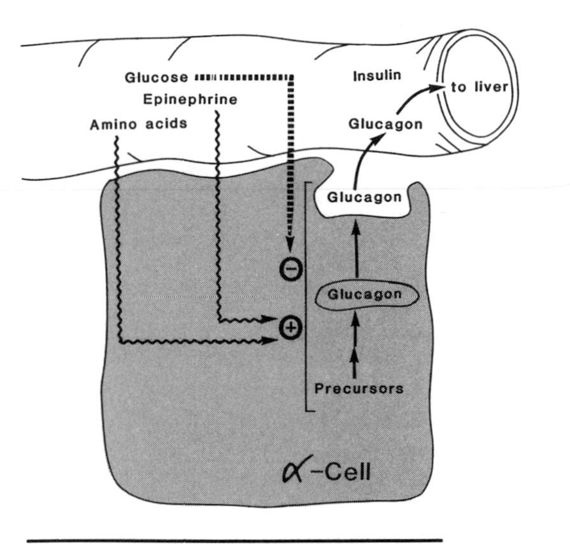

Figure 23.6
Regulation of glucagon and insulin release.

D. Metabolic effects of glucagon

1. ***Effects on carbohydrate metabolism:*** The intravenous administration of glucagon leads to an immediate rise in blood sugar, which results from an increase in the breakdown of liver (not muscle) glycogen (see p. 74) and an increase in gluconeogenesis (see p. 129).
2. ***Effects on lipid metabolism:*** Glucagon favors the hepatic oxidation of fatty acids and the subsequent formation of ketones from acetyl CoA. Glucagon also stimulates *hormone-sensitive lipase* of adipose tissue.

3. ***Effects on protein metabolism:*** Glucagon increases the uptake of amino acids by the liver, resulting in the increased availability of carbon skeletons for gluconeogenesis. As a consequence, plasma levels of amino acids are decreased.

E. Mechanism of action of glucagon

1. Glucagon binds to high-affinity receptors on the cell membrane of target cells such as the hepatocyte or adipocyte. The receptors for glucagon are distinct from those that bind insulin or epinephrine.
2. Glucagon binding results in activation of *adenyl cyclase* in the plasma membrane. This causes a rise in cAMP (the second messenger) which in turn activates *protein kinase* and increases the phosphorylation of specific enzymes. This cascade of increasing enzymatic activities results in the phosphorylation-mediated activation or inhibition of key regulatory enzymes involved in carbohydrate and lipid metabolism. An example of such a cascade is presented for the case of glycogen degradation on p. 74 and Figure 7.7.

F. Prevention of hypoglycemia

1. ***Glucoregulatory systems:*** Humans have two, overlapping glucose regulating systems that are activated by hypoglycemia (low levels of blood sugar): (1) the islets of Langerhans, which release glucagon, and (2) receptors in the hypothalamus, which respond to abnormally low concentrations of blood glucose. The hypothalamic glucoreceptors can trigger the secretion of epinephrine (mediated by the autonomic nervous system) and induce release of ACTH and growth hormone (GH) by the pituitary (Figure 23.7).
2. ***Counter-regulatory hormones:*** Hypoglycemia in normal individuals causes a secretion of four hormones: glucagon, epinephrine, cortisol, and GH (Figure 23.7). These are sometimes called the "counter-regulatory" hormones because each opposes the action of insulin on glucose use. Of these counter-regulatory hormones, glucagon and epinephrine are most important in the acute, short-term regulation of blood glucose levels. Epinephrine inhibits insulin secretion, promotes lipolysis, and inhibits the insulin-mediated uptake of glucose by peripheral tissues. Cortisol and growth hormone are less important in the short-term maintenance of blood glucose concentrations; rather, these hormones play a role in the long-term management of glucose metabolism (Figure 23.7).

IV. OTHER HORMONES

A. Hypothalamic hormones

1. ***Releasing hormones:*** The ***hypothalamus,*** located at the base of the brain just above the pituitary gland, is the control center for many of the regulatory functions of the autonomic nervous system. Specialized hypothalamic neurons respond to stimulation by secreting polypeptide hormones into a network of capillaries that descend into the ***anterior pituitary*** (Figure 23.8). These hormones either promote the release of anterior pituitary hormones (thyrotropin, gonadotropin, corticotropin, growth hor-

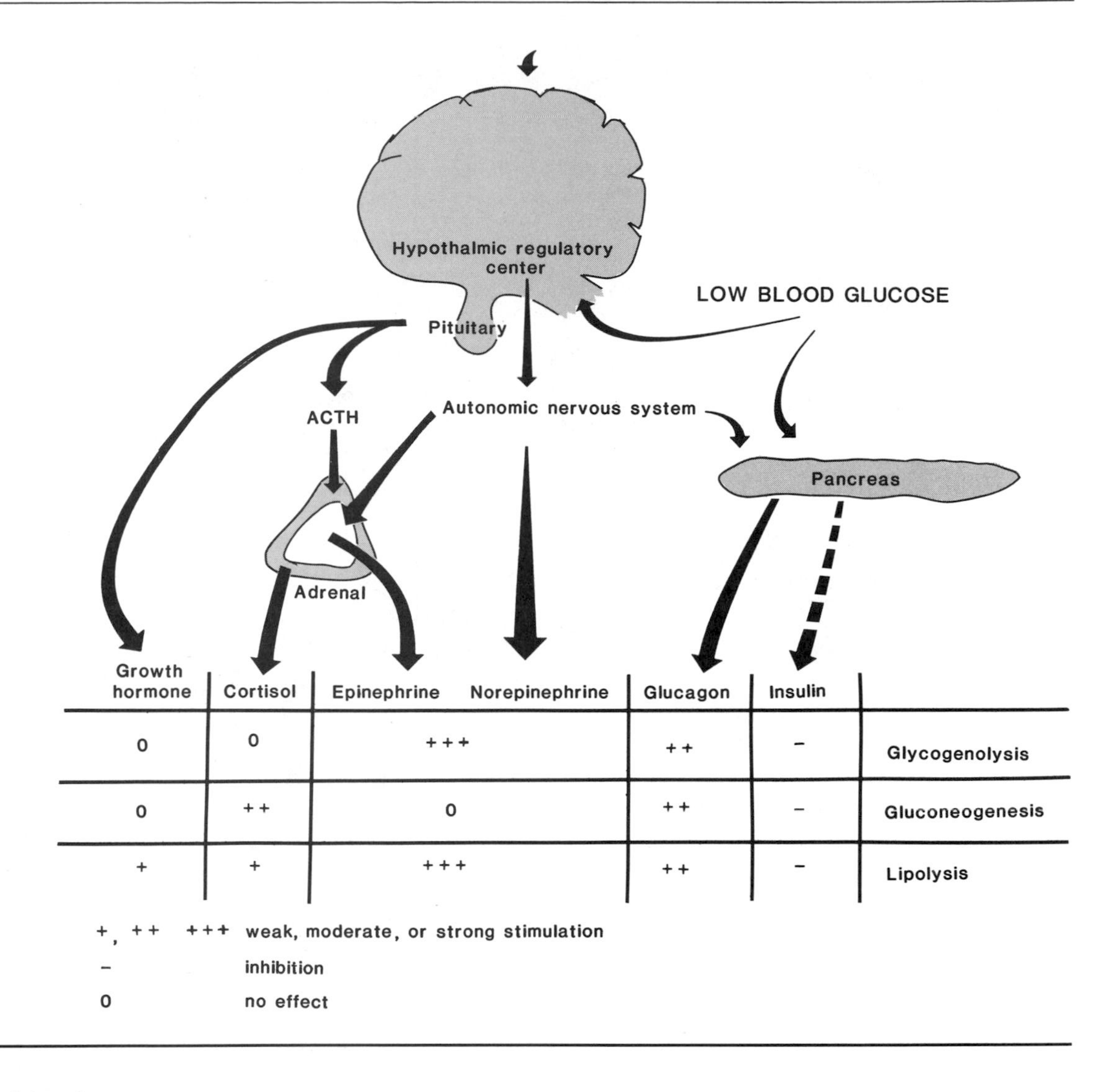

Growth hormone	Cortisol	Epinephrine Norepinephrine	Glucagon	Insulin	
0	0	+++	++	–	Glycogenolysis
0	++	0	++	–	Gluconeogenesis
+	+	+++	++	–	Lipolysis

Figure 23.7
Actions of the glucoregulatory hormones.

mone, prolactin) or inhibit the secretion of pituitary hormones (somatostatin or prolactin).

2. ***Vasopressin and oxytocin:*** Precursors of these hormones are synthesized in specialized neurons in the hypothalamus and incorporated into neurosecretory vesicles that travel from the hypothalamus through axons that terminate in the posterior lobe of the pituitary. Before secretion the larger precursor molecules are cleaved to yield the peptide hormones vasopressin (also called antidiuretic hormone) or oxytocin. The actions of these hormones are summarized in Figure 23.8.

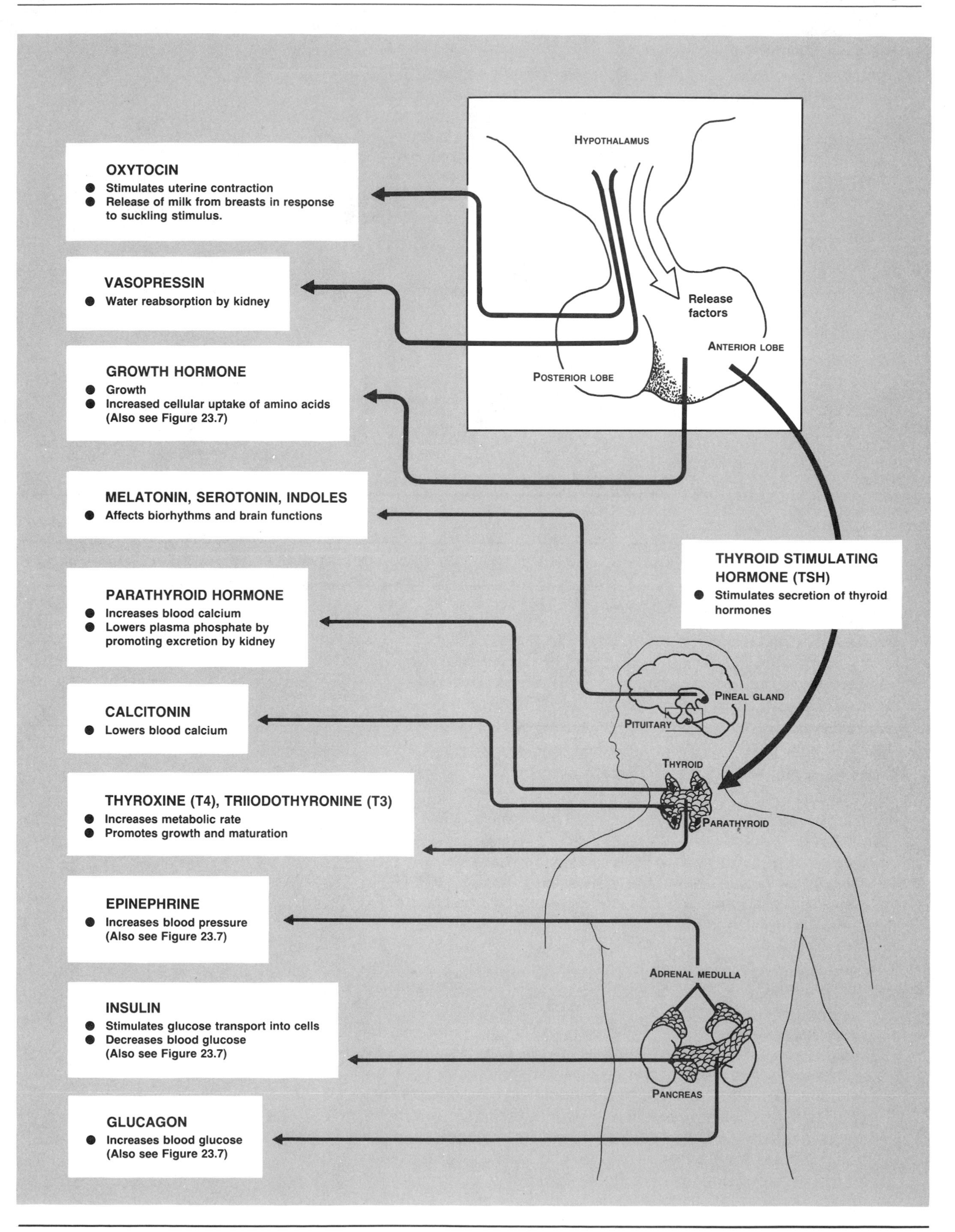

Figure 23.8
Major hormones secreted in the human.

B. Pituitary hormones

The ***anterior pituitary,*** in response to elevated levels of hypothalamic releasing hormones, secretes ***trophic hormones,*** which in turn stimulate the production of additional hormones by other endocrine glands, such as the adrenal, testes, ovary, or the thyroid (Figures 19.19 and 23.8). See the following pages for further discussion of these hormones:

Luteinizing hormone (LH)	p. 222
Follicle-stimulating hormone (FSH)	p. 222
Adrenocorticotropin (ACTH)	pp. 219-222, 270
Thyroid-stimulating hormone (TSH)	p. 263
Growth hormone (GH)	pp. 268, 270

A summary of nonsteroidal hormone secretion in humans is shown in Figure 23.8.

Study questions

Choose the ONE best answer:

23.1 In which of the following tissues is glucose transport into the cell enhanced by insulin?

A. Brain
B. Lens
C. Red blood cell
D. Adipose tissue
E. Nerve

23.2 Insulin does all of the following EXCEPT

A. enhance glucose transport into muscle.
B. enhance glycogen formation by liver.
C. decrease lipolysis in adipose tissue.
D. enhance gluconeogenesis in liver.
E. enhance amino acid transport into muscle.

23.3 Which one of the following statements about glucagon is INCORRECT?

A. High levels of blood glucose decrease the release of glucagon from the α-cells of the pancreas.
B. Glucagon levels increase after ingestion of a protein-rich meal.
C. Glucagon increases the intracellular levels of cAMP in liver cells, causing an increase in glycogen breakdown.
D. Glucagon and insulin are produced by the β-cells of the islets of Langerhans in the pancreas.
E. Glucagon stimulates the formation of ketone bodies by the liver.

23.4 Insulin causes the deposition of triacylglycerols in adipose tissue because it

A. inhibits glycolysis in adipose tissue.
B. increases the concentration of blood glucose
C. stimulates gluconeogenesis, providing glucose that can serve as a precursor for triacylglycerol synthesis.
D. inhibits the activation of the hormone-sensitive lipase in adipose tissue.
E. stimulates the uptake of glycerol by adipose tissue.

The Well-fed or Absorptive State

24

I. OVERVIEW

The absorptive state is the 2- to 4-hour period after ingestion of a normal meal. During this interval there occurs a transient increase in plasma glucose, amino acids, and triacylglycerol, the last found primarily as components of chylomicra synthesized by the intestinal mucosal cells (see p. 208). Islet tissue of the pancreas responds to the elevated levels of glucose and amino acids with an increased secretion of insulin and a drop in the release of glucagon (Figure 24.1). The elevated insulin:glucagon ratio and the ready availability of circulating substrates make the 2 to 4 hours after ingestion of a meal into an ***anabolic period*** characterized by increased synthesis of triacylglycerol, glycogen, and protein. During this absorptive period virtually all tissues use glucose as a fuel.

During the absorptive period the metabolic response of the body is dominated by alterations in the metabolism of four major tissues: liver, adipose, muscle, and brain. In this chapter, the roles these tissues play in the metabolism of dietary nutrients will be discussed.

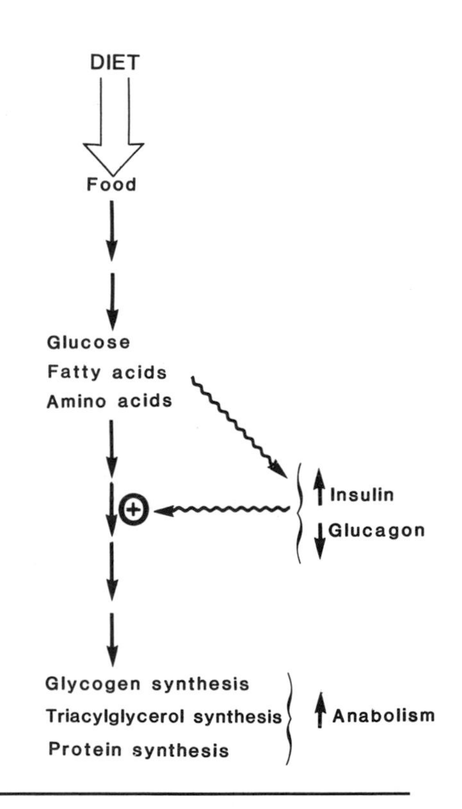

Figure 24.1
Metabolic responses during the absorptive period.

II. LIVER: THE NUTRIENT DISTRIBUTION CENTER

The liver is uniquely situated to process and distribute nutrients because the venous drainage of the gut and pancreas first passes through the hepatic portal vein before entry into the general circulation. Thus the liver is bathed in blood containing nutrients from the diet and elevated levels of insulin secreted by the pancreas. During the absorptive period the liver takes up carbohydrates, lipids, and most amino acids. These nutrients are then metabolized, stored, or routed to other tissues. Thus the liver smooths out potentially broad fluctuations in the availability of nutrients for the peripheral tissues.

A. Carbohydrate metabolism

Liver is normally a glucose-producing rather than a glucose-using tissue. However, after a meal containing carbohydrate, the liver becomes a net consumer of glucose, retaining roughly 60 of every 100 g of glucose presented by the portal system. This increased use of glucose is not a result of stimulated glucose transport into the hepatocyte because this process is normally rapid and not influenced by insulin. Rather, hepatic metabolism of glucose is

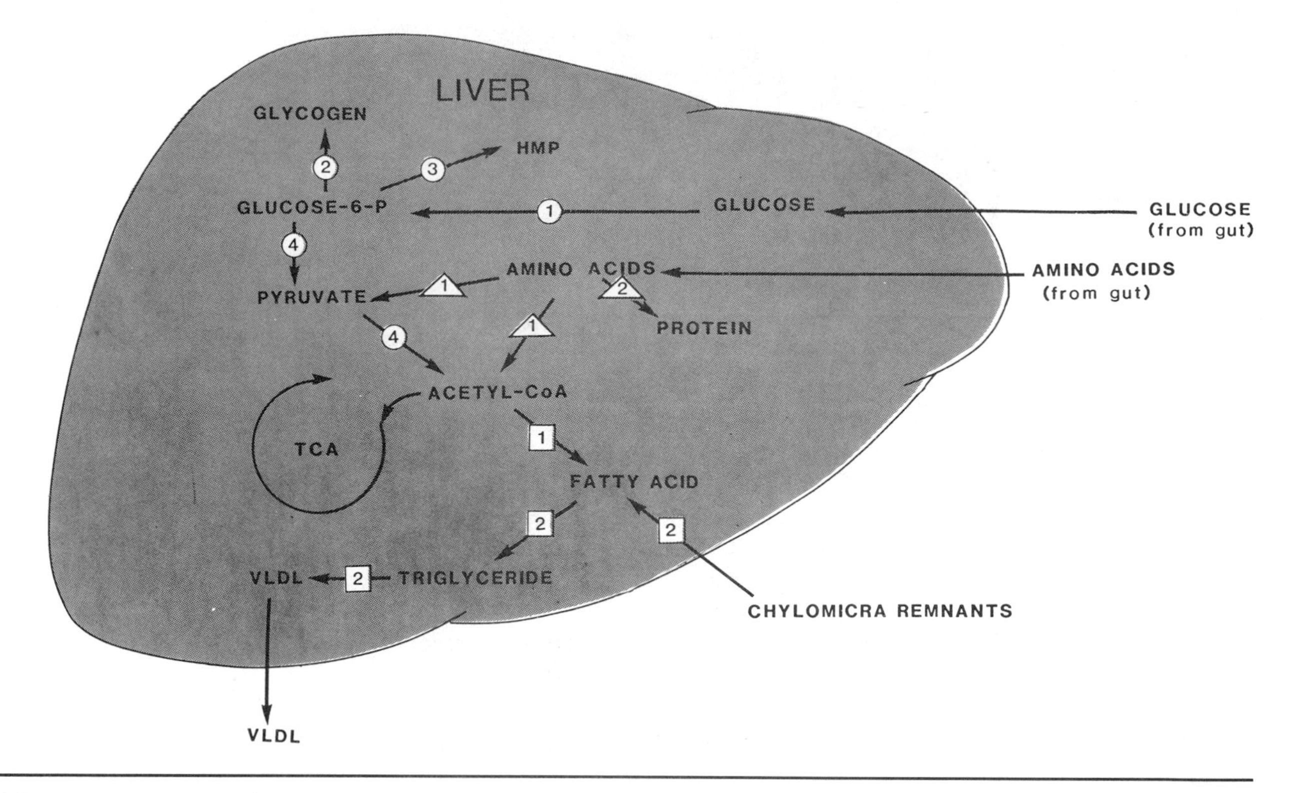

Figure 24.2
Major metabolic pathways in liver in the absorptive state. The numbers in circles, squares, or triangles that appear both on the figure and in the text indicate important pathways for carbohydrate, fat, or protein respectively.

increased by the following mechanisms: (Note: the numbers in circles in text refer to Figure 24.2.)

1. ***Increased phosphorylation of glucose:*** Elevated levels of intracellular glucose in the hepatocyte allow *glucokinase* to actively phosphorylate glucose to glucose 6-phosphate (see p. 111). This contrasts with the postabsorptive state in which hepatic glucose levels are lower and *glucokinase* is largely dormant because of its low affinity (high K_m) for glucose. *Hexokinase* has a high affinity (low K_m) for glucose and functions close to maximal velocity under most conditions (Figure 24.2, ①).
2. ***Increased glycogen synthesis:*** The conversion of glucose 6-phosphate to glycogen is favored by insulin-mediated inactivation of *glycogen phosphorylase* and activation of *glycogen synthase* (see p. 74 and Figure 24.2, ②).
3. ***Increased activity of the hexosemonophosphate pathway (HMP):*** The increased availability of glucose 6-phosphate in the well-fed state, combined with the active use of NADPH in hepatic lipogenesis, stimulates the HMP (see Chapter 14). This pathway typically accounts for 5% to 10% of the glucose metabolized by the liver (Figure 24.2, ③).
4. ***Increased glycolysis:*** In liver, glycolytic metabolism of glucose is significant only during the absorptive period following a carbohydrate-rich meal. The conversion of glucose to acetyl CoA is stimulated by the elevated insulin:glucagon ratio that activates

the rate-limiting enzymes of glycolysis, for example, *phosphofructokinase* and *pyruvate kinase* (see p. 113). Acetyl CoA either is used as a building block for fatty acid synthesis or provides energy by its oxidation by the TCA cycle (Figure 24.2, ④).

5. ***Decreased gluconeogenesis:*** Although glycolysis is stimulated in the absorptive state, gluconeogenesis is decreased. *Pyruvate carboxylase,* which catalyzes the first step in gluconeogenesis, is largely inactive due to low levels of acetyl CoA—an allosteric effector essential for enzyme activity (see p. 125). In the hepatocyte the concentration of acetyl CoA is kept low as a result of its consumption in fatty acid synthesis. The high insulin:glucagon ratio observed in the absorptive period also favors inactivation of other enzymes unique to gluconeogenesis, such as *fructose 1,6-bisphosphatase* (see p. 129).

B. Fat metabolism

1. ***Increased fatty acid synthesis:*** Liver is the primary tissue for *de novo* synthesis of fatty acids (Figure 24.2, 1). This pathway occurs in the absorptive period, since the dietary energy intake exceeds energy expenditure by the body. Fatty acid synthesis is favored by the availability of substrates (acetyl CoA and NADPH derived from the metabolism of glucose) and by the activation of *acetyl CoA carboxylase*. This enzyme catalyzes the formation of malonyl CoA from acetyl CoA, a reaction that is rate-limiting in fatty acid synthesis (see p. 162).

2. ***Increased triacylglycerol synthesis:*** Triacylglycerol synthesis is favored because fatty acyl CoA is available (a) from *de novo* synthesis from acetyl CoA and (b) from hydrolysis of the triacylglycerol component of chylomicron remnants removed from the blood by hepatocytes (see p. 208). Glycerol 3-phosphate, the backbone for triacylglycerol synthesis, is provided by the glycolytic metabolism of glucose. The liver packages triacylglycerol as very low-density lipoprotein (VLDL) particles that are secreted into the blood for use by extrahepatic tissues, particularly adipose and muscle tissue (Figure 24.2, 2)(see p. 210).

C. Amino acid metabolism

1. ***Increased amino acid degradation:*** In the absorptive period, more amino acids are present than the liver can use in the synthesis of proteins and other nitrogen-containing molecules. The surplus amino acids are either released into the blood for all tissues to use in protein synthesis or are deaminated, with the resulting carbon skeletons being degraded by the liver to pyruvate, acetyl CoA, or TCA cycle intermediates. These metabolites can be oxidized for energy or used in fatty acid synthesis (Figure 24.2, A). The liver has limited capacity to degrade the branched-chain amino acids leucine, isoleucine, and valine; they pass through the liver essentially unchanged and are preferentially metabolized in muscle (see p. 244).

2. ***Increased protein synthesis:*** The body cannot store protein in the same way that it maintains glycogen or triacylglycerol reserves. However, a transient increase in the synthesis of hepatic proteins does occur in the absorptive state, resulting in replacement of

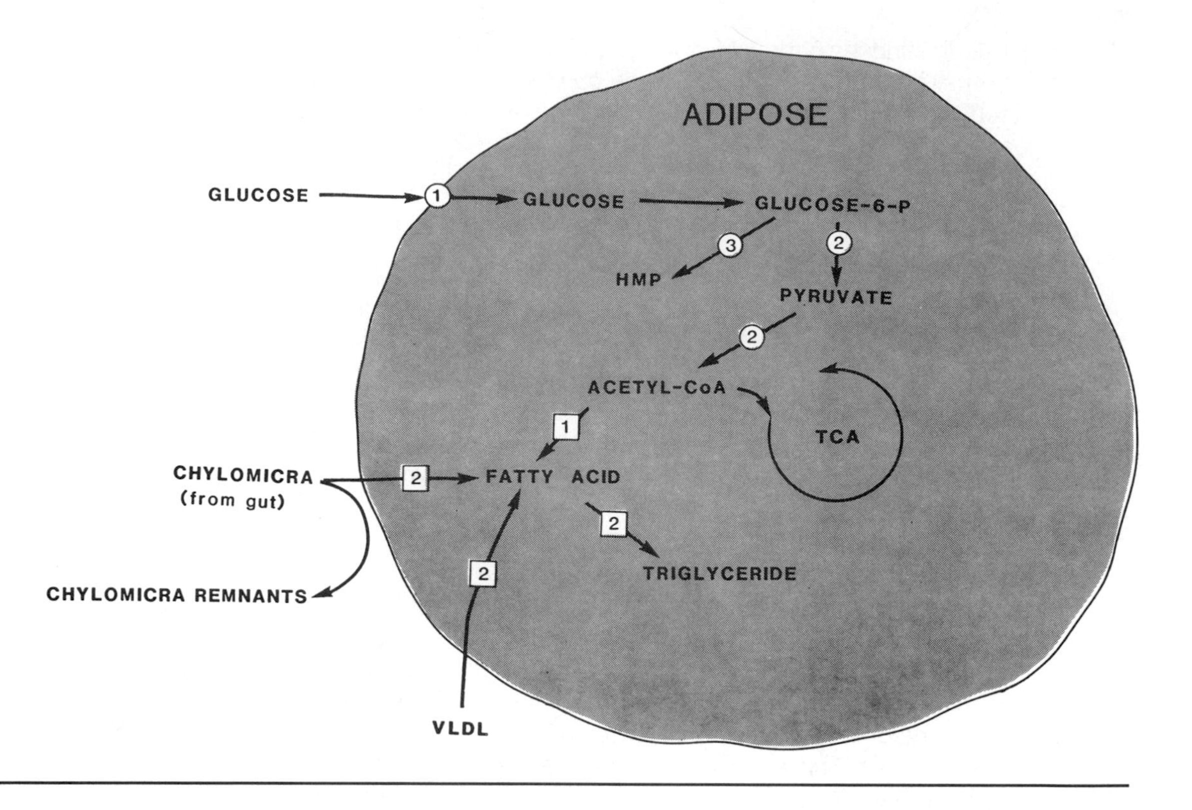

Figure 24.3
Major metabolic pathways in adipose tissue in the absorptive state. The numbers in circles or squares that appear both on the figure and in the text indicate important pathways for carbohydrate and fat, respectively.

any proteins that may have been degraded during the previous postabsorptive period (Figure 24.2, △2).

III. ADIPOSE TISSUE: NUTRIENT STORAGE DEPOT

Adipose tissue is second only to the liver in its ability to distribute fuel molecules. In a 70-kg man, adipose tissues weighs about 14 kg or about half as much as the total muscle mass. In obese individuals adipose tissue can constitute up to 70% of body weight. Nearly the entire volume of each adipocyte can be occupied by a droplet of triacylglycerol.

A. Carbohydrate metabolism

1. ***Increased glucose transport:*** Glucose transport into the adipocyte is very sensitive to the concentration of insulin in the blood. Circulating insulin levels are elevated in the absorptive state, resulting in an influx of glucose into the adipocyte (Figure 24.3, ①).
2. ***Increased glycolysis:*** The increased intracellular availability of glucose results in an enhanced rate of glycolysis. In adipose tissue, glycolysis serves a synthetic function by supplying glycerol 3-phosphate and acetyl CoA for triacylglycerol synthesis (see p. 167 and Figure 24.3, ②).
3. ***Increased activity in the hexosemonophosphate pathway (HMP):*** Adipose tissue can metabolize glucose by means of the HMP, producing

NADPH, essential for fat synthesis (see p. 165). The pathway is active in the well-fed state and metabolizes about 30% to 50% of the total available glucose (Figure 24.3, ③).

B. Fat metabolism

1. ***Increased synthesis of fatty acids:*** *De novo* synthesis of fatty acids from acetyl CoA in adipose tissue occurs primarily during high carbohydrate intake. At other times, fatty acid synthesis in adipose tissue is not a major pathway in humans (Figure 24.3, [1]). Instead, most of the triacylglycerol added to the adipocytes' lipid stores is provided by the liver via VLDL (see p. 210).

2. ***Increased triacylglycerol synthesis:*** Hydrolysis of the triacylglycerol component of chylomicrons (from the intestine) and VLDL (from the liver) provide adipose tissue with fatty acids after consumption of a lipid-containing meal. These exogenous fatty acids are released by the action of *lipoprotein lipase,* an extracellular enzyme attached to the capillary walls in many tissues—particularly adipose and muscle. Adipose tissue lacks the enzyme *glycerol kinase,* so that glycerol 3-phosphate used in triacylglycerol synthesis must come from the metabolism of glucose (see p. 167). Thus, in the well-fed state, elevated levels of glucose and insulin favor storage of triacylglycerol (Figure 24.3, [2]).

3. ***Decreased triacylglycerol degradation:*** The elevated insulin:glucagon ratio depresses the activity of *hormone-sensitive lipase*. Triacylglycerol degradation is thus inhibited in the well-fed state.

IV. SKELETAL MUSCLE

The energy metabolism of muscle is unique in being able to respond to substantial changes in the demand for ATP that accompany muscle contraction. At rest, muscle accounts for about 30% of the oxygen consumption of the body; during vigorous exercise it is responsible for up to 90% of the total oxygen consumption. This graphically illustrates the fact that skeletal muscle, despite its potential for transient periods of anaerobic glycolysis, is an ***oxidative tissue***.

A. Carbohydrate metabolism

1. ***Increased glucose transport:*** The transient increase in plasma glucose and insulin after a carbohydrate-rich meal leads to an increase in glucose transport into the cell. Glucose is phosphorylated to glucose 6-phosphate and metabolized to provide the basal energy needs of the cell (Figure 24.4, ①). This contrasts with the postabsorptive state in which ketones and fatty acids are the major fuels of resting muscle.

2. ***Increased glycogen synthesis:*** The increased insulin:glucagon ratio and the availability of glucose 6-phosphate favor glycogen synthesis, particularly if glycogen stores have been depleted as a result of exercise (Figure 24.4, ②).

B. Fat metabolism

1. Fatty acids are released from chylomicra and VLDL by the action of *lipoprotein lipase* (see p. 209). However, fatty acids are of secondary importance as a fuel for muscle in the well-fed state in which glucose is the primary source of energy.

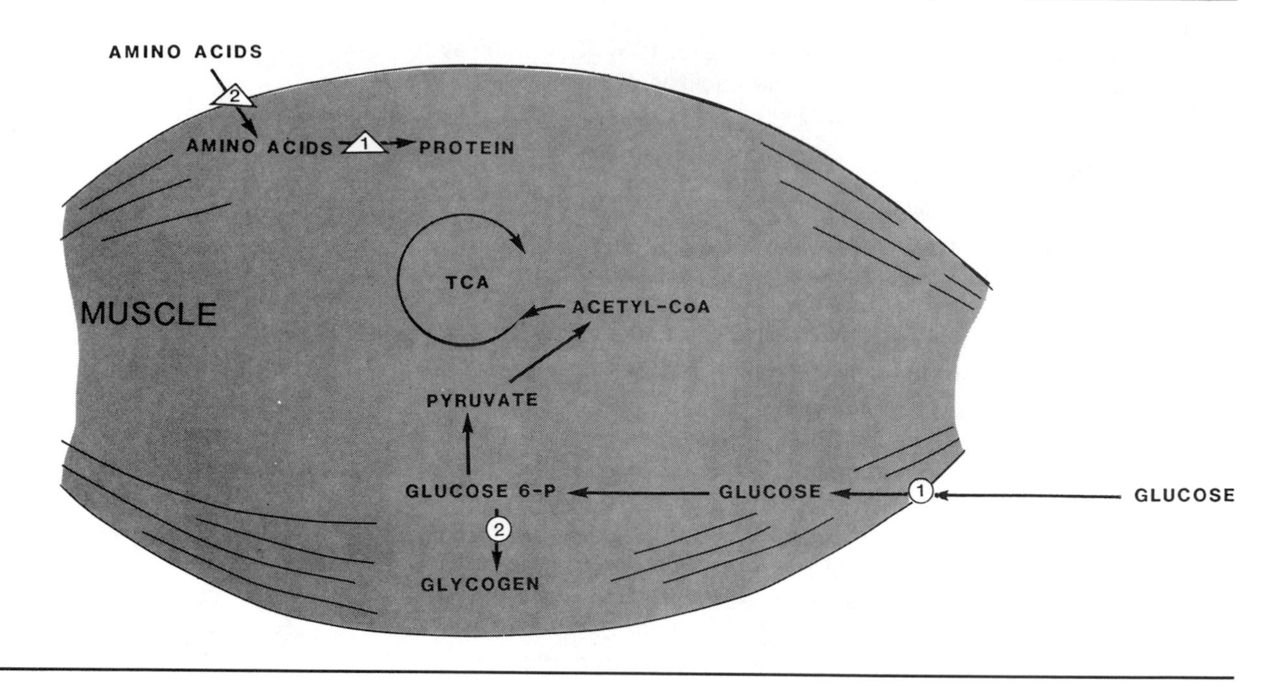

Figure 24.4
Major metabolic pathways in skeletal muscle in the absorptive state. The numbers in circles and triangles that appear both on the figure and in the text indicate important pathways for carbohydrate or protein, respectively.

C. Amino acid metabolism

1. ***Increased protein synthesis:*** A spurt in amino acid uptake and protein synthesis occurs in the absorptive period after ingestion of a meal containing protein. This synthesis replaces protein degraded since the previous meal to provide gluconeogenic precursors (Figure 24.4, △1).
2. ***Increased uptake of branched-chain amino acids:*** Muscle is the principal site for degradation of branched-chain amino acids (see p. 244). Leucine, isoleucine, and valine escape metabolism by the liver and are taken up by muscle, where they are used for protein synthesis and as sources of energy (Figure 24.4, △2).

V. BRAIN

Although contributing only 2% of the adult weight, the brain accounts for 20% of the basal oxygen consumption of the body at rest. Brain uses energy at a constant rate. Because brain is vital to the proper functioning of all organs of the body, special priority is given to its fuel needs. To provide energy, substrates must be able to cross the endothelial cells that line the blood vessels in the brain (sometimes called the "blood–brain barrier"). Normally glucose serves as the primary fuel, since in the fed state the concentration of ketones is too low to serve as an alternate energy source. Note, however, that ketones play a significant role during prolonged starvation (see p. 288).

A. Carbohydrate metabolism

1. In the well-fed state, brain uses glucose exclusively as a fuel, completely oxidizing about 140 g per day to carbon dioxide and

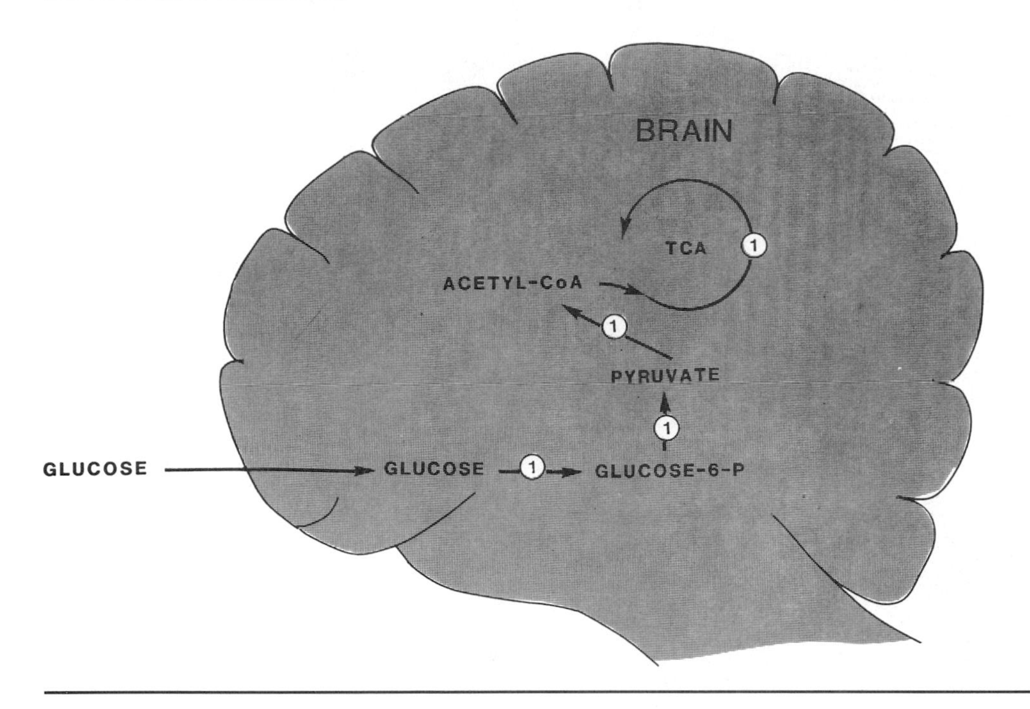

Figure 24.5
Major metabolic pathways in brain in the absorptive state. The numbers in circles that appear both on the figure and in the text indicate important pathways for carbohydrate metabolism.

water. Brain contains no significant stores of glycogen and is therefore completely dependent on the availability of blood glucose (Figure 24.5, ①).

B. Fat metabolism

1. Brain has no significant stores of triacylglycerol, and the oxidation of fatty acids obtained from blood makes little contribution to energy production because fatty acids do not efficiently cross the blood–brain barrier.

VI. SUMMARY OF ABSORPTIVE STATE

For several hours after ingestion of a meal, there is an abundance of circulating nutrients that triggers the secretion of insulin and inhibits the release of glucagon. The intertissue exchanges characteristic of the absorptive period are summarized in Figure 24.6.

Study Questions

Answer A if 1, 2, and 3 are correct
B if 1 and 3 are correct
C if 2 and 4 are correct
D if only 4 is correct
E if all are correct

24.1 Which of the following is(are) elevated in plasma during the absorptive period (compared to the postabsorptive state)?

1. Insulin
2. VLDL
3. Chylomicra
4. Free fatty acids

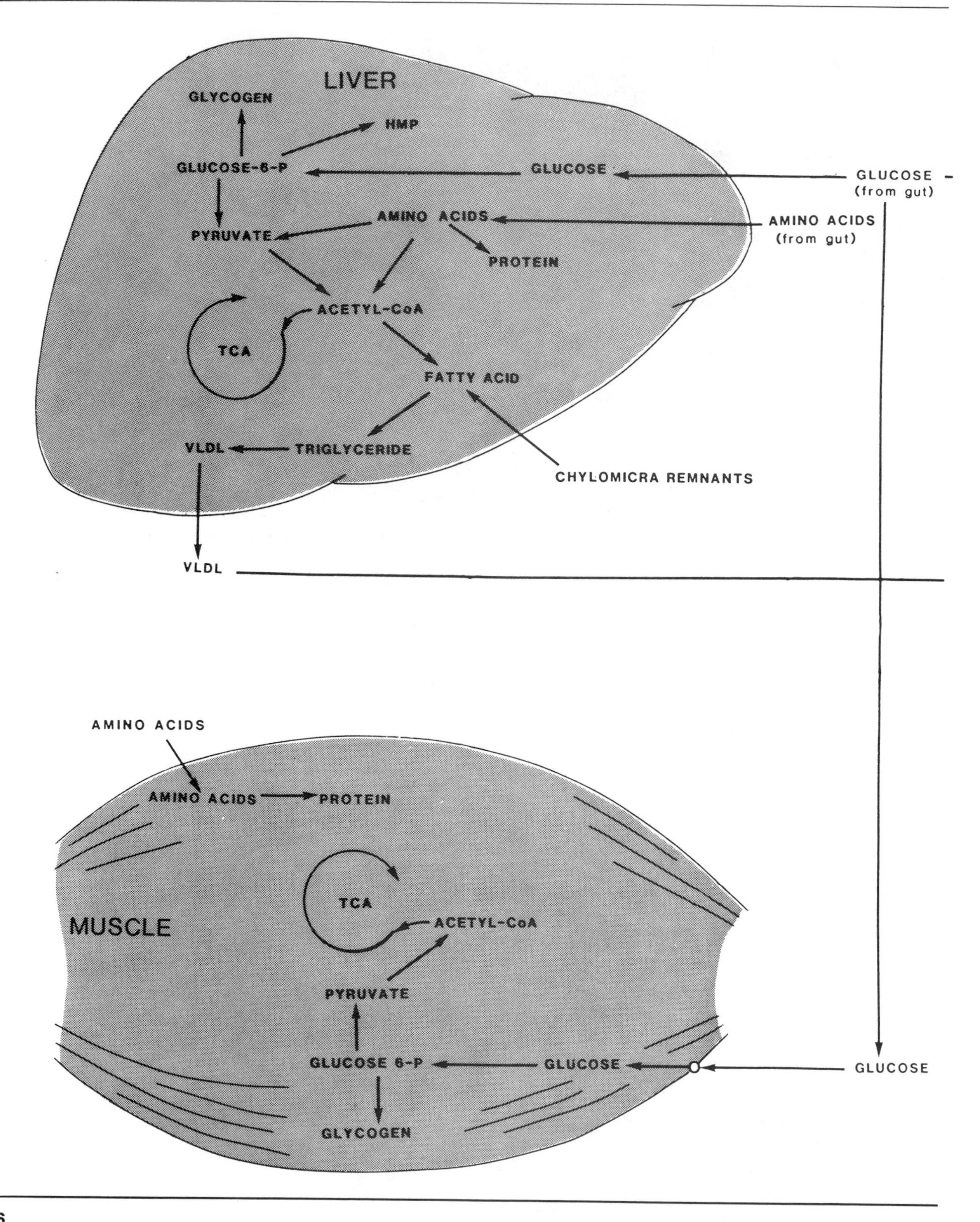

Figure 24.6
Intertissue relationships in the absorptive state. Small circles on perimeter of tissues indicate transport systems.

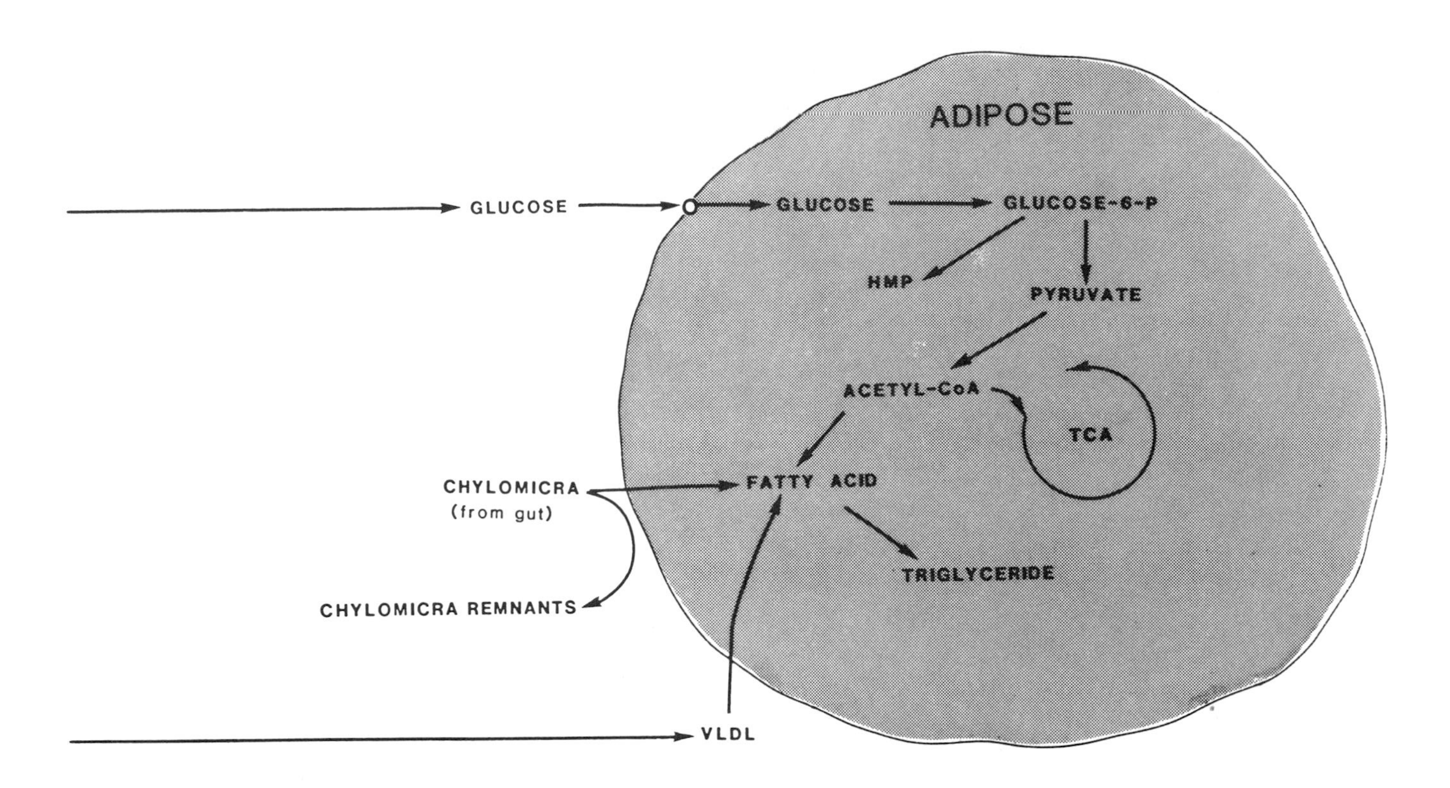
ADIPOSE
GLUCOSE
GLUCOSE
GLUCOSE-6-P
HMP
PYRUVATE
ACETYL-CoA
TCA
CHYLOMICRA
(from gut)
FATTY ACID
TRIGLYCERIDE
CHYLOMICRA REMNANTS
VLDL

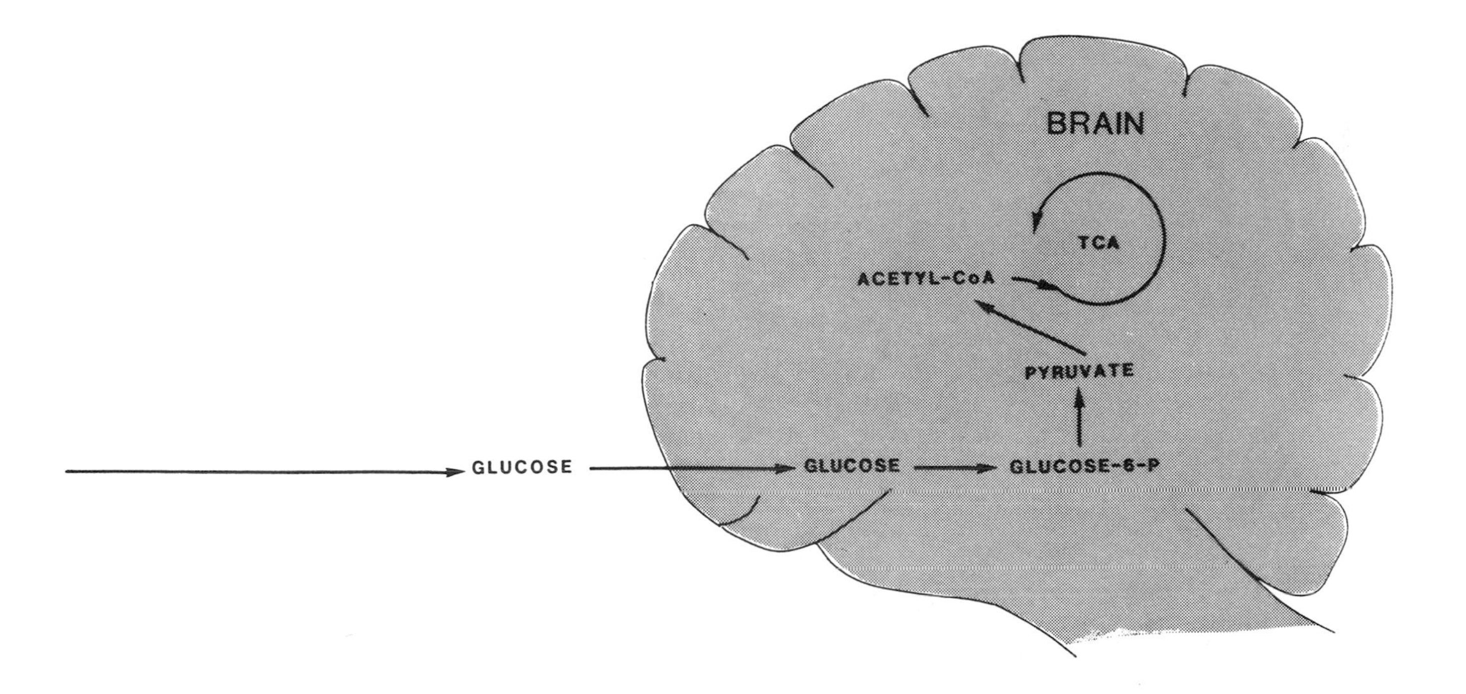
BRAIN
TCA
ACETYL-CoA
PYRUVATE
GLUCOSE
GLUCOSE
GLUCOSE-6-P

24.2 Which of the following fuel molecules is(are) used by the brain in the absorptive period?

1. β-Hydroxybutyrate
2. Free fatty acids
3. Amino acids
4. Glucose

24.3 Ingestion of a meal consisting exclusively of protein would result in which of the following?

1. An increased release of insulin
2. Hypoglycemia
3. An increased release of glucagon
4. Ketoacidosis caused by the metabolism of ketogenic amino acids

24.4 In the absorptive period (as compared to the postabsorptive state), the adipose tissue shows

1. increased transport of glucose into the adipocyte.
2. increased production of NADPH.
3. increased rate of glycolysis.
4. decreased activity of hormone-sensitive lipase.

Starvation and Diabetes

25

I. OVERVIEW

Starvation may result from an inability to obtain food, from the desire to lose weight rapidly, or in clinical situations in which an individual cannot eat because of trauma (surgery, burns, and so forth). In the absence of food, plasma levels of glucose, amino acids, and triacylglycerol fall, triggering a decline in insulin secretion and an increase in glucagon release. This sets into motion an exchange of substrates among liver, adipose, muscle, and brain that is guided by two priorities: (a) the need to maintain adequate plasma levels of glucose to sustain energy metabolism of the brain and other glucose-requiring tissues, and (b) the need to mobilize fatty acids from adipose tissue and ketones from liver to supply energy to all other tissues.

II. FUEL STORES

The metabolic fuels available in a normal 70-kg man at the beginning of a fast are shown in Figure 25.1. Note the enormous caloric stores available in the form of triacylglycerols compared to those contained in glycogen. Although it is listed as an energy source, protein does not exist solely as a fuel depot. Rather, each protein molecule has a function, for example, as structural components of the body, enzymes, and so forth. Only about one third of the body's protein can be used for energy production without fatally compromising vital functions.

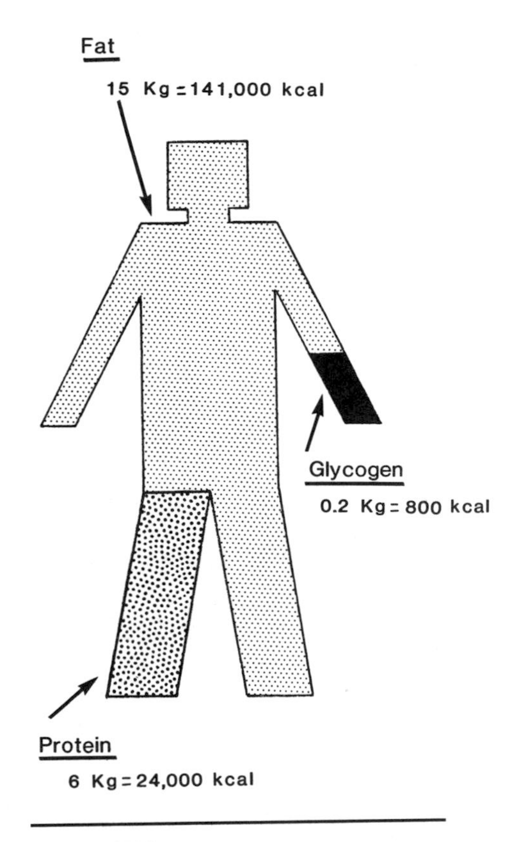

Figure 25.1
Metabolic fuels available in a 70-kg man at the beginning of a fast.

III. LIVER

A. *Carbohydrate metabolism:* The liver first uses glycogen degradation, then gluconeogenesis, to maintain blood glucose levels.

1. ***Increased glycogen degradation:*** Figure 25.2 shows the sources of blood glucose after ingestion of 100 g of glucose. During the absorptive period, glucose from the diet is the major source of blood sugar. Several hours after the meal, blood glucose levels have declined sufficiently to cause an increased secretion of glucagon and decreased release of insulin. The increased glucagon:insulin ratio causes a rapid mobilization of liver glycogen stores (which contain about 100 g in the well-fed state). Note that liver glycogen is nearly exhausted after 6 to 12 hours of

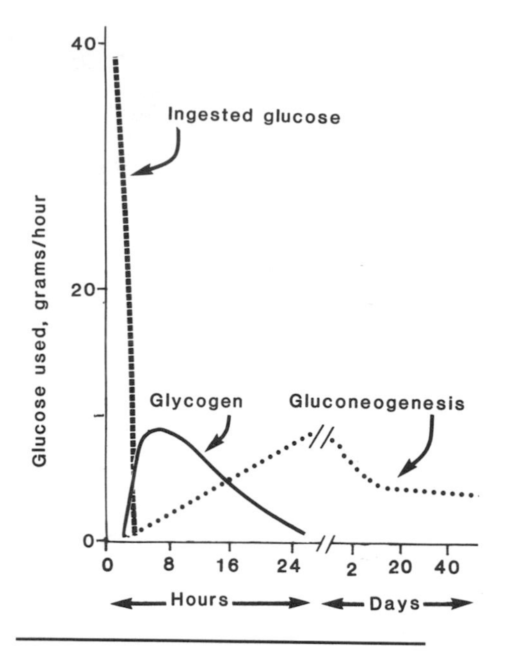

Figure 25.2
Sources of blood glucose after ingestion of 100 g of glucose.

fasting, and therefore hepatic glycogenolysis is a transient response to early starvation. Figure 25.3, ①, shows glycogen degradation as part of the overall metabolic response of the liver during starvation.

2. ***Increased gluconeogenesis:*** The synthesis of glucose and its subsequent release into the circulation are vital hepatic functions during starvation (Figure 25.3, ②). The carbon skeletons for gluconeogenesis are derived primarily from amino acids, glycerol, and lactate. Gluconeogenesis begins 4 to 6 hours after the last meal and becomes fully active as stores of liver glycogen are depleted (see Figure 25.2). Gluconeogenesis plays an essential role in maintaining blood glucose during both overnight and prolonged fasting.

B. Fat metabolism

1. ***Increased fatty acid oxidation:*** The oxidation of fatty acids derived from adipose tissue is the major source of energy in hepatic tissue in the postabsorptive state (Figure 25.3, [1]).
2. ***Increased synthesis of ketones:*** Liver is unique in being able to synthesize and release ketone bodies (primarily β-hydroxybutyrate) for use as fuels by peripheral tissues (see p. 179). Ketone synthesis is favored when the concentration of acetyl CoA,

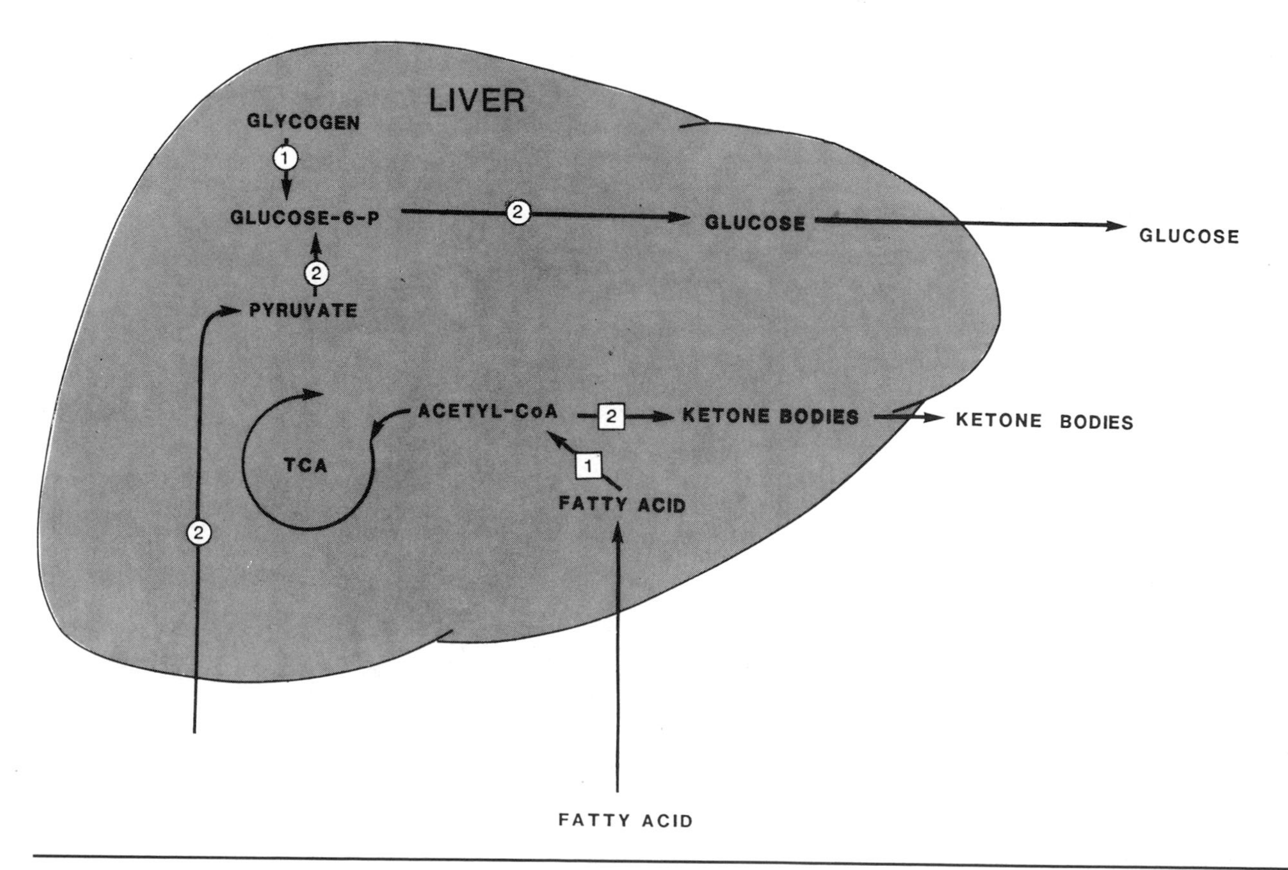

Figure 25.3
Major metabolic pathways in liver during starvation. The numbers in circles or squares that appear both on the figure and in the corresponding citation in the text indicate important pathways for carbohydrate or fat, respectively.

produced from fatty acid metabolism, exceeds the oxidative capacity of the TCA cycle. Synthesis of ketones starts during the first days of starvation (Figure 25.4). The availability of circulating ketones is important in starvation because they can be used for fuel by most tissues, including brain, once their level in the blood is sufficiently high. This reduces the need for gluconeogenesis from amino acid carbon skeletons, thus slowing the loss of essential protein. Ketone synthesis as part of the overall hepatic response to starvation is shown in Figure 25.3, [2].

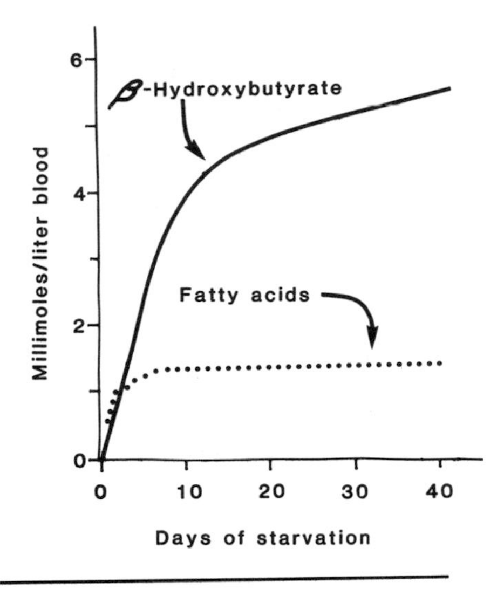

Figure 25.4
Concentrations of fatty acids and β-hydroxybutyrate in the blood during starvation.

IV. ADIPOSE TISSUE

A. Carbohydrate metabolism

1. Glucose transport into the adipocyte and its subsequent metabolism are depressed owing to low levels of circulating insulin. This leads to a decrease in fatty acid and triacylglycerol synthesis.

B. Fat metabolism

1. ***Increased degradation of triacylglycerols:*** The activation of *hormone-sensitive lipase* (see p. 170) and subsequently hydrolysis of stored triacylglycerol are enhanced by the elevated glucagon:insulin ratio. Epinephrine and, particularly, norepinephrine released from the sympathetic nerve endings in adipose tissue are also physiologically important activators of *hormone-sensitive lipase* (Figure 25.5, [1]).
2. ***Increased release of fatty acids:*** Fatty acids obtained from hydrolysis of stored triacylglycerol are released into the blood. Bound to albumin, they are transported to various tissues for use as fuel. The glycerol produced after triacylglycerol degradation is used as a gluconeogenic precursor by the liver (Figure 25.5, [2]).

V. SKELETAL MUSCLE

A. Carbohydrate metabolism

1. Glucose transport into muscle cells and its subsequent metabolism are depressed owing to low levels of circulating insulin.

B. Lipid metabolism

1. During the first two weeks of starvation, muscle uses fatty acids from adipose tissue and ketones from the liver as fuels (Figure 25.6, [1]). After about 3 weeks of starvation, muscle decreases its use of ketones and oxidizes fatty acids almost exclusively. This leads to a further increase in the already elevated level of circulating ketone bodies.

C. Protein metabolism

1. During the first few days of starvation there is a rapid breakdown of muscle protein, providing amino acids that are used by the liver for gluconeogenesis (Figure 25.6, [A]). After several weeks of starvation the rate of muscle proteolysis decreases owing to a decline in the need for glucose as a fuel for brain.

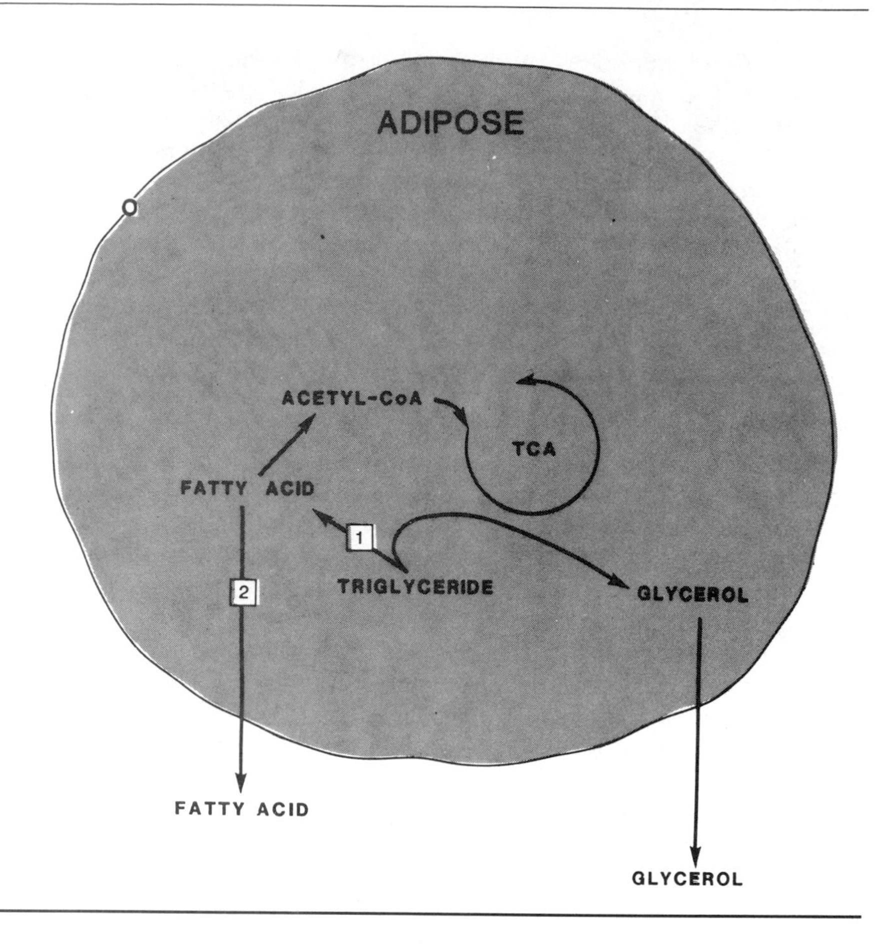

Figure 25.5
Major metabolic pathways in adipose tissue during starvation. The numbers in the squares, which appear both on the figure and in the corresponding citation in the text, indicate important pathways for fat metabolism.

VI. BRAIN

A. Metabolism of fuels

1. During the first days of starvation, the brain continues to use glucose exclusively. Blood sugar is maintained by hepatic gluconeogenesis from amino acids provided by the rapid breakdown of muscle protein (Figure 25.7, ①).
2. In prolonged starvation (greater than 2–3 weeks), plasma ketones reach markedly elevated levels and are used as a fuel by the brain (Figure 25.7, [1]). This reduces the need for protein catabolism for gluconeogenesis.

VII. SUMMARY OF STARVATION

The metabolic changes that occur during starvation ensure that all tissues have an adequate supply of fuel molecules. The response of the major tissues involved in energy metabolism is summarized in Figure 25.8.

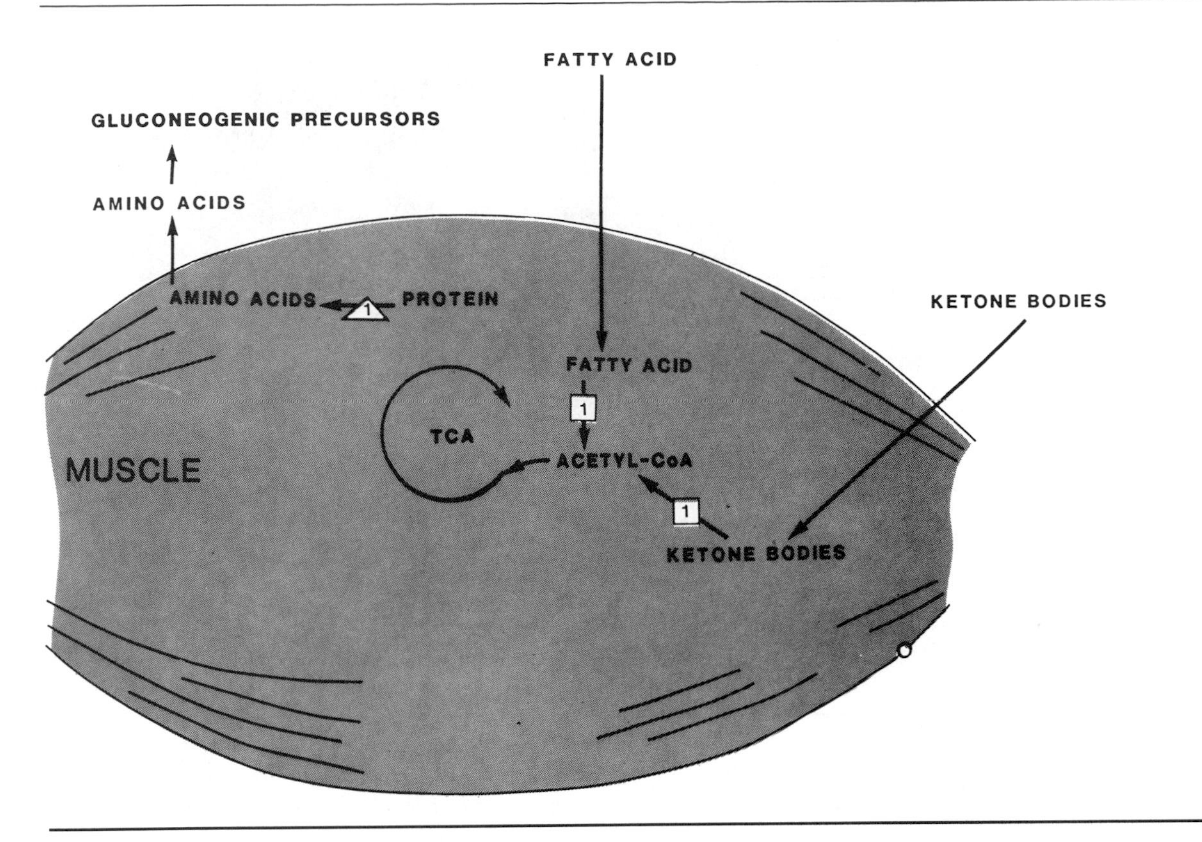

Figure 25.6
Major metabolic pathways in skeletal muscle during starvation. The numbers in squares or triangles, which appear both on the figure and in the corresponding citations in the text, indicate important pathways for fat or protein metabolism, respectively.

Study Questions

Choose the ONE best answer:

25.1 Increased formation of ketone bodies during starvation is due to

A. mobilization of high-density lipoproteins.
B. formation of acetyl CoA in amounts that exceed the oxidative capacity of the liver.
C. decreased levels of free fatty acids in serum.
D. inhibition of β-oxidation of fatty acids in the liver.
E. a decreased mobilization of triacylglycerols from adipose tissue.

25.2 Which one of the following is the most important source of blood glucose during the ***last*** hours of a 48-hour fast?

A. Muscle glycogen
B. Fatty acids
C. Liver glycogen
D. Amino acids
E. Acetyl CoA

25.3 Starvation results in all of the following EXCEPT

A. decreased levels of VLDL.
B. stimulation of adipose tissue hormone-sensitive lipase.
C. increased levels of ketone bodies in the blood.
D. increased fatty acid oxidation.
E. increased synthesis of fatty acids in adipose tissue.

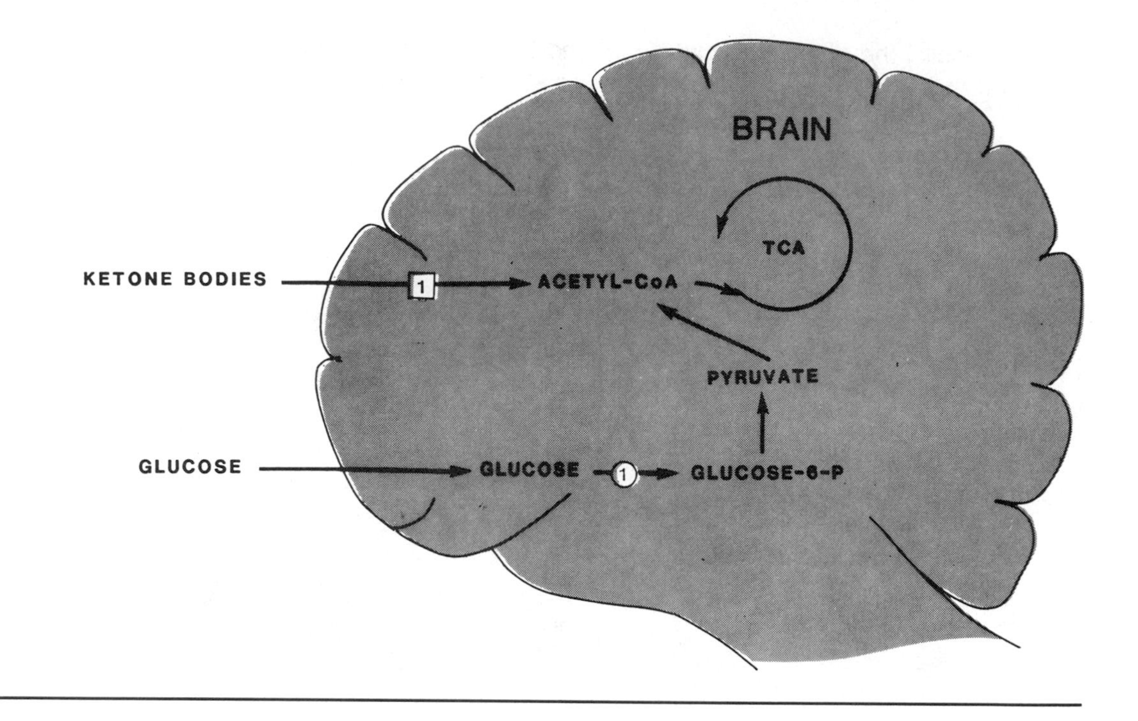

Figure 25.7
Major metabolic pathways in brain during starvation. The numbers in squares or circles, which appear both on the figure and in the corresponding citations in the text, indicate important pathways for fat or carbohydrate, respectively.

25.4 Which one of the following series best describes the chronological sequence of events that occurs during the first week of starvation?

A. Glycogenolysis, gluconeogenesis, ketogenesis, hypoglycemia.
B. Gluconeogenesis, glycogenolysis, fatty acid mobilization, ketogenesis
C. Glycogenolysis, gluconeogenesis, fatty acid mobilization, ketogenesis.
D. Gluconeogenesis, glycogenolysis, ketogenesis, fatty acid mobilization.
E. Glycogenolysis, fat mobilization, gluconeogenesis, hypoglycemia.

VIII. DIABETES MELLITUS

Diabetes is not one disease but rather is a heterogeneous group of syndromes all characterized by an elevation of blood glucose caused by a ***relative or absolute deficiency in insulin***. Frequently the inadequate release of insulin is aggravated by an excess of glucagon. Diabetics can be conveniently divided into two groups, based on their requirements for insulin.

A. Insulin-dependent diabetes

1. Insulin-dependent or ***type I diabetics*** require insulin to avoid ketoacidosis. Insulin-dependent diabetes is characterized by an absolute deficiency of insulin caused by massive β-cell lesions or necrosis. Loss of β-cell function may be due to invasion by viruses, the action of chemical toxins, or autoimmune antibodies directed against the β-cell. Destruction of the β-cells by host antibodies usually requires a synergistic stimulus from the environment, such as a viral infection. As a result of the destruction

of β-cells, the pancreas fails to respond to ingestion of glucose, and the type I diabetic shows symptoms of insulin deficiency.

2. Insulin-dependent diabetics constitute 10% to 20% of the 60 million diabetics in the United States.

B. Noninsulin-dependent diabetes

1. In non-insulin-dependent or ***type II diabetes***, the pancreas retains some β-cell capacity, resulting in insulin levels that vary from below normal to above normal, but in all cases are less than that required to maintain glucose homeostasis.
2. Type II diabetes is frequently accompanied by target organ ***insulin resistance*** which results in a decreased responsiveness to both endogenous and exogenous insulin. In some cases, insulin resistance can be due to a decreased number of insulin receptors. Other patients show an as yet undefined defect in the events that occur after insulin binds to its receptor on the cell membrane.
3. The occurrence of the type II disease is almost completely determined by ***genetic factors***. There appears to be no involvement of viruses or autoimmune antibodies. The metabolic alterations observed are milder than those described for the insulin-dependent form of the disease.

C. Diagnosis of diabetes

1. The diagnosis of diabetes depends on a test that demonstrates an intolerance for glucose. An ***elevated*** level of ***blood glucose,*** together with an increase in the concentration of ***blood ketones,*** is strongly indicative of the presence of diabetes.
2. The ***glucose tolerance test*** is a commonly used diagnostic test in which the patient is given 100 g of glucose orally after an overnight fast. Blood glucose concentrations are determined at 30-minute intervals for the next 3 hours. Figure 25.9 shows typical results for normal and diabetic individuals. Fasting blood glucose is initially high (greater than 140 mg/dl) in the diabetic and rises to concentrations greater than 200 mg/dl after the oral administration of glucose. The rate of glomerular filtration of glucose exceeds that of tubular reabsorption in the kidney, and glucose appears in the urine. In contrast, normal individuals show fasting blood glucose of 70 to 90 mg/dl and a rise to only 140 mg/dl after a glucose load. However, the glucose tolerance test gives many false-positive results primarily as a result of stress-induced epinephrine release that impairs the response to a glucose load.

D. Metabolic changes in diabetes

1. The metabolic changes observed in untreated type 1 diabetes resemble those described for starvation, except they are more exaggerated. The metabolic differences between diabetes and starvation include the following:
   a. ***Insulin levels:*** Insulin is virtually absent in the blood of type I diabetics, rather than merely low as in the case of starvation. Thus, the metabolic effects of glucagon are virtually unopposed in the diabetic.
   b. ***Blood glucose levels:*** Diabetics exhibit a characteristic hypergly-

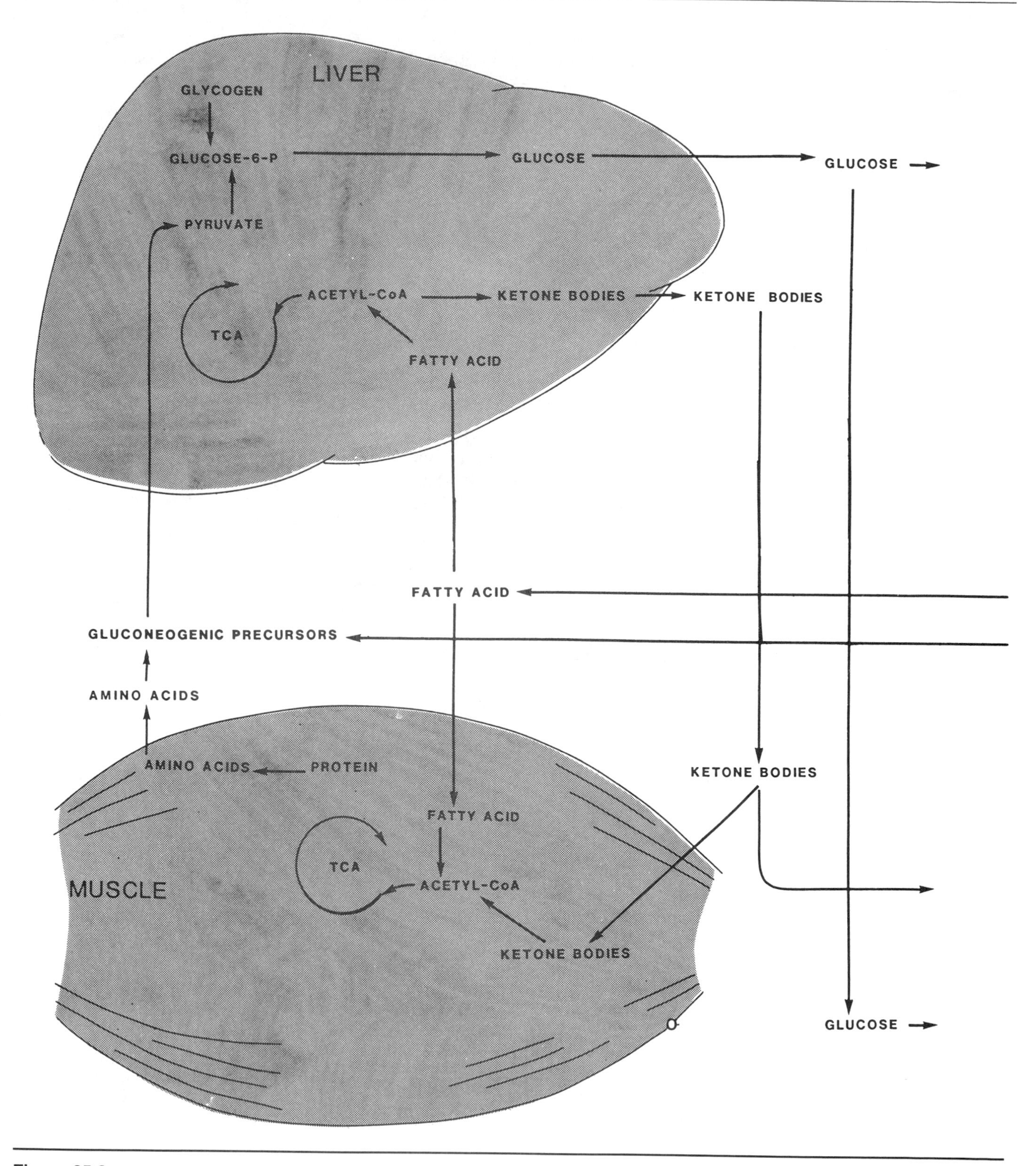

Figure 25.8
Intertissue relationships during starvation.

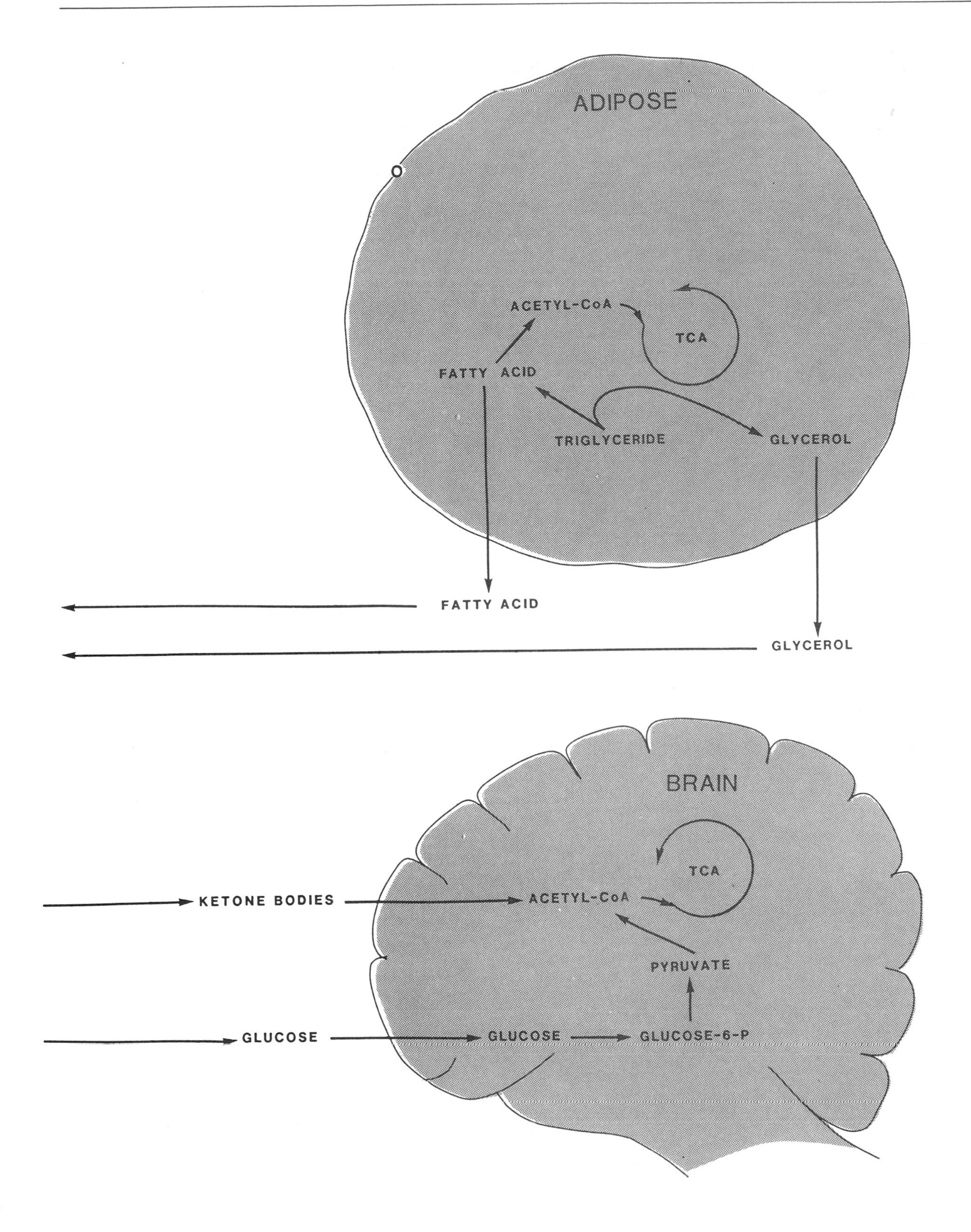
ADIPOSE
ACETYL-CoA
TCA
FATTY ACID
TRIGLYCERIDE
GLYCEROL
FATTY ACID
GLYCEROL
BRAIN
TCA
KETONE BODIES
ACETYL-CoA
PYRUVATE
GLUCOSE
GLUCOSE
GLUCOSE-6-P

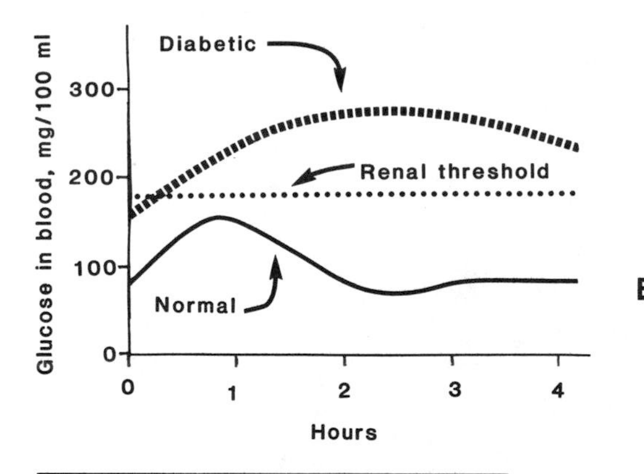

Figure 25.9
Blood glucose levels after ingestion of glucose in normal and diabetic individuals.

cemia, whereas individuals deprived of food maintain a blood glucose level near normal.

c. ***Ketosis:*** The mobilization of fatty acids from adipose tissue and hepatic ketogenesis are greater in diabetes than in starvation. As a result, the ketoacidosis observed in diabetes is much more severe than that during starvation.

E. Treatment of type I diabetes

1. ***Insulin replacement:*** After ingestion of a meal, a burst of insulin secretion occurs in normal individuals as a response to transient increases in the levels of circulating glucose and amino acids. In the postabsorptive period, β-cell secretion maintains low, basal levels of circulating insulin. However, the type I diabetic has virtually no functional β-cells and can neither respond to variations in circulating fuels nor maintain even a basal secretion of insulin. The diabetic must rely on ***exogenous (injected) insulin*** injected intramuscularly in order to control the hyperglycemia and ketoacidosis.
2. ***Exercise:*** Sustained muscular activity increases the use of glucose by muscle even without insulin. This can decrease both the hyperglycemia characteristic of diabetes and the patient's requirement for insulin.

F. Treatment of type II diabetes

1. In the overweight patient, non-insulin-dependent diabetes is dramatically improved when the individual reduces his weight to the normal range. Sulfonylurea drugs, such as ***tolbutamide,*** also may decrease blood glucose and may be used to supplement diet therapy in some patients.

Study Questions

Choose the ONE best answer:

25.5 Relative or absolute lack of insulin in humans would result in which one of the following reactions in the liver?

A. Increased glycogen synthesis
B. Increased gluconeogenesis from lactate
C. Decrease glycogenolysis
D. Decreased formation of acetoacetate
E. Increased action of hormone-sensitive lipase

25.6 Which one of the following is always found in patients with diabetes mellitus?

A. An inability to metabolize glucose appropriately
B. Extremely low levels of insulin synthesis and secretion
C. Synthesis of an insulin with an abnormal amino acid sequence
D. A simple pattern of genetic inheritance
E. Microangiopathy

25.7 An individual with obesity-associated diabetes (type II)

A. usually has a normal glucose tolerance test.
B. usually has a lower plasma level of insulin than a normal individual.
C. usually develops a normal glucose tolerance test if his weight returns to normal.
D. usually benefits from receiving insulin about 6 hours after a meal.
E. usually has lower plasma levels of glucagon than a normal individual.

25.8 Relative or absolute lack of insulin in humans would result in which one of the following reactions in the skeletal muscle?

A. Increased use of muscle proteins for production of amino acids
B. Increased glycogen synthesis
C. Increased uptake of glucose from the blood
D. Increase gluconeogenesis from amino acids
E. Increased rate of glucose 6-phosphate oxidation in the pentose phosphate pathway

Nutrition

26

I. OVERVIEW

Nutrients are the constituents of food necessary to sustain the normal functions of the body. These compounds provide both energy and "essential" molecules that either cannot be synthesized by the tissues or cannot be synthesized at a rate sufficient to meet the needs for growth and maintenance. These essential nutrients include certain amino acids, fatty acids, vitamins, and minerals (Figure 26.1). This chapter describes the nutrients that must be supplied in the diet, reviews the food sources of these compounds, and discusses the consequences of dietary deficiencies and excesses of the essential nutrients.

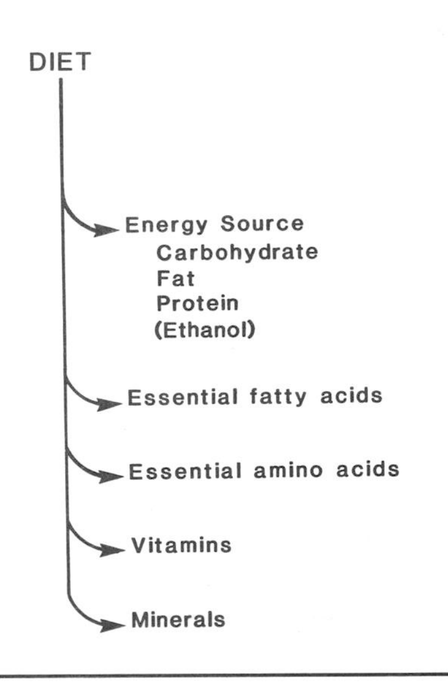

Figure 26.1
Essential nutrients obtained from the diet. Ethanol is not considered an essential component of the diet but may provide a significant contribution to the daily caloric intake of some individuals.

II. NUTRIENT REQUIREMENTS IN HUMANS

Enough food must be eaten to provide the minimum quantity of every nutrient needed by a given individual. It is frequently difficult to determine these minimal nutrient requirements because they are influenced by a variety of genetic and environmental factors unique to each individual. However, it is possible to estimate the ***Recommended Dietary Allowance*** (RDA), which is the quantity of each nutrient that amply meets the needs of most healthy Americans.

A. Recommended Dietary Allowances

1. The RDA is an estimate of the amount of a nutrient required to meet the needs of 95% of the U.S. population. The RDA is ***not*** the minimal requirement for individuals; rather it is intentionally set to provide a margin of safety for most individuals. RDAs for selected nutrients are shown in Figure 26.2.

B. Factors that influence the RDA

1. ***Age:*** The total amount of each nutrient recommended generally increases from infancy to adulthood. However, when expressed per unit of body weight, the allowances are frequently higher in children than in adults owing to the demands of rapid growth. For example, adults require about 0.8 g of protein per kilogram of body weight, whereas infants need more than 2.0 g per kilogram of body weight per day.
2. ***Sex:*** The dietary allowances for men are approximately 20% greater than those for women, reflecting the generally larger body

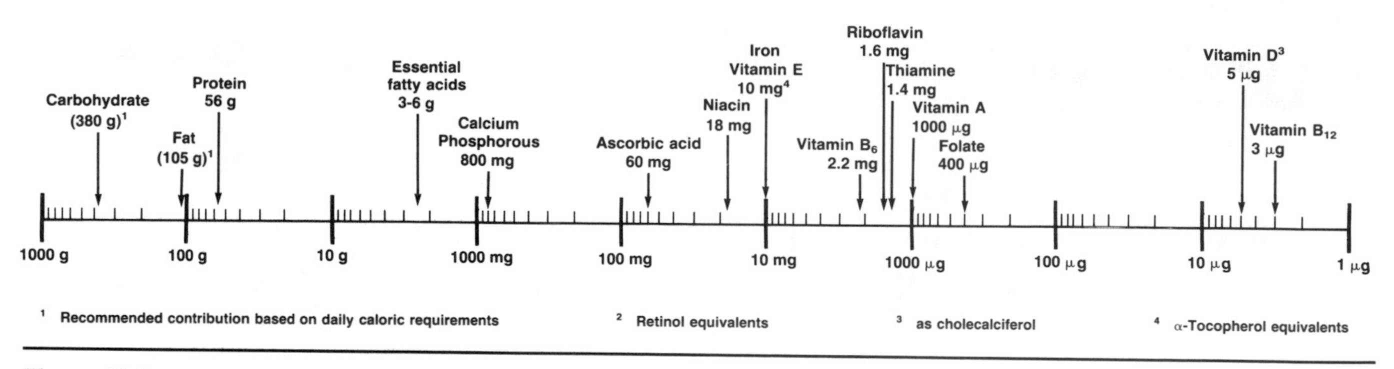

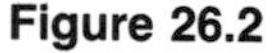
Figure 26.2
Recommended Dietary Allowances for selected nutrients.

mass of men. The allowance for iron is an exception, since women must replace iron lost during menstruation.

3. ***Other factors:*** Pregnant or lactating women have recommended allowances for most nutrients that are increased about 20% to 30% above normal. Patients with injury or illness also show an increased requirement for some nutrients.

	Kcal/g
Carbohydrate	4
Protein	4
Fat	9

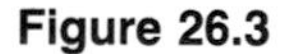
Figure 26.3
Energy available from the major food components.

III. ENERGY REQUIREMENTS OF HUMANS

A. Energy content of food

1. The energy content of food is calculated from the heat released by the total combustion of food in a calorimeter. It is expressed in ***kilocalories*** (kcal or C; see p. 96).
2. The standard conversion factors for determining the caloric content of fat, protein, and carbohydrate are shown in Figure 26.3. Note that the energy content of fat is more than twice that of carbohydrate or protein, whereas the energy contained in ethanol is intermediate to fat and carbohydrate. In some individuals, ethanol provides a significant fraction of the daily caloric intake. For example, consumption of two 8-oz glasses of wine (12% alcohol) provides approximately 300 calories. This represents more than 10% of the daily energy needs of a sedentary individual.

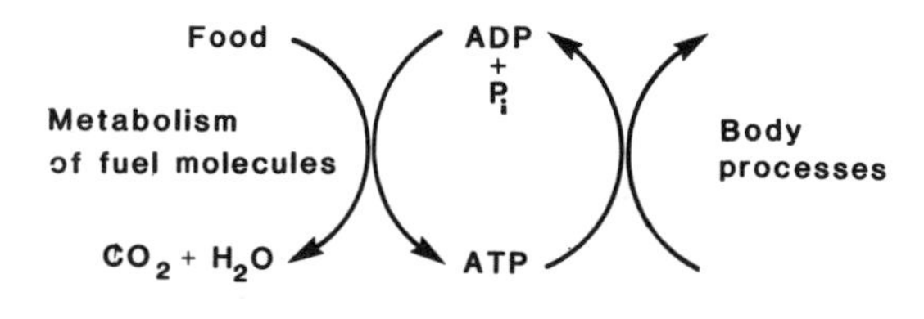

Figure 26.4
The cyclic interconversion of ATP and ADP allows energy to be transferred from food (fuel oxidation) to energy-requiring processes in the cell.

B. How energy is used in the body

1. Part of the chemical energy released by the oxidation of fuel molecules is dissipated as ***heat,*** which in part is used to maintain body temperature. About 40% of the energy in food is captured in synthesis of ***ATP*** from ADP and P_i (Figure 26.4).
2. Cleavage of the high-energy phosphate of the ATP molecule is coupled to energy-requiring processes, such as biosynthetic reactions, muscular contraction, and the propagation of nerve impulses (Figure 26.4).

C. RDA for energy

Assuming light activity levels typical for most Americans, the recommended dietary energy intake for a 70-kg adult man is approximately 2900 kcal and for a 50-kg adult woman, about 2100 kcal. Unlike other allowances, the RDA for energy is not intentionally overestimated, but closely approximates the minimal energy intake consistent with good health. The total energy required by an individual is the sum of three energy-requiring processes that occur in the body: ***basal metabolism, specific dynamic action,*** and ***physical activity.***

1. ***Basal metabolic rate:*** The basal metabolic rate (BMR) is the energy expended by an individual in a resting, postabsorptive state. It represents the energy required to carry out the normal body functions, such as respiration, blood flow, and maintenance of neuromuscular integrity. In an adult, the BMR is roughly 1800 kcal for men (70 kg) and 1300 kcal for women (55 kg). From 50% to 70% of the daily energy expenditure in sedentary individuals is attributable to the BMR (Figure 26.5).
2. ***Specific dynamic action:*** The production of heat by the body increases as much as 30% above the basal level during the digestion and absorption of food. This effect is called the specific dynamic action or ***diet-induced thermogenesis.*** Over a 24-hour period the thermogenic response to food intake may amount to 5% to 10% of the total energy expenditure.
3. ***Physical activity:*** Muscular activity provides the greatest variation in energy expenditure. The amount of energy consumed depends on the time and intensity of the exercise. The daily expenditure of energy can be determined by carefully recording the type and duration of all the activities. In general, a sedentary person requires about 30% to 50% more than the basal caloric requirement for energy balance (Figure 26.5), whereas a highly active individual may require 100% or more calories above the BMR.

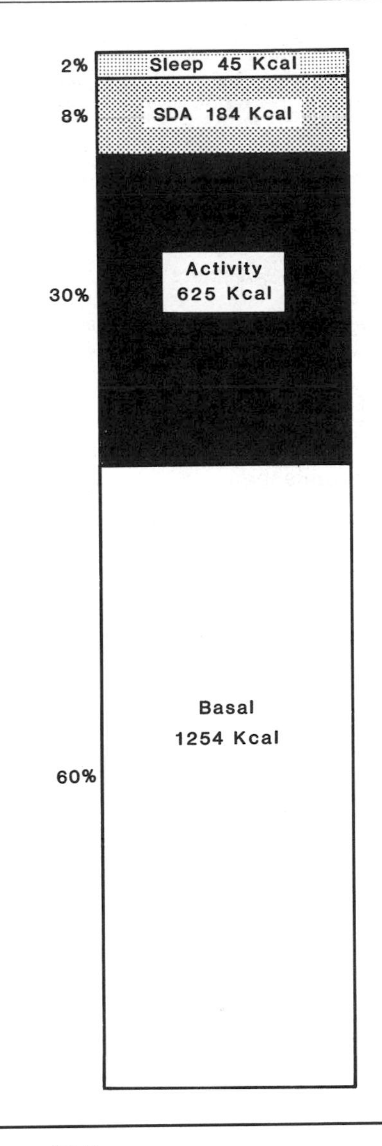

Figure 26.5
Estimated energy consumption in a typical 20-year-old woman, 165 cm (5′6″) tall, weighing 55 kg, and engaged in light activity,

IV. MAJOR NUTRIENTS: SOURCES OF ENERGY

All energy in the diet is provided by three nutrients: carbohydrate, protein, and fat (and ethanol if it is present in the diet). The intake of these fuel molecules is larger than that of the other dietary nutrients. Therefore, carbohydrate, fat, and protein are called the ***major nutrients*** and are described in detail in the next section. Those nutrients needed in lesser amounts, such as vitamins and minerals, are called the ***minor nutrients.***

A. Carbohydrates

Carbohydrates in the diet are classified as either monosaccharides and disaccharides (simple sugars), polysaccharides (complex sugars), or fiber. The metabolism of carbohydrates is discussed in Unit II.

1. ***Monosaccharides:*** Glucose and fructose are the principal monosaccharides found in food (see p. 55). Glucose is abundant in fruits, sweet corn, corn syrup, and honey, whereas free fructose is found with free glucose and sucrose in honey and fruit.
2. ***Disaccharides:*** The most abundant disaccharides are sucrose (glucose + fructose), lactose (glucose + galactose), and maltose (glucose + glucose) (see p. 65). Sucrose is ordinary "table sugar" and is abundant in molasses, maple syrup, and maple

Natural sugars	Relative sweetness
Sucrose	1.0
Glucose	0.7
Fructose	1.7
Maltose	0.3
Lactose	0.2
Artificial sweetners	
Aspartame	180
Saccharin	400

Figure 26.6
Relative sweetness of sugars, and artificial sweeteneers.

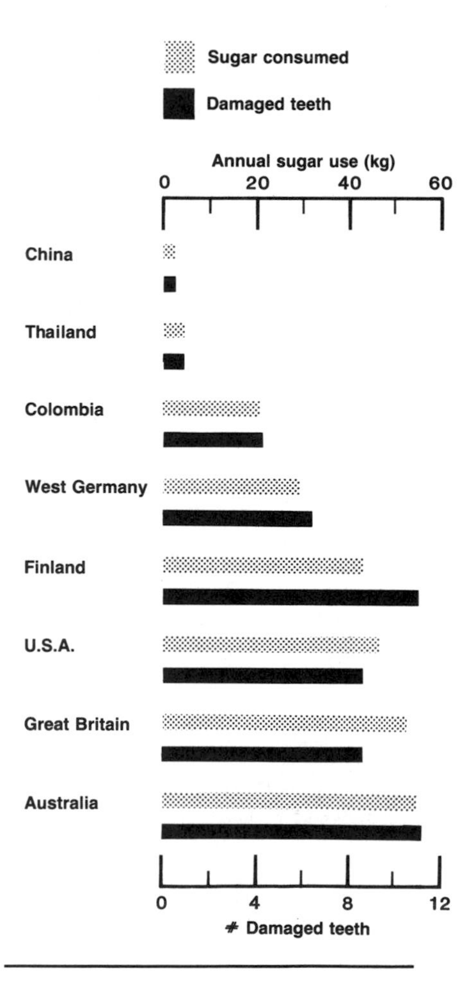

Figure 26.7
Correlation of sucrose consumption and the incidence of dental caries.

sugar. Lactose is the principal sugar found in milk. Maltose is not a naturally occurring sugar but is a product of enzymic digestion of polysaccharides. It is found in significant quantities in beer and malt liquors. Whereas simple carbohydrates generally have a sweet taste, the intensity of the sweetness varies widely (Figure 26.6).

3. ***Polysaccharides:*** Complex carbohydrates are composed of polysaccharides, most often polymers of glucose, and do not have a sweet taste. Starch is an example of a complex carbohydrate that is found in abundance in plants (see p. 51). Common sources include wheat and other grains, potatoes, dried peas and beans (legumes), and vegetables.

4. ***Fiber:*** Dietary fiber is a family of nondigestible carbohydrates, including cellulose, lignin, and pectin. Dietary fiber provides no energy but has several beneficial effects. First, it adds bulk to the diet. Fiber can absorb 10 to 15 times its own weight in water, drawing fluid into the lumen of the intestine and increasing bowel motility. Second, the binding properties of fiber can result in decreased absorption of toxic compounds, including certain carcinogens. Also, fiber in the diet decreases the risk for ***diverticulosis*** and ***colon cancer.*** However, dietary fiber can bind trace elements (e.g., Zn^{+2}) and decrease the absorption of fat-soluble vitamins. Thus supplementation of the diet with excess fiber is not recommended; rather, moderate amounts of fiber should be obtained naturally from whole-grain cereals and breads, fruits, and legumes.

5. ***Requirements for carbohydrate:*** Carbohydrate is not an essential nutrient, since the carbon skeletons of amino acids can be converted into glucose (see pp. 129 and 239). However, the absence of dietary carbohydrate leads to (1) ketone body production and (2) an excessive degradation of body protein, whose constituent amino acids provide carbon skeletons required for gluconeogenesis.

6. ***Simple sugars and disease:*** There is no direct evidence that the consumption of simple sugars is harmful. Contrary to folklore, diets high in sucrose do not lead to diabetes or hypoglycemia (see p. 272 for a discussion of hypoglycemia). However, some individuals do transiently show the symptoms of hypoglycemia (sweating, weakness, hunger, tachycardia) in response to the consumption of simple sugars (see p. 272). This "reactive" hypoglycemia is rare and typically results from abnormalities in the release of insulin in response to ingested sugar. In the absence of other disease processes (e.g., a pancreatic tumor), treatment consists of minimizing simple sugars in the diet. Also contrary to popular belief, carbohydrates are not inherently fattening. They yield 4 cal/g (the same as protein and less than half that of fat; see Figure 26.3) and will result in fat synthesis only when consumed in excess of the body's energy needs. However, it is well established that the incidence of dental caries shows a strong correlation with the amount of sucrose consumed (Figure 26.7). Further, foods high in sucrose tend to lack essential nutrients and contribute "empty calories" to the diet.

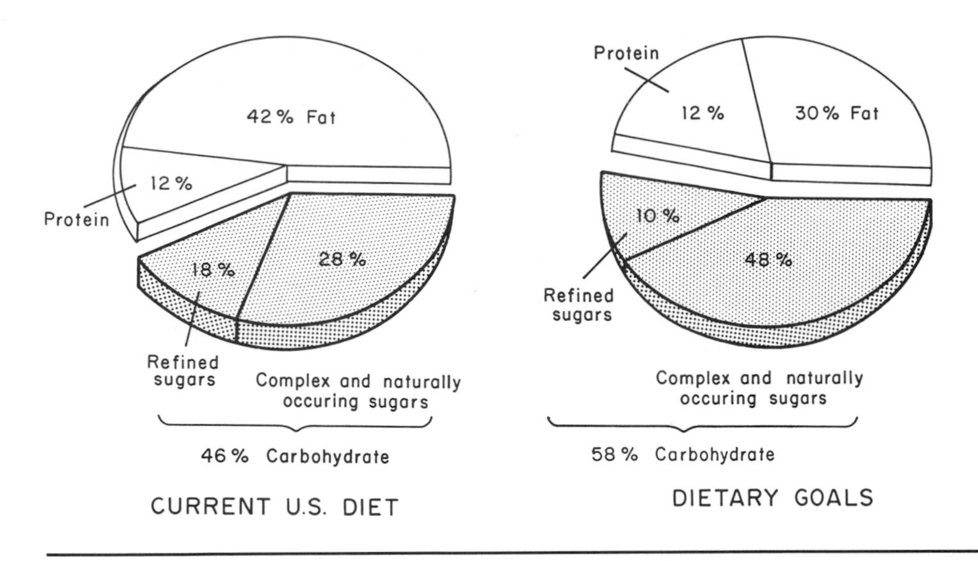

Figure 26.8
Current and recommended contribution of carbohydrate to the total caloric intake.

7. ***Dietary goals:*** Dietary goals designed to decrease diet-related disease in the U.S. population have been developed by various academic groups and government agencies. Although differing in detail, most of these plans are similar to the widely accepted recommendations of the U.S. Senate Select Committee on Nutrition and Human Needs. These dietary goals call for an increase in carbohydrate intake from the present 46% of total calories to 58%, most of which should be supplied by complex carbohydrate (Figure 26.8).

B. Fat

1. ***Triacylglycerol:*** The most important class of dietary fats from an energy perspective is triacylglycerol, constituting more than 90% of total dietary lipid. These compounds also supply the essential fatty acids required by the body.
2. ***Fats from plant sources:*** Triacylglycerols obtained from plants generally contain more unsaturated fatty acids than those from animals (Figure 26.9). Coconut oil and palm oil are exceptions in that these vegetable oils are primarily saturated. Unsaturated fatty acids found in food lipids may be monounsaturated or polyunsaturated and, in general, are liquid at room temperature. Corn oil, soybean oil, and olive oil are examples of unsaturated oils. Margarine is almost always made from pure vegetable oil but is subjected to varying degrees of hydrogenation or saturation to make it more solid and stable as a spread.
3. ***Fat from animal sources:*** Triacylglycerols obtained from animals generally contain a higher proportion of ***saturated fat*** than do those contained in plants, with the exception of fish, whose fat is largely unsaturated.
4. ***Requirements for dietary fat:*** Dietary fat provides the ***essential fatty acids*** (EFA), ***linoleic acid,*** and ***linolenic acid. Arachidonic acid*** becomes

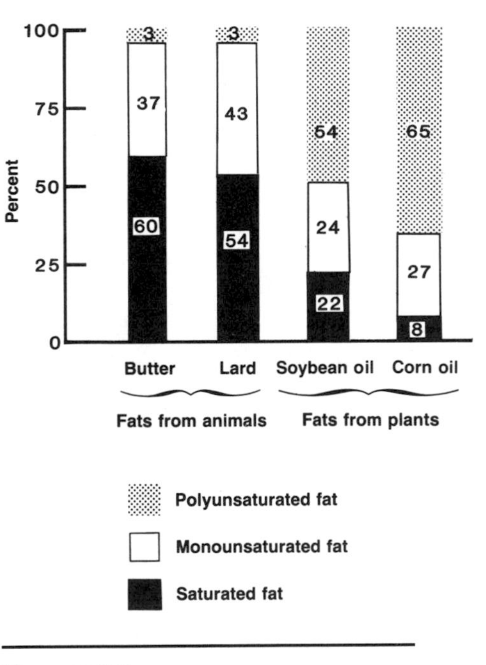

Figure 26.9
Composition of commonly encountered dietary lipids.

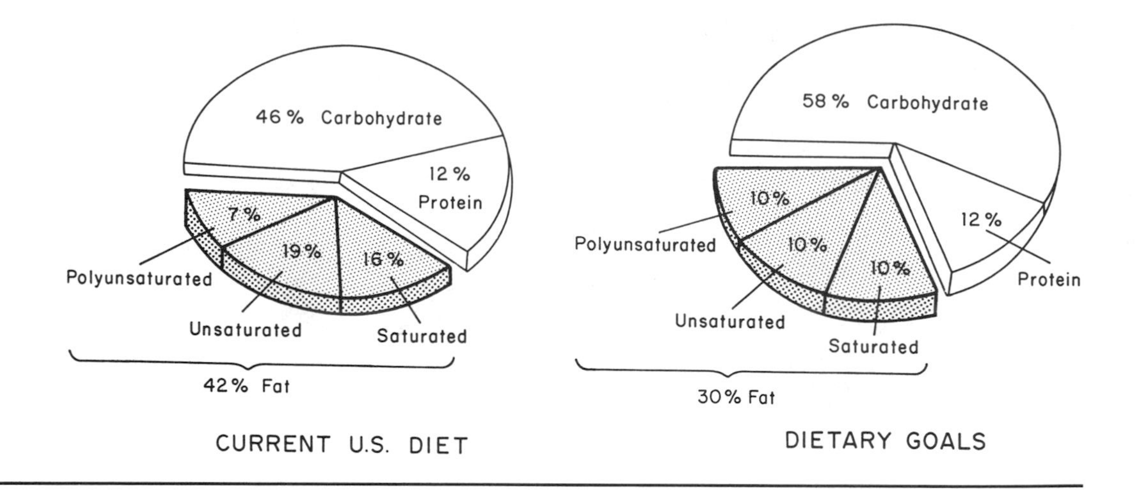

Figure 26.10
Current and recommended contribution of fat to the daily caloric intake.

essential if there is an insufficient amount of linoleic acid, from which it is synthesized, in the diet (see p. 160). The EFAs are required for the fluidity of membrane structure and for prostaglandin synthesis (see p. 175). In addition, dietary fat increases the palatability of food, producing a feeling of satiety. The presence of fat in the diet is also required for the absorption of fat-soluble vitamins.

5. ***Essential fatty acid deficiency:*** A deficiency of essential fatty acids is characterized by scaly dermatitis, hair loss, and poor wound healing. Because EFAs are widely distributed in nature, a deficiency is rare. Synthetic diets should include about 2% of calories as linoleic acid.

6. ***Dietary goals:*** The U.S. Senate Select Committee on Nutrition and Human Needs recommends a reduction in fat consumption, particularly saturated fats; cholesterol consumption should be cut in half from the current average intake of 600 mg/day to 300 mg/day (Figure 26.10).

C. Protein

1. Humans have no dietary requirement for protein, per se; rather the protein in food provides ***essential amino acids*** that cannot be synthesized by humans (see Chapter 21). These amino acids are used for the synthesis of tissue protein and as precursors for the synthesis of nonprotein compounds.

2. ***Essential amino acids:*** Ten of the 20 amino acids needed for the synthesis of body proteins are essential, that is, they cannot be synthesized in man at an adequate rate (see p. 241). Of these ten, eight are essential at all times, whereas two are required only during periods of rapid tissue growth characteristic of childhood. Figure 26.11 shows the requirement for the essential amino acids.

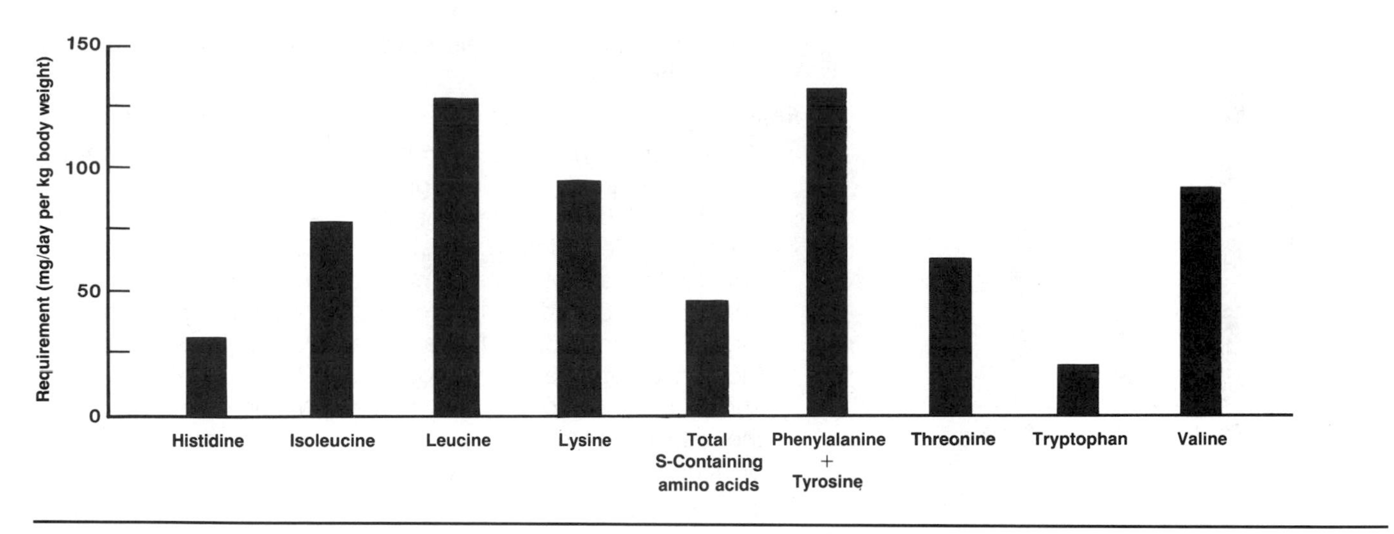

Figure 26.11
Requirements for the essential amino acids in humans.

3. ***Biological value of proteins***

   a. The biological value of a dietary protein is a measure of its ability to provide the essential amino acids required for tissue maintenance. Proteins from animal sources (meat, poultry, milk, fish) have a high biological value because they contain all the essential amino acids in the proportions similar to those required for synthesis of human tissue proteins (Figure 26.12).

   b. Proteins from plant sources (wheat, corn, rice, beans) typically have a lower biological value than animal proteins. However, proteins from different plant sources may be combined in such a way that the result is equivalent in nutritional value to animal protein. For example, corn (lysine-deficient but methionine-rich) may be combined with kidney beans (methionine-poor but lysine-rich) to produce a complete protein of high biological value. Thus, eating foods with different limiting amino acids at the same meal results in a dietary combination with a higher biological value than either of the component proteins (Figure 26.13). The ***limiting amino acid*** is defined as the essential amino acid present in the lowest amount compared with the optimal amount required.

Source	Biological value
Animal proteins	
Eggs	100
Beef	100
Fish	87
Milk	85
Plant proteins	
Soybean meal	67
Potatoes	67
Whole wheat bread	30

Figure 26.12
Biological value of some common dietary proteins.

4. ***Nitrogen balance:*** Nitrogen balance occurs when the amount of nitrogren consumed ***equals*** the nitrogen excreted in the urine, sweat, and feces. Most healthy adults are normally in nitrogen balance.

   a. ***Positive nitrogen balance:*** Positive nitrogen balance occurs when nitrogen intake exceeds nitrogen excretion. It is observed in situations in which tissue growth occurs, for example, in children, pregnancy, or during recovery from an emaciating illness.

   b. ***Negative nitrogen balance:*** Negative nitrogen balance occurs when nitrogen losses are greater than nitrogen intake. It is associated with inadequate dietary protein, lack of an essential amino

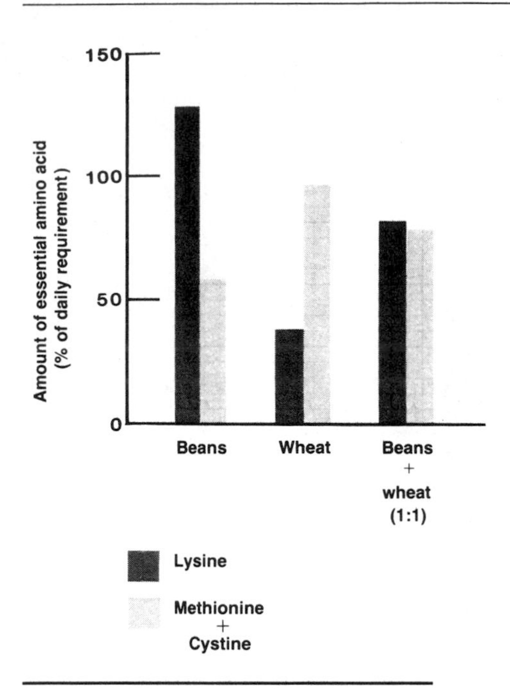

Figure 26.13
Combining two incomplete proteins that have complementary amino acid deficiencies results in a mixture with a higher biological value.

acid, or during physiologic stresses such as trauma, burns, illness, or surgery.

5. ***Requirement for protein in humans***
   a. The amount of dietary protein that is required in the diet varies with its ***biological value***. The greater the proportion of animal protein included in the diet, the less protein is required. Recommended Dietary Allowance (RDA) for protein is computed in terms of proteins of mixed biological value at 0.8 gram per kilogram of body weight for adults, or about 56 g of protein for a 70-kg individual. There is no physiologic advantage to the consumption of more protein than the RDA. Protein consumed in excess of the body's needs will be deaminated and the resulting carbon skeletons metabolized to provide energy or acetyl CoA for fatty acid synthesis.
   b. The dietary protein requirement is influenced by the carbohydrate content of the diet. When the intake of carbohydrate is low, amino acids are deaminated to provide carbon skeletons for the synthesis of glucose for use as a fuel by the central nervous system. If carbohydrate intake is less than 150 g a day, substantial amounts of protein will be metabolized to provide precursors for gluconeogenesis. Therefore, carbohydrate is considered to be "protein-sparing" because it allows amino acids to be used for repair and maintenance of tissue protein rather than for gluconeogenesis.
6. ***Dietary recommendations:*** The U.S. Senate Select Committee on Nutrition and Human Needs has called for protein consumption to be maintained at the present level of 12% of total calories (Figure 26.14).

V. CHOLESTEROL

Cholesterol performs a number of vital functions in the body, such as providing essential components of cell membranes and serving as a precursor of bile acids, steroid hormones, and vitamin D (see pp. 204, 219, and 326). However, when present in excess in the blood, cholesterol can pose a serious threat to health. For example, cholesterol is a principal ingredient in lipid-containing plaques that can be deposited in the walls of arteries. These lipid deposits can accumulate until they block the normal flow of blood.

A. Blood cholesterol and atherosclerosis

1. Individuals with elevated levels of blood cholesterol have a high incidence of ***atherosclerosis,*** a chronic disease in which deposits of cholesterol, cholesterol esters, and cellular debris accumulate on the inner surfaces of the large and medium-sized arteries (Figure 26.15). As the disease progresses, the deposits reduce or even stop the flow of blood. The cells normally irrigated by the affected artery are deprived of oxygen and nutrients and rapidly die. If this interruption of blood flow occurs in an artery of the heart, a ***myocardial infarction,*** or ***heart attack,*** occurs. As a result, part of the heart muscle becomes nonfunctional and death may result.

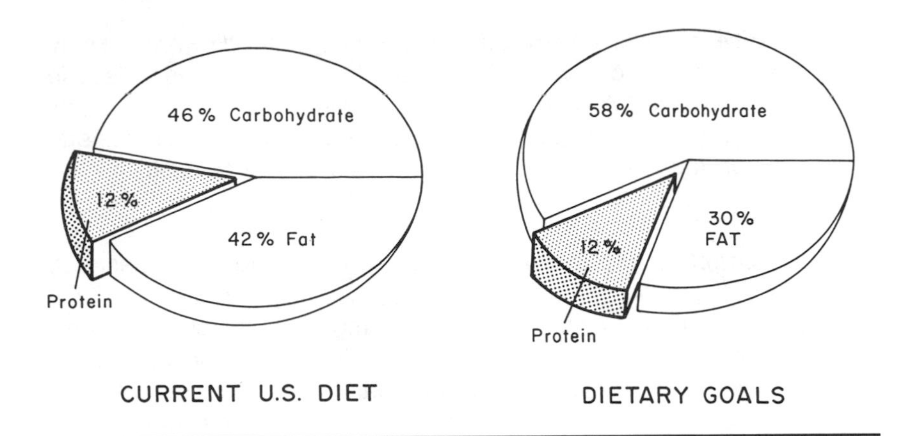

Figure 26.14
Current and recommended contribution of protein to the daily caloric intake.

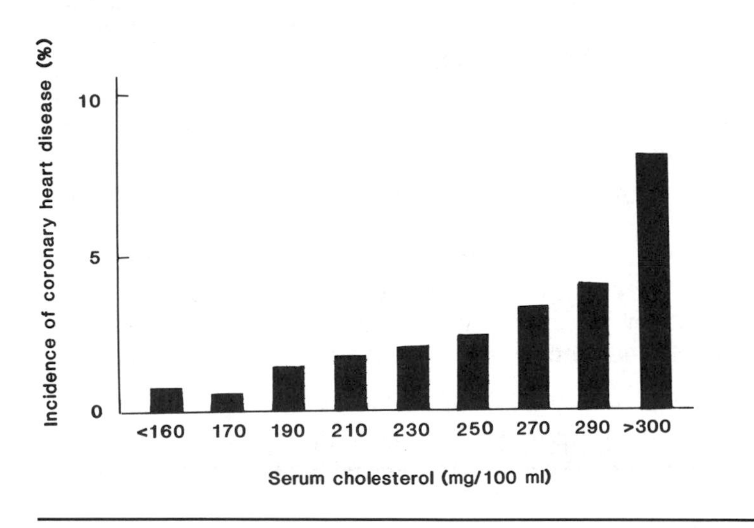

Figure 26.15
Correlation of deaths caused by coronary heart disease and blood cholesterol.

2. Although there is an association of high total plasma cholesterol with heart disease, a much stronger correlation exists between the levels of ***LDL-cholesterol*** in the blood and heart disease; approximately 80% of the cholesterol in the blood is carried as LDL (see p. 213). In contrast, high levels of HDL cholesterol have been associated with a ***decreased*** risk for heart disease. Obese, inactive individuals tend to have higher levels of LDL, whereas athletes have higher levels of HDL. In general, women have higher levels of HDL than men, which may, in part, account for the lower incidence of heart disease in women. (See p. 208 for a discussion of these serum lipoproteins.)
3. Although there is clearly an association between blood cholesterol levels and heart disease, it remains an open question as to whether the reduction of blood cholesterol can actually reduce heart disease. However, it has recently been shown that ***choles-***

tyramine, a cholesterol-lowering drug, substantially lowers not only blood cholesterol levels, but also the incidence of heart disease in middle-aged men who started out with very high cholesterol levels. These results strongly suggest that lowering of cholesterol through modification of the diet may also be beneficial.

B. Blood cholesterol and diet

1. ***Influence of dietary cholesterol:*** All tissues can synthesize cholesterol. Thus this lipid is not an essential nutrient. In addition, the average American ingests about 600 mg of cholesterol each day. This cholesterol from the diet causes a decrease in the rate of cholesterol synthesis by the tissues, particularly the liver. However, the reduction in cholesterol formation in response to ingested cholesterol does not fully compensate for the increased dietary intake. As a result, the levels of cholesterol in the blood are often elevated by diets high in cholesterol and are decreased 10% to 20% when low cholesterol diets are consumed. Thus, it is important to identify and limit foods that are rich in cholesterol. For example, cholesterol is found only in foods from animal sources. Certain foods such as egg yolks and organ meats are very rich in cholesterol. In contrast, plant products, including margarine and vegetable oils, contain no cholesterol.
2. ***Influence of dietary fats:*** The amount of cholesterol in the blood is also influenced by the amounts and kinds of fats consumed. For example, diets rich in triacylglycerols that contain saturated fatty acids tend to raise blood cholesterol levels, whereas polyunsaturated fats in the diet lead to reduced circulating levels of cholesterol. The mechanism for these effects is not known.

VI. PROTEIN-CALORIE MALNUTRITION

A. Occurrence

1. ***Developed countries:*** In the developed countries, protein-calorie malnutrition is seen most frequently in hospital patients with chronic illness or in individuals who suffer from major trauma, severe infection, or the effects of major surgery. Such highly catabolic patients frequently require intravenous administration of nutrients.
2. ***Underdeveloped countries:*** Inadequate intake of protein or energy is commonly observed in the populations of developing countries. Affected individuals show a variety of symptoms, including a depressed immune system with a reduced ability to resist infection. Death from secondary infection is common. Two extreme forms of malnutrition are kwashiorkor and marasmus.

B. Kwashiorkor

1. Kwashiorkor is a disease caused by an ***inadequate intake of protein*** in the presence of adequate intake of calories.
2. Kwashiorkor is frequently seen in children after weaning at about 1 year of age when their diet is shifted to predominantly carbohydrates. Typical symptoms include edema, skin lesions, de-

pigmented hair, anorexia, enlarged fatty liver, and decreased serum albumin.

3. Edema results from the lack of adequate serum proteins to maintain the distribution of water between blood and tissues. A child with kwashiorkor will frequently show a deceptively plump belly caused by edema.

C. Marasmus

1. Marasmus, also known as protein calorie malnutrition, results from a ***chronic deficiency of calories*** and can occur in the presence of adequate intake of protein.
2. Marasmus usually occurs in children under 1 year of age when the mothers' breast milk is supplemented with thin watery gruels of native cereals which are usually deficient in protein and calories. Typical symptoms include arrested growth, extreme muscle wasting (emaciation), weakness, and anemia.
3. Victims of marasmus do not show the edema or changes in serum proteins observed in kwashiorkor.

VII. MINERALS

Minerals are ***inorganic*** elements that serve a variety of functions such as cofactors in enzyme-catalyzed reactions, in the regulation of acid–base balance, in nerve conduction and muscle irritability, and as structural elements in the body. Each mineral is required in specific amounts ranging from micrograms to grams per day (see Figure 26.2). Some of the more important of these are calcium, phosphorus, sodium, potassium, and iron.

A. Calcium and phosphorus

1. Calcium and phosphorus are the ***most abundant*** minerals in the body. Calcium exists in two forms that have quite different functions. Most of the calcium in the body is found as calcium phosphate crystals in the bones and teeth, forming the cement that contributes to the physical strength of these structures. Calcium is also found in an unbound ionic form (Ca^{+2}) that performs critical functions in muscle contraction, nerve impulse transmission, ion transport, and transmission of signals across membranes. The concentration of extracellular calcium is tightly regulated.
2. A ***fall*** in the extracellular calcium levels triggers the release of ***parathyroid hormone*** (PTH), which increases the absorption of calcium from the glomerular filtrate in the kidney and decreases the absorption of phosphate. PTH also increases the synthesis of ***1,25-dihydroxycholecalciferol,*** the active form of vitamin D (see p. 328). In turn, 1,25-dihydroxycholecalciferol stimulates release of calcium from bone and increases the active transport of calcium from the intestine to the blood.
3. A ***rise*** in the extracellular calcium levels triggers the secretion of ***calcitonin*** by specialized cells found among the follicular cells of the thyroid gland (see p. 327). Calcitonin decreases the resorption

of bone and increases the loss of both calcium and phosphate ions in the urine.

4. A chronic deficiency in dietary calcium appears to accelerate the net loss of bone mass seen in most individuals after the age of about 35. This resorption of bone, which is often pronounced in postmenopausal women and in the elderly, can lead to ***osteoporosis***. Osteoporosis is characterized by frequent bone fractures, which are a major cause of disability among the elderly. Although treatment of the disease is controversial, recent evidence suggests that dietary calcium in excess of the RDA of 800 mg/day may be beneficial. The current average calcium intake for postmenopausal women in the United States is 540 mg/day.
5. Dietary calcium can be obtained from milk, milk products, and calcium supplements, typically in the form of $CaCO_3$, calcium gluconate, or calcium lactate.

B. Sodium, potassium, and chloride

1. Sodium, potassium, and chloride function together to regulate pH and maintain the osmolarity of both the intracellular and extracellular fluid.
2. Although a dietary supply of sodium is essential for life, the RDA has not been established. However, a deficiency of sodium is not a public health problem because Americans daily consume about 12 g of salt (NaCl)—about 8 g in food and 4 g from salt added at the table.
3. A complex relationship exists between sodium intake and ***hypertension*** (high blood pressure). Most of the U.S. population appears not to be genetically predisposed to hypertension. Of the remaining population who may develop high blood pressure, about a third respond with a decrease in blood pressure when the sodium in the diet is reduced. However, no causal relationship has been shown between hypertension and the consumption of sodium at levels found in the typical American diet.

C. Iron

1. Most of the iron in the body is found either in the heme component of hemeproteins (mostly hemoglobin, p. 21, and cytochromes, p. 105) or in storage forms (ferritin and hemosiderin). Serum iron and the various iron-containing enzymes represent less than 1% of total body iron.
2. A deficiency of iron causes a reduction in the rate of hemoglobin synthesis and ultimately can result in ***iron-deficiency anemia***. Iron deficiency is most commonly seen in premenopausal women as a result of blood loss during menstruation and in men with undetected bleeding from the gastrointestinal tract. Iron deficiency can also be caused by a diet poor in iron or by impaired intestinal absorption of iron.
3. The total iron content of the diet is not a reliable indicator of the adequacy of the diet, since the availability of dietary iron depends on the nature of the diet, particularly whether iron is present as heme-iron (more rapidly absorbed) or non-heme-iron (less rapidly absorbed). Iron deficiency is treated by the addition of any of

several ferrous salts (such as ferrous sulfate, ferrous gluconate, or ferrous fumarate) to the diet.

Study Questions

Answer A if 1, 2, and 3 are correct
B if 1 and 3 are correct
C if 2 and 4 are correct
D if only 4 is correct
E if all are correct

26.1 Kwashiorkor

1. is characterized by growth retardation, anemia, hypoproteinemia, edema, and fatty infiltration of the liver.
2. symptoms respond therapeutically to a high protein diet containing meat and milk products.
3. affects populations largely dependent on cereals and grains or other products of low biological value.
4. is a disease observed primarily in highly developed industrial areas.

26.2 You are to design a new formula diet "Ultima Plus!," taking into account established nutritional guidelines. Which of the following statements about the composition of "Ultima Plus!" is INCORRECT?

1. The quantity of protein should be 0.8 g/kg/day, or about 50 to 75 g/day.
2. About 30% of calories should come from fat.
3. A 100 g/day of carbohydrate should be included to avoid ketosis.
4. To maintain the weight of a normally active 70-kg individual, the formula should contain 1200 to 1500 calories per day.

26.3 Given the information that a 70-kg man is consuming a daily average of 275 g of carbohydrate, 75 g of protein, and 65 g of lipid, one can draw the following conclusions:

1. Total energy intake per day is about 3000 kcal.
2. About 30% of the calories are derived from lipid.
3. The diet does not contain a sufficient amount of dietary fiber.
4. The proportions of carbohydrate, protein, and lipid in the diet conform to the recommendations of the Senate Select Committee on Nutrition.

Vitamins

27

I. OVERVIEW

Vitamins are ***organic compounds*** required by the body in trace amounts to perform specific cellular functions. They cannot be synthesized by humans, and therefore must be supplied by the diet. Nine vitamins (thiamine, riboflavin, pyridoxine, cyanocobalamin, niacin, pantothenic acid, biotin, folic acid, and ascorbic acid) are classified as ***water-soluble***, while four vitamins (vitamins A, D, E, and K) are termed ***fat-soluble***. Many of the water-soluble vitamins provide cofactors for the enzymes of intermediary metabolism (Figure 27.1). Except as noted, the water-soluble vitamins are not toxic, and the amounts stored in the body are usually small. When ingested in excess of the body's needs, they are readily excreted in the urine, and therefore must be continually supplied in the diet. In contrast, significant quantities of the fat-soluble vitamins are stored in the liver and adipose tissue and can accumulate to toxic levels. The fat-soluble vitamins are digested, absorbed, and transported with the fat in the diet and are not readily excreted in the urine.

II. THIAMINE (VITAMIN B_1)

A. Structure of thiamine pyrophosphate

1. ***Thiamine pyrophosphate*** (TPP) is the biologically active form of the vitamin, formed by the transfer of a pyrophosphate group from ATP to thiamine (Figure 27.2).

B. Functions of thiamine pyrophosphate

1. TPP serves as a cofactor in the ***oxidative decarboxylation*** of α-keto acids (see pp. 131, 137, 244 and Figure 27.1).
2. TPP is also required as a cofactor in the formation or degradation of α-ketols by *transketolase* (see p. 146 and Figure 27.1).

C. Distribution of thiamine

1. Pork, whole grains, and legumes are the richest sources of thiamine. Outer layers of seeds are particularly rich in thiamine. Thus, whole wheat bread is a good source of the vitamin, whereas white bread prepared from milled grain is low in thiamine.

D. Requirement for thiamine

1. The requirement for thiamine increases with the caloric intake. The RDA is 0.5 mg for each 1000 kcal in the diet, or about

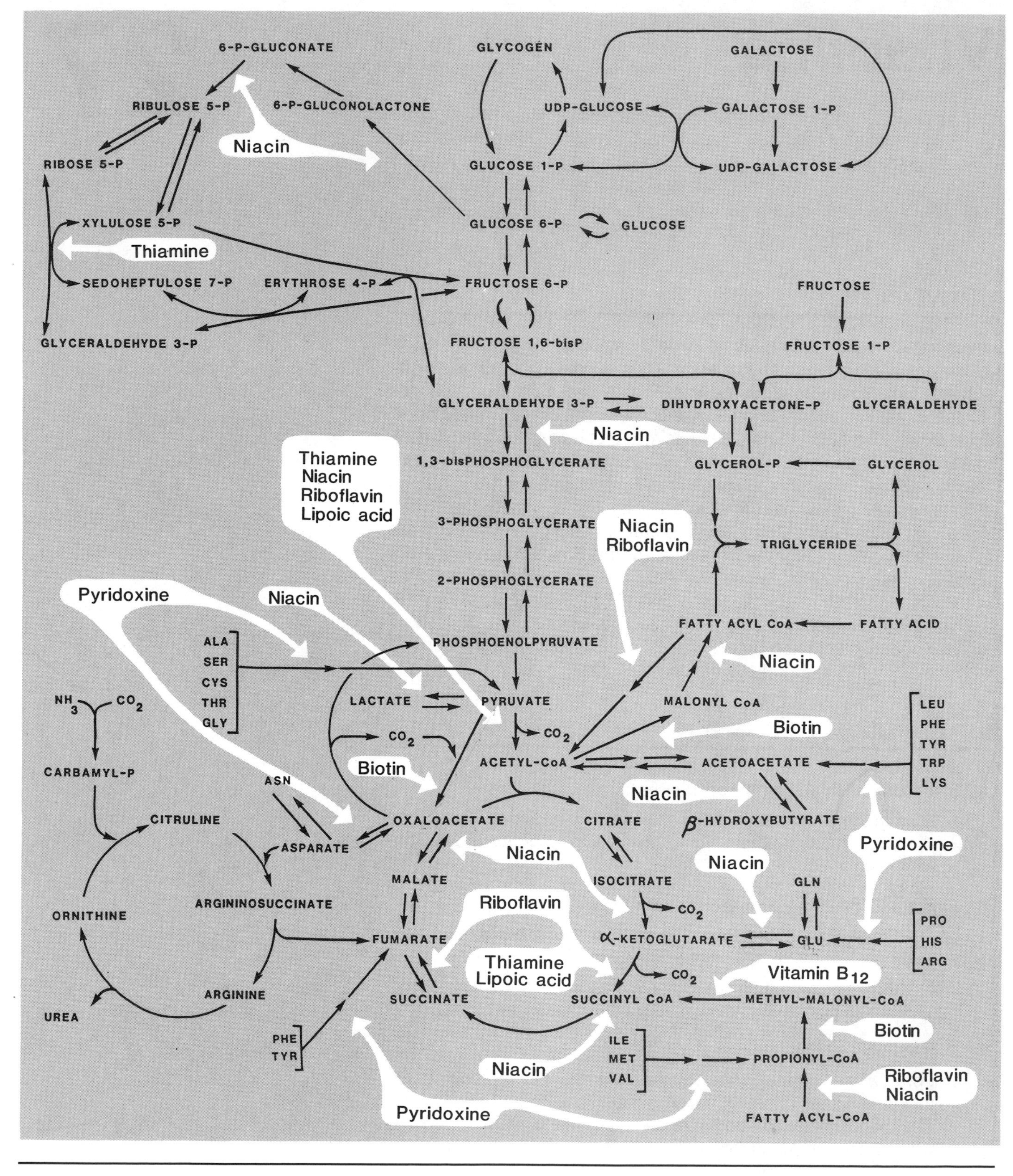

Figure 27.1
Summary of reactions involving cofactors derived from water-soluble vitamins.

1.5 mg for the normal adult male. A minimum of 1 mg/day is recommended for adults and the elderly, even when the energy intake is less than 2000 kcal. The thiamine content of a typical American diet is marginal, providing less than 0.8 mg/day

2. The requirement for thiamine increases in individuals who consume a high carbohydrate diet or who have elevated metabolic needs because of pregnancy, lactation, fever, or hyperthyroidism.

E. Thiamine deficiency

1. The oxidation of pyruvate and α-ketoglutarate plays a key role in ***energy metabolism*** of most tissues. In thiamine deficiency the activity of these two dehydrogenase reactions is decreased, resulting in a decreased production of ATP, and thus impaired cellular function.

2. ***Beri-beri:*** Beri-beri is a severe thiamine-deficiency syndrome found in areas where polished rice is the major component of the diet. Signs of infantile beri-beri include tachycardia, vomiting, convulsion, and, if not treated, death. The deficiency syndrome can have a rapid onset in nursing infants whose mothers are deficient in thiamine. Adult beri-beri is characterized by dry skin, irritability, disorderly thinking, and progressive paralysis.

3. ***Wernicke-Korsakoff syndrome:*** In the United States, thiamine deficiency is seen primarily in association with chronic alcoholism and is due to dietary insufficiency or impaired intestinal absorption of the vitamin. Some alcoholics develop the Wernicke–Korsakoff syndrome, a deficiency state characterized by apathy, loss of memory, and a rhythmical to-and-fro motion of the eyeballs. The condition is a medical emergency since coma, irreversible brain damage, and death can occur if the individual is not treated with intravenous thiamine.

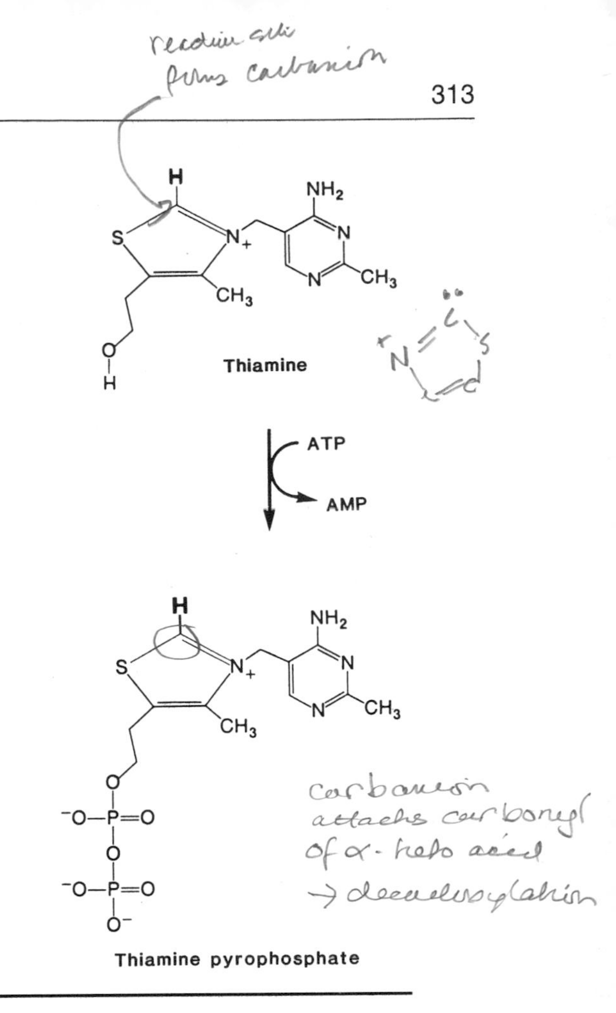

Figure 27.2
Structure of thiamine and its cofactor form, thiamine pyrophosphate.

III. RIBOFLAVIN (VITAMIN B_2)

A. Structure of riboflavin and its cofactor forms FAD and FMN

1. The two biologically active forms are ***flavin mononucleotide*** (FMN) and ***flavin adenine dinucleotide*** (FAD), formed by the transfer of an AMP moiety from ATP to FMN (Figure 27.3)

B. Functions of FMN and FAD

1. FMN and FAD are each capable of reversibly binding two hydrogen atoms, forming $FMNH_2$ or $FADH_2$. (Both flavin nucleotides accept hydrogen atoms at the positions shown on the isoalloxazine ring in Figure 27.4.)

2. FMN and FAD are bound tightly—sometimes covalently—to flavoenzymes that catalyze the oxidation or reduction of a substrate.

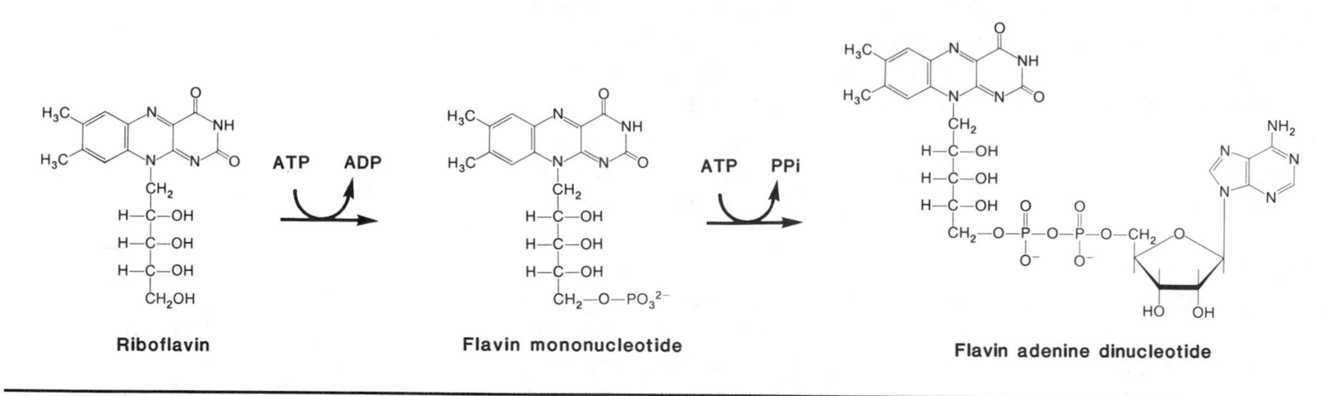

Figure 27.3
Structure and biosynthesis of flavin mononucleotide (FMN) and flavin adenine dinucleotide (FAD).

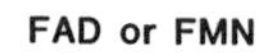

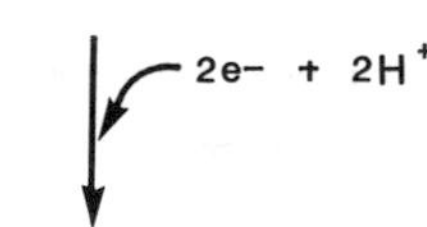

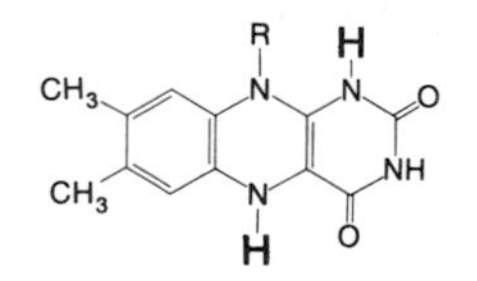

Figure 27.4
Reduction of FAD (or FMN) to $FADH_2$ (or $FMNH_2$).

C. Distribution of riboflavin

1. Milk, eggs, liver, and green leafy vegetables are good sources of riboflavin. Strict vegetarians who exclude milk from their diet may have a marginal intake of riboflavin. The vitamin is readily destroyed by ultraviolet components of sunlight.

D. Requirement for riboflavin

1. Riboflavin requirements are based on energy intake, that is, 0.6 mg/1000 kcal of dietary intake, or approximately 1.5 mg/day for normal adults. A minimum of 1.2 mg/day is recommended for adults and the elderly.

E. Deficiency of riboflavin

1. Riboflavin deficiency is not associated with a major human disease, although it frequently accompanies other vitamin deficiencies. Deficiency symptoms include dermatis, cheilosis (fissuring at the corners of the mouth), and glossitis (the tongue appearing smooth and purplish).

IV. NIACIN

A. Structure of niacin and its cofactor forms, NAD^+, and $NADP^+$

1. ***Niacin,*** or ***nicotinic acid,*** is a substituted pyridine derivative. The biologically active cofactor forms are ***nicotinamide adenine dinucleotide*** (NAD^+) and its phosphorylated derivative, ***nicotinamide adenine dinucleotide phosphate*** ($NADP^+$; see Figure 27.5).
2. ***Nicotinamide,*** a derivative of nicotinic acid that contains an amide instead of a carboxyl group, also occurs in the diet. Nicotinamide is readily deaminated in the body and therefore is nutritionally equivalent to nicotinic acid.

B. Functions of niacin

1. NAD^+ and $NADP^+$ serve as coenzymes in oxidation-reduction reactions in which the coenzyme undergoes reduction of the pyridine ring by accepting a hydride ion (hydrogen atom plus

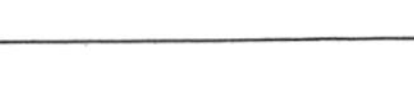

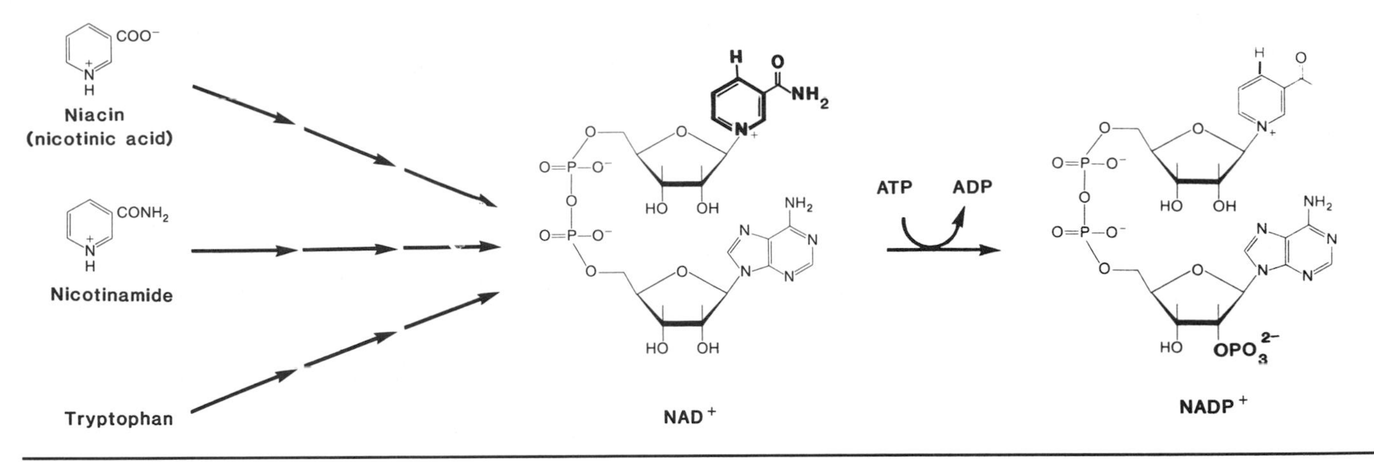

Figure 27.5
Structure and biosynthesis of NAD^+ and $NADP^+$.

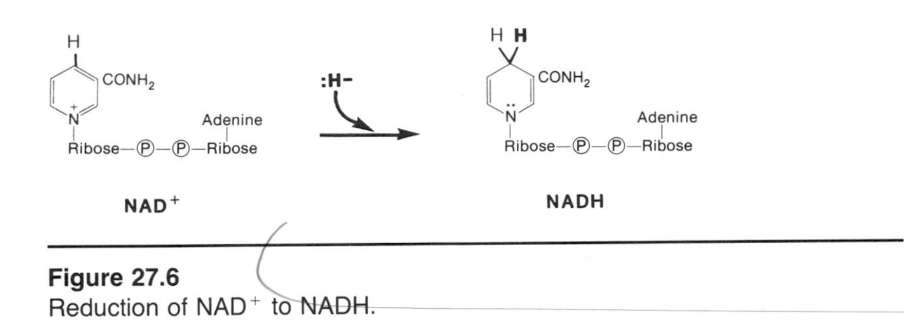

Figure 27.6
Reduction of NAD^+ to NADH.

one electron). The reduced forms of NAD^+ and $NADP^+$ are NADH and NADPH, respectively (Figure 27.6). NADH and NADPH can then be used to reduce substrates in other reactions.

2. Examples of pathways that require either the oxidized or reduced form of a niacin-containing cofactor include, among many others, glycolysis, gluconeogenesis, the tricarboxylic acid cycle, the hexose monophosphate pathway, and fatty acid synthesis and degradation.
3. These reduced nicotinamide-containing compounds show a characteristic absorption of light at 340 nm that is not observed with the oxidized cofactors (Figure 27.7). Therefore, the progress of a reaction involving NADH as a substrate or a product can be monitored by measuring the rate of increase or decrease of absorption at 340 nm of a reaction mixture.

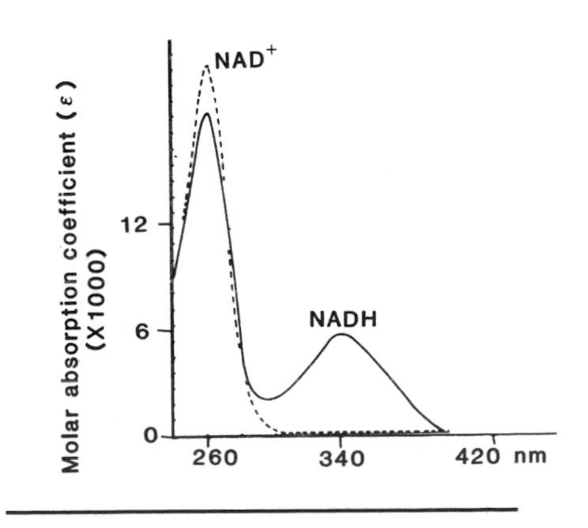

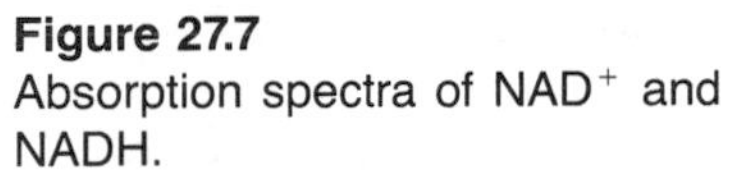

Figure 27.7
Absorption spectra of NAD^+ and NADH.

C. Distribution of niacin

1. Niacin is found in unrefined grains and cereal, milk, and lean meats, especially liver.
2. Limited quantities of niacin can also be obtained from the metabolism of tryptophan. The pathway is inefficient in that only about 1 mg of nicotinic acid is formed from 60 mg of tryptophan. Further, tryptophan is metabolized to niacin only when there is

a relative abundance of the amino acid, that is, after the needs for protein synthesis and energy production have been met.

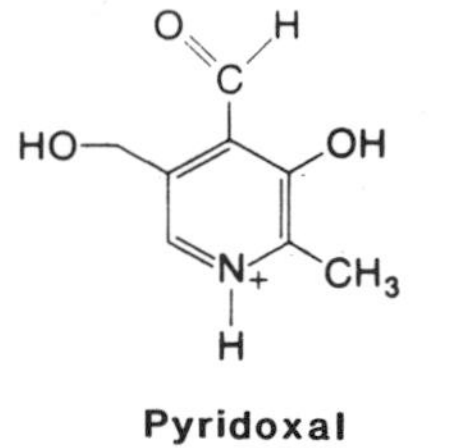

Pyridoxal

D. Requirement for niacin

1. The requirement for niacin is measured in niacin equivalents (NE) that take into account the contribution of dietary tryptophan as a source of niacin. One niacin equivalent is defined as 1 mg of niacin or 60 mg of tryptophan. Adults should ingest 13 NE/ 1000 kcal in the diet, or a minimum of 13 NE/day.

E. Deficiency of niacin

1. Deficiency of niacin causes ***pellagra,*** a disease involving the skin, gastrointestinal tract, and central nervous system. The symptoms of pellagra progress through the three D's: dermatitis, diarrhea, and dementia—and, if untreated, death.

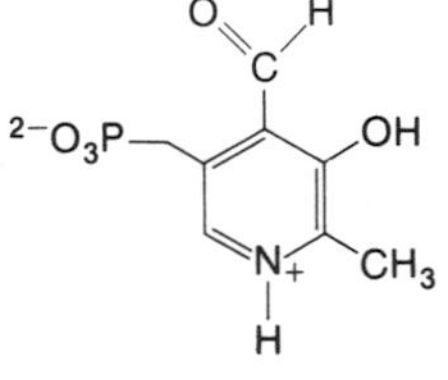

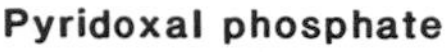
Pyridoxal phosphate

V. PYRIDOXINE (VITAMIN B_6)

A. Structure of pyridoxine and its cofactor form, pyridoxal phosphate

1. ***Vitamin B_6*** is a collective term for ***pyridoxine, pyridoxal,*** and ***pyridoxamine,*** all derivatives of pyridine, differing only in the nature of the functional group attached to the ring. Pyridoxine occurs primarily in plants, whereas pyridoxal and pyridoxamine are found in foods obtained from animals. All three compounds can serve as precursors of the biologically active coenzyme, ***pyridoxal phosphate.***

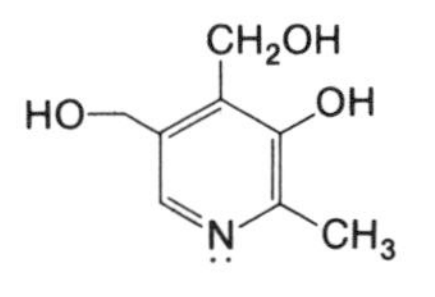

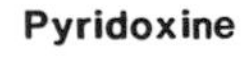
Pyridoxine

B. Functions of pyridoxine

1. Pyridoxal phosphate functions as a coenzyme for a large number of enzymes, particularly those that catalyze reactions involving amino acids.

Reaction type	Example
Transamination (p. 228)	Oxaloacetate + glutamate ⇄ aspartate + α-ketoglutarate
Deamination (p. 241)	Serine → pyruvate + NH_3
Decarboxylation (p. 261)	Histidine → histamine + CO_2
Condensation (p. 257)	Glycine + succinyl CoA → δ-amino-levulinic acid

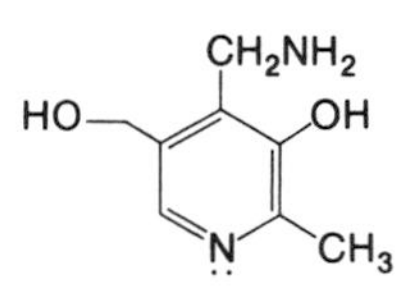

Pyridoxamine

C. Distribution of pyridoxine

1. Good sources of the vitamin are wheat, corn, egg yolk, liver, and muscle meats.

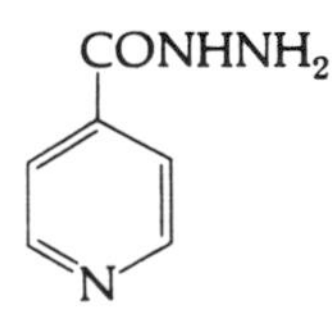

Isoniazid

D. Requirement for pyridoxine

1. The requirement for pyridoxine is increased by a high intake of protein. The RDA is 2.2 mg for adult men and 2.0 mg for adult women, based on an intake of approximately 100 g of protein per day.

E. Deficiency of pyridoxine

1. ***Isoniazid*** (isonicotinic acid hydrazide), a drug frequently used to treat tuberculosis, can induce a B_6 deficiency by forming an inactive derivative with pyridoxal phosphate.
2. Dietary deficiencies in pyridoxine are rare but have been observed in newborn infants fed formulas low in vitamin B_6, in women taking oral contraceptives, and in alcoholics. Although a deficiency of pyridoxine alone is rarely seen, inadequate supplies of the vitamin frequently accompany other vitamin deficiencies.

F. Toxicity of pyridoxine

1. Neurologic symptoms have been observed at intakes of greater than 2 g/day.

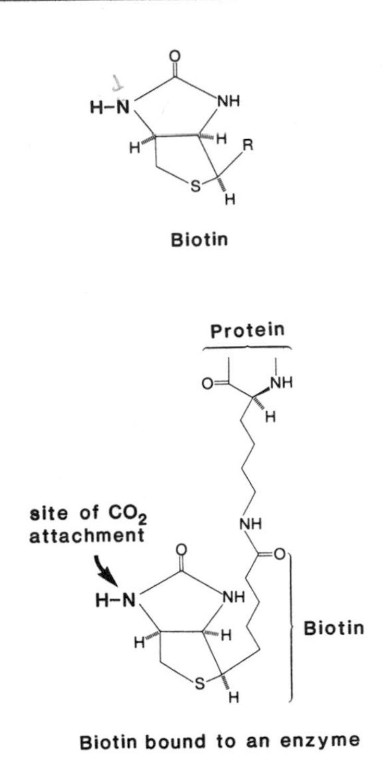

Figure 27.8
Structure of biotin and biotin covalently bound to a lysyl-residue of an enzyme.

VI. BIOTIN

A. Structure of biotin

1. Biotin is an imidazole derivative that in its biologically active form is covalently bound to the ε-amino groups of lysine residues of biotin-dependent apoenzymes (see p. 127 and Figure 27.8).

B. Function of biotin

1. Biotin is a cofactor in carboxylation reactions serving as a carrier of activated carbon dioxide (see Figure 27.1). (See p. 127 for the mechanism of biotin-dependent carboxylations.)

C. Distribution of biotin

1. Biotin is present in almost all foods, particularly liver, milk, and egg yolk.

D. Requirement for biotin

1. Adequate levels are estimated at 100 to 200 μg/day. Most American diets are adequate in biotin.

E. Deficiency of biotin

1. Biotin deficiency does not occur naturally because the vitamin is widely distributed in food. Also, a large percentage of the biotin requirement in humans is supplied by intestinal bacteria.
2. The addition of raw egg white to the diet as a source of protein will induce symptoms of biotin deficiency, namely, dermatitis, glossitis, loss of appetite, and nausea. Raw egg white contains a glycoprotein, ***avidin,*** that tightly binds biotin and prevents its absorption from the intestine. However, with a normal diet, it has been estimated that 20 eggs per day would be required to induce a deficiency syndrome. Thus, inclusion of an occasional raw egg in the diet is not harmful.

VII. FOLIC ACID

A. Structure of folic acid

1. Folic acid is composed of a ***pterin ring*** attached to a ***p-aminobenzoic acid*** (PABA) and conjugated with one or more glutamic acid

residues. Humans cannot synthesize PABA or attach the first glutamic acid (Figure 27.9).

2. The biologically active form of folic acid is ***tetrahydrofolic acid*** (THF), produced by the two-step reduction of folate by *dihydrofolate reductase* (Figure 27.9).

   a. *Dihydrofolate reductase* is competitively inhibited by ***methotrexate*** and ***aminopterin,*** folic acid analogues that have been used to effect the remission of acute leukemia in children (Figure 27.9).

   b. ***Sulfanilamide*** and its derivatives are structural analogues of p-aminobenzoic acid (Figure 27.9). These drugs competitively inhibit the synthesis of folic acid, and thereby decrease the synthesis of critical nucleotides needed for the replication of DNA and RNA. Sulfa drugs do not affect human DNA or RNA synthesis because mammalian cells cannot synthesize folic acid.

B. Function of folic acid

1. Tetrahydrofolic acid receives ***one-carbon fragments*** from donors such as serine, glycine, and histidine and transfers them to intermediates in the synthesis of amino acids (see p. 247), purines (see p. 347), and thymidylic acid—the characteristic pyrimidine of DNA (see p. 358).

C. Distribution of folic acid

1. Folic acid is found in green leafy vegetables, liver, lima beans, and whole grain cereals.

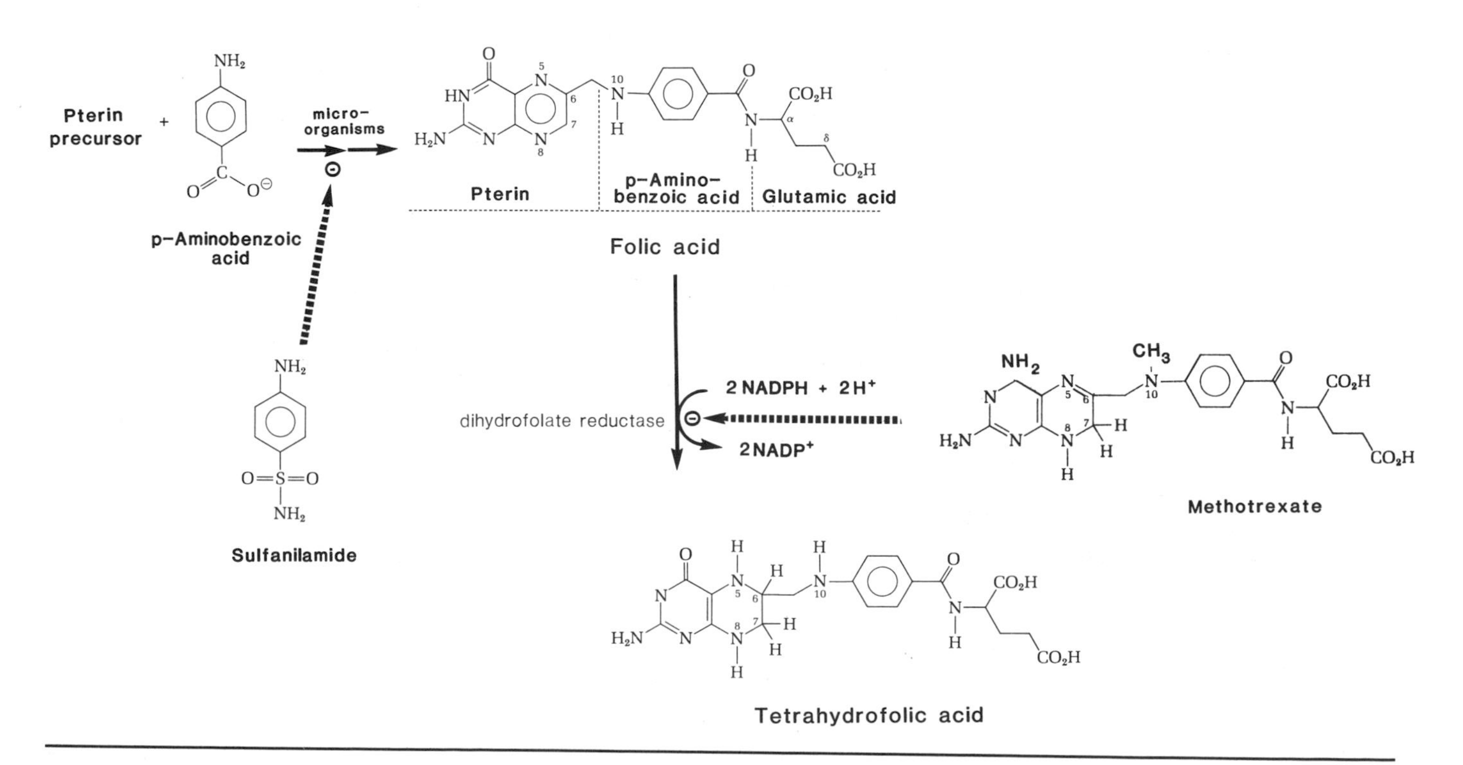

Figure 27.9
Conversion of folic acid to dihydrofolate and tetrahydrofolate.

D. Requirement for folic acid

1. The RDA for folic acid is 100 μg. Because of the role of folic acid in nucleic acid synthesis, its requirement increases during periods of rapid tissue growth; the RDA during pregnancy and lactation are 800 and 500 μg per day, respectively.

E. Deficiency of folic acid

1. Folic acid deficiency is characterized by growth failure and ***megaloblastic anemia***. The anemia is a result of diminished DNA synthesis that requires tetrahydrofolate derivatives. Folic acid deficiency is probably the most common vitamin deficiency in the United States, particularly among pregnant women and alcoholics.

VIII. COBALAMIN (VITAMIN B_{12})

CO B ALT

A. Structure of cobalamin and its cofactor forms

1. ***Cobalamin*** contains a ***corrin ring system*** that differs from the porphyrins in that two of the pyrrole rings are linked directly rather than through a methene bridge. ***Cobalt*** is held in the center of the corrin ring by four coordinate bonds from the nitrogens of the pyrrole groups. The remaining coordinate bonds of the cobalt are with the nitrogen of 5,6-dimethylbenzimidazole and with cyanide in commercial preparations of the vitamin, producing ***cyanocobalamin*** (Figure 27.10).

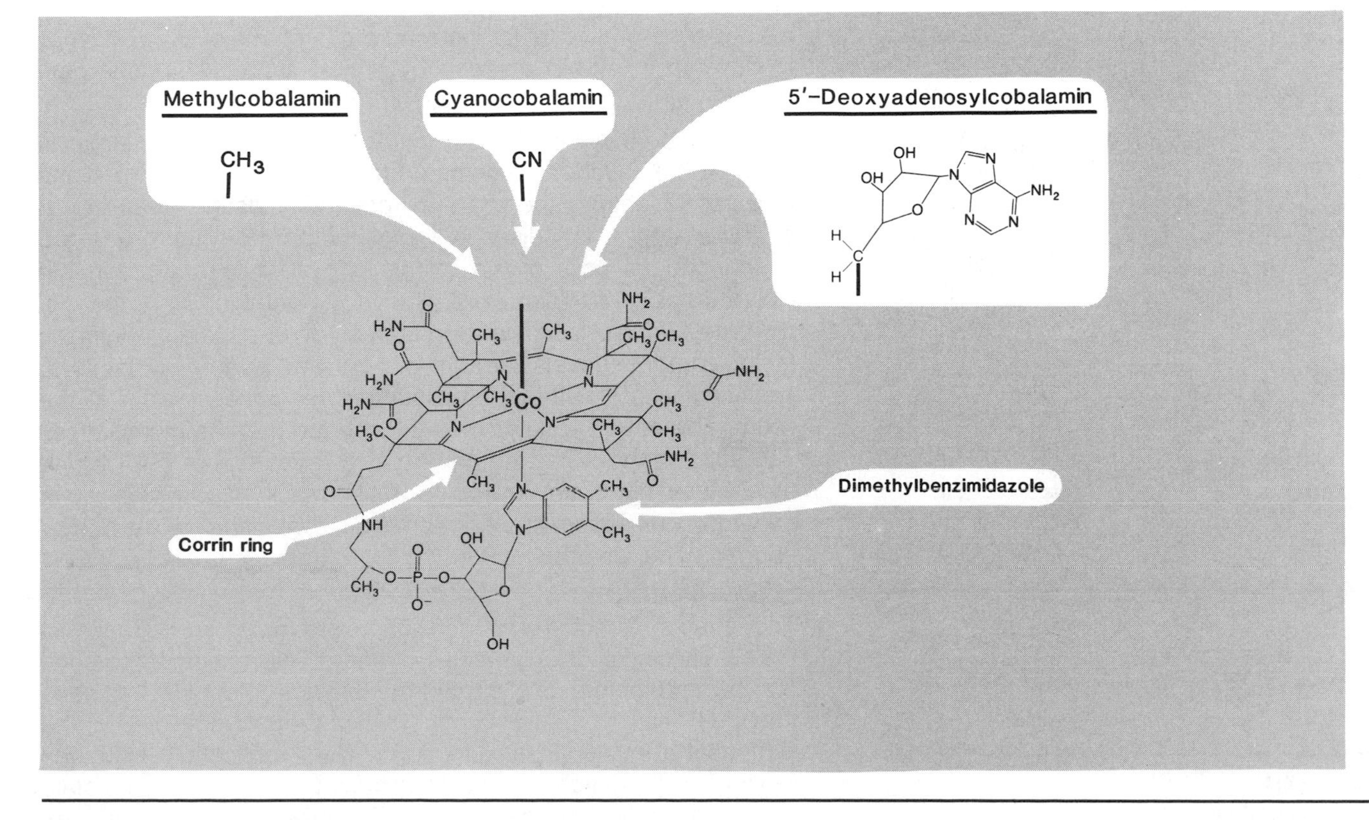

Figure 27.10
Structure of cobalamin and its coenzyme forms.

2. The ***coenzyme forms*** of cobalamin are ***5′-deoxyadenosylcobalamin***, in which cyanide is replaced with 5′-deoxyadenosine (forming an unusual carbon-cobalt bond), and ***methylcobalamin,*** in which cyanide is replaced by a methyl group (Figure 27.10).

B. Functions of cobalamin

1. In humans, only two reactions are known to require cobalamin coenzymes:
   a. The synthesis of methionine from homocysteine requires methylcobalamin (see p. 243).
   b. The rearrangement of carbon atoms in methylmalonyl CoA to produce succinyl CoA requires deoxyadenosylcobalamin (see p. 173).

C. Distribution of cobalamin

1. Vitamin B_{12} is synthesized only by microorganisms; it is not present in plants. Animals obtain the vitamin preformed from their natural bacterial flora or by eating foods derived from other animals. Cobalamin is present in appreciable amounts in liver, whole milk, eggs, oysters, fresh shrimp, pork, and chicken.

D. Requirement for cobalamin

1. The RDA is 3 μg/day, increasing to approximately 6 μg/day during pregnancy and lactation.

E. Deficiency of cobalamin

1. In contrast to other water-soluble vitamins, significant amounts (4–5 mg) of vitamin B_{12} are stored in the body. As a result, it may take several years for the clinical symptoms of B_{12} deficiency to develop in individuals who have had a partial or total gastrectomy and can no longer absorb the vitamin.
2. Vitamin B_{12} deficiency is rarely due to a lack of the vitamin in the diet. It is much more common to find deficiencies in patients who fail to absorb the vitamin from the intestine, resulting in ***pernicious anemia***. The disease is most commonly due to a failure of the parietal cells of the stomach to secrete a glycoprotein called ***intrinsic factor***. Normally, vitamin B_{12} obtained from the diet binds to intrinsic factor in the stomach. The cobalamin-intrinsic factor complex travels through the gut and eventually binds to specific receptor sites on the surface of mucosal cells of the ileum. The bound cobalamin is transported into the mucosal cell and subsequently into the general circulation where it is carried by B_{12}-binding proteins (Figure 27.11). Lack of intrinsic factor prevents the absorption of vitamin B_{12}, resulting in pernicious anemia. The disease is treated by intramuscular injection of cyanocobalamin.
3. The effects of cobalamin deficiency are most pronounced in rapidly dividing cells such as the erythropoietic tissue of the bone marrow and the mucosal cells of the intestine. Such tissues need the N^5-N^{10}-methyl and N^{10}-formyl forms of tetrahydrofolate for the synthesis of nucleotides required for DNA replication. However, in vitamin B_{12} deficiency, the N^5-methyl form of tetrahydrofolate is not efficiently used (see p. 243). Because the methylated form

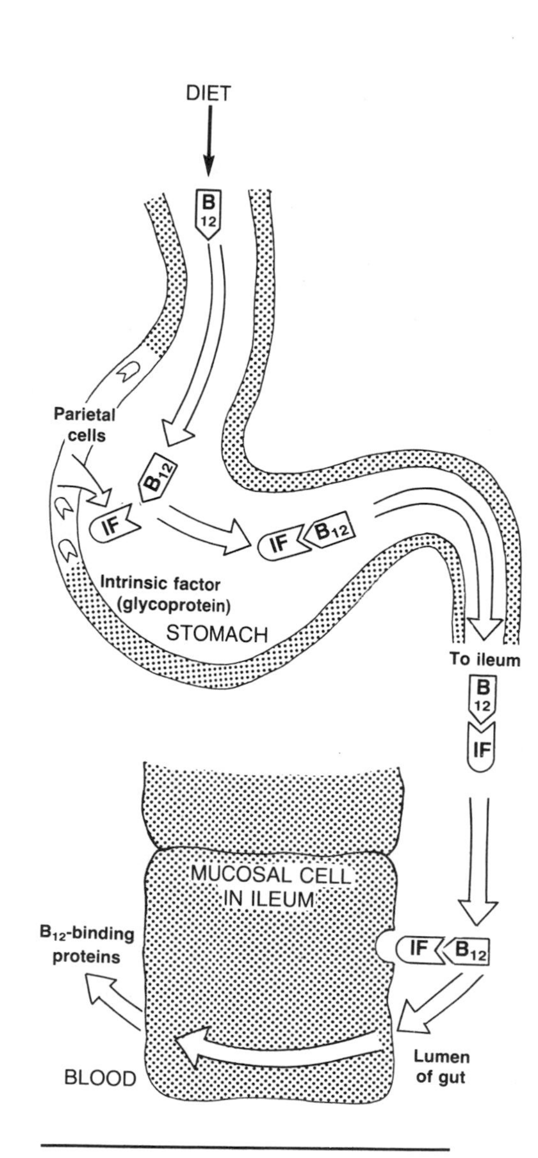

Figure 27.11
Metabolism of vitamin B_{12}.

cannot be converted directly to other forms of tetrahydrofolate, the N^5-methyl form accumulates while the levels of the other forms decrease. Thus, cobalamin deficiency leads to a deficiency of the tetrahydrofolate forms needed in purine and thymine synthesis, resulting in the symptoms of megaloblastic anemia.

4. Vitamin B_{12} deficiency also leads to a degeneration of nerve fibers in the spinal cord and peripheral nerves. These effects are irreversible and occur by mechanisms that appear to be different from those described for megaloblastic anemia.

IX. ASCORBIC ACID (VITAMIN C)

A. Structure of ascorbic acid

1. Ascorbic acid is a reducing agent that is readily oxidized by oxygen, particularly in the presence of metal ions. At physiologic pH, the carboxyl group on the ascorbic acid is ionized.

Ascorbic acid

B. Functions of ascorbic acid

1. Ascorbic acid is essential to a variety of hydroxylation processes, including the hydroxylation of prolyl- and lysyl-residues of collagen (see p. 32).
2. Ascorbic acid also facilitates the absorption of iron by reducing it to the ferrous state in the stomach.

C. Distribution of ascorbic acid

1. Citrus fruits, potatoes (particularly in their skins), tomatoes, and green vegetables are good sources of vitamin C.

D. Requirements for ascorbic acid

1. Although 10 mg/day will prevent scurvy, the RDA has been set at 60 mg/day for adults.

E. Deficiency of ascorbic acid

1. A deficiency in ascorbic acid results in ***scurvy,*** a disease characterized by sore, spongy gums, loose teeth, fragile blood vessels, swollen joints, and anemia. Many of the deficiency symptoms can be explained by a deficiency in the hydroxylation of collagen, resulting in defective connective tissue (see p. 32 for a discussion of collagen synthesis).

F. Toxicity of ascorbic acid

1. No acute toxicity has been observed with ascorbic acid. Most of the vitamin is excreted unaltered, although a small portion is oxidized to dehydroascorbic acid and metabolized to ***oxalate***. The calcium salts of oxalate are one of the major constituents of ***kidney stones***. Thus chronic massive doses of ascorbic acid should be avoided, particularly in individuals with a tendency to form kidney stones.
2. Pharmacologic doses of ascorbic acid (1–4 g/day) appear to decrease the severity or duration of colds slightly but do not alter their frequency significantly. Other claims about the beneficial effects of massive doses of vitamin C remain unproven.

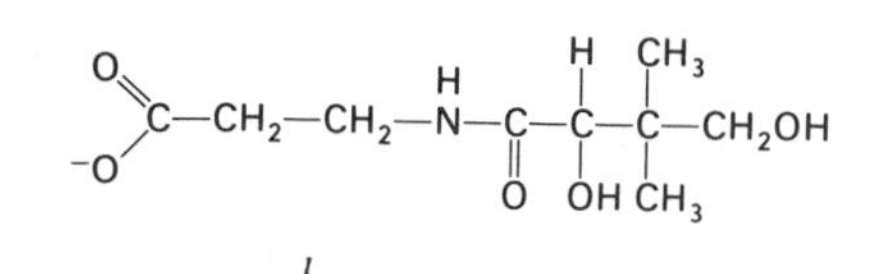

Pantothenic acid

X. PANTOTHENIC ACID

A. Structure of pantothenic acid

1. Pantothenic acid consists of a dihydroxydimethylbutyric acid joined to β-alanine by a peptide bond.

B. Functions of pantothenic acid

1. Pantothenic acid is a component of ***coenzyme A*** that functions in the transfer of acyl groups. Coenzyme A contains a thiol group that carries acyl compounds as activated thiol esters. Examples of such structures are succinyl CoA (see p. 139), fatty acyl CoA (see p. 172), and acetyl CoA (see p. 135).
2. Pantothenic acid is also a component of *fatty acid synthase* (see p. 163).

C. Distribution of pantothenic acid

1. Eggs, liver, and yeast are the most important sources of pantothenic acid, although the vitamin is widely distributed.

D. Requirement for pantothenic acid

1. The RDA for pantothenic acid is estimated at 4 to 7 mg per day.

E. Deficiency of pantothenic acid

1. Pantothenic acid deficiency is not well characterized in humans.

Study Questions

Choose the ONE best answer:

27.1 The coenzyme required in oxidative decarboxylation is

A. biotin.
B. vitamin B_{12}.
C. pyridoxal phosphate.
D. ascorbic acid.
E. thiamine pyrophosphate.

27.2 Which one of the following compounds is synthesized from glutamic acid, p-aminobenzoic acid, and a pteridine nucleus?

A. Vitamin B_{12}
B. Cyanocobalamin
C. Folic acid
D. Biotin
E. Coenzyme A

27.3 Which one of the following statements about vitamin B_{12} is INCORRECT?

A. It can be converted to cofactor forms containing a 5′-deoxyadenosine or methyl group attached to cobalt.
B. It can serve as a source of a cofactor required for the conversion of methylmalonyl CoA to succinyl CoA.
C. It requires a specific glycoprotein for its absorption.
D. It may be present in inadequate quantities in a strictly vegetarian diet.
E. It contains a heme group.

27.4 Which one of the following statements about ascorbic acid is INCORRECT?

A. It is readily oxidized, particularly in the presence of divalent metal ions.
B. It is a cofactor required for the hydroxylation of proline and lysine.
C. Its requirement varies with the caloric intake.

D. It is metabolized in part to oxalate, which can form an insoluble salt with calcium.
E. It facilitates the absorption of dietary iron.

Answer A if 1, 2, and 3 are correct
B if 1 and 3 are correct
C if 2 and 4 are correct
D if only 4 is correct
E if all are correct

27.5 The nutritional requirement for niacin in humans is

1. increased when the diet includes large amounts of raw egg white.
2. decreased when the diet is supplemented with commercial "liquid protein" consisting largely of hydrolyzed collagen (which does not contain tryptophan).
3. independent of the composition of the diet.
4. decreased when the diet contains large amounts of animal protein.

27.6 A deficiency of biotin in a higher animal is likely to be accompanied by

1. defective oxidation of fatty acids to acetyl CoA.
2. decreased formation of lactate in skeletal muscular contraction.
3. decreased oxidation of succinate by mitochondria isolated from the liver of such animals.
4. defective synthesis of fatty acids.

27.7 Which of the following reactions involve the participation of thiamine?

1. Lactate → pyruvate
2. α-ketoglutarate → succinyl CoA
3. Acetyl CoA → malonyl CoA
4. Ribose 5-phosphate → sedoheptulose 7-phosphate

27.8 Which of the following statements about niacin is(are) true?

1. Niacin forms part of the structure of $NADP^+$.
2. Niacin is derived from the degradation of tryptophan.
3. Niacin is involved as a cofactor in oxidation-reduction reactions.
4. Niacin is a constituent of FAD.

27.9 Vitamin B_{12}

1. participates in the conversion of homocysteine to methionine.
2. contains cobalt.
3. when injected into patients with pernicious anemia overcomes the lack of intrinsic factor.
4. can be obtained in the diet from peas and carrots.

XI. VITAMIN A

A. Structure of vitamin A

1. Vitamin A is a collective term for three biologically active molecules (Figure 27.12)
   a. ***Retinol:*** A primary alcohol containing a β-ionone ring with an unsaturated side chain. Retinol is found in animal tissues as a retinyl ester with long-chain fatty acids.
   b. ***Retinal:*** The aldehyde derived from the oxidation of retinol. Retinal and retinol can readily be interconverted.
   c. ***Retinoic acid:*** The acid derived from the oxidation of retinal. Retinoic acid cannot be reduced in the body and therefore cannot give rise to either retinal or retinol. However, retinoic acid is active in the maintenance of epithelial cells.

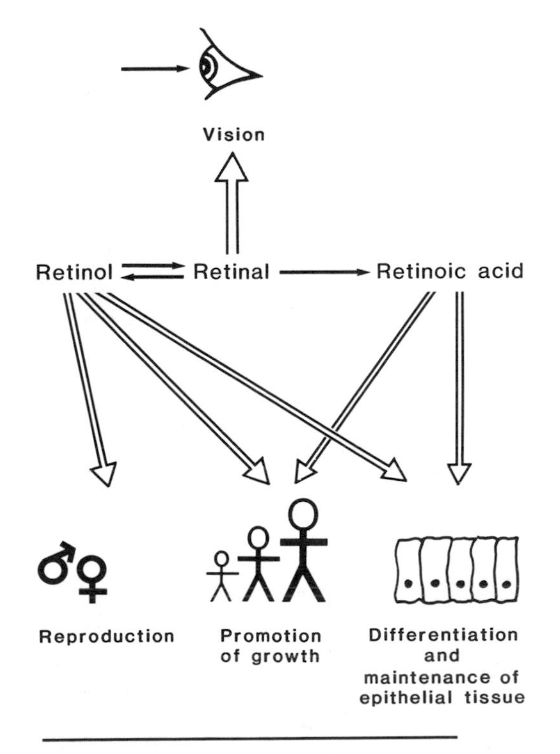

Figure 27.12
Interconversion of compounds showing vitamin A activity.

2. Plant foods contain **β-*carotene,*** which can be oxidatively cleaved in the intestine to yield two molecules of retinal (Figure 27.13). In humans, the conversion is inefficient, and β-carotene is only about one sixth as active as retinol.

B. Absorption and transport of vitamin A

1. Retinyl esters present in the diet are hydrolyzed in the intestinal mucosa, releasing retinol and free fatty acids (Figure 27.13).
2. Retinol derived from esters and from the cleavage and reduction of carotenes is reesterified to long-chain fatty acids in the intestinal mucosa and secreted as a component of chylomicra into the lymphatic system (see Figure 27.13 and p. 208)
3. Retinyl esters contained in chylomicrons are taken up by, and stored in, the liver (Figure 27.13).
4. When needed, retinol is released from the liver and transported to extrahepatic tissues by the plasma ***retinol-binding protein*** (RBP). The retinol-RBP complex attaches to specific receptors on the surface of the cells of peripheral tissues, permitting retinol to enter.
5. Many tissues contain a cellular retinol-binding protein that carries retinol to sites in the nucleus where the vitamin may act in a manner analogous to steroid hormones.

C. Functions of vitamin A

1. ***Visual Cycle:*** Vitamin A is a component of the visual pigment, rhodopsin.
   a. ***Rhodopsin,*** the visual pigment of the rod cells in the retina, consists of Δ^{11}-cis-retinal specifically bound to the protein ***opsin***. When rhodopsin is exposed to light, a series of photochemical isomerizations occurs, resulting in the bleaching of the visual pigment and dissociation of all-trans-retinal and opsin. This process triggers a nerve impulse that is transmitted by the optic nerve to the brain (Figure 27.13).
   b. Regeneration of rhodopsin requires isomerization of all-trans-retinal back to Δ^{11}-cis-retinal. Trans-retinal, after being released from rhodopsin, is first reduced to trans-retinol in the retina and then transported to the liver, where it is isomerized to 11-cis-retinol (Figure 27.13).
   c. 11-Cis-retinol is transported back to the retina where it is oxidized to 11-cis-retinal, which spontaneously combines with opsin to form rhodopsin, thus completing the cycle (Figure 27.13).
2. ***Growth:***
   a. Animals deprived of vitamin A initially lose their appetites, possibly because of keratinization of the taste buds.
   b. Bone growth is slow and fails to keep pace with growth of the nervous system, leading to central nervous system damage.
3. ***Reproduction:***
   a. Retinol and retinal are essential for normal reproduction, supporting spermatogenesis in the male and preventing fetal resorption in the female.

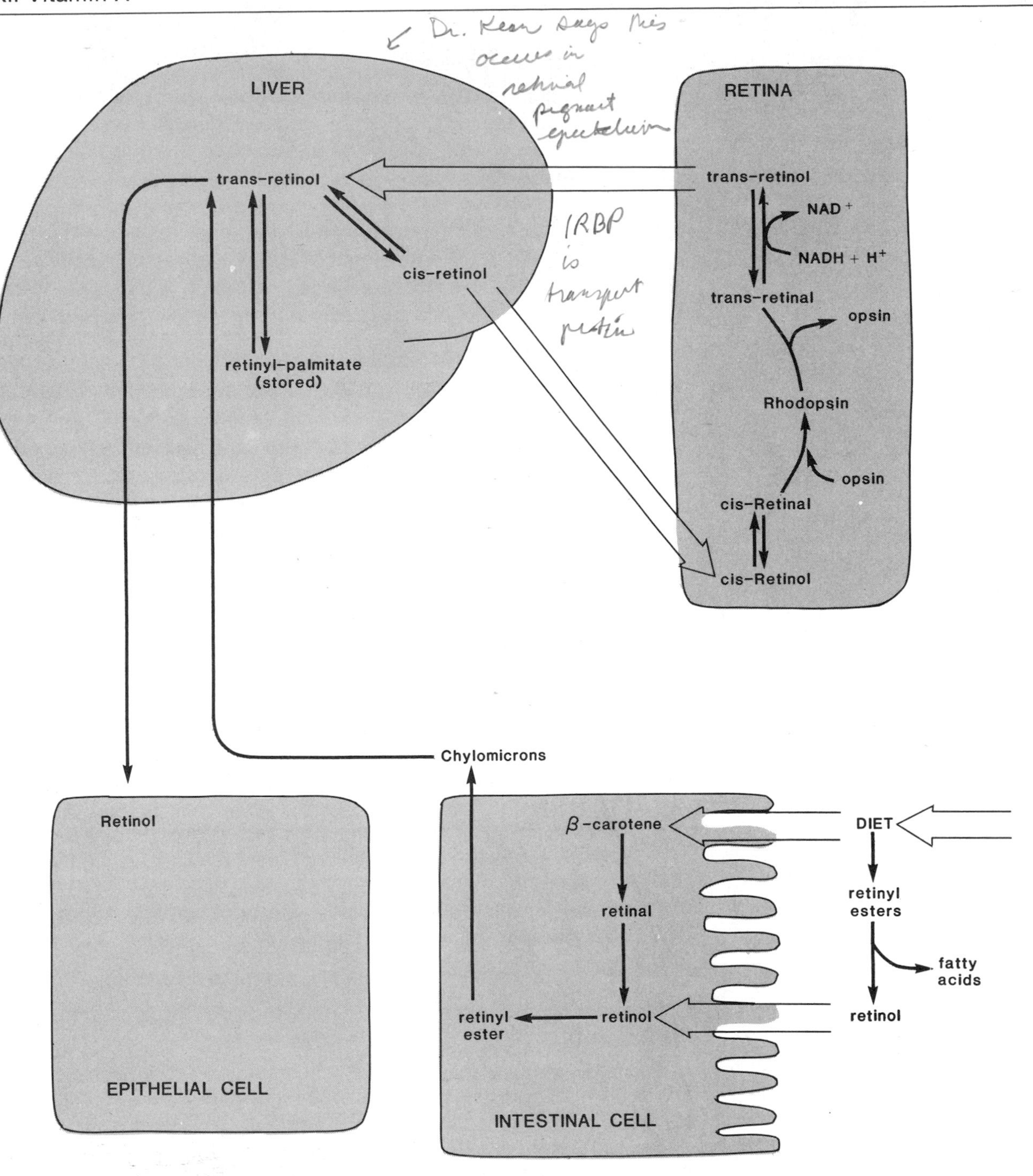

Figure 27.13
Absorption, transport, and storage of vitamin A and its derivatives.

b. Retinoic acid is inactive in maintaining reproduction and in the visual cycle; thus, animals given vitamin A only as retinoic acid from birth are blind and sterile.

4. ***Maintenance of epithelial cells:***

a. Vitamin A is essential for normal differentiation and mucus secretion of epithelial tissues.

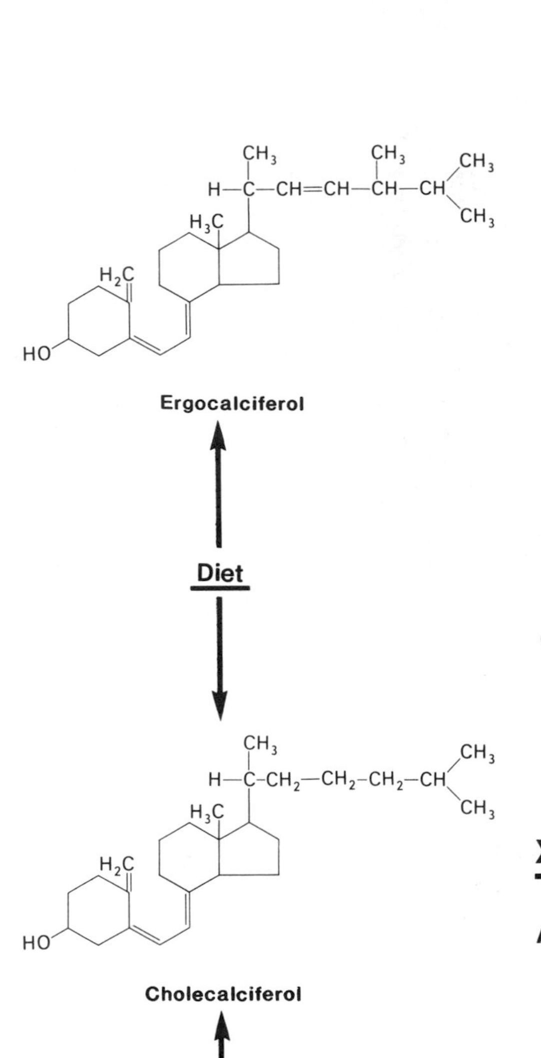

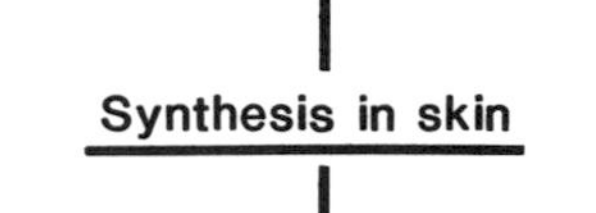

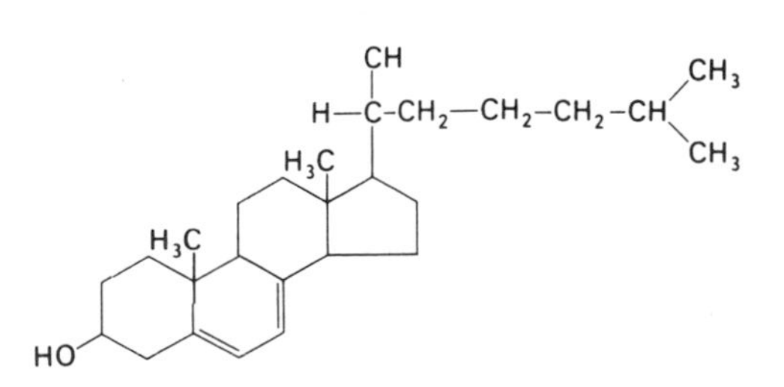

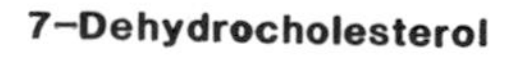

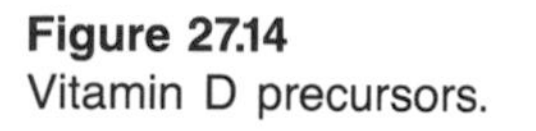

Figure 27.14
Vitamin D precursors.

D. Distribution of vitamin A

1. Liver, kidney, cream, butter, and egg yolk are good sources of preformed vitamin A. Yellow and green vegetables and fruits are good dietary sources of the carotenes, which serve as precursors of vitamin A.

E. Requirement for vitamin A

1. The RDA for adults is 1000 retinol equivalents (RE) for males and 800 RE for females (one RE = 1 μg of retinol, 6 μg of β-carotene, or 12 μg of other carotenoids).

F. Deficiency of vitamin A

1. Night blindness ***(nyctalopia)*** is one of the earliest signs of vitamin A deficiency. The visual threshold is increased, making it difficult to see in dim light. Prolonged deficiency leads to an irreversible loss in the number of visual cells.
2. Severe vitamin A deficiency leads to ***xerophthalmia,*** a pathologic dryness of the conjunctiva and cornea. If untreated, xerophthalmia leads to ulceration and ultimately to blindness. The condition is most frequently seen in children in developing tropical countries.

G. Toxicity of vitamin A

1. Vitamin A toxicity has been observed at daily doses of 25,000 international units (IU) (3.33 IU = 1 μg of retinol). Symptoms include headache, drowsines, nausea, diarrhea, and scaly dermatitis.

XII. VITAMIN D

A. Structure of vitamin D

1. The D vitamins are a group of compounds resembling steroids in which the B-ring has been opened at the 9,10 position (Figure 27.14).

B. Distribution of vitamin D: Humans have two sources of vitamin D

1. ***Diet: Ergocalciferol*** (vitamin D_2), found in plants, and ***cholecalciferol*** (vitamin D_3), found in animal tissues, are sources of preformed vitamin D activity. Ergocalciferol and cholecalciferol differ chemically only in presence of an additional double bond and methyl group in the plant sterol (Figure 27.14).
2. ***Endogenous vitamin precursor: 7-Dehydrocholesterol,*** an intermediate in cholesterol synthesis, is converted to ***cholecalciferol*** in the dermis and epidermis of humans exposed to sunlight. Preformed vitamin D is a dietary requirement only in individuals not exposed to sunlight.

C. Metabolism of vitamin D

1. Vitamins D_2 and D_3 are not biologically active but are converted *in vivo* to the active form of the D vitamin by two sequential hydroxylation reactions (Figure 27.15):
   a. Hydroxylation of vitamin D_3 at the 25-position by a specific *hydroxylase* in the liver results in the formation of ***25-hydroxy-***

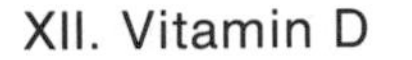

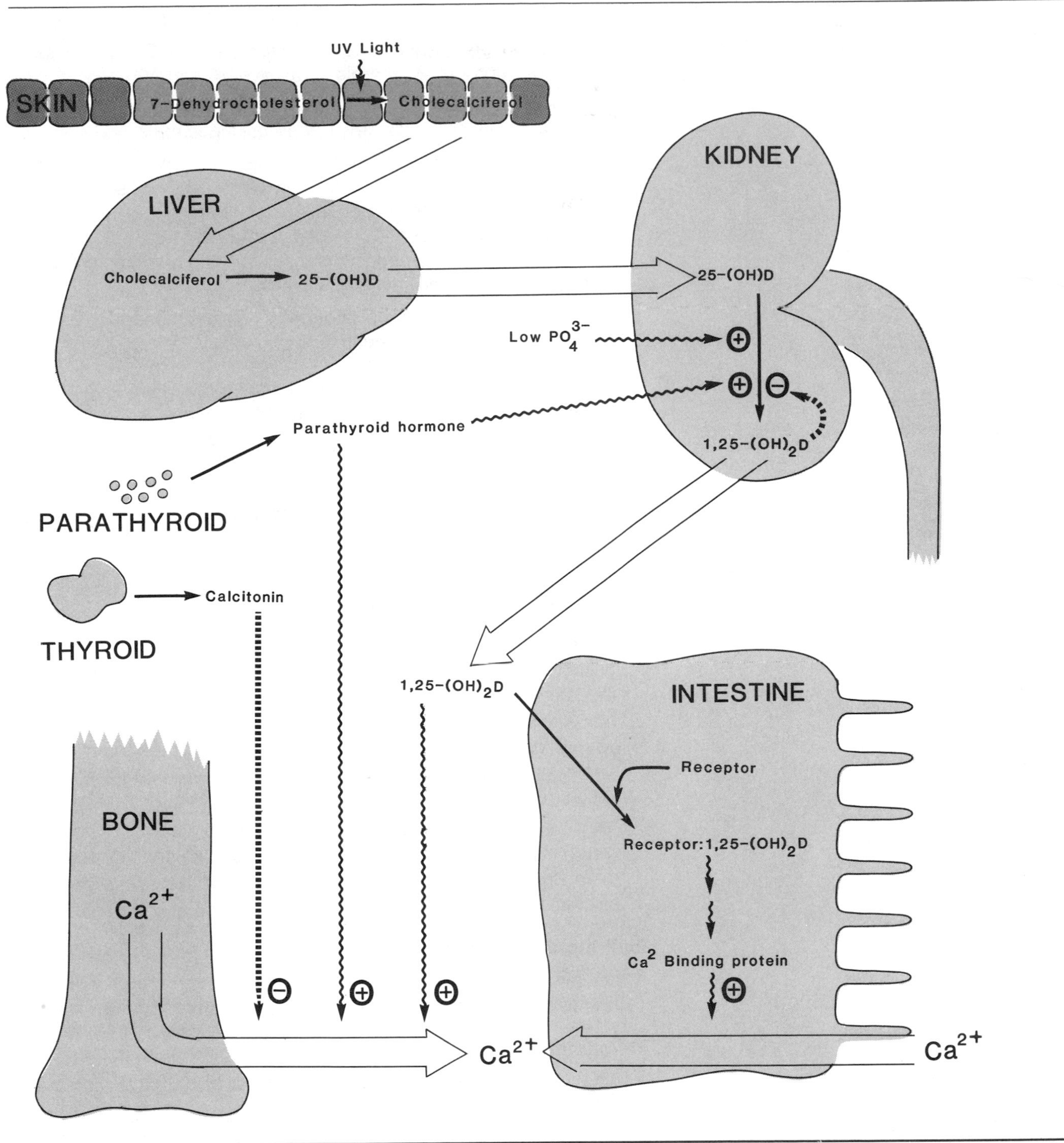

Figure 27.15
Metabolism and actions of vitamin D.

cholecalciferol, or 25-OH D_3. 25-OH D_3 is the predominant form of vitamin D in the plasma and is the major storage form of the vitamin.

b. 25-OH D_3 is further hydroxylated at the 1 position by a specific *25-hydroxycholecalciferol 1-hydroxylase* found primarily in the kidney, resulting in the formation of ***1,25-dihydroxycholecalciferol***

(1,25-diOH D_3). This *hydroxylase* and the liver *25-hydroxylase* use cytochrome P_{450}, molecular oxygen, and NADPH.

2. 1,25-diOH D_3 is the most potent vitamin D metabolite. Its formation is tightly regulated by the level of serum phosphate and calcium ions:

   a. *25-Hydroxycholecalciferol 1-hydroxylase* activity is increased directly by low serum phosphate or indirectly by low serum calcium, which triggers the release of ***parathyroid hormone*** (PTH). Hypocalcemia caused by insufficient dietary calcium thus results in elevated levels of plasma 1,25-diOH D_3.

   b. *1-Hydroxylase* activity is thought to be decreased by excess 1,25-diOH D_3, the product of the reaction.

D. Function of vitamin D: The overall function of 1,25-diOH D_3 is to maintain adequate serum levels of calcium. It performs this function by (1) increasing uptake of calcium by the intestine, 2) minimizing losses of calcium by the kidney, and (3) stimulating resorption of bone when necessary (Figure 27.15).

1. ***Effect of vitamin D on the intestine:*** 1,25-diOH D_3 stimulates the intestinal absorption of calcium and phosphate. 1,25-DiOH D_3 enters the intestinal cell and binds to a cytoplasmic receptor. The 1,25-DiOH D_3 complex then moves to the nucleus where it selectively interacts with the cellular DNA by mechanisms that are not understood. As a result, calcium uptake is enhanced by an increased synthesis of a specific calcium-binding protein. Thus, the mechanism of action of 1,25-diOH D_3 is typical of steroid hormones.

2. ***Effect of vitamin D on bone:*** 1,25-diOH D_3 stimulates the mobilization of calcium and phosphate from bone by a process that requires protein synthesis and the presence of parathyroid hormone. The result is an increase in serum calcium and phosphate. Thus bone is an important reservoir of calcium that can be mobilized to maintain serum levels (see p. 307 for role of calcitonin in regulating calcium levels).

E. Distribution of vitamin D

1. Vitamin D occurs naturally in fatty fish, eggs, liver, egg yolk, and butter. Milk, unless fortified, is not a good source of the vitamin.

F. Requirement for vitamin D

1. The RDA for adults is 5 μg of cholecalciferol or 200 IU of vitamin D.

G. Deficiency of vitamin D

1. Vitamin D deficiency causes a net demineralization of bone, resulting in ***rickets*** in children and ***osteomalacia*** in adults. Rickets is characterized by the continued formation of the collagen matrix of bone but incomplete mineralization, resulting in soft, pliable bones. In osteomalacia, demineralization of preexisting bones increases their susceptibility to fracture.

H. Toxicity of vitamin D

1. Vitamin D is the most toxic of all vitamins. Like all the fat-soluble vitamins, vitamin D can be stored in the body and is only slowly

metabolized. High doses (100,000 IU for weeks or months) can cause loss of appetite, nausea, thirst, and stupor.

2. Enhanced calcium absorption and bone resorption results in ***hypercalcemia***, which can lead to calcium deposits in many of the organs, particularly the arteries and kidneys.

XIII. VITAMIN K

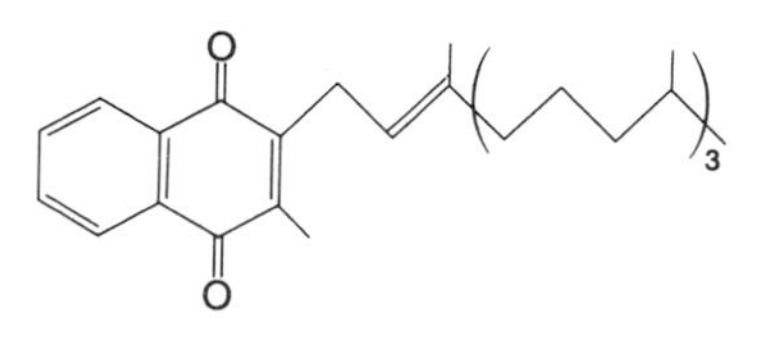

Vitamin K

A. Structure of vitamin K

1. The K vitamins are polyisoprenoid substituted naphthoquinones.

B. Function of vitamin K

1. Vitamin K is required in the hepatic synthesis of ***prothrombin*** and the ***blood clotting factors II, VII, IX, and X:***
   a. These proteins are synthesized as inactive precursor molecules. Formation of the active clotting factors requires the vitamin-K-dependent carboxylation of glutamic acid residues, forming a mature clotting factor that contains γ-carboxyglutamic acid (Gla). The reaction requires O_2, CO_2, and the hydroquinone form of vitamin K (Figure 27.16).
   b. The formation of Gla is sensitive to inhibition by ***dicumarol,*** a naturally occurring anticoagulant.
2. The Gla residues of prothrombin are good chelators of positively charged calcium ions because of the two adjacent, negatively charged carboxylate groups. The prothrombin-calcium complex is then able to bind to essential phospholipids on the surface of platelets. Attachment to the platelet increases the rate at which the proteolytic conversion of prothrombin to thrombin can occur (Figure 27.17).
3. Gla is also present in other proteins unrelated to the clotting process. However, the physiologic role of these proteins and the function of vitamin K in their synthesis are not known.

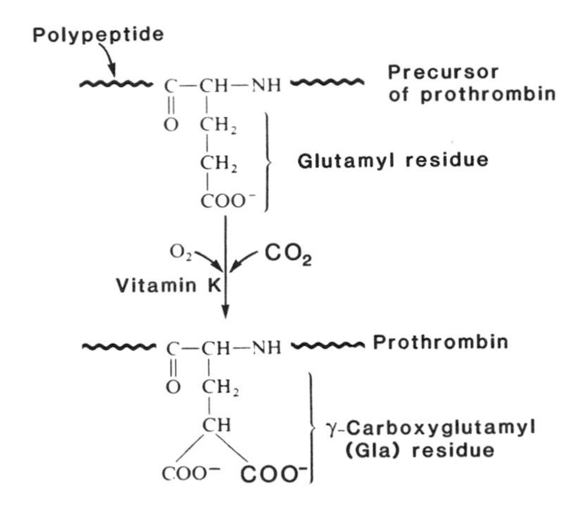

Figure 27.16
Carboxylation of glutamate to form γ-carboxyglutamate (Gla).

C. Distribution of vitamin K

1. Vitamin K is found in cabbage, cauliflower, spinach, egg yolk, and liver. There is also extensive synthesis of the vitamin by the bacteria in the gut.

D. Requirement for vitamin K

1. There is no RDA for vitamin K, but 70 to 140 μg/day is recommended as an adequate level. The lower level assumes that one half of the estimated requirement comes from bacterial synthesis, whereas the upper figure assumes no bacterial synthesis.

E. Deficiency of vitamin K

1. A deficiency in the adult is unlikely, due to the synthesis of the vitamin by the intestinal flora because it is widely distributed in food.
2. A prolonged coagulation time, characteristic of vitamin K deficiency, is sometimes observed in newborn infants. The intestinal tract of the newborn infant is sterile for the first several days

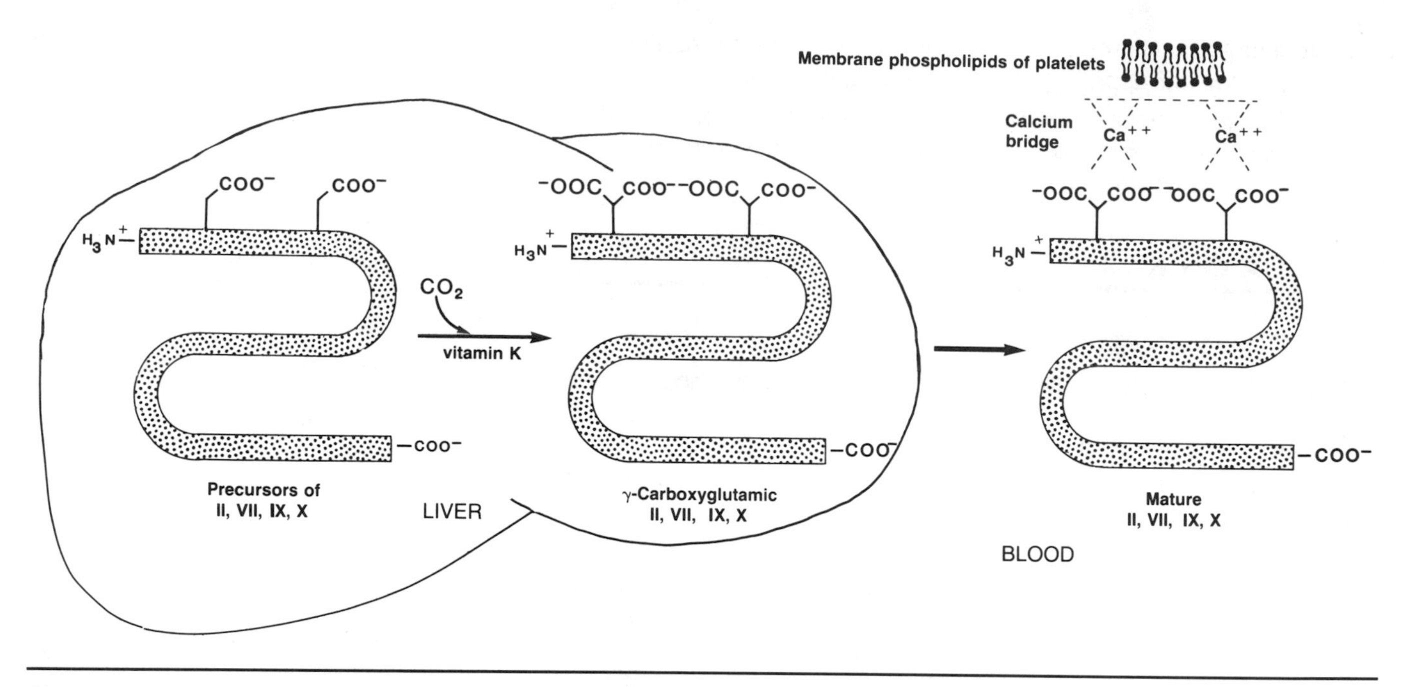

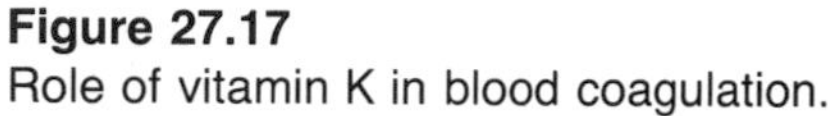

Figure 27.17
Role of vitamin K in blood coagulation.

after birth and is therefore not a source of vitamin K. Further, breast and cow's milk are low in vitamin K. Supplementation of the diet at birth with 1 mg of vitamin K is usually sufficient to prevent hemorrhagic disease.

F. Toxicity of vitamin K

1. Prolonged administration of large doses of vitamin K can produce hemolytic anemia and jaundice in the infant because of toxic effects on the membrane of red blood cells.

IV. VITAMIN E

A. Structure of vitamin E

1. The E vitamins consist of eight naturally occurring tocopherols, of which ***α-tocopherol*** is the most active.

B. Function of vitamin E

1. The primary function of vitamin E is as an antioxidant—preventing the nonenzymic oxidation of polyunsaturated fatty acids by molecular oxygen and free radicals.

C. Distribution of vitamin E

1. Vegetable oils are rich sources of vitamin E; liver and eggs contain moderate amounts.

D. Requirement for vitamin E

1. The RDA for α-tocopherol is 10 mg for men and 8 mg for women. The vitamin E requirement increases as the intake of polyunsaturated fatty acid increases.

E. Deficiency of vitamin E

1. Vitamin E deficiency is almost entirely restricted to premature infants. When observed in adults it is usually associated with defective lipid absorption or transport. The signs of human vitamin E deficiency include sensitivity of erythrocytes to peroxide and the appearance of abnormal cellular membranes.

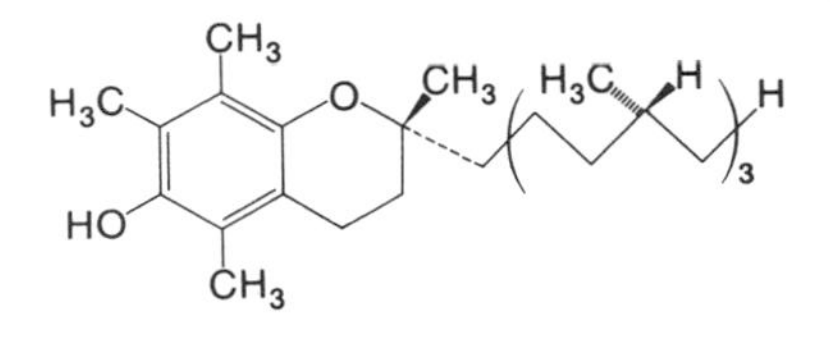

Vitamin E

F. Toxicity of vitamin E

1. Vitamin E is the least toxic of the fat-soluble vitamins; no toxicity has been observed at doses of 300 mg/day.

Study Questions

Answer A if 1, 2, and 3 are correct
B if 1 and 3 are correct
C if 2 and 4 are correct
D if only 4 is correct
E if all are correct

27.10 Vitamin A (or one of its derivatives)

1. can be enzymically formed from dietary β-carotene.
2. is transported from the intestine to the liver in chylomicrons.
3. is the light-absorbing portion of rhodopsin.
4. is phosphorylated and dephosphorylated during the visual cycle.

27.11 Prolonged deficiency of vitamin D will result in

1. increased secretion of calcitonin.
2. increased urinary excretion of calcium.
3. increased density of bone.
4. increased secretion of parathyroid hormone.

27.12 Vitamin D

1. increases absorption of calcium from the intestine.
2. is not required in the diet of individuals exposed to sunlight.
3. is not really a vitamin because the active form, 1,25-dihydroxycholecalciferol, can be synthesized in humans.
4. opposes the effect of parathyroid hormone.

27.13 Vitamin K

1. plays an essential role in preventing thrombosis.
2. decreases the coagulation time in newborn infants with hemorrhagic disease.
3. is present in high concentration in cow's or breast milk.
4. is synthesized by intestinal bacteria.

27.14 α-Tocopherol

1. functions primarily as an antioxidant.
2. deficiency is commonly found in adults.
3. requirements increase with the amount of polyunsaturated fatty acids in the diet.
4. is found in high concentrations in whole grains and cereals.

Structure of Nucleic Acids

28

I. OVERVIEW

Unlike carbohydrates, lipids, and proteins, nucleic acids are not used primarily for either cellular energy or the structural integrity of the cell. Instead, they are used for the ***storage*** and ***expression*** of genetic information. There are two chemically distinct types of nucleic acids: ***deoxyribonucleic acid*** (DNA) and ***ribonucleic acid*** (RNA). The DNA contained in a single fertilized egg encodes the information that directs the development of an organism. This development may ultimately require the production of billions of cells. Each of these cells is specialized, expressing only those functions that are required for it to perform its role in maintaining the organism. Therefore, the DNA must be able not only to ***replicate precisely*** each time a cell divides, but also to have the information that it contains be ***selectively expressed***.

Members of the second class of nucleic acids, the RNAs, participate in the process of selective expression of the genetic information stored in the DNA. DNA is found not only in chromosomes in the nucleus of eukaryotic organisms, but also in mitochondria and in the chloroplasts of plants. RNA synthesized in the nucleus performs its function in the cytoplasm, whereas RNA synthesized in the mitochondria or chloroplasts remains within these organelles. Prokaryotic cells, which lack nuclei, have a single chromosome but may also contain nonchromosomal DNA in the form of plasmids.

II. NUCLEOTIDE STRUCTURE

Nucleotides are the building blocks of both DNA and RNA. They also serve as the energy currency of the cell (see p. 99) and as structural components of a number of essential cofactors (see Chapter 27). Nucleotides are composed of a nitrogenous base, a monosaccharide, and one, two, or three phosphate groups.

A. Purines and pyrimidines

1. The bases belong to two families of compounds: the ***purines*** and the ***pyrimidines*** (Figure 28.1).
2. Both DNA and RNA contain the same purine bases: ***adenine*** (A) and ***guanine*** (G).
3. Both DNA and RNA contain the pyrimidine ***cytosine*** (C), but they ***differ*** in their second pyrimidine bases: DNA contains ***thymine*** (T),

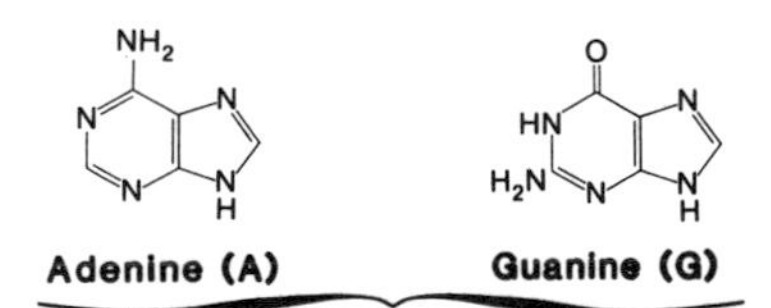

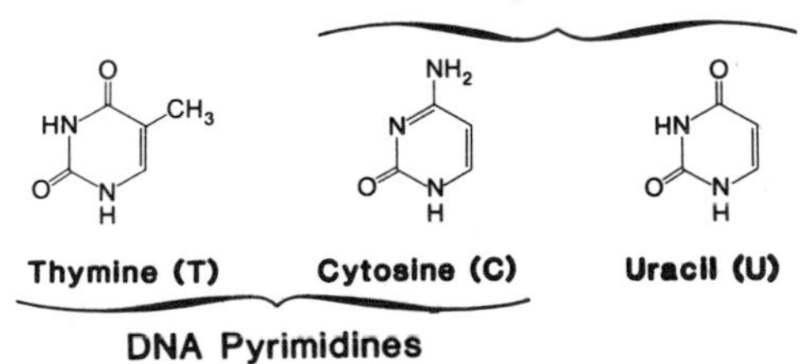

Figure 28.1
Purines and pyrimidines commonly found in DNA and RNA.

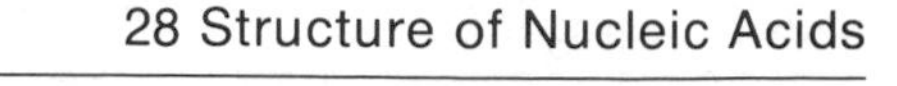

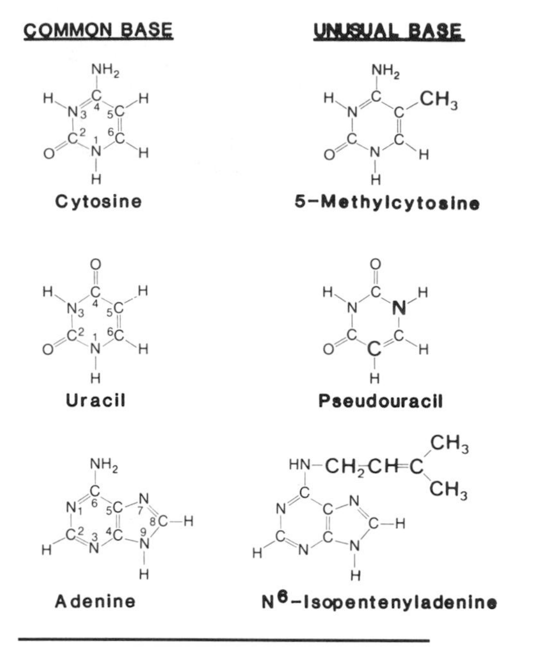

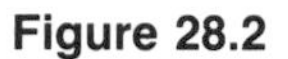

Figure 28.2
Examples of unusual bases found in nucleic acids.

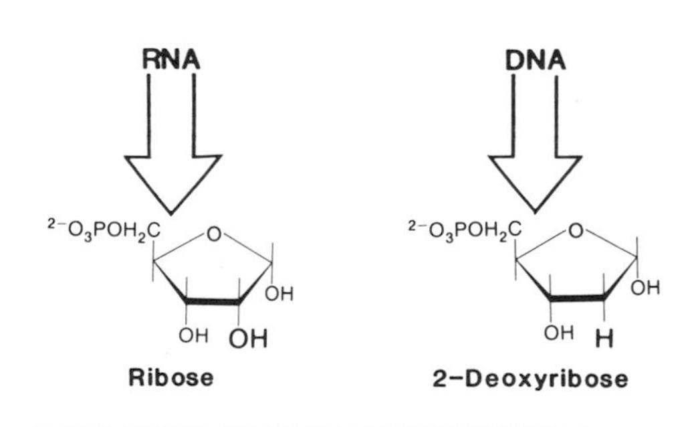

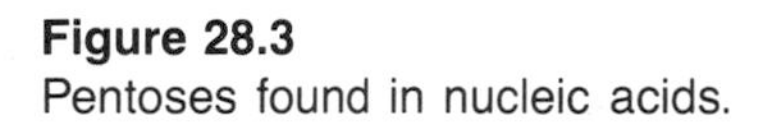

Figure 28.3
Pentoses found in nucleic acids.

whereas RNA contains ***uracil*** (U). (Note that T and U differ only by one methyl group present on T but absent on U; see Figure 28.1.)

4. ***Unusual bases*** are found occasionally in some species of DNA and RNA, for example, in some viral DNA and in transfer RNA (Figure 28.2). These include the following:

   DNA: 5-methylcytosine, 5-hydroxymethylcytosine, glucosylated 5-hydroxymethylcytosine, hydroxymethyluracil

   RNA: Hypoxanthine, thymine, methylated purines and pyrimidines, thiouracil, dihydrouracil, isopentenyl adenine, acetyl cytosine, pseudouracil

   The presence of an unusual base in a nucleotide sequence may aid in its recognition by specific enzymes or protect it from being degraded by nucleases.

B. Nucleosides

1. The addition of a pentose sugar to a base produces a nucleoside.
2. If the sugar is ribose, a ***ribonucleoside*** is produced. If the sugar is 2-deoxyribose, a ***deoxyribonucleoside*** is produced (see Figure 28.3). (The mechanism for removing the hydroxyl group from ribose to form deoxyribose is discussed on p. 354.)
3. The carbon and nitrogen atoms in the ring(s) of the base and the sugar ring are numbered separately (Figure 28.4). Note that the atoms in the rings of the bases are numbered 1–6 in pyrimidines, and 1–9 in purines, while the carbons in the pentose are numbered 1′–5′. Thus, when you refer to the 5′-carbon, you are specifying a carbon atom in the pentose rather than an atom in the base.
4. The major deoxyribonucleosides are shown in Figure 28.4

C. Nucleotides

1. Nucleotides are phosphate esters of nucleosides.
2. The phosphate group is usually attached by an ester linkage to the 5′-OH of the pentose. Such a compound is called a nucleoside 5′-phosphate or a 5′-nucleotide. (Note: The type of pentose is

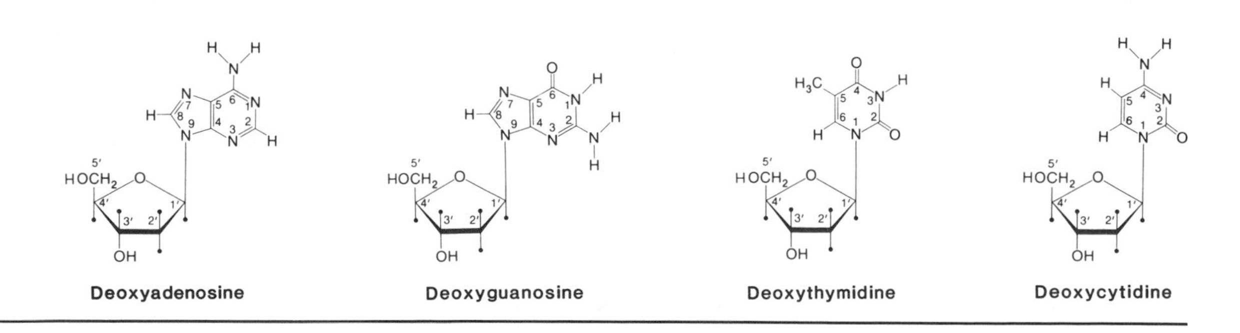

Figure 28.4
Major ***deoxy***ribonucleosides. (If an —OH were present at carbon #2′ of the sugar, the structure would be a ***ribo***nucleoside.)

denoted by the prefix in the names "5′- ***ribo***nucleotide" and "5′- ***deoxyribo***nucleotide.")

3. If one phosphate group is attached to the 5′-carbon of the pentose, the structure is a ***nucleoside monophosphate*** (NMP) like AMP or CMP. If a second or third phosphate is added to the nucleotide, a nucleoside diphosphate or triphosphate results (Figure 28.5).
4. The dissociation of hydrogen from the phosphate groups at neutral pHs is responsible for the ***acidic nature*** of nucleotides and nucleic acids (Figure 28.5).

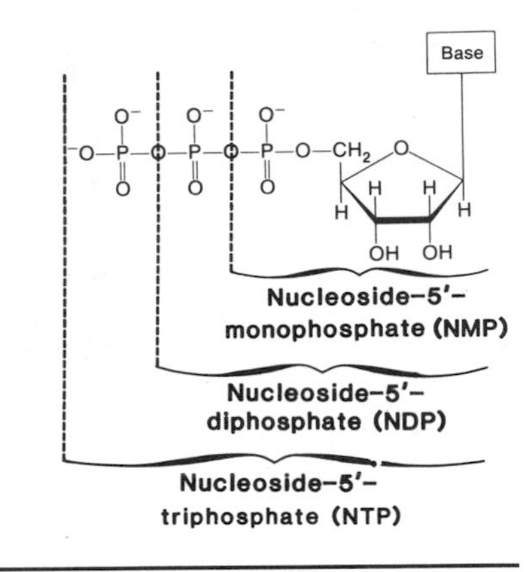

Figure 28.5
Mono-, di-, and triphosphates.

III. STRUCTURE OF DNA

A. Building blocks of DNA

1. DNA is a polynucleotide that contains many mononucleotides covalently linked to each other by ***3′,5′-phosphodiester bonds.***
2. These bonds join the 5′-hydroxyl group of the pentose of one nucleotide to the 3′-hydroxyl group of the pentose of another nucleotide through a phosphate group (Figure 28.6).
3. The resulting long, unbranched chain has ***polarity,*** with a 5′-end that is not attached to another nucleotide and a 3′-end that is also unattached (Figure 28.6). The bases located along the resulting ***ribose-phosphate backbone*** are, by convention, always written in sequence from the 5′-end of the chain to the 3′-end. For example, the sequence of nucleotides shown in Figure 28.6 is read "thymine, adenine, cytosine, guanine."
4. Phosphodiester linkages between nucleotides (in both DNA and RNA) can be cleaved hydrolytically by chemicals or can be enzymatically hydrolyzed by a family of nucleases, for example, *deoxyribonucleases* for DNA and *ribonucleases* for RNA.
   a. Nucleases that cleave the nucleotide chain at positions in the interior of the chain are called ***endo****nucleases.* Those that cleave the chain only by removing individual nucleotides from one of the two ends are called ***exo****nucleases.*
   b. A special group of nucleases produced by microorganisms are called *restriction endonucleases.* These enzymes recognize short stretches of DNA (generally 4 or 6 base pairs) that contain specific base sequences. These sequences, which differ for each *restriction endonuclease,* have twofold rotational symmetry (Figure 28.7). This means that within a short region of the double helix, the nucleotide sequence on the "top" strand, read 5′→3′, is identical to that of the "bottom" strand, also read in the 5′→3′ direction. Therefore, if you turn the page upside down, that is, ***rotate*** it 180°, the structure remains the same. Because they cleave the DNA at specific positions, these enzymes are used experimentally to obtain precisely defined DNA segments and are among the most important tools in the ***cloning*** of genes, a brief introduction to which is given in Figure 28.13.

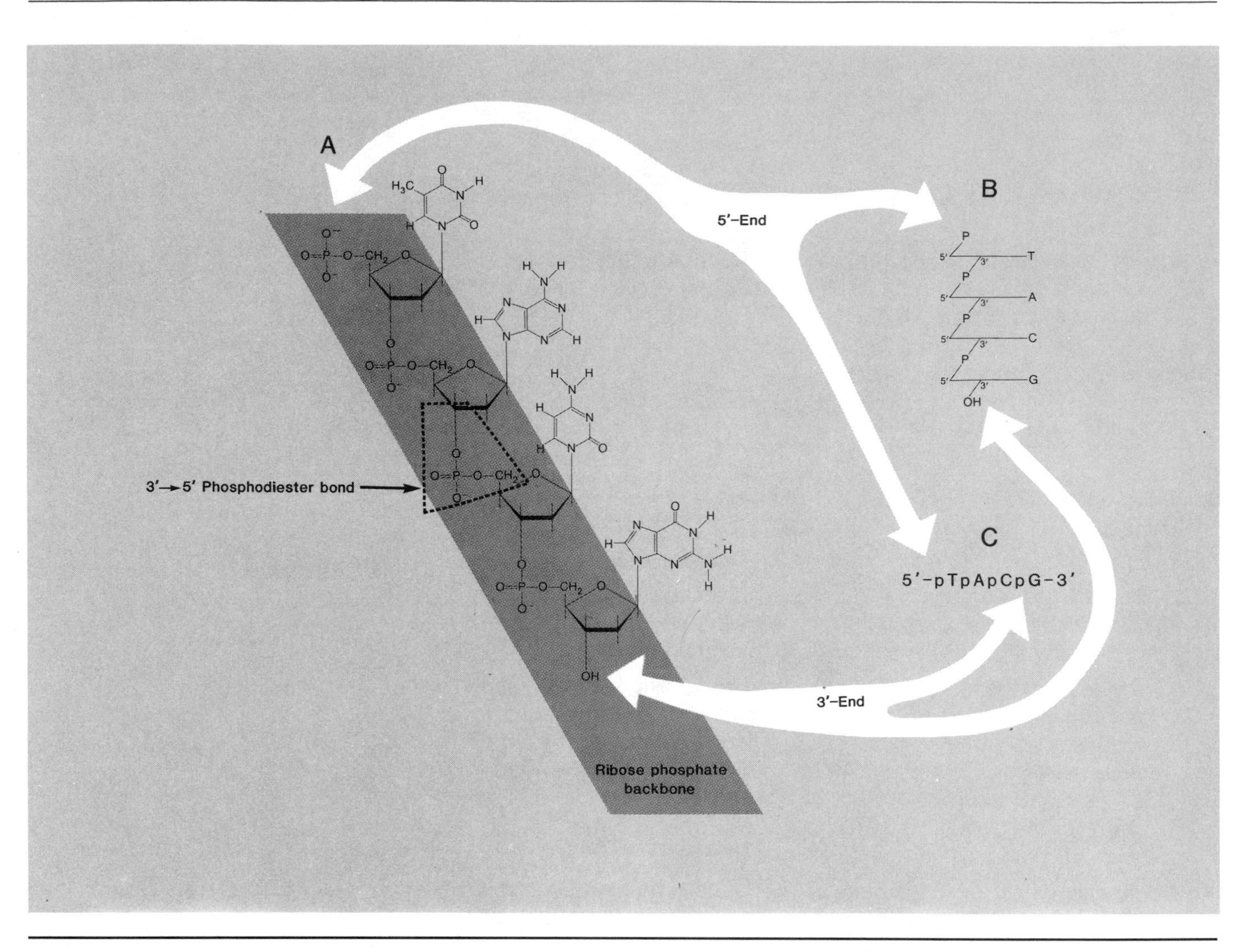

Figure 28.6
Panel A: DNA chain with the nucleotide sequence shown written in the 5′ → 3′ direction. A 3′ → 5′ phosphodiester bond is shown highlighted, and the ribose-phosphate backbone is shaded. ***Panel B:*** The DNA chain written in a more stylized form, emphasizing the ribose–phosphate backbone. ***Panel C:*** A simple representation of the nucleotide sequence.

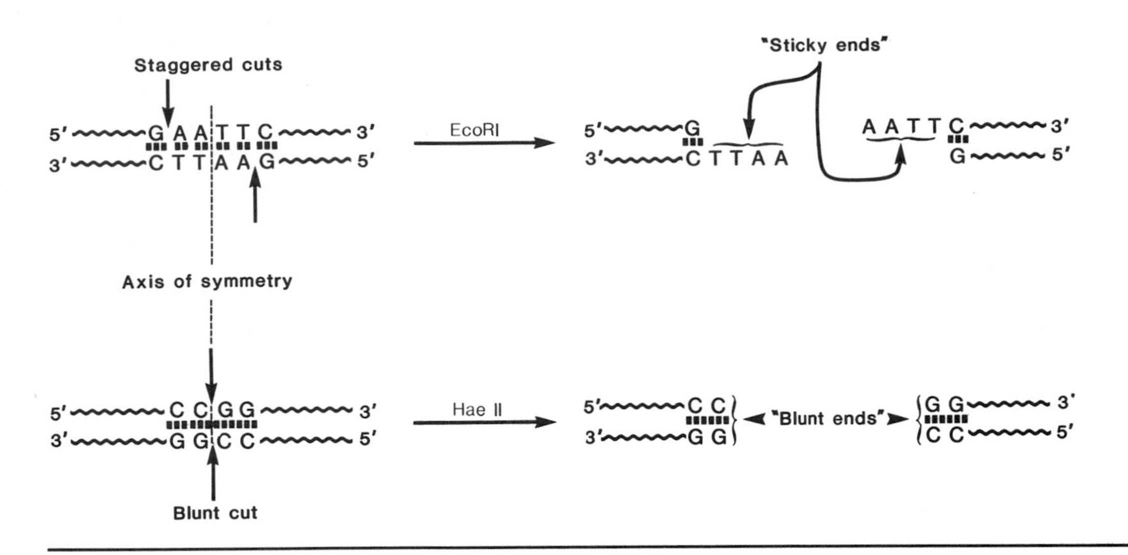

Figure 28.7
Examples of *restriction endonuclease* cleavage sites on DNA showing twofold, rotational symmetry. (Cleavage sites shown are those of the restriction endonucleases *Eco R1* and *Hae II*). The cleavage sites are found at the arrows. The axes of symmetry are marked by dotted lines.

B. Structure of DNA

1. With the exception of a few viruses that contain single-stranded DNA, DNA exists as a double-stranded molecule in which the two strands wind around each other forming a ***double helix***.
2. The two chains are coiled around a ***common axis*** (Figure 28.8).
3. The chains are paired in an ***antiparallel*** manner, that is, the 5′-end of one strand is paired with the 3′-end of the other strand (Figure 28.8).
4. In the most common type of DNA helix, the classic "B" form, the hydrophilic deoxyribose-phosphate backbones of each chain are on the outside of the molecule, whereas the hydrophobic bases are stacked inside, ***perpendicular*** to the axis of the helix. The overall structure resembles a twisted ladder (Figure 28.8). The spatial relationship between the two strands in the helix creates a major (wide) groove and a minor (narrow) groove.
5. The bases of one strand are ***paired*** with the bases of the second strand so that an adenine is always paired with a thymine, while a cytosine is always paired with a guanine. Therefore, one polynucleotide chain of the DNA double helix is always the ***complement*** of the other. Given the sequence of bases on one chain, the sequence of bases on the complementary chain is determined (Figure 28.9).
   a. The base pairs are held together by hydrogen bonds: two between A and T, and three between G and C (Figure 28.10). These hydrogen bonds, plus the hydrophobic interactions between the stacked bases, stabilize the structure of the double helix.
   b. The two strands of the double helix separate when the hydrogen bonds between the paired bases are disrupted. Disruption can

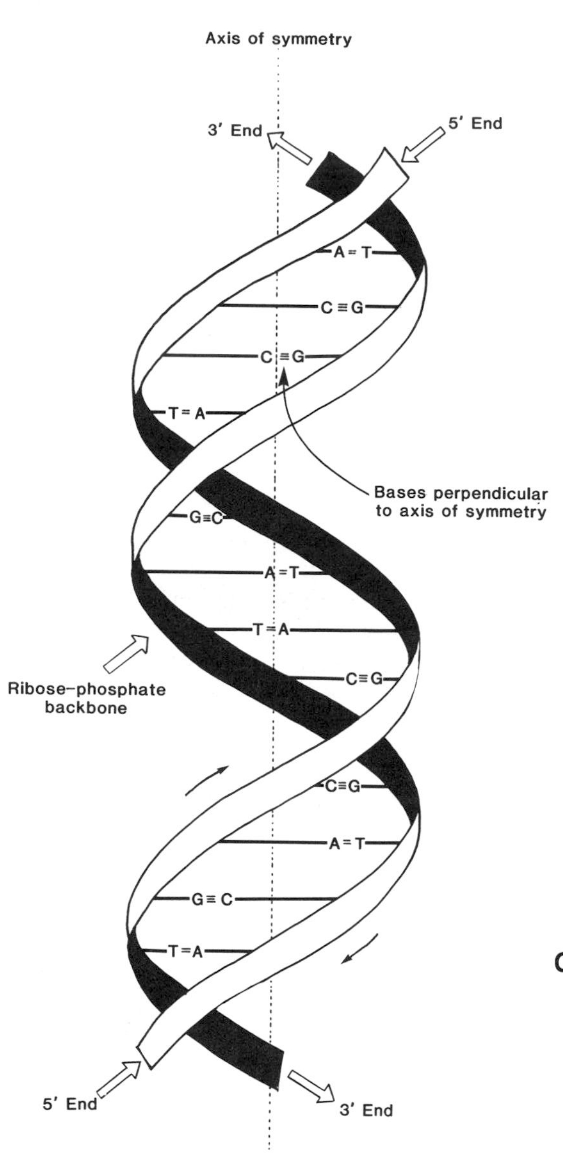

Figure 28.8
DNA double-helix illustrating some of its major structural features.

occur if the pH of the DNA solution is altered so that the nucleotide bases ionize or if the solution is heated.

c. When DNA is heated, the temperature at which half of the helical structure is lost is defined as the ***melting temperature*** (T_m). The loss of helical structure in DNA is called ***denaturation*** and can be monitored by measuring its absorbance at 260 nm. Because there are three hydrogen bonds between G and C but only two between A and T, DNA that contains high concentrations of A and T will denature at a lower temperature than G- and C-rich DNA (Figure 28.11).

6. Three structural forms of DNA have been described: the B form, described by Watson and Crick in 1953, the A form, and the Z form:

   a. The ***B form*** is a ***right-handed helix*** with ten residues per 360° turn of the helix, and with the planes of the bases perpendicular to the helical axis (Figure 28.12). Chromosomal DNA is thought to consist primarily of B DNA.

   b. The ***A form*** is produced by moderately dehydrating the B form. It is also a ***right-handed helix,*** but there are 11 base pairs per turn, and the planes of the base pairs are tilted 20° away from the perpendicular to the helical axis. The conformation found in DNA–RNA hybrids or RNA–RNA double-stranded regions is probably very close to the A form.

   c. ***Z DNA*** is a ***left-handed helix*** that contains about 12 base pairs per turn (Figure 28.12). It appears to occur naturally in specific regions of DNA and may play an important role in regulating gene expression.

C. Plasmids

1. ***Prokaryotic organisms*** contain single, large, circular chromosomes. In addition, most species of bacteria also contain small, circular, extrachromosomal DNA molecules called plasmids.

2. ***Plasmid DNA*** carries genetic information and undergoes replication that may or may not be synchronized to chromosomal division. Plasmids may carry genes that convey ***antibiotic resistance*** to the host bacterium and may facilitate the transfer of genetic information from one bacterium to another. A description of these processes can be found in a microbiology textbook.

3. Plasmids can be readily isolated from bacterial cells, their circular DNA cleaved at specific sites by *restriction endonucleases,* and foreign genes inserted into the circle. This hybrid plasmid can be reintroduced into a bacterium and large numbers of copies of the plasmid containing the foreign DNA produced (Figure 28.13). This DNA can then be further studied. The method of amplification of specific genetic material by a microorganism is called ***gene cloning,*** and is another important tool for ***"genetic engineering."***

4. When double-helical DNA is converted to a closed, circular molecule, it can itself be twisted to form a right- or left-handed ***supercoil*** (also called "supertwist" or "superhelix").

   a. Energy is required to introduce supertwists, since it introduces a strain in the DNA double helix.

   b. Supertwisting is of biological significance because superhelical

DNA has a more compact shape than its relaxed precursor (Figure 28.14). Also, negative supertwists result in a partial unwinding of the double helix, which is important in DNA replication (see p. 257).

c. Supertwists can also occur in linear DNA. They are caused by the unwinding of the double helix or can be enzymatically introduced. A further discussion of these supertwists is presented on p. 257.

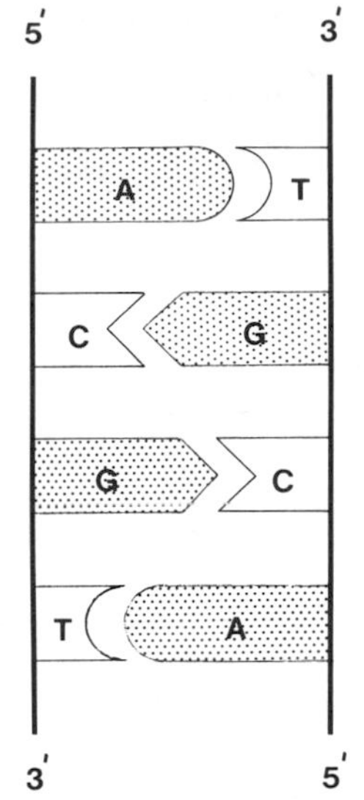

IV. ORGANIZATION OF EUKARYOTIC DNA

A. Histones

1. A typical human cell contains 46 chromosomes, each of which probably contains a single molecule of DNA. Eukaryotic DNA, however, is not "bare," but rather is associated with tightly bound proteins, including the ***histones,*** which serve to order the DNA into structural units called ***nucleosomes*** that resemble beads on a string (Figure 28.15).
2. The histones are small proteins and are positively charged at physiologic pH owing to their high content of ***lysine*** and ***arginine***. Because of their ***positive charge,*** the histones form ionic bonds with the negatively charged DNA.
3. The five major classes of histones, designated H1, H2A, H2B, H3, and H4, fall into two main groups:
   a. The first group of histones form the structural core of the individual nucleosome "beads." Two molecules each of H2A, H2B, H3, and H4 associate to form the nucleosome core, around which a segment of the DNA double helix is wound, forming a negatively supertwisted helix (Figure 28.15).
   b. Histone H1, of which there are several related species that form the second group of histones, is not found in the nucleosome core but appears to bind to the DNA chain ***between*** the nucleosome beads (the ***linker DNA***). H1 appears to aid the packing of nucleosomes into a more compact structure called the ***chromatin fiber.*** During cell division, the chromatin condenses further to form the ***chromosomes*** that are visible in the light microscope.
4. In addition to the histones, small nonhistone proteins called ***protamines*** bind to the DNA. Numerous enzymes and regulatory proteins also associate with the chromatin through sequence-specific interactions that may facilitate or inhibit DNA replication or RNA transcription.

Figure 28.9
Two complementary DNA sequences.

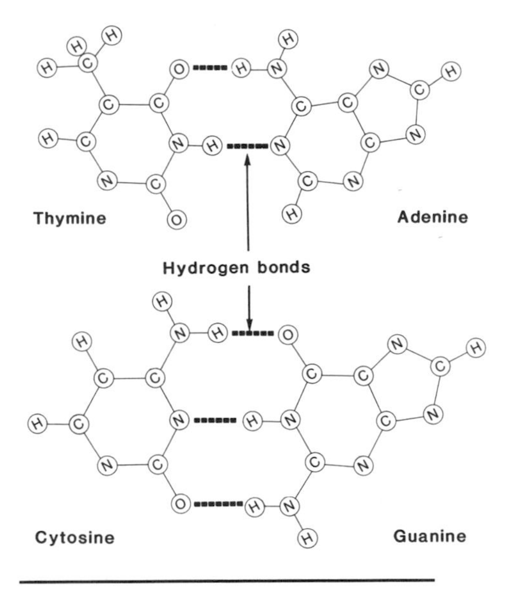

Figure 28.10
Hydrogen bonds between complementary bases.

V. STRUCTURE OF RNA

There are three major types of RNA: ribosomal RNA (rRNA), transfer RNA (tRNA), and messenger RNA (mRNA). Like DNA, all three types of RNA are long, unbranched molecules composed of mononucleotides joined together by phosphodiester bonds. They differ as a group from DNA in several ways, however; for example, they are considerably smaller than DNA and, as previously discussed, contain ***ribose*** instead

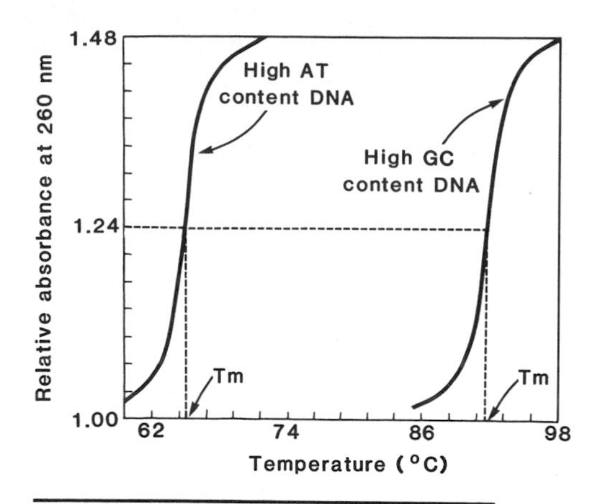

Figure 28.11
Melting temperature of DNA molecules with different nucleotide compositions. (At a wavelength of 260 nm, single-stranded DNA has a higher relative absorbence than does double-stranded DNA.)

of deoxyribose and ***uracil*** instead of thymine. The three types of RNA also differ from each other in terms of size, function, and special structural modifications.

A. Ribosomal RNA

1. There are three distinct size species of rRNA (23S, 16S, and 5S) in prokaryotic cells and eukaryotic mitochondria. In the eukaryotic cytosol, there are four rRNA size species (5S, 5.8S, 18S, and 28S). (Note: "S" is the ***Svedberg unit,*** which is related to the molecular weight of the compound.) Together, they make up about 80% of the RNA in the cell.
2. Ribosomal RNA is found in association with a number of different proteins as components of the ribosomes—the complex structures that serve as the sites for protein synthesis (see p. 380).

B. Transfer RNA

1. The smallest of the RNA molecules (4S), transfer RNA has between 73 and 93 nucleotide residues. There is at least one specific type of tRNA molecule for each of the 20 amino acids

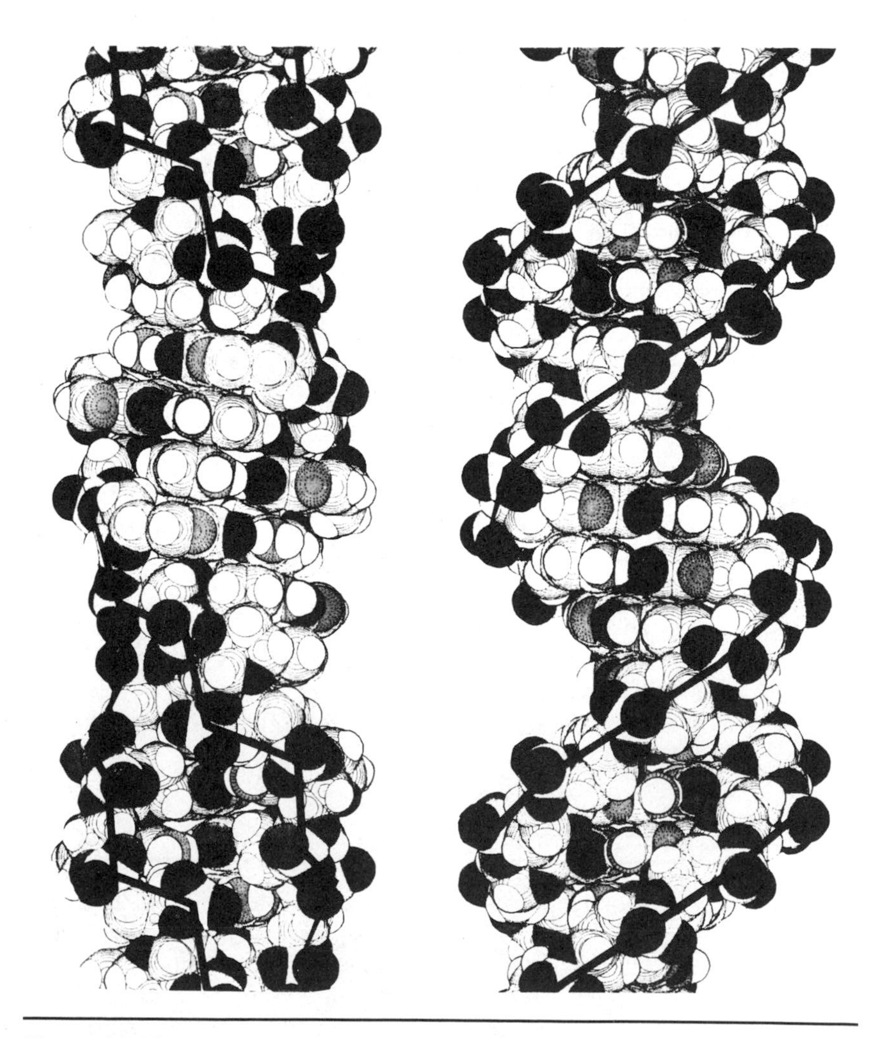

Figure 28.12
Comparison of the structures of Z DNA (left) and B DNA (right).

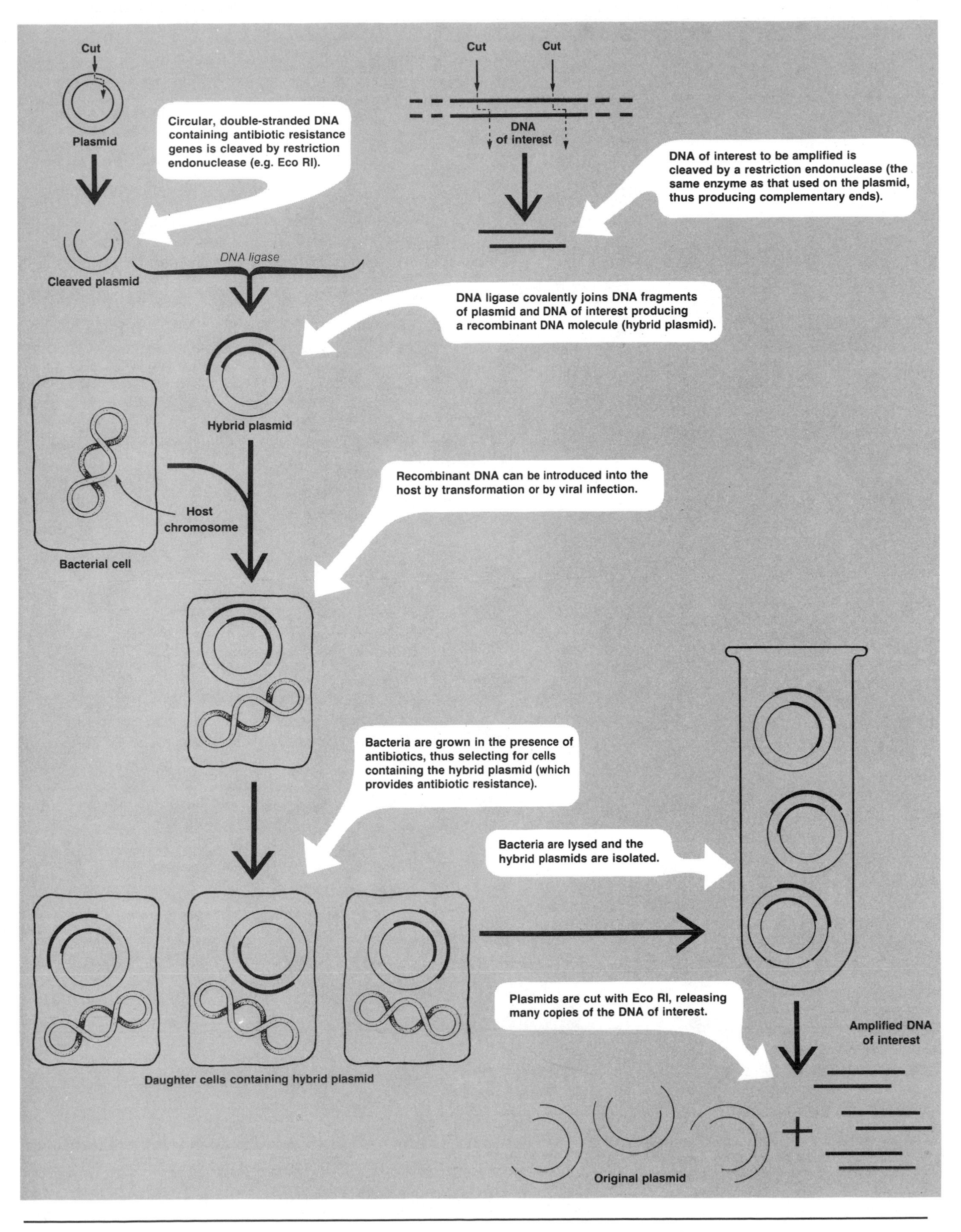

Figure 28.13
Summary of gene cloning.

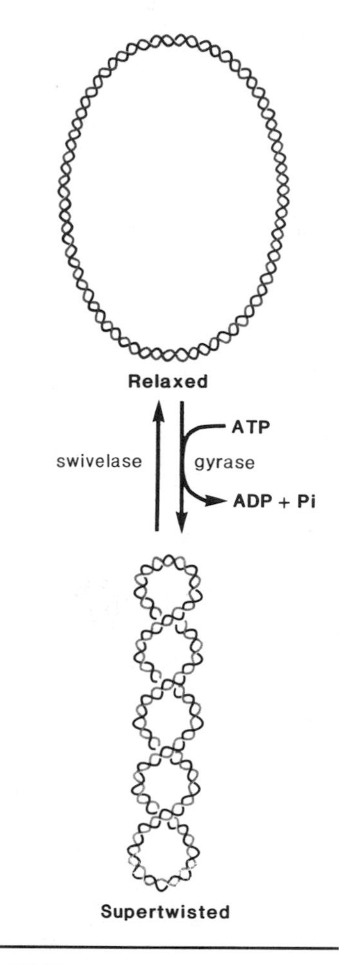

Figure 28.14
Introduction of supertwists in a double-helical DNA molecule.

commonly found in proteins. Together they make up about 15% of the RNA in the cell.

2. The tRNA molecules contain many unusual bases (see p. 334) and have extensive intrachain base pairing, as shown in Figure 28.16. Additional features of this structure are also identified in Figure 28.16.
3. Each tRNA serves as an "adaptor" molecule that carries its specific amino acid to the site of protein synthesis. There, it recognizes the genetic code word that specifies the addition of its amino acid to the growing peptide chain (see p. 381).

C. Messenger RNA

1. mRNA composes only about 5% of the RNA in the cell yet is by far the most heterogeneous type of RNA in terms of size. The mRNA carries the genetic information from the DNA and is used as the ***template*** for protein synthesis.
2. Special structural characteristics of eukaryotic mRNA include a long sequence of adenines (a "poly-A tail") on the 3′-end of the RNA chain, plus a "cap" on the 5′-end consisting of a molecule

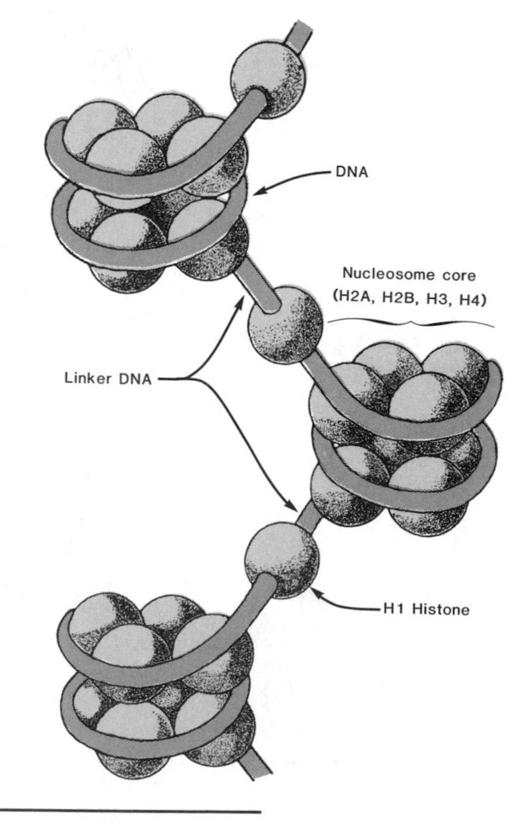

Figure 28.15
Organization of human DNA, illustrating the structure of nucleosomes.

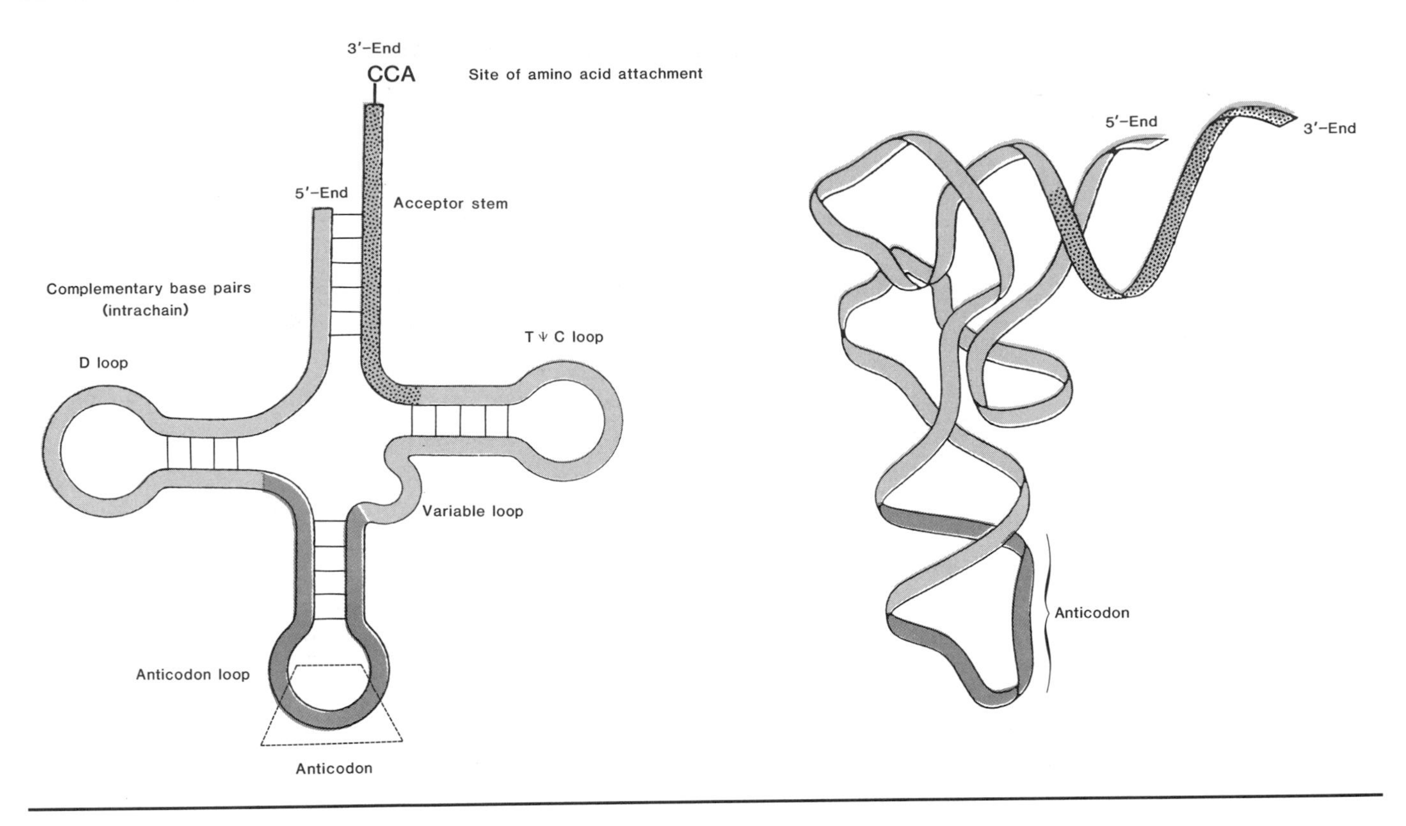

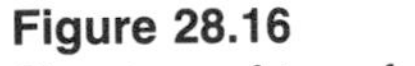

Figure 28.16
Structure of transfer RNA.

of 7-methylguanosine attached "backward" through a triphosphate linkage, as shown in Figure 28.17. (The mechanisms for modifying mRNA to give it these special structural characteristics are discussed on p. 373.)

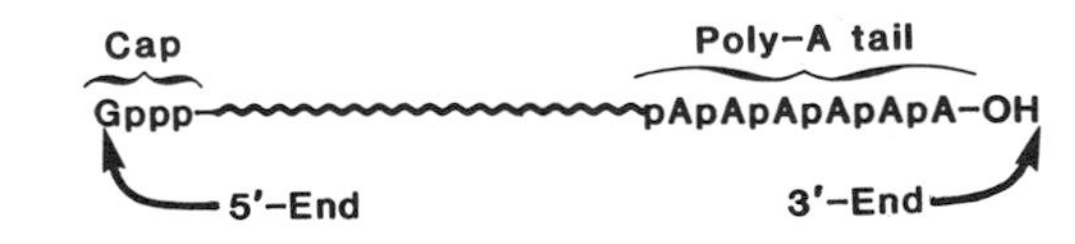

Figure 28.17
Structure of messenger RNA.

Study Questions

Choose the ONE best answer:

28.1 Which ***one*** of the following statements about the structure of double-helical DNA is INCORRECT?

A. Within the double-helix there are ten base pairs per turn of the helix.
B. The forces that stabilize the DNA double-helix are hydrogen bonds between complementary bases and stacking interactions between bases.
C. Separation of the two strands of the double-helix requires untwisting of the helix.
D. The double-helix contains antiparallel chains that form a major and a minor groove on the surface of the helix.
E. The molar amount of adenine plus thymine equals the molar amount of guanine plus cytosine.

28.2 Complete acid hydrolysis of nucleic acids yields all of the following ***except***

A. phosphoric acid.
B. purines.
C. pentoses.
D. adenosine.
E. cytosine.

28.3 Which one of the following choices best completes the following sentence? Transfer RNA...

A. contains the information necessary for the synthesis of a specific protein.
B. must exist in at least 20 different forms, one for each amino acid.
C. is the largest of the RNA species.
D. has little or no secondary structure.
E. exists in the cytoplasm associated with histones.

28.4 Which one of the following choices best completes the following sentence? Histones...

A. are basic proteins rich in lysine or arginine, or both.
B. are bound covalently to DNA.
C. have relatively high molecular weights (200,000 daltons or higher).
D. are identical to protamines.
E. are found in high concentrations in ribosomes.

28.5 Which one of the following statements about most eukaryotic messenger RNA is INCORRECT?

A. The pentose found in mRNA is D-ribose.
B. mRNA exists as a single-stranded molecule.
C. mRNA has a long sequence of adenine nucleotides on its 3′-end.
D. mRNA has a molecule of 7-methylguanosine at its 5′-end.
E. The mRNA chain is longer than that of DNA.

Nucleotide Metabolism

29

I. OVERVIEW

Ribonucleoside and deoxyribonucleoside triphosphates (nucleotides) are essential for all cells. Without these compounds, neither DNA nor RNA can be produced, proteins cannot be synthesized, and therefore cells cannot proliferate. In addition, nucleotides play an extremely important role as "energy currency" in the cell. Nucleotides serve as carriers of activated intermediates in the synthesis of some carbohydrates, lipids, and proteins and are structural components of a number of essential cofactors such as coenzyme A, FAD, NAD^+, and $NADP^+$. Finally, nucleotides are important regulatory compounds for many of the pathways of intermediary metabolism, inhibiting or activating key enzymes.

The purine and pyrimidine bases found in nucleotides can be synthesized *de novo* or can be obtained through salvage pathways that allow the reuse of the preformed bases resulting from normal cell turnover or from the diet.

II. *DE NOVO* PURINE NUCLEOTIDE SYNTHESIS

A. Sources of atoms in the purine ring

1. The atoms of the purine ring are contributed by a number of compounds, including the amino acids aspartic acid, glycine, and glutamine, CO_2, and derivatives of tetrahydrofolic acid (Figure 29.1).
2. The purine ring is constructed by a series of reactions that add the donated carbons and nitrogens to a preformed ribose 5-phosphate.

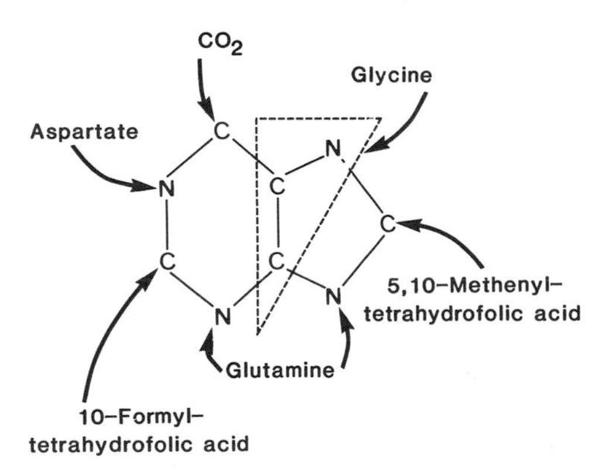

Figure 29.1
Sources of the individual atoms in the purine ring.

B. Synthesis of 5′-phosphoribosyl-1′-pyrophosphate (PRPP)

1. The synthesis of PRPP from ATP and ribose 5′-phosphate is shown in Figure 29.2. (Note that the sugar moiety is ***ribose***. In synthesizing nucleotides, ***ribo***nucleotides are first produced and may subsequently be reduced to ***deoxyribo***nucleotides.)
2. PRPP also participates in the synthesis of pyrimidines (see p. 351) and in the salvage reactions of purine and pyrimidine bases (see p. 351).

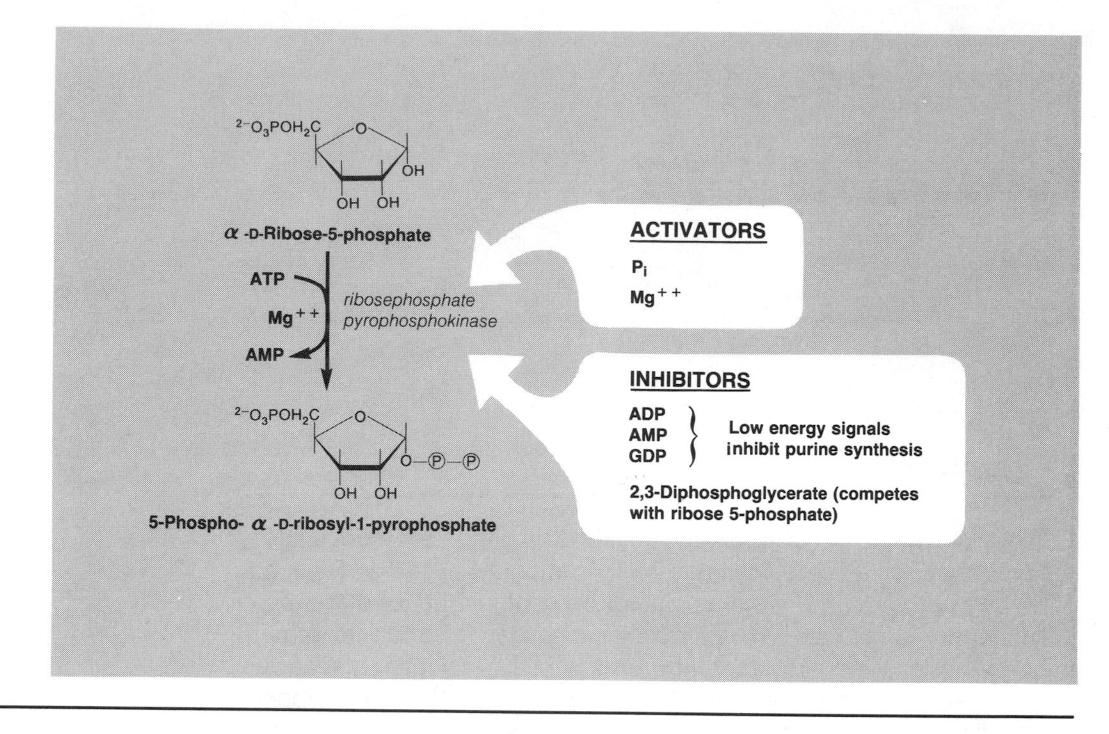

Figure 29.2
Synthesis of 5′-phosphoribosyl-1′-pyrophosphate (PRPP) showing activators and inhibitors of the pathway.

C. Synthesis of 5′-phosphoribosylamine

1. The synthesis of 5′-phosphoribosylamine from PRPP and glutamine is shown in Figure 29.3. The amide group of glutamine replaces the pyrophosphate group attached to carbon #1 of PRPP.
2. The enzyme *glutamine phosphoribosyl pyrophosphate amidotransferase* is inhibited by purine 5′-nucleotides—the end-products of this pathway—including AMP, GMP, and IMP. Nucleoside diphosphates and triphosphates also have some inhibitory effect. This is the ***committed step*** in purine nucleotide biosynthesis.
3. The rate of the reaction is also controlled by the intracellular concentrations of the substrates glutamine and PRPP.

   a. The intracellular concentration of PRPP is normally 10^{-5} to 10^{-6}M, whereas the K_m for the *amidotransferase* is 3×10^{-4}M. Therefore, since the substrate concentration is far below the K_m, any small change in the PRPP concentration will cause a proportional change in the rate of the reaction.

D. Synthesis of inosine monophosphate (IPP), the "parent" purine

1. The next nine steps in purine nucleotide biosynthesis leading to the synthesis of IPP are illustrated in Figure 29.3.
2. This pathway requires four ATP molecules as the major energy source.

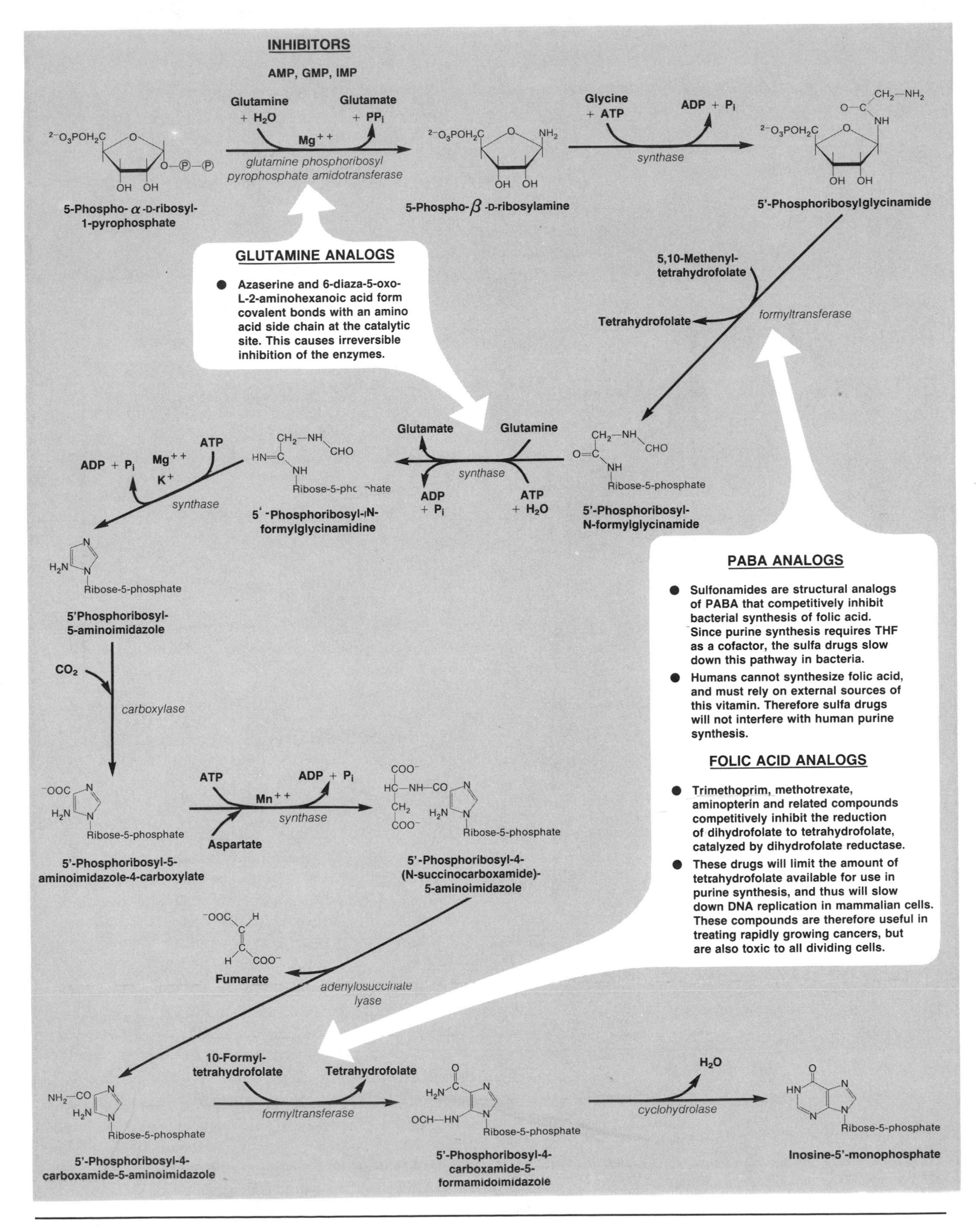

Figure 29.3
Synthesis of purine nucleotides showing inhibitory effect of structural analogues.

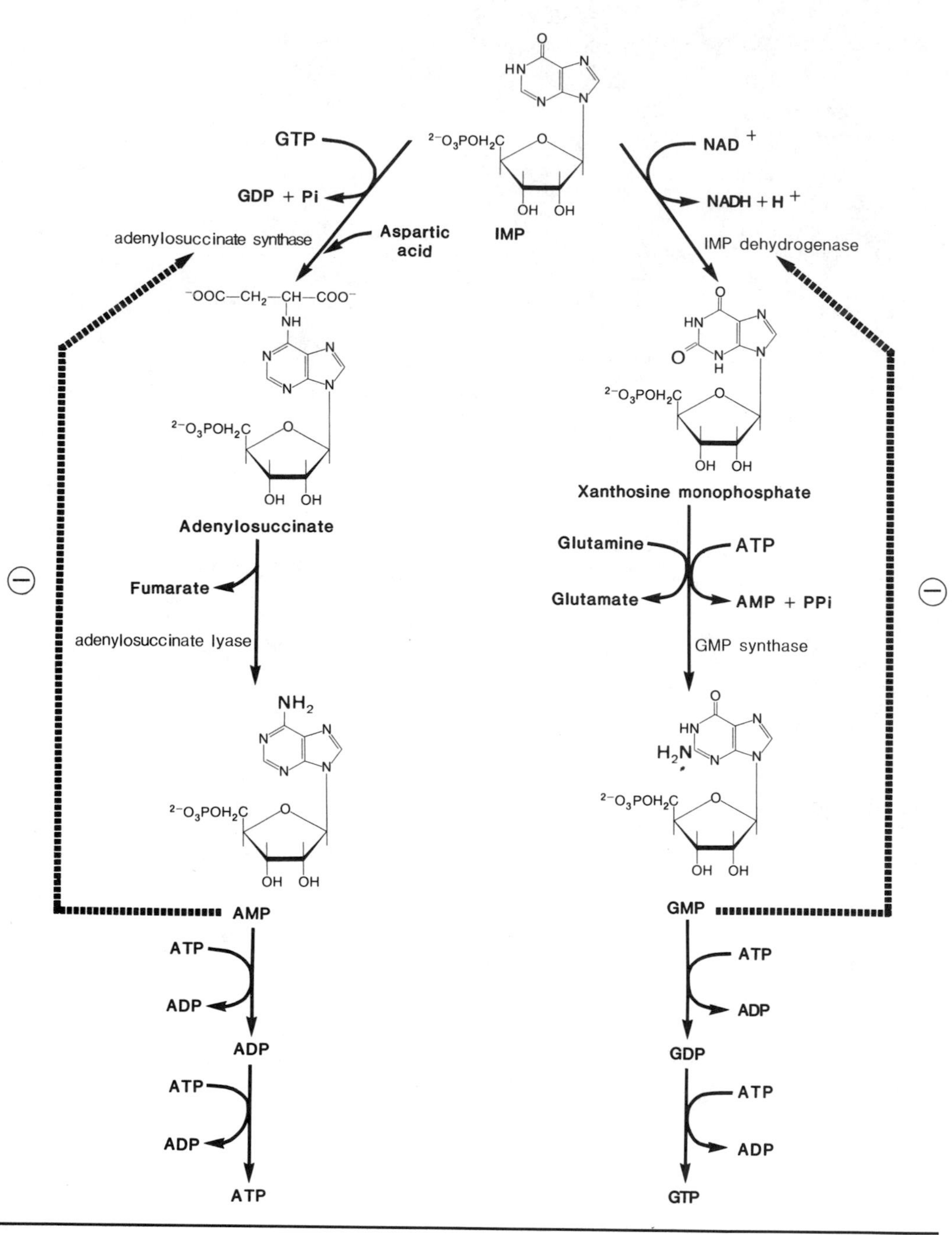

Figure 29.4
Conversion of IMP to AMP and GMP showing feedback inhibition.

E. Conversion of IMP to AMP and GMP

1. The conversion of IMP to either AMP or GMP utilizes a two-step, energy-requiring pathway (Figure 29.4). Note that the synthesis of AMP requires GTP as an energy source, whereas the synthesis of GMP requires ATP. Also, the first reaction in each pathway is inhibited by the end-product of that pathway.

F. Inhibitors of purine synthesis

1. Inhibitors of purine synthesis are extremely toxic, especially to rapidly growing microorganisms, tumor cells, or developing structures such as in a fetus.
2. ***Structural analogues*** of glutamine and folic acid are used pharmacologically to control the spread of cancer or infections by interfering with the synthesis of nucleotides, and therefore of DNA and RNA. Examples of these structural analogues and the sites of their inhibitory activities are illustrated in Figure 29.3.

III. DEGRADATION OF PURINE NUCLEOTIDES

A. Formation of uric acid

Purine nucleotides are sequentially degraded by the removal or alteration of portions of the nucleotide. The end-product of this pathway in humans is uric acid. A summary of the steps in the production of uric acid is shown in Figure 29.5:

[1] An amino group is removed from AMP to produce IMP, or from adenosine to produce inosine.

[2] IMP and GMP are converted into their nucleoside forms—inosine and guanosine—by the action of *5′-nucleotidase.*

[3] *Purine nucleoside phosphorylase* converts inosine and guanosine into their respective purine bases, hypoxanthine and guanine.

[4] Guanine is deaminated to produce xanthine.

[5] Hypoxanthine is oxidized by *xanthine oxidase,* producing xanthine, which is further oxidized to ***uric acid,*** the final product of human purine degradation. Uric acid is excreted in the urine.

Mammals other than primates oxidize uric acid further to allantoin, which, in some animals other than mammals, may be further degraded to urea or even ammonia.

B. Degradation of dietary nucleic acids in the small intestine

1. *Ribonucleases and deoxyribonucleases,* secreted in pancreatic juice, hydrolyze RNA and DNA primarily to oligonucleotides.
2. Oligonucleotides are further hydrolyzed by pancreatic *phosphodiesterases,* producing a mixture of 3′- and 5′-mononucleotides.
3. A family of *nucleotidases* removes the phosphate groups hydrolytically, releasing nucleosides that may be absorbed by the intestinal mucosal cells or further degraded to free bases before uptake.
4. The dietary purines and pyrimidines are not used to a large extent for the synthesis of tissue nucleic acids but are largely catabolized in the intestinal mucosal cells.
5. A summary of this pathway is shown in Figure 29.6.

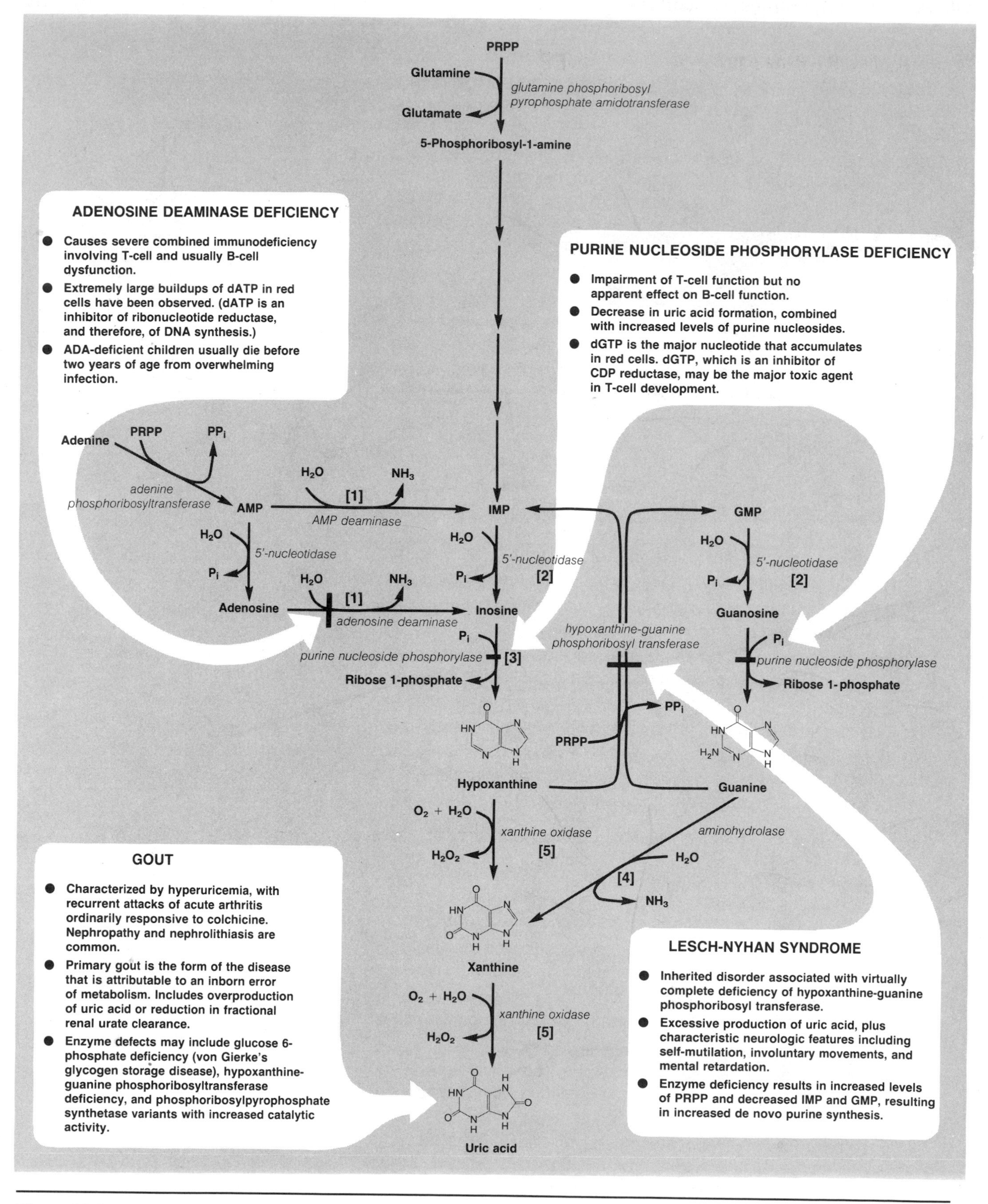

Figure 29.5

Degradation of purine nucleotides to uric acid and salvage pathways of free bases, illustrating some of the genetic diseases associated with these pathways. The numbers in brackets refer to the correspondingly numbered text.

IV. SALVAGE PATHWAY FOR PURINES

A. Purines that either result from the normal turnover of cellular nucleic acids or are obtained from the diet and not degraded can be reconverted into nucleoside triphosphates and used by the body. This is referred to as the "salvage pathway" for purines.

1. Although *de novo* synthesis of purines occurs primarily in the liver, the salvage pathway occurs primarily in extrahepatic tissues. A summary of the purine "salvage" pathway is shown in Figure 29.5.
2. Two enzymes are involved: *adenine phosphoribosyltransferase* (APRT) and *hypoxanthine-guanine phosphoribosyltransferase* (HGPRT). Both enzymes use PRPP as the source of the ribose 5-phosphate group. The release of pyrophosphate makes these reactions irreversible.
3. A deficiency of HGPRT causes the ***Lesch–Nyhan Syndrome*** (see Figure 29.5).

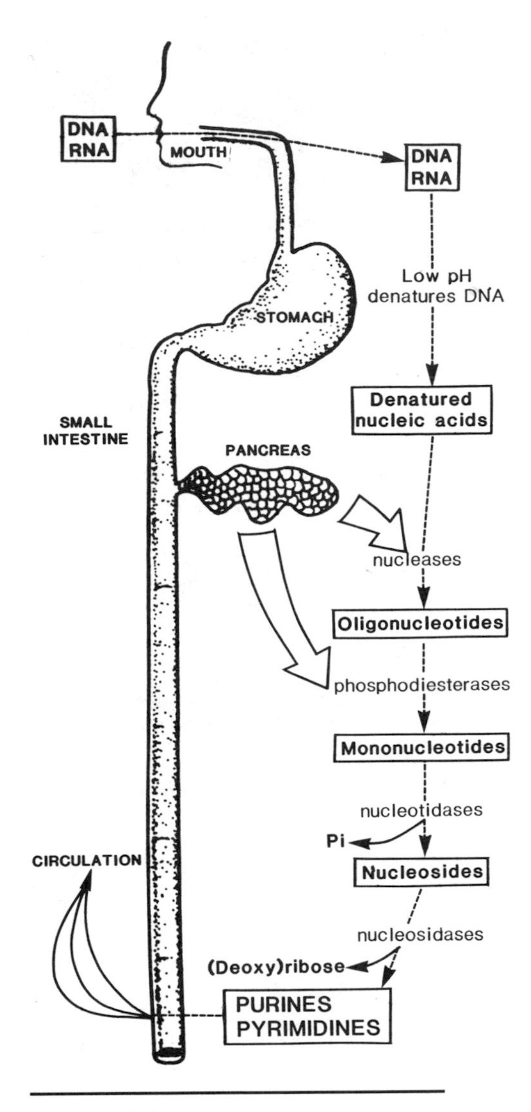

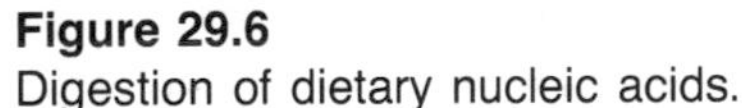
Figure 29.6
Digestion of dietary nucleic acids.

V. PYRIMIDINE SYNTHESIS

A. Formation of the pyrimidine ring

1. Unlike the purine ring, the pyrimidine ring is synthesized before being attached to ribose 5-phosphate, which is donated by PRPP (Figure 29.7).
   a. Sources of the carbon and nitrogen atoms are ***carbamoyl phosphate*** and ***aspartic acid*** (Figure 29.8). Carbamoyl phosphate is also a precursor of urea, but, in the pyrimidine synthetic pathway, carbamoyl phosphate is made in the cytoplasm by *carbamoyl phosphate synthetase II (CPS II)*. (Note: Carbamoyl phosphate processed through the urea cycle is synthesized in the mitochondria by *carbamoyl phosphate synthetase I*; see p. 231). *CPS I* uses ammonia as the source of nitrogen, whereas *CPS II* uses the γ-amino group of glutamine. Thus ***glutamine*** is required for both purine and pyrimidine synthesis (see Table 29.1 for a summary of the differences between these two enzymes.)

TABLE 29.1

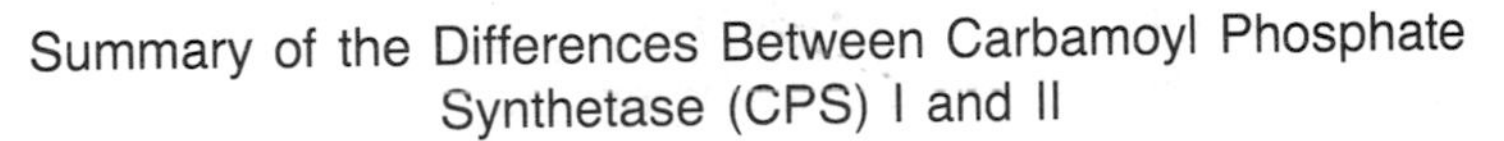
Summary of the Differences Between Carbamoyl Phosphate Synthetase (CPS) I and II

	CPS I	CPS II
Cellular location:	Mitochondria	Cytoplasm
Pathway involved:	Urea cycle	Pyrimidine synthesis
Source of nitrogen:	Ammonia	γ-Amino group of glutamine

   b. The committed step in this pathway is catalyzed by *aspartate transcarbamoylase,* an extensively studied regulatory enzyme

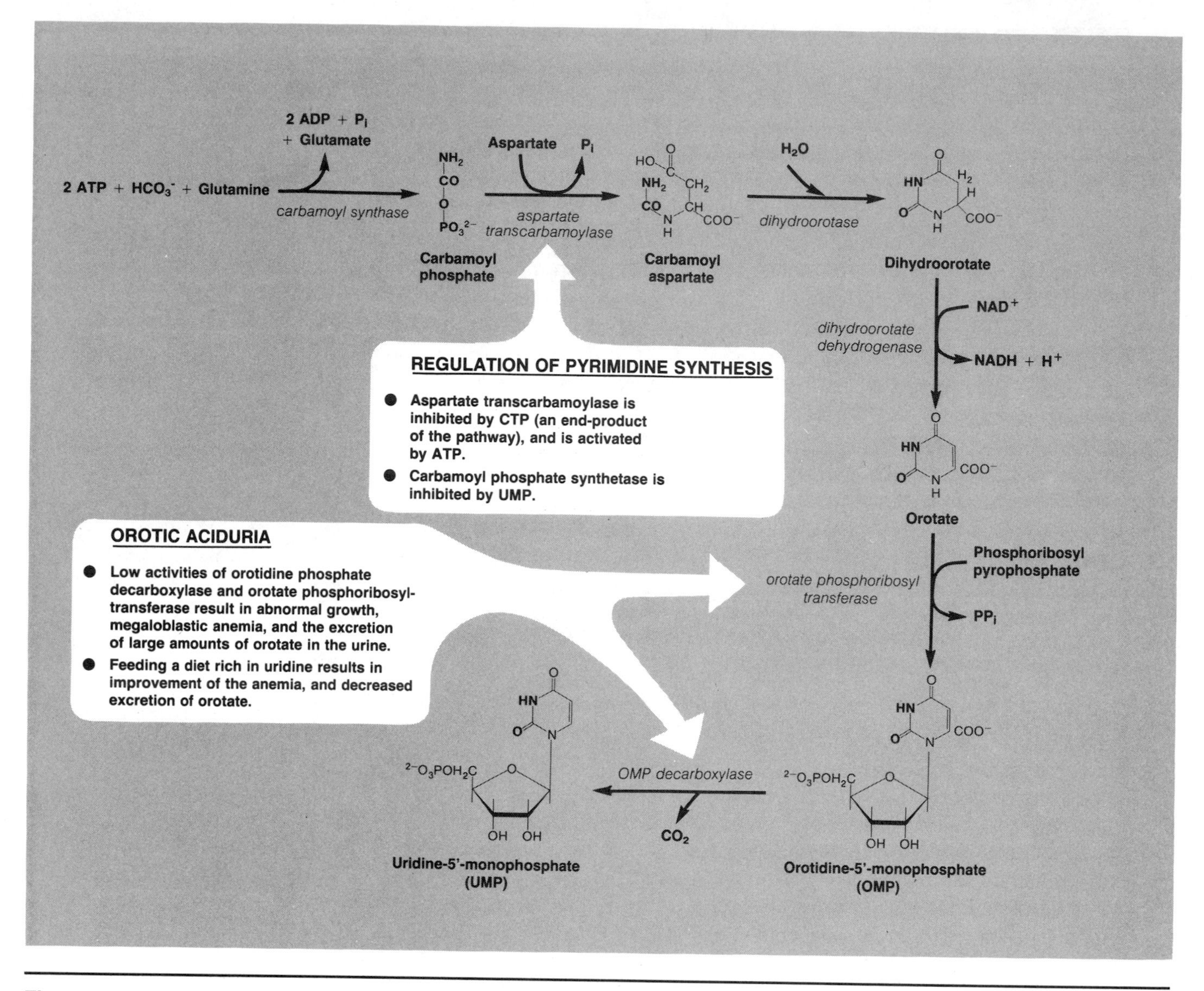

Figure 29.7
Pyrimidine synthesis, illustrating enzyme complexes and genetic diseases associated with this pathway.

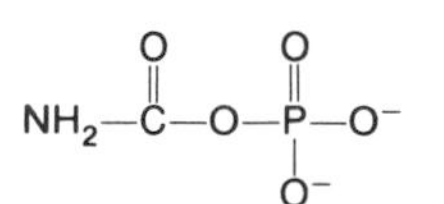

(see Figure 29.7). It produces ***N*-carbamoylaspartate** from carbamoyl phosphate and aspartic acid.

c. The pyrimidine ring is closed hydrolytically by *dihydroorotase*. The resulting dihydroorotate is oxidized to produce ***orotic acid*** (see Figure 29.7).

d. The first three enzymes in this pathway (*CPS II, aspartate transcarbamoylase,* and *dihydroorotase*) are all domains of the same polypeptide chain (see p. 18 for a discussion of domains). This is an example of a ***multienzyme complex*** that facilitates the ordered synthesis of an important compound.

2. The completed pyrimidine ring is converted to the nucleotide ***orotidine 5'-monophosphate*** (OMP) in the second stage of pyrimidine nucleotide synthesis (see Figure 29.7):

a. PRPP is again the ribose 5-phosphate donor. The enzyme *orotate phosphoribosyl transferase* produces the nucleotide

(OMP) with the release of pyrophosphate, making the reaction biologically irreversible.

b. Thus, both purine and pyrimidine synthesis require glutamine and PRPP as essential precursors.

3. OMP, the parent pyrimidine mononucleotide, is converted to ***uridine monophosphate*** (UMP) by *orotidylate decarboxylase*, which removes the acidic carboxyl group (see Figure 29.7).

4. The *orotate phosphoribosyl transferase* and *orotidylate decarboxylase* are also domains of a single polypeptide chain. ***Orotic aciduria*** results from a deficiency of this bifunctional enzyme, resulting in orotic acid in the urine.

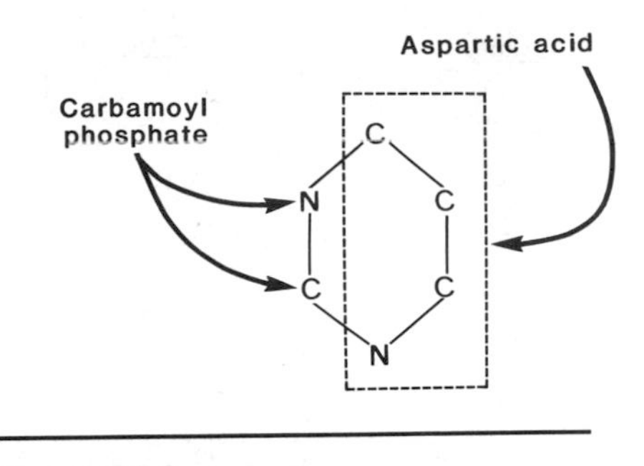

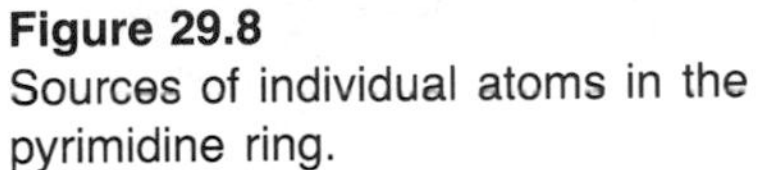

Figure 29.8
Sources of individual atoms in the pyrimidine ring.

B. Synthesis of cytidine triphosphate

1. Cytidine triphosphate (CTP) is produced by the amination of UTP (Figure 29.9). The nitrogen is provided by glutamine—another example of a reaction in nucleotide biosynthesis in which this amino acid is required.

C. Synthesis of thymidine monophosphate (dTMP) from dUMP

1. dUMP is converted to dTMP by *thymidylate synthetase* (Figure 29.10), which uses ***5,10-methylene tetrahydrofolic acid*** as the source of the methyl group (see p. 318 for a discussion of this cofactor).

   a. This is an unusual reaction in that the tetrahydrofolic acid (THF) contributes not only a carbon unit but also a hydrogen atom from the pteridine ring, resulting in the oxidation of THF to dihydrofolic acid (DHF).

   b. DHF can be reduced to THF by *dihydrofolate reductase*, the enzyme that is inhibited in the presence of drugs such as ***aminopterin*** and ***methotrexate***. By decreasing the supply of THF, these folic acid analogues not only inhibit purine synthesis (see Figure 29.3), but also, by preventing the methylation of dUMP to dTMP, lower the cellular concentration of this essential component of DNA. DNA synthesis is therefore inhibited by these agents and cell growth slowed. Because of their ability to slow the replication of DNA due to a lowered supply of nucleotide precursors, these drugs are used to decrease the growth rate of cancer cells.

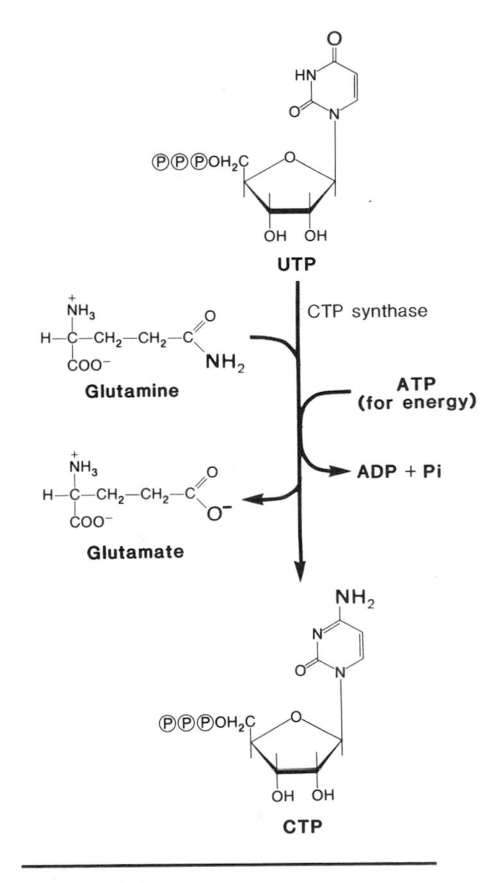

Figure 29.9
Synthesis of CTP from UTP.

D. Regulation of pyrimidine synthesis

1. Pyrimidine synthesis is ***inhibited*** by the end-product of the pathway, UMP (and UTP), and also by the "low energy signal" AMP (see Figure 29.7).

2. Pyrimidine synthesis is ***activated*** by the "high-energy signal" ATP. Phosphoribosylpyrophosphate (PRPP), also an allosteric activator of the pathway, is itself synthesized only in the absence of low-energy signals (see Figure 29.3).

E. Formation of nucleoside trinucleotides

1. The formation of diphosphates from monophosphates is catalyzed by a family of kinases, each of which is specific for a particular base but nonspecific for the sugar portion of the nucleotide (i.e., ribose versus deoxyribose). ATP is the source of the added phosphate.

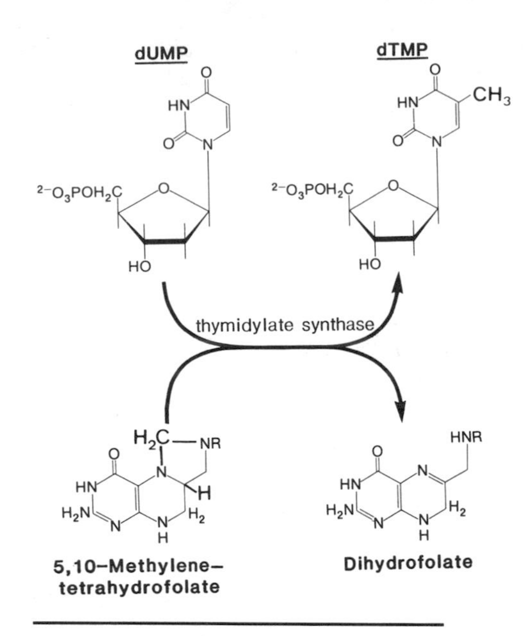

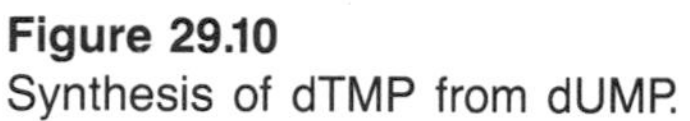

Figure 29.10
Synthesis of dTMP from dUMP.

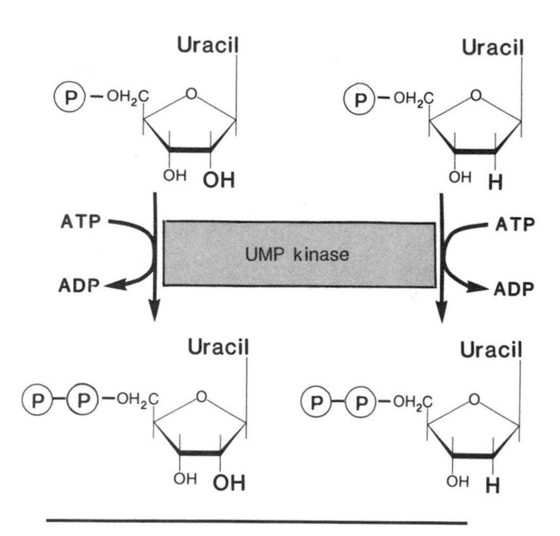

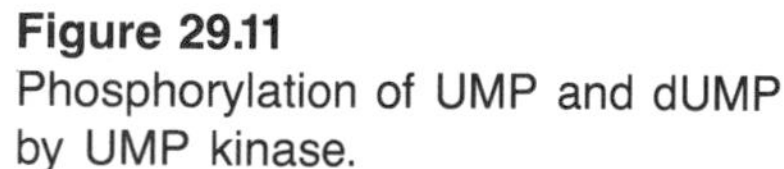

Figure 29.11
Phosphorylation of UMP and dUMP by UMP kinase.

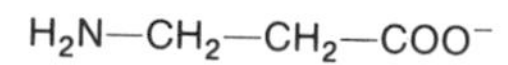

$H_2N{-}CH_2{-}CH_2{-}COO^-$

β-Alanine

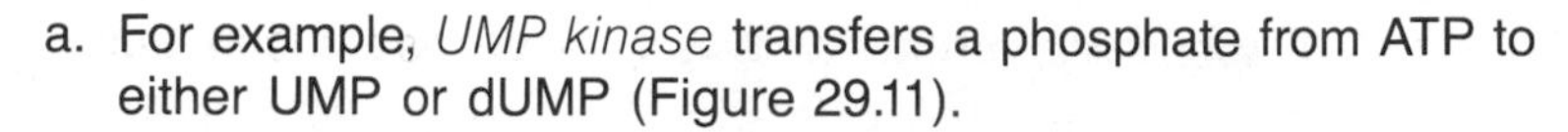

a. For example, *UMP kinase* transfers a phosphate from ATP to either UMP or dUMP (Figure 29.11).

b. A specialized enzyme, *adenylate kinase,* is particularly active in tissues such as the liver and muscle, where the turnover of energy from ATP is high. Its function is to maintain an equilibrium among AMP, ADP, and ATP:

$$2ADP \rightleftarrows AMP + ATP$$

2. Nucleoside diphosphates and triphosphates are interconverted by *nucleoside diphosphate kinase*—an enzyme that, unlike the monophosphate kinases, has a broad specificity.

VI. DEGRADATION OF PYRIMIDINE NUCLEOTIDES

A. Unlike the purine rings, which are not cleaved in human cells, the pyrimidine ring can be opened and the resulting structure further utilized by the body. A summary of the pathway for the degradation of thymine is shown in Figure 29.12.

B. The degradation pathway for uracil is very similar, with the end-product being β-alanine instead of β-aminoisobutyrate.

VII. CONVERSION OF RIBONUCLEOTIDES TO DEOXYRIBONUCLEOTIDES

The nucleotides synthesized by the pathways described thus far in this chapter are all ***ribo***nucleotides. These can be used as building blocks in RNA synthesis or as nucleotide carriers of other compounds such as sugars (see Unit II for a number of examples of nucleotides in this role). The nucleotides required for DNA synthesis are ***2′-deoxyribo***nucleotides, which are produced from ribonucleotide ***di***phosphates (see Figure 29.13 for a summary of the pathway for conversion of ribonucleotides to deoxyribonucleotides).

A. Ribonucleoside reductase

1. *Ribonucleoside reductase* is a multi-subunit enzyme that is specific for the reduction of nucleoside diphosphates (ADP, GDP, CDP, and UDP).

2. The immediate donor of the hydrogen atoms needed for the reduction is the small protein ***thioredoxin,*** which contains two cysteine residues separated by two amino acids in the peptide chain. The two sulfhydryl groups donate their hydrogen atoms, forming a disulfide bond (cystine; see p. 18). The two hydrogen atoms are used by the enzyme to reduce the ribonucleotide to a ***deoxyribonucleotide,*** and produce water (Figure 29.13).

3. Thioredoxin must be converted back into its reduced form in order to continue to perform its function. The necessary reducing equivalents are provided by NADPH + H^+, and the reaction is catalyzed by *thioredoxin reductase* (Figure 29.13).

4. The regulation of *ribonucleotide reductase* is complex.
   a. The binding of dATP to an allosteric site on the enzyme decreases the overall catalytic activity of the enzyme.
   b. The binding of ***deoxyribo***nucleoside ***tri***phosphates to additional allosteric sites on the enzyme regulates ***substrate specificity,*** causing an ***increase*** in the conversion of different species of ribonucleotides to deoxyribonucleotides as they are required for DNA synthesis.

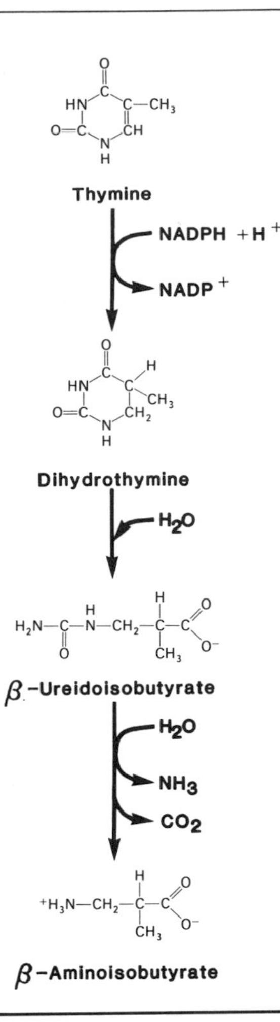

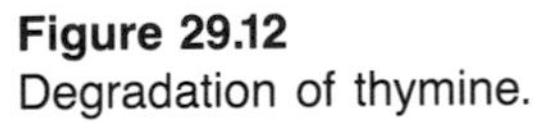
Figure 29.12
Degradation of thymine.

Study Questions

Choose the ONE BEST answer:

29.1 The formation of uric acid from purines is catalyzed by
A. adenylate deaminase.
B. uricase.
C. allantoinase.
D. urease.
E. xanthine oxidase.

29.2 The committed step in pyrimidine biosynthesis
A. provides a classic example of positive feedback control.
B. results in the formation of dihydroorotic acid.
C. is the formation of N-carbamoylaspartic acid.
D. is catalyzed by orotate decarboxylase.
E. requires ATP.

29.3 The four nitrogen atoms of the purine ring are derived from
A. aspartate, glutamine, and glycine.
B. glutamine, ammonia, and aspartate.
C. glycine and aspartate.
D. ammonia, glycine, and glutamate.
E. urea and ammonia.

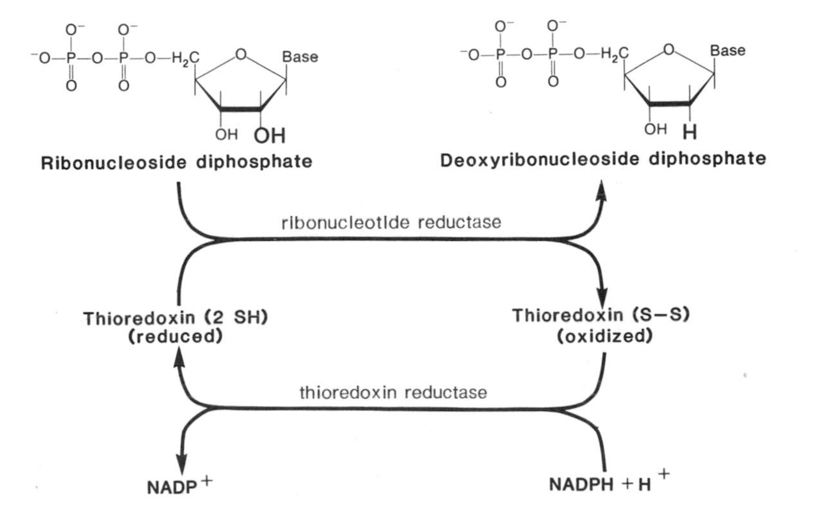

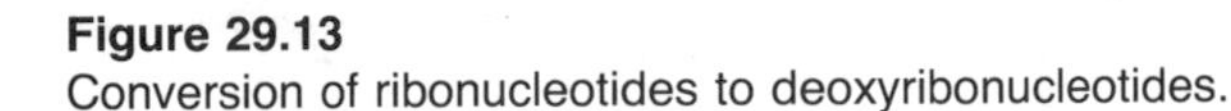
Figure 29.13
Conversion of ribonucleotides to deoxyribonucleotides.

29.4 The absence of which enzyme involved in the "salvage pathways" of nucleotide metabolism results in the genetic disease Lesch-Nyhan Syndrome?

A. Hypoxanthine-guanine phosphoribosyl transferase
B. Aspartate transcarbamoylase
C. Thymidylate kinase
D. Adenylate deaminase
E. Xanthine oxidase

29.5 6-Mercaptopurine, which has been used to treat acute leukemia, is converted to the nucleotide 6-mercaptopurine-9-ribose-5′-phosphate in the body. This nucleotide interferes with the conversion of inosine 5′-phosphate (IMP) to adenosine 5′-phosphate (AMP). Which one of the following compounds is the immediate source of the amino group that is introduced into IMP during this conversion?

A. Aspartate
B. NH_4^+
C. S-Adenosylmethionine
D. Glutamine
E. Asparagine

Answer A if 1, 2, and 3 are correct
B if 1 and 3 are correct
C if 2 and 4 are correct
D if only 4 is correct
E if all are correct

29.6 In the formation of purine and pyrimidine nucleotides,

1. both pathways require ATP.
2. all intermediates of the pyrimidine nucleotides are derivatives of ribose 5′-phosphate.
3. all intermediates of the purine nucleotides are derivatives of ribose 5′-phosphate.
4. 5-phosphoribosyl-1-pyrophosphate is not involved in the synthesis of pyrimidine nucleotides.

29.7 Uric acid is a breakdown product of

1. AMP.
2. IMP.
3. GMP.
4. CMP.

29.8 Which of the following statements about purine and pyrimidine biosynthesis is(are) CORRECT?

1. The formation of 5-phosphoribosyl-1-amine is an important regulatory step in purine biosynthesis.
2. The *de novo* synthesis of purines requires the participation of tetrahydrofolate-derivatives.
3. 5-Phosphoribosyl-1-pyrophosphate (PRPP) is used for the synthesis of uridine 5′-phosphate (UMP) from orotate.
4. Thymidine 5′-phosphate is formed in a reaction involving the direct participation of PRPP and thymidine.

DNA Synthesis

30

I. OVERVIEW

If adenine (A) is present on one strand of a DNA double-helix, it must be paired with thymine (T) on the complementary strand; similarly, guanine (G) must be paired with cytosine (C) as discussed on p. 337. Therefore, the information contained in the sequence of one strand is also present, although in a complementary form, in the second strand. When the two sister strands are separated, each can serve as a ***template*** for the replication of a new, complementary strand. This process is called ***semiconservative replication*** since, although the parental duplex is separated into two halves (and therefore not "conserved" as an entity), each of the individual parental strands is left intact in one of the two new duplexes (Figure 30.1).

The enzymes involved in the replicative process are template-directed polymerases that can synthesize the complementary sequence of each strand with extraordinary fidelity. The reactions described in this section are best known from studies on the bacterium *Escherichia coli (E. coli)*, and therefore the enzyme names used below in general refer to the process in that microorganism. DNA synthesis in higher organisms is less well understood but involves the same types of mechanisms.

II. STEPS IN DNA SYNTHESIS

A. Strand separation

1. In order for the two individual strands of the parental double helical DNA to be replicated, they must first separate, at least in a small region, since the polymerases use only single-stranded DNA as a template.
2. In prokaryotic organisms, DNA replication begins at a single, discrete site—the ***origin of replication*** (Figure 30.2). In eukaryotes, replication begins at multiple sites along the DNA helix. This provides a mechanism for rapidly replicating the great length of the eukaryotic DNA molecules.
3. As the two strands unwind and separate they form a "V" where active synthesis occurs (Figure 30.2). This region is called the ***replication fork***. The replication fork moves along the DNA molecule as synthesis occurs. Replication of double-stranded DNA is bidirectional, that is, replication forks move in both directions away from the origin (Figure 30.2).

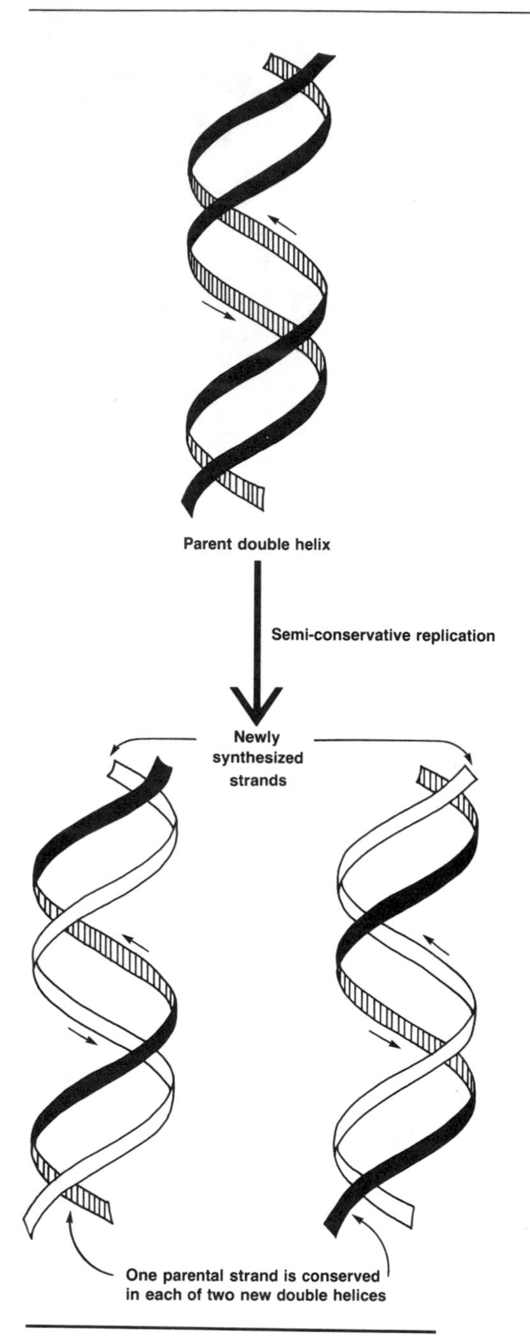

Figure 30.1
Semiconservative replication of DNA.

4. A special group of proteins is responsible for maintaining the separation of the parental strands and for unwinding the double-helix ahead of the advancing replication fork (Figure 30.3). These proteins include the following:

   a. ***Helix-destabilizing (HD) proteins,*** also called single-stranded DNA-binding (SSB) proteins, bind ***nonenzymatically*** to single-stranded DNA. They bind ***cooperatively,*** that is, the binding of one molecule of HD protein makes it easier for additional molecules of HD protein to bind to the DNA strand. The HD proteins are not enzymes, but rather serve to shift the equilibrium between double- and single-stranded DNA in the direction of the single-stranded species. These proteins not only keep the two strands of DNA separated in the area of the replication origin, thus providing the necessary single-stranded template, but also protect the DNA from nucleases that cleave single-stranded DNA.

   b. ***DNA helix-unwinding proteins,*** also called *DNA helicases,* bind to single-stranded DNA near the replication fork and then move into the neighboring double-stranded region, forcing the strands apart. These enzymes require energy provided by ATP. Once the strands separate, HD proteins bind, preventing double-helix reformation. The functions of these proteins are summarized in Figure 30.3.

5. As the two strands of the double-helix are separated, the entire chromosome ahead of the replicating fork would either have to rotate or accumulate positive supertwists if a second group of enzymes were not available to introduce "swivel" points along the double-helix. (The rotation can be demonstrated by tying the ends of two ropes together, twisting them to form a double-helix, and then pulling the two ropes apart in the center of the "helix," as shown in Figure 30.4. To demonstrate the supertwisting, have a colleague hold the two ends of your rope "double-helix" in a fixed position as you pull the two strands apart.) The rotation of an entire chromosome would require the input of large amounts of energy and possibly cause extensive "tangling" of the DNA molecule, while positive supertwists interfere with further unwinding of the double-helix.

   a. The class of enzymes responsible for forming the "swivels" in the helix are called *DNA topoisomerases.*

   b. *Type I DNA topoisomerases* (e.g., *DNA swivelases*) reversibly cut a single strand of the double-helix. Therefore they have both nuclease (strand-cutting) and ligase (strand-resealing) activities. They do not require ATP, but rather appear to store the energy from the phosphodiester bond they cleave, reusing the energy to reseal the strand (Figure 30.5).

   c. By creating a transient "nick," the DNA helix on either side of the nick is allowed to rotate at the phosphodiester bond ***opposite*** the nick, thus relieving accumulated supertwists (see p. 360 for a discussion of supertwists).

   d. *Type II DNA topoisomerases* (e.g., *DNA gyrase*) bind tightly to both strands of the DNA and make transient breaks in both strands of the DNA helix. The enzyme then causes a second

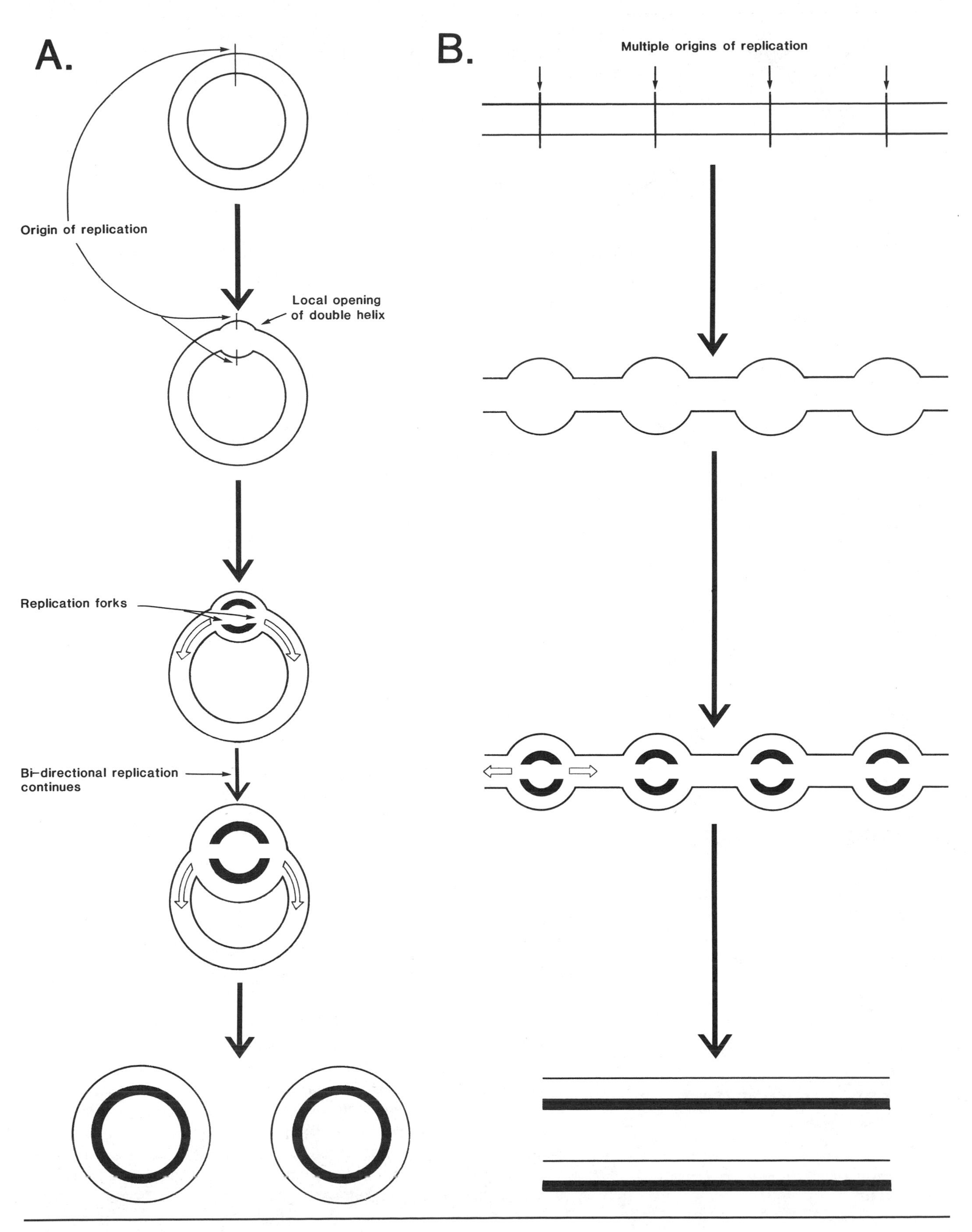

Figure 30.2
Replication of DNA: origin(s) and replication forks. **(A)** Small circular DNA. **(B)** Very long eukaryotic DNA.

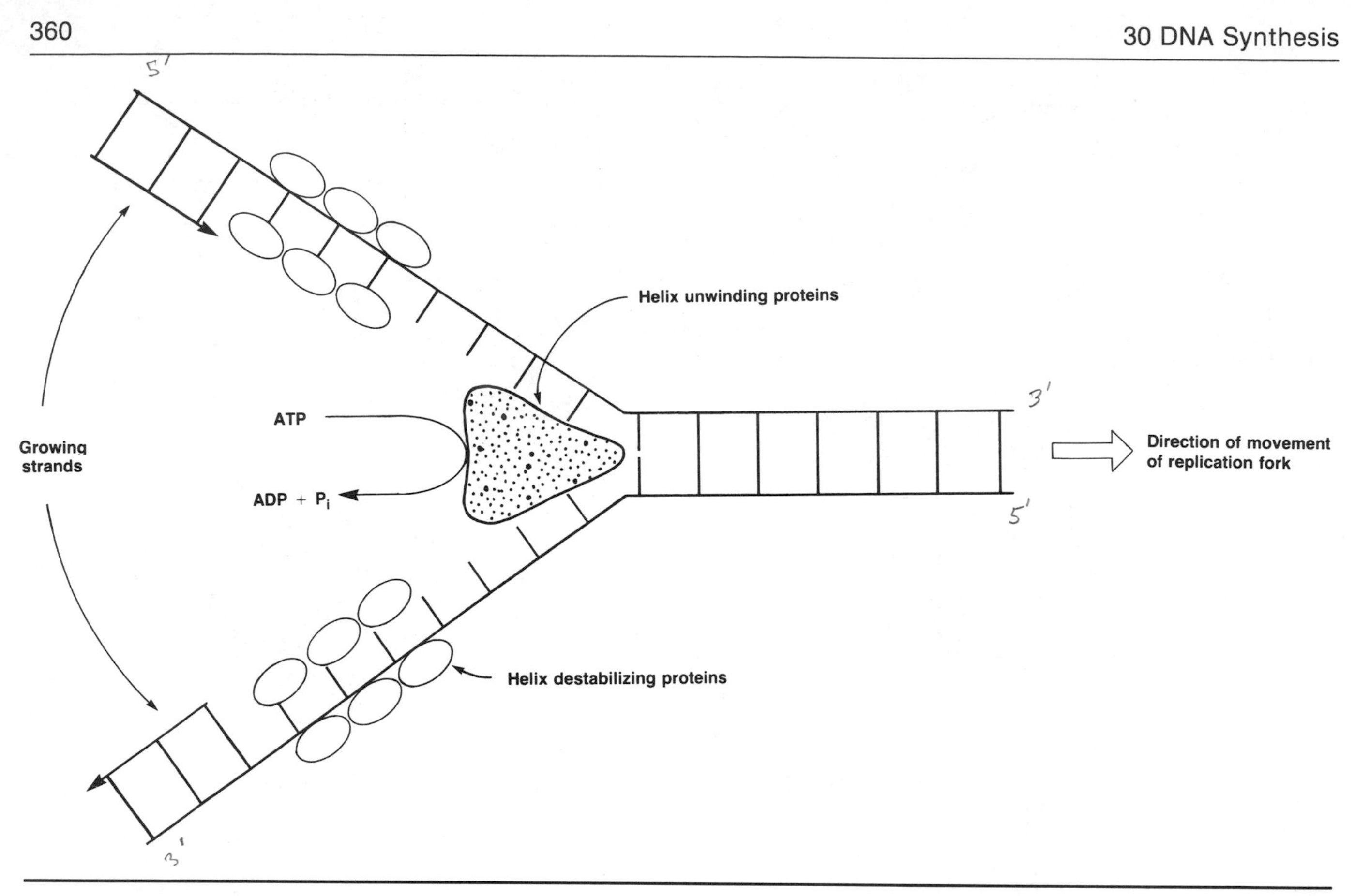

Figure 30.3
Proteins responsible for maintaining the separation of the parental strands and unwinding the double-helix ahead of the advancing replication fork.

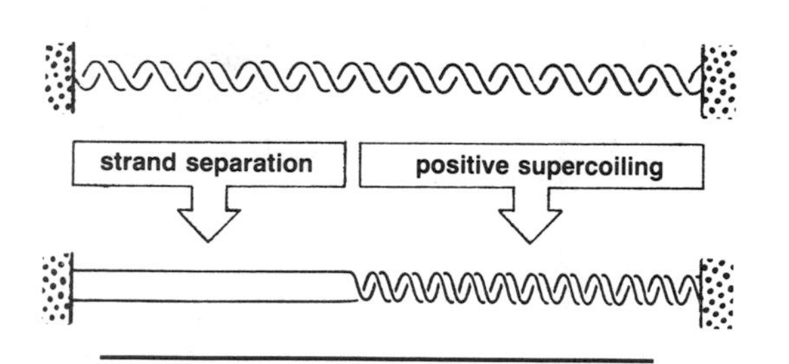

Figure 30.4
Supertwisting resulting from unwinding of the double-helix.

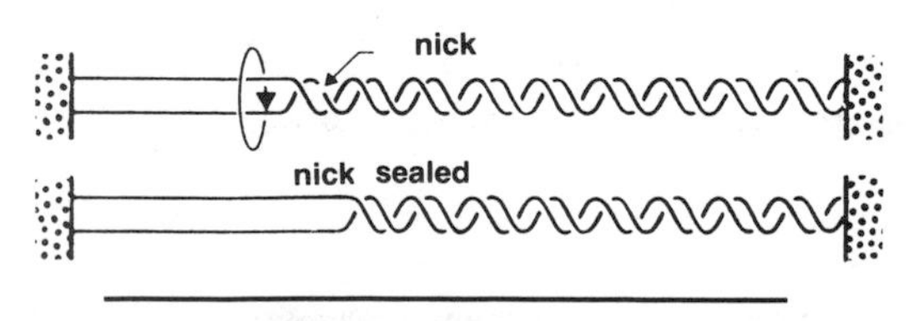

Figure 30.5
Action of *type I DNA topoisomerases* (e.g., *DNA swivelase*).

stretch of the DNA double-helix to pass through the break and finally reseals the break (Figure 30.6). As a result, ***negative supertwists*** can be introduced that allow easier unwinding of the DNA double-helix.

e. Both types of *topoisomerases* can also be used to separate two interlocked molecules of circular DNA or knot or unknot a circular DNA molecule.

B. Both DNA strands serve as templates for DNA synthesis

1. Both parental strands serve as templates for DNA synthesis at the replication fork, producing two daughter molecules, each of which contains two DNA strands with an antiparallel orientation (see p. 337).
2. The *DNA polymerases* responsible for copying these templates are only able to "read" the parental nucleotide sequences in the $3' \rightarrow 5'$ direction and synthesize the new DNA strands in the $5' \rightarrow 3'$ direction. Therefore, beginning with one parental double-helix, the two newly synthesized stretches of nucleotide chains must grow in opposite directions—one in the $5' \rightarrow 3'$ direction ***toward*** the replication fork, and one in the $5' \rightarrow 3'$ direction ***away*** from the replication fork (see Figure 30.7). This feat is accomplished by a slightly different mechanism on each strand:

a. The strand that is being copied in the direction of the advancing replication fork is called the ***leading strand*** and is synthesized almost continuously (see Figure 30.7).

b. The strand that is being copied in the direction away from the replication fork is synthesized discontinuously, with small fragments of DNA being copied near the replication fork. These short stretches of discontinuous DNA, termed ***Okazaki fragments,*** are eventually joined to become a single, continuous strand. The new strand of DNA produced by this mechanism is termed the ***lagging strand*** (see Figure 30.7).

C. RNA primer

1. *DNA polymerases* cannot initiate synthesis of a complementary strand of DNA on a totally single-stranded template. Rather, they require a ***primer,*** that is, a short, double-stranded region with a free hydroxyl group on the 3′-end of the shorter strand (see Figure 30.7). This hydroxyl group serves as the first acceptor of a nucleotide from *DNA polymerase.* In *de novo* DNA synthesis, that free 3′-hydroxyl is provided by a short stretch of ***RNA*** rather than DNA.
2. A specific RNA polymerase, *primase,* synthesizes short stretches of RNA (approximately ten nucleotides in length) that are complementary and antiparallel to the DNA template. As shown in Figure 30.7, these short RNA sequences are constantly being synthesized at the replication fork on the lagging strand, but very few are required on the leading strand. The building blocks for this process are 5′-***ribo***nucleoside triphosphates, and ***pyrophosphate*** is released as each phosphodiester bond is made.
3. Before RNA primer synthesis begins on the lagging strand, a prepriming complex of several proteins is assembled and binds to the single strand of DNA, displacing some of the single-stranded DNA-binding protein. This protein complex plus the *primase* is called the ***primosome***. It initiates Okazaki fragments by moving along the lagging strand in the 5′→3′ direction, periodically synthesizing RNA primer. Thus, the primosome moves in the ***opposite direction*** from that of DNA synthesis of the lagging strand.
4. The RNA primer is later removed as described on p. 363.

E. Chain elongation

1. DNA chain elongation is catalyzed by *DNA polymerase III* (see Figure 30.7).
2. Using the 3′-hydroxyl group of the RNA primer as the acceptor of the first deoxyribonucleotide, *DNA polymerase III* begins to add nucleotides along the single-stranded template, which specifies the sequence of bases in the newly synthesized chain. The new strand grows in the 5′→3′ direction, ***antiparallel*** to the parental strand (see Figure 30.7).

   a. The nucleotide building blocks are ***5′-deoxy***ribonucleoside triphosphates. Pyrophosphate (PP_i) is released when each new nucleotide is added to the growing chain (Figure 30.8).

   b. All four deoxyribonucleoside triphosphates (dATP, dTTP, dCTP, and dGTP) must be present for DNA elongation to occur. If

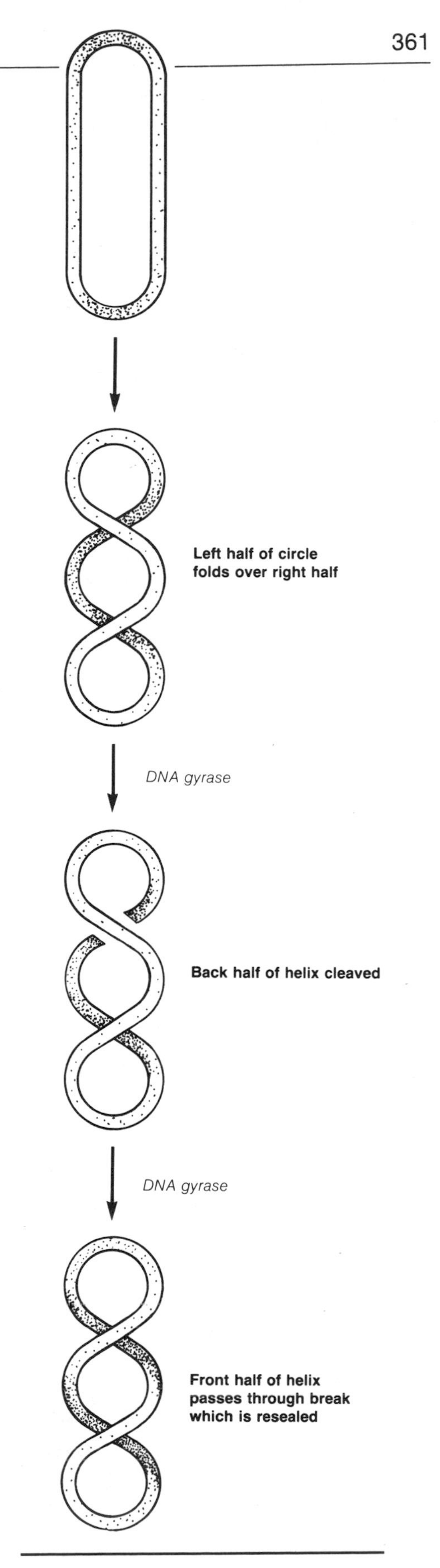

Figure 30.6
Action of *type II DNA topoisomerase* (e.g., *DNA gyrase*).

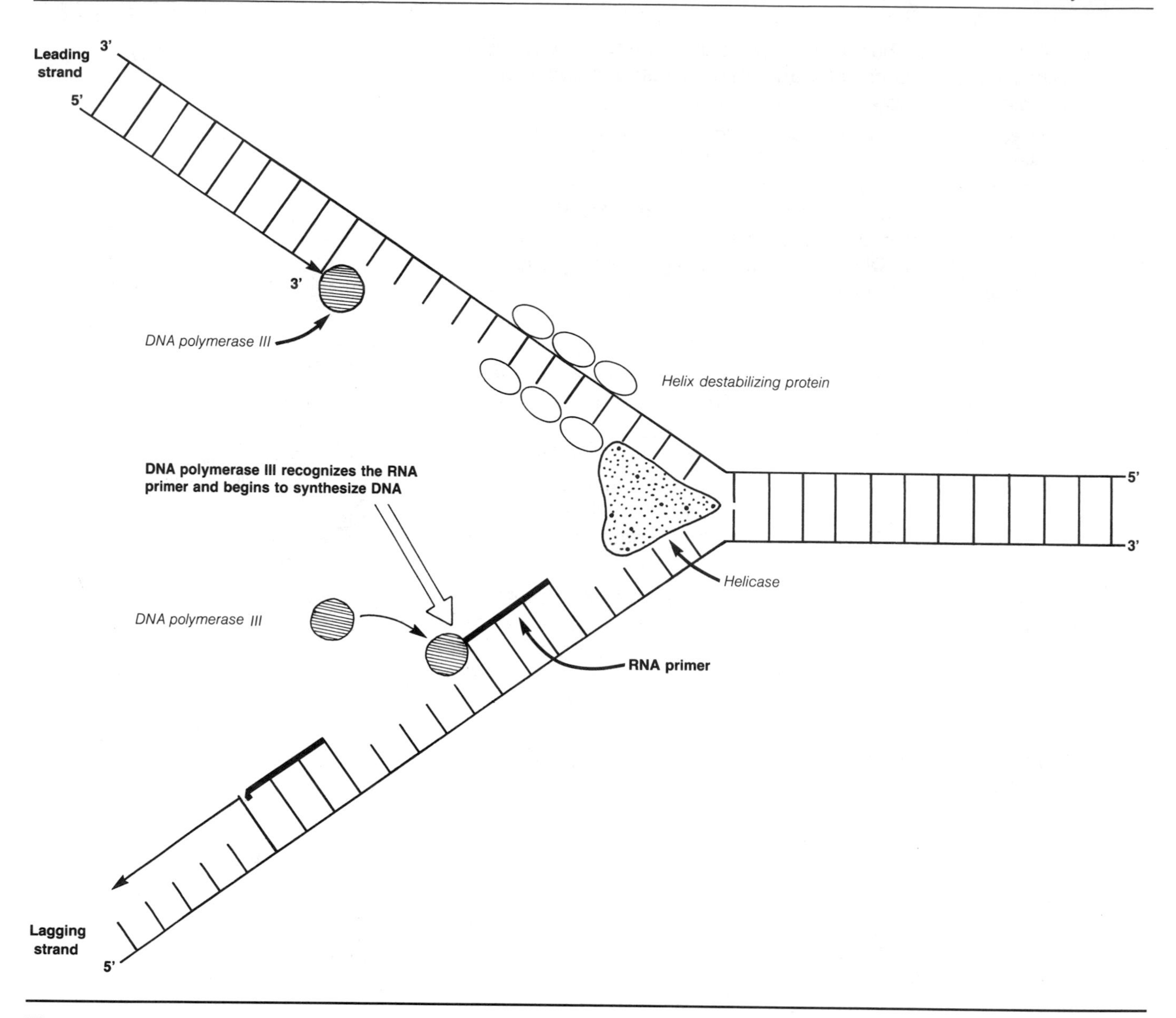

Figure 30.7
Elongation of the leading and lagging strands.

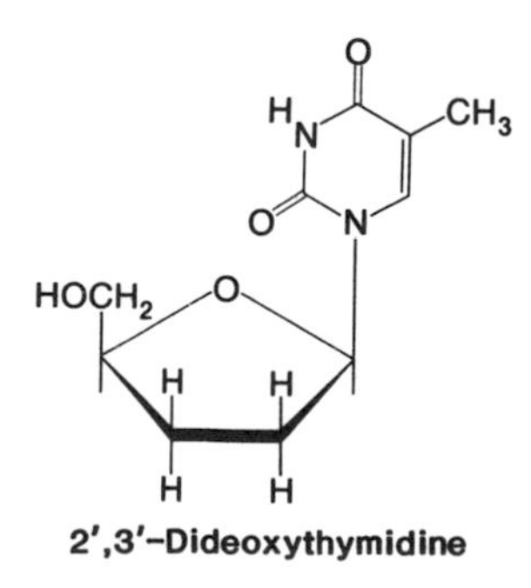

one of the four is in short supply, DNA synthesis will stop when that nucleotide is depleted.

c. DNA chain growth can be blocked by the incorporation of certain nucleotide analogues that have been modified in the sugar portion of the nucleotide. For example, removal of the hydroxyl group from the 3′-carbon of the deoxyribose ring (i.e., 2′,3′-dideoxynucleoside) or conversion of the deoxyribose to arabinose (i.e., arabinosylnucleoside) prevents further chain elongation. By blocking DNA replication, these compounds slow the division of rapidly growing cells and viruses. Therefore, cytosine arabinoside (araC) has been used in anticancer chemotherapy, whereas adenine arabinoside (araA) is an antiviral agent.

3. It is highly important for the survival of the organism that the nucleotide sequence of DNA be replicated with as few errors as possible. Misreading of the template sequence could result in deleterious, perhaps lethal, mutations. To ensure replication fidelity, *DNA polymerase III* has, in addition to its *5′→3′ polymerase* activity, a "proofreading" activity (*3′→5′-exonuclease*, Figure 30.9).

   a. As each nucleotide is added to the chain, *DNA polymerase III* checks to make sure the added nucleotide is, in fact, correctly matched to its complementary base on the template and edits its mistakes. For example, if the template base is adenine and the enzyme mistakenly inserts a cytosine instead of thymine into the new chain, *DNA polymerase III* hydrolytically removes the misplaced nucleotide and replaces it with the correct nucleotide containing thymine (Figure 30.9).

   b. This additional enzyme activity is a *3′→5′-exonuclease* (NOT 5′→3′ like the *polymerase* activity, since the excision is done in the reverse direction from that of synthesis). It is an ***exo**nuclease* because it degrades the DNA chain only from the end rather than cleaving it internally as do the ***endo**nucleases* (Figure 30.10).

   c. This *3′→5′-exonuclease* requires an ***improperly*** base-paired 3′-hydroxy terminus. It does not degrade correctly paired nucleotides.

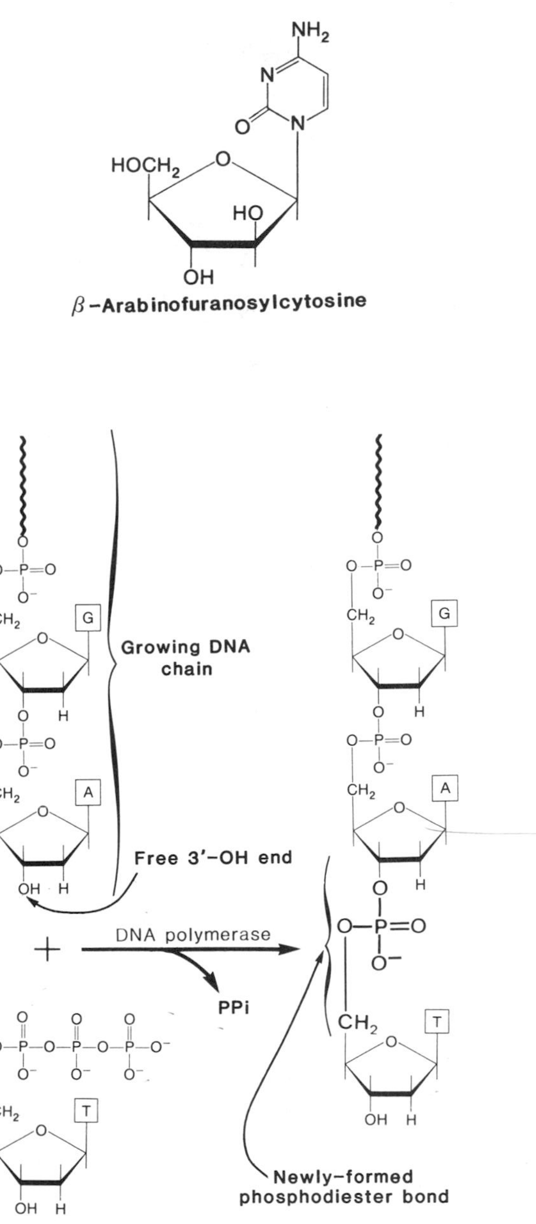

Figure 30.8
DNA synthesis: addition of a nucleotide to the 3′-OH end of the growing chain.

F. Excision of RNA primer and its replacement with DNA

1. *DNA polymerase III* continues to synthesize DNA until it is blocked by a stretch of the RNA primer. When this occurs, the RNA is excised and the gap filled by *DNA polymerase I* (Figure 30.11).

2. In addition to having the *5′→3′-polymerase* activity that synthesizes DNA and the *3′→5′-exonuclease* activity that proofreads the newly synthesized DNA chain like *polymerase III*, *DNA polymerase I* also has a *5′→3′-exonuclease* activity that can hydrolytically remove the RNA primer.

   a. First, *DNA polymerase I* locates the space ("nick") between the 3′-end of the DNA newly synthesized by *DNA polymerase III* and the 5′-end of the adjacent RNA primer (Figure 30.11).

   b. Next, *DNA polymerase I* hydrolytically removes the RNA nucleotides "ahead" of itself, moving in the 5′→3′ direction.

   c. As it removes the RNA, *DNA polymerase I* replaces it with ***deoxy**ribonucleotides*, synthesizing DNA in the 5′→3′ direction (*5′→3′ polymerase* activity). As it synthesizes the DNA, it also "proofreads" the new chain using the *3′→5′ exonuclease* activity.

   d. This removal/synthesis/proofreading continues until the RNA is totally degraded and the gap is filled with DNA (Figure 30.11).

3. The *5′→3′-exonuclease* activity of *DNA polymerase I* differs from the *3′→5′-exonuclease* used by both *DNA polymerase I* and *DNA polymerase III* for proofreading in several important ways:

   a. *5′→3′-Exonuclease* can remove one nucleotide at a time from a region of DNA that is properly base-paired. The

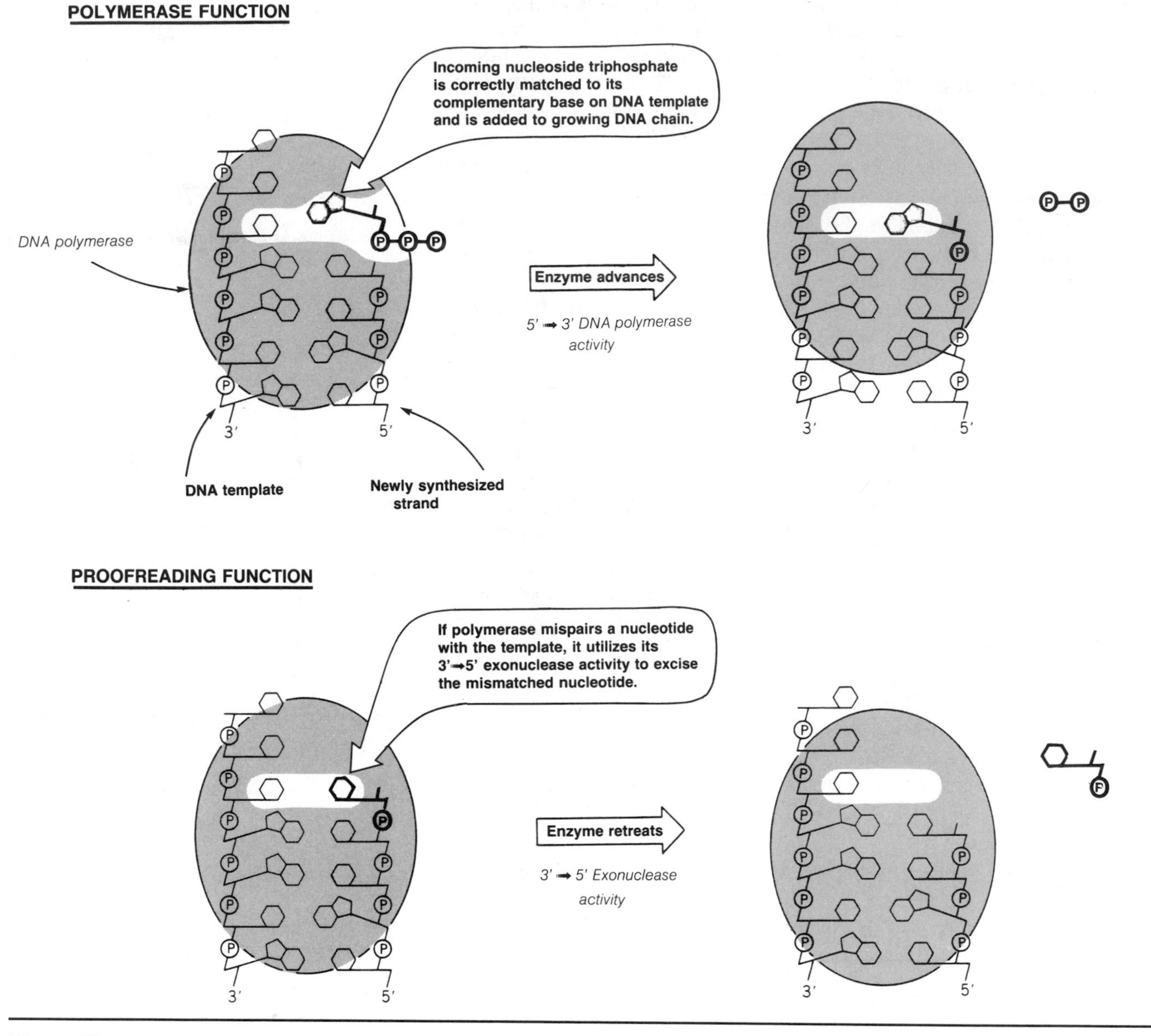

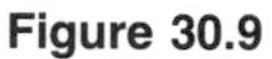

Figure 30.9
3′ → 5′-Exonuclease activity enables *DNA polymerase III* to "proofread" the newly synthesized DNA strand.

nucleotides it removes can be either ribonucleotides or deoxyribonucleotides.

b. *5′→3′-Exonuclease* can also remove mismatched ends in the 5′→3′ direction, removing from one to ten nucleotides at a time. This ability is important for the removal of pyrimidine dimers, described on p. 365.

G. DNA ligase

1. The final phosphodiester linkage between the 5′-phosphate group on the DNA chain synthesized by *DNA polymerase III* and the 3′-hydroxyl group on the chain made by *DNA polymerase I* is catalyzed by *DNA ligase* (Figure 30.12).

2. The joining of these two stretches of DNA requires energy, which in humans is provided by the cleavage of ATP to AMP + PP_i.

H. Eukaryotic DNA replication

1. Three classes of eukaryotic *DNA polymerases* have been identified and categorized on the basis of molecular weight, cellular location, sensitivity to inhibitors, and the templates or substrates on which they act. They have been named *DNA polymerase* α, β, and γ.
2. Eukaryotic helix-destabilizing proteins and ATP-dependent DNA-unwinding enzymes have been identified, whose functions are analogous to those of the prokaryotic enzymes previously discussed.
3. After DNA replication, nucleosomes are formed, and the resulting structure is assembled into ***chromatin***.

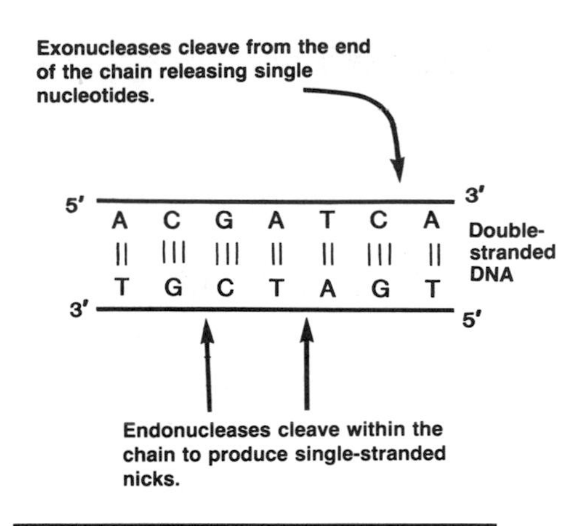

Figure 30.10
Endonuclease versus *exonuclease* activity.

III. DNA REPAIR

DNA is constantly being subjected to environmental insults that cause the alteration or removal of the nucleotide bases. The damaging agents can be either radiation or chemicals. If the damage is not repaired, a permanent mutation may be introduced that can result in any of a number of deleterious effects, including loss of control over the proliferation of the mutated cell, leading to cancer. Spontaneous alteration or loss of bases also occurs regularly in cells. Luckily, cells are remarkably efficient at repairing the damage done to their DNA. Most of these repair mechanisms involve recognizing the lesion, removing the damaged section of the DNA strand, and, using the sister strand as a template, filling the gap left by the excision of the abnormal DNA (see Figure 30.13 for a summary of this process).

A. Repair of damage caused by ultraviolet light

1. Exposure of a cell to ultraviolet light can result in the covalent joining of two adjacent pyrimidines (usually thymines), producing a dimer. These thymine dimers prevent *DNA polymerase* from replicating the DNA strand beyond the site of dimer formation. The thymine dimers are excised in bacteria as illustrated in Figure 30.13. (A similar pathway is present in humans).
   a. First, a specialized *UV-specific endonuclease* recognizes the dimer and cleaves the damaged strand at a phosphodiester bond at the 5′-side of the dimer.
   b. Next, an *excision exonuclease* recognizes the incision made by the *endonuclease*. In *E. coli*, this 5′→3′ exonuclease activity is associated with *DNA polymerase I*. In other organisms, the *excision exonucleases* may or may not be tightly coupled to replication enzymatic activity.
   c. The gap left by the removal of the stretch of DNA containing the thymine dimer is filled, using the sister strand as a template, by a *5′→3′ DNA polymerase* (*polymerase I* in *E. coli*).
   d. The 3′-hydroxyl of the newly synthesized DNA is spliced to the 5′-phosphate of the remaining stretch of the original DNA strand by *DNA ligase*.

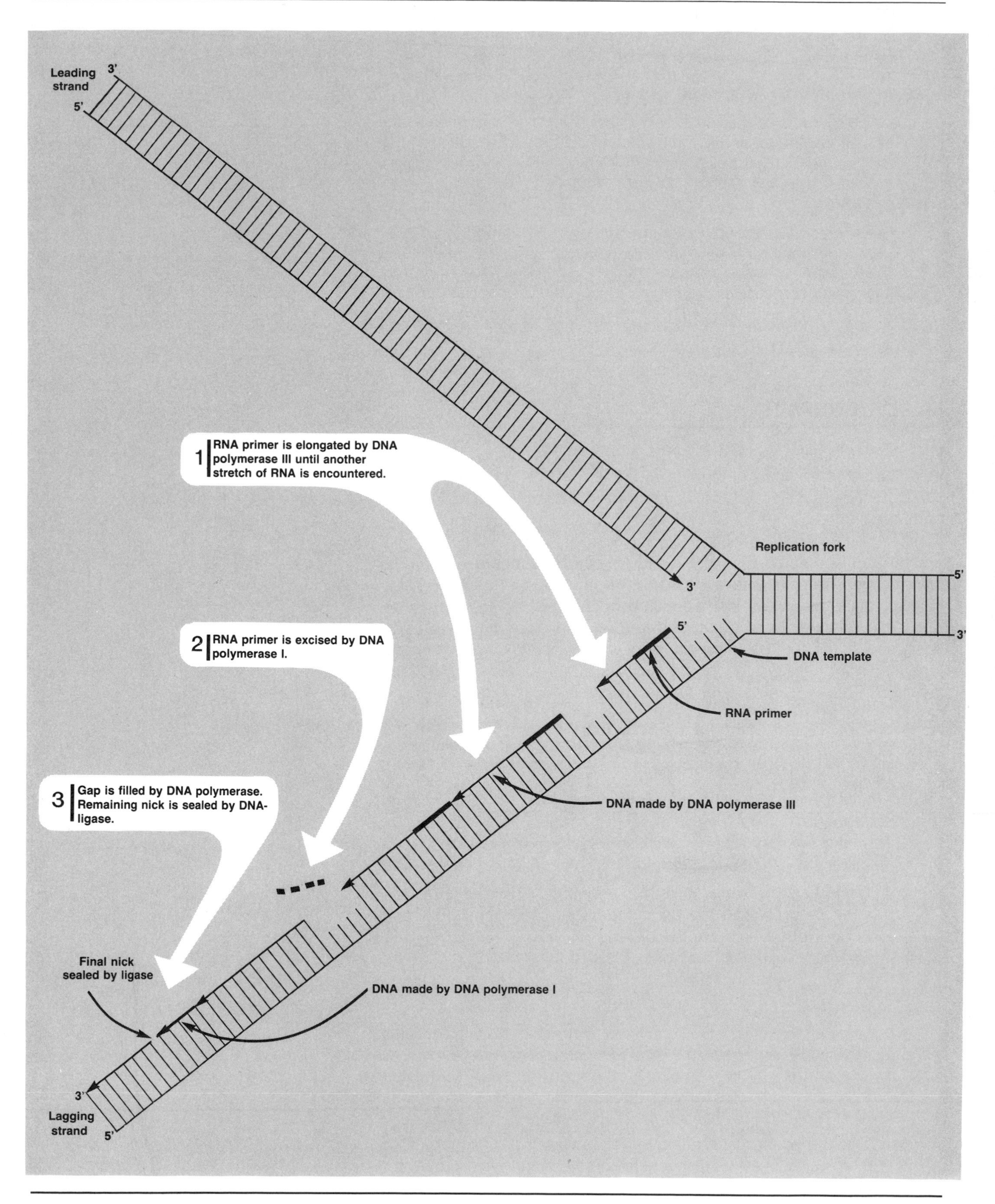

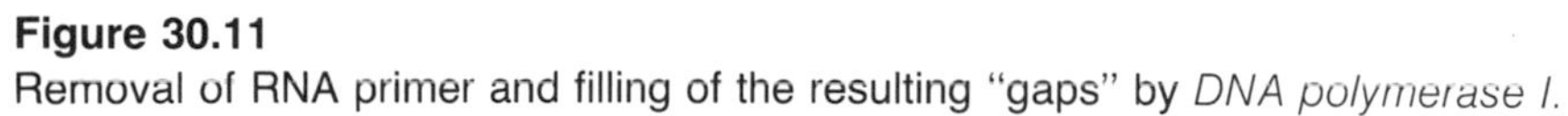

Figure 30.11
Removal of RNA primer and filling of the resulting "gaps" by *DNA polymerase I*.

2. Ultraviolet radiation causes pyrimidine dimers in the skin cells of people exposed to unfiltered sunlight. In the rare genetic disease ***xeroderma pigmentosum,*** the cells cannot repair the damaged DNA, resulting in extensive accumulation of mutations and, consequently, skin cancer. The most common form of this disease is caused by the absence of the *UV-specific endonuclease* described above (Figure 30.13).

B. Correction of base alterations

1. The bases of DNA can be altered, either spontaneously, as is the case with cytosine, which slowly undergoes the loss of its amino group to form uracil, or by the action of deaminating or alkylating compounds. For example, ***nitrous acid,*** which is formed by the cell from precursors such as the nitrosamines, nitrites, and nitrates, is a potent compound that removes the amino group (i.e., deaminates) from cytosine, adenine, and guanine. Bases may also be lost spontaneously; for example, about 10,000 purine bases are lost spontaneously per cell per day. Lesions involving base alterations or loss can be corrected by the following mechanisms:
   a. Abnormal bases are recognized by specific *glycosidases* that hydrolytically cleave the base from the deoxyribose-phosphate backbone of the strand.
   b. Specific *endonucleases* recognize that a base is missing and initiate the process of excision and gap filling, as described above for thymine dimers.
   c. In addition, other *endonucleases* recognize abnormal bases in the DNA but initiate the ***nucleotide*** excision process without requiring that the defective base be cleaved from its sugar before the *endonuclease* action.
2. Thus a family of enzymes, each of which is highly specific for recognizing defective DNA, is responsible for excising the lesion and replacing it with the proper base sequence as defined by the template of the sister strand.

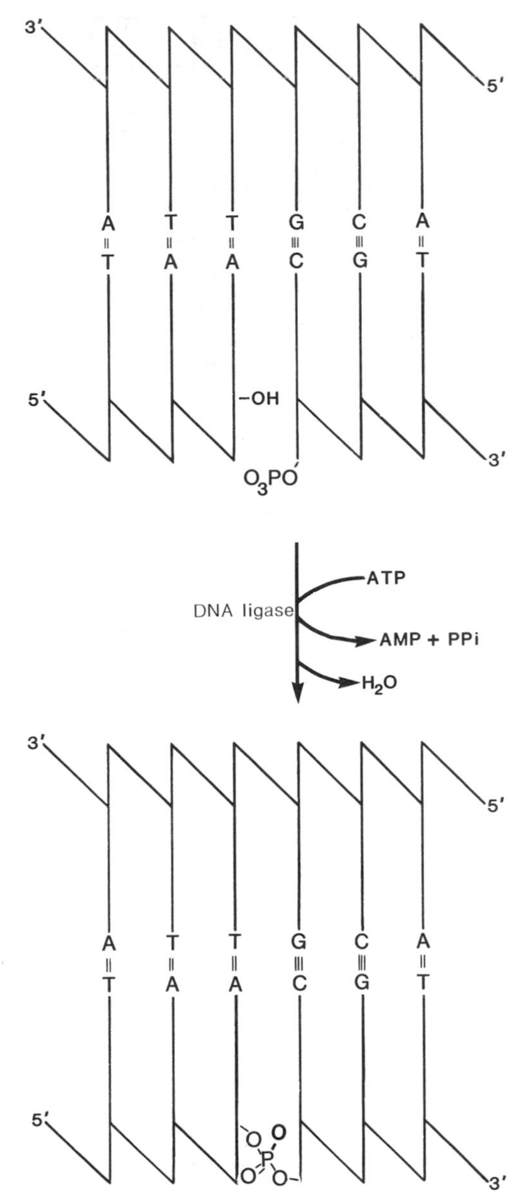

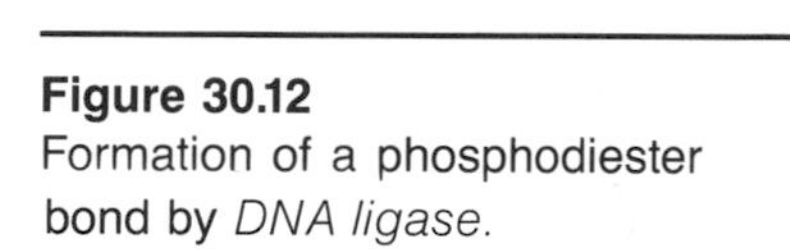

Figure 30.12
Formation of a phosphodiester bond by *DNA ligase.*

Study Questions

Choose the ONE best answer:

30.1 Which one of the choices below BEST completes the statement: The fact that DNA polymerase I from *E. coli* has a 5′→3′ exonuclease activity...

A. ...implies that the enzyme has multiple subunits.
B. ...implies that DNA polymerase I can use both RNA and DNA as primers.
C. ...makes the enzyme able to detect thymine-dimers in double-stranded DNA.
D. ...enables the enzyme to play an important role in DNA replication.
E. ...makes the enzyme able to correct errors during elongation of a primer.

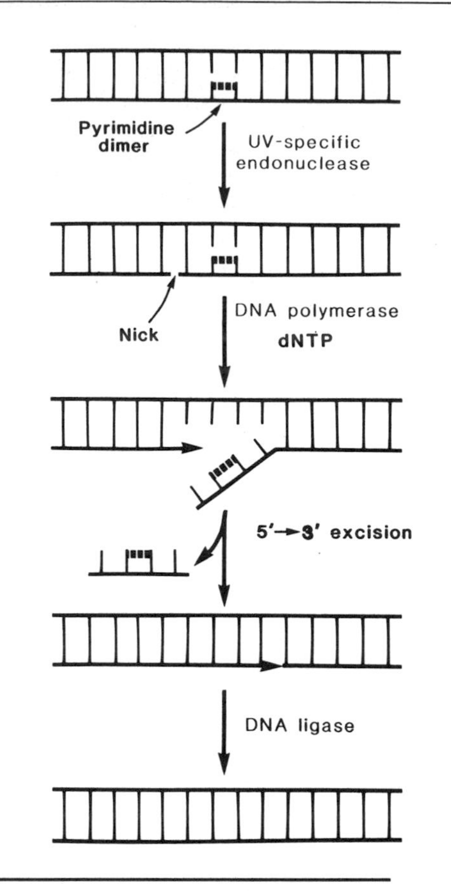

Figure 30.13
Excision repair of pyrimidine dimers in DNA.

30.2 During DNA replication, the sequence 5′-TpApGpAp-3′ would produce which of the following complementary structures:

A. 5′-TpCpTpAp-3′
B. 5′-ApTpCpTp-3′
C. 5′-UpCpUpAp-3′
D. 5′-GpCpGpAp-3′
E. 3′-TpCpTpAp-3′

Answer A if 1, 2, and 3 are correct
B if 1 and 3 are correct
C if 2 and 4 are correct
D if only 4 is correct
E if all are correct

30.3 Which of the following statements about DNA polymerases is(are) CORRECT?

1. DNA polymerases require primers.
2. DNA polymerases can add nucleotides at both the 3′- and the 5′-ends of the growing polynucleotide chain.
3. In addition to their polymerizing activity, DNA polymerases have a 3′→5′-exonuclease activity.
4. DNA polymerases can synthesize DNA only in the presence of an RNA template.

30.4 Which of the following statements about DNA ligase is(are) CORRECT?

1. DNA ligase is an important enzyme in replication of DNA because it seals the gaps between RNA primers and the growing DNA strands.
2. DNA ligase requires free 3′- and 5′-hydroxyl ends plus ATP. The terminal phosphate group of ATP is used to form the phosphodiester bond between the two DNA strands that are joined.
3. DNA ligase fills in gaps in double-helical DNA.
4. DNA ligase participates in the process of excision-repair of damaged DNA.

RNA Synthesis

31

I. OVERVIEW

The genetic master plan of an organism is contained in the sequence of deoxyribonucleotides that constitute the DNA. However, it is through the ribonucleic acid (RNA) "working copies" of the DNA that the master plan is expressed. The copying process, which uses one of the two DNA strands as a template, is called ***transcription***. The messenger RNAs, which are transcripts of certain regions of the DNA, are ***translated*** into a sequence of amino acids—the polypeptide chain. Ribosomal RNAs, transfer RNAs, and additional small RNA molecules perform specialized functions without translation.

A central feature of transcription is that it is highly selective: For some regions of the DNA, many transcripts are made. For other regions, few or no transcripts are made. This selectivity is due, at least in part, to signals embedded in the nucleotide sequence of the DNA. These signals instruct the *RNA polymerase* where to start transcription, how often to start transcription, and where to stop transcription. The biochemical differentiation of different tissues of an organism is ultimately due to the selectivity of the transcription process.

A second important feature of transcription is that the RNA transcripts, which initially are faithful copies of one of the two DNA strands, undergo various modifications (terminal additions, base modifications, trimming, internal segment removal, and splicing) that convert the inactive primary transcript into a functional molecule.

The structure of the *RNA polymerase,* the signals that control transcription, and the varieties of modification differ from organism to organism, and particularly from prokaryotes to eukaryotes. For convenience, in the following chapter we shall distinguish between transcription in prokaryotes, for which our understanding is more extensive, and transcription in eukaryotes.

II. TRANSCRIPTION OF PROKARYOTIC GENES

A. Properties of prokaryotic RNA polymerase

1. This multi-subunit enzyme recognizes nucleotide sequences (the ***promoter region***) at the ***beginning*** of a stretch of DNA that is to be transcribed, makes a complementary RNA copy of the DNA template, and then recognizes the ***end*** of the DNA sequence to

be transcribed (the ***terminator region***). The ***transcription unit*** extends from the promoter to the terminator.

a. Four of the peptide subunits, 2 α, 1 β, and 1 β', are responsible for the $5' \rightarrow 3'$ *RNA polymerase* activity. However, this ***core enzyme*** lacks specificity—it cannot recognize the promoter region on the DNA template.

b. The σ-subunit ("factor") enables the polymerase to recognize promoter regions on the DNA. The ***σ-factor*** plus the core enzyme compose the ***holoenzyme***.

c. Some regions on the DNA that signal the termination of transcription are recognized by the *RNA polymerase* itself. Others are recognized by specific termination factors, an example of which is the ***ρ-factor*** of *E. coli*.

B. Steps in RNA synthesis.

The transcription of a typical gene of *E. coli* is summarized in Figure 31.1.

1. ***Initiation:*** Initiation of transcription involves the binding of *RNA polymerase* to a ***promoter region*** on the DNA. The general, characteristic nucleotide sequences of the promoter region that are recognized by *RNA polymerase* (Figure 31.2) include the following:

   a. ***The Pribnow box:*** This is a stretch of seven nucleotides centered around ten nucleotides to the left of the initial base of the mRNA.

   b. ***A second nucleotide sequence, TGTTG:*** This sequence, located about 35 bases to the left of the initial base of the mRNA, is also recognized by the *RNA polymerase*.

   c. The structure of eukaryotic promoters is much more complex and variable.

2. ***Elongation:*** Once the promoter region has been recognized, the RNA polymerase begins to synthesize a transcript of the DNA sequence:

   a. Unlike *DNA polymerase, RNA polymerase* does not require a primer and has no known endonuclease or exonuclease activity.

   b. The binding of the enzyme to the DNA template results in a local unwinding of the DNA helix. Therefore, *RNA polymerase* does not require additional unwinding enzymes or helix-destabilizing enzymes as does *DNA polymerase*.

   c. Like *DNA polymerase, RNA polymerase* uses ***nucleoside triphosphates*** and releases pyrophosphate each time a nucleotide is added to the growing chain.

   d. The RNA is synthesized from its 5′-end to its 3′-end, antiparallel to its DNA template. The template is copied as it is in DNA synthesis, where a G on the DNA specifies a C in the RNA, a C specifies a G, a T on the DNA template specifies an A in the RNA, but an A on the template specifies a ***U*** (instead of a T) on the RNA.

   e. The process of ***elongation*** of the RNA chain continues until a termination signal is reached.

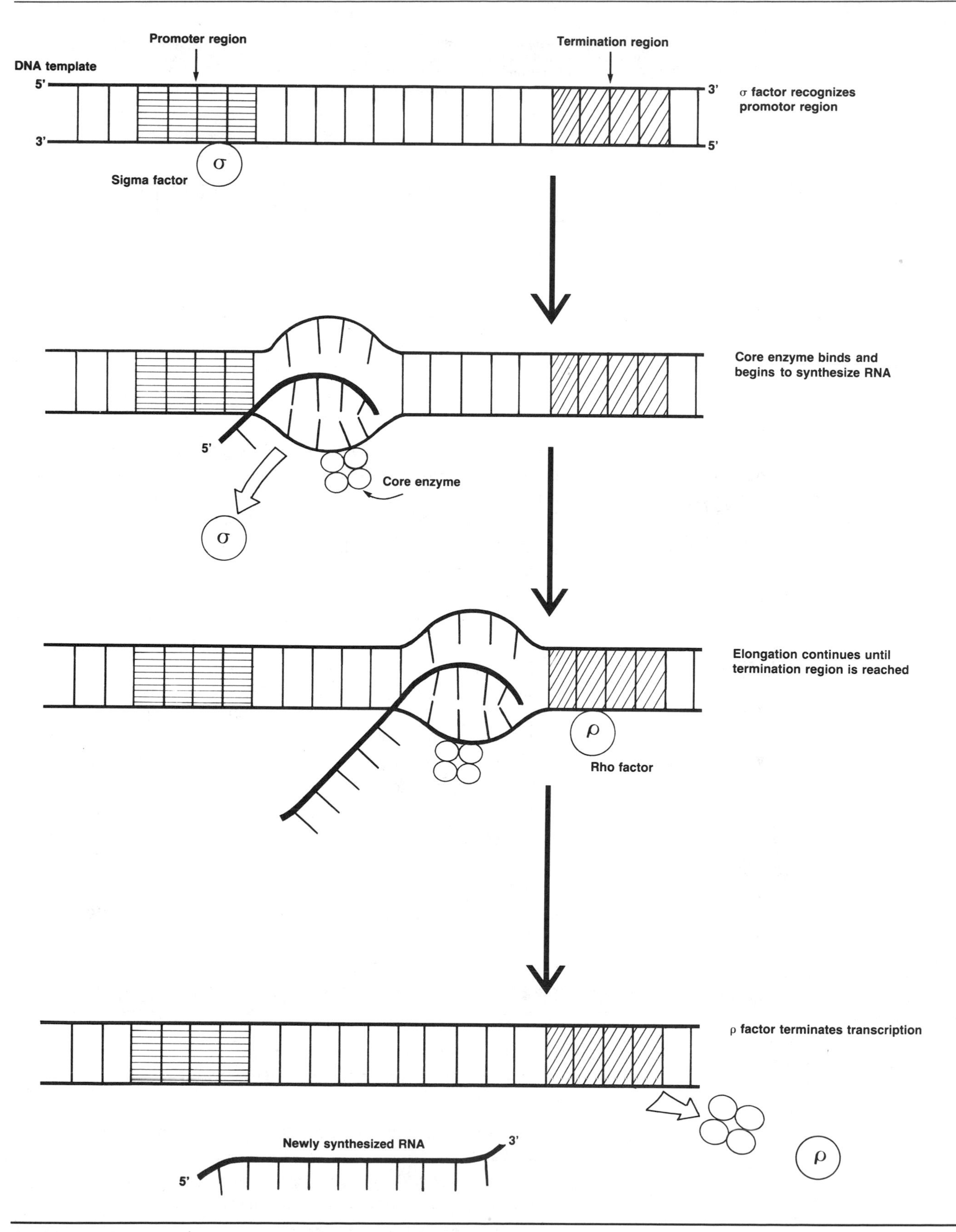

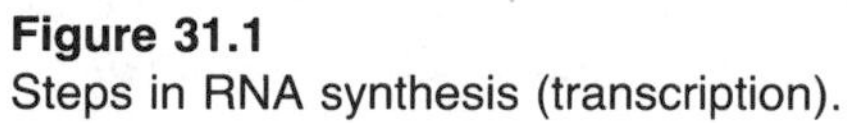

Figure 31.1
Steps in RNA synthesis (transcription).

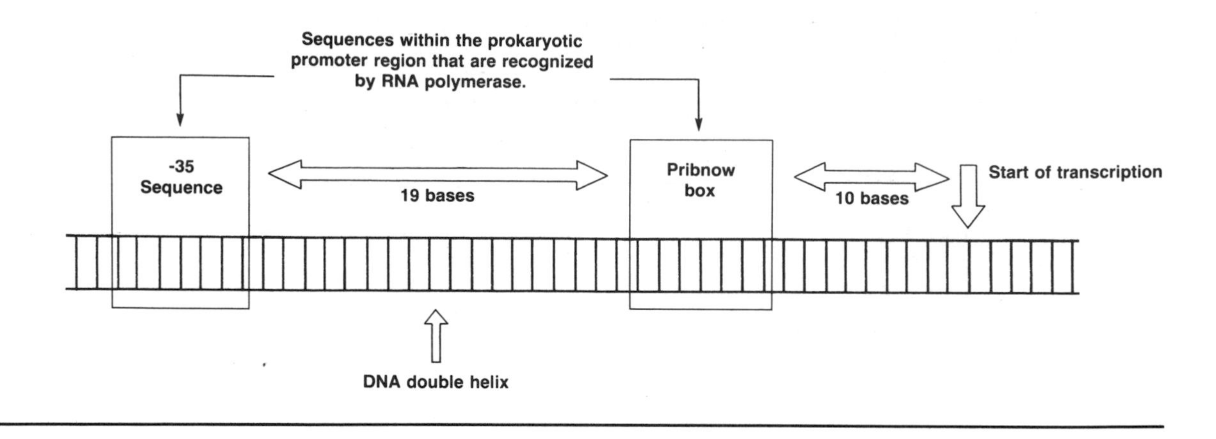

Figure 31.2
Structure of the prokaryotic promoter region.

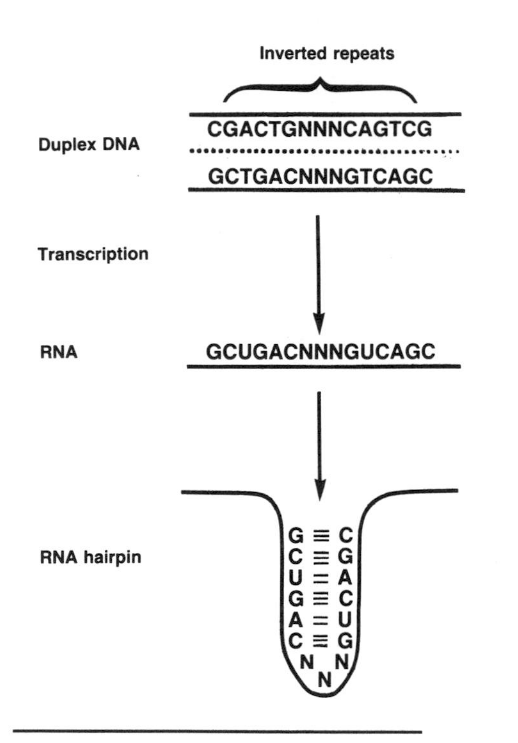

Figure 31.3
An example of a palindrome. A palindrome is a region of double-stranded DNA in which each of the two strands has the same sequence when read in the same direction (e.g., in the 5′→3′ direction).

3. ***Termination:*** *RNA polymerase* can, in some instances, recognize ***termination regions*** on the DNA template ***(σ-independent termination).*** Alternatively the *ρ-factor* may be required for the release of the RNA product and *RNA polymerase* ***(ρ-dependent termination).***
   a. Termination regions of the DNA exhibit twofold symmetry owing to the presence of palindromes (Figure 31.3). The RNA transcript of the DNA palindrome can form a stable ***hairpin turn*** that slows down the progress of the *RNA polymerase* at this terminator site.
   b. Meanwhile, ρ factor binds to the 5′-end of the RNA transcript and moves along the RNA, following the polymerase. When the polymerase pauses at the terminator site, ρ-factor catches up to the polymerase and causes termination (see Figure 31.1).
4. Some antibiotics prevent cell growth by inhibiting RNA synthesis. Some examples include the following:
   a. The antibiotics ***rifamycin*** and ***rifampicin*** inhibit the initiation of transcription by binding to the β-subunit of prokaryotic *RNA polymerase,* thus interfering with the formation of the first phosphodiester bond.
   b. ***Actinomycin D*** binds to the DNA template and interferes with the movement of *RNA polymerase* along the DNA.

III. TRANSCRIPTION OF EUKARYOTIC GENES

A. RNA polymerases of eukaryotic cells

There are three distinct species of *RNA polymerase* in eukaryotic cells:

1. *RNA polymerase I* synthesizes the large ribosomal RNAs in the ***nucleolus.***
2. *RNA polymerase II* synthesizes the precursors of ***messenger RNAs*** that will be translated to produce proteins.
   a. A sequence of nucleotides that is almost identical to that of the Pribnow box is found centered about 25 nucleotides to

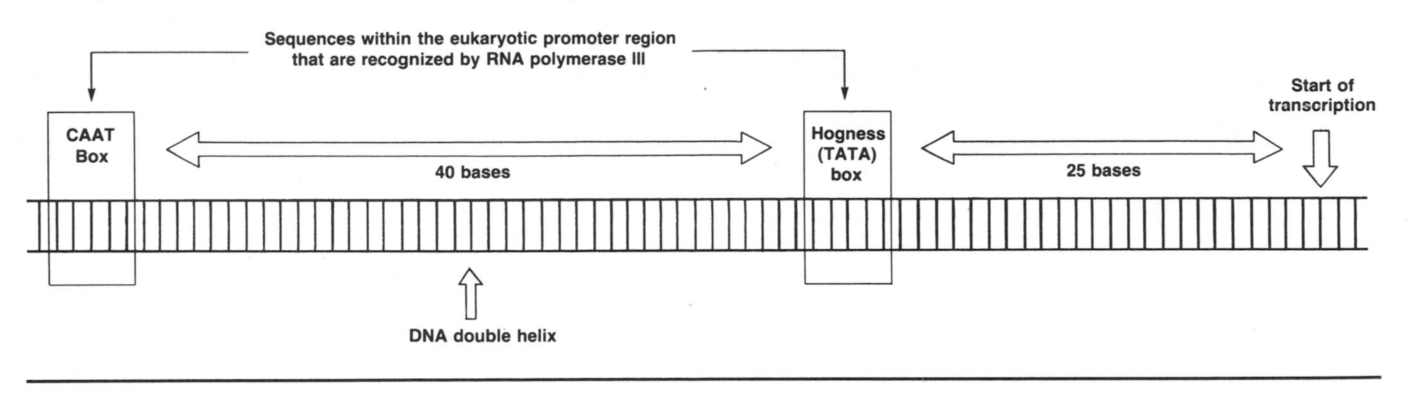

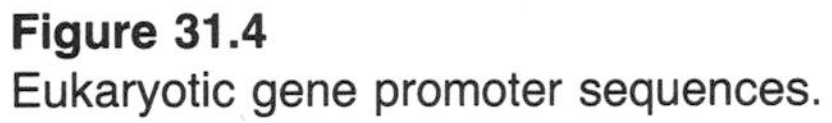
Figure 31.4
Eukaryotic gene promoter sequences.

the left of the initial base of the DNA strand coding for an mRNA molecule. This ***consensus sequence*** is called the ***TATA*** or ***Hogness box***. Between 70 and 80 nucleotides to the left of the initial base of the mRNA is a second consensus sequence known as the ***CAAT*** box (Figure 31.4). One or both of these sequences may serve as recognition sites in eukaryotic promoters.

b. *RNA polymerase II* is inhibited by ***α-amanitin,*** a potent toxin produced by the poisonous mushroom ***Amanita phalloides***.

3. *RNA polymerase III* produces the ***small RNAs,*** including the tRNAs, and the small 5S ribosomal RNA.

IV. POST-TRANSCRIPTIONAL MODIFICATION OF RNA

A. Eukaryotic messenger RNA

The RNA molecule synthesized by *RNA polymerase* (the ***primary transcript,*** sometimes called "hnRNA" for heterogeneous nuclear RNA) contains the sequences that will be found in cytoplasmic mRNA. This primary transcript is extensively modified after transcription. These modifications may include

1. ***5′ "Capping":*** This process occurs as the first of the processing reactions for hn RNA (Figure 31.5). The ***cap*** is a 7-methyl-guanosine attached "backward" through a triphosphate linkage to the 5′ terminal end of the mRNA. The addition of the guanosine triphosphate part of the cap is catalyzed by the nuclear enzyme *guanylyl transferase*. Methylation of this terminal guanine occurs in the cytoplasm and is catalyzed by *guanine-7-methyl-transferase*. S-Adenosylmethionine is the source of the methyl group (see p. 243). Additional methylation steps may occur. The addition of this 7-methylguanosine "cap" through the unusual 5′→5′ triphosphate linkage appears to facilitate the initiation of translation and helps stabilize the mRNA. Eukaryotic mRNAs lacking the cap are not translated efficiently.
2. ***Addition of a poly(A) tail:*** Most eukaryotic mRNAs (with several

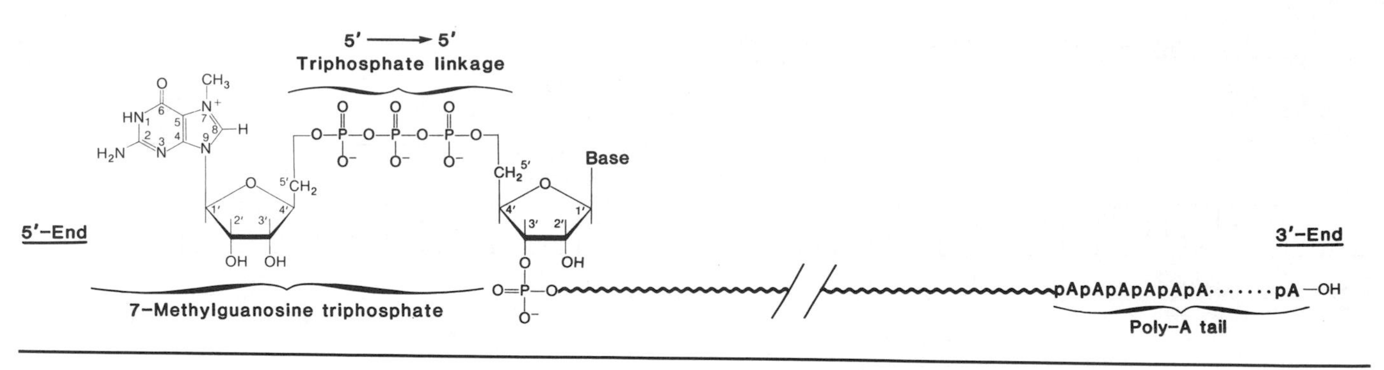

Figure 31.5
Post-transcriptional modification of mRNA showing the 7-methylguanosine cap and poly(A)-tail.

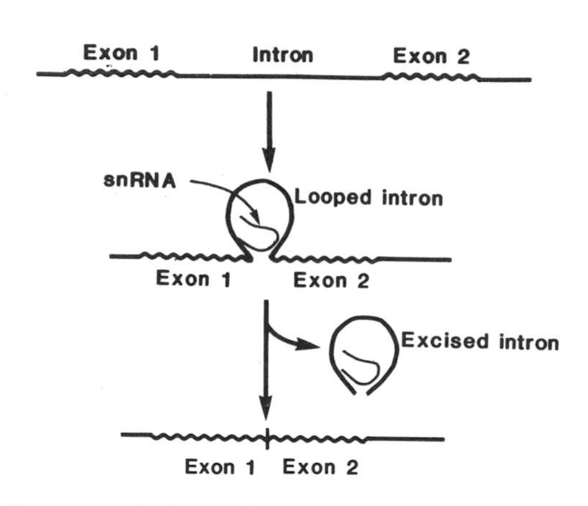

Figure 31.6
Excision of introns and splicing of exons in eukaryotic RNA.

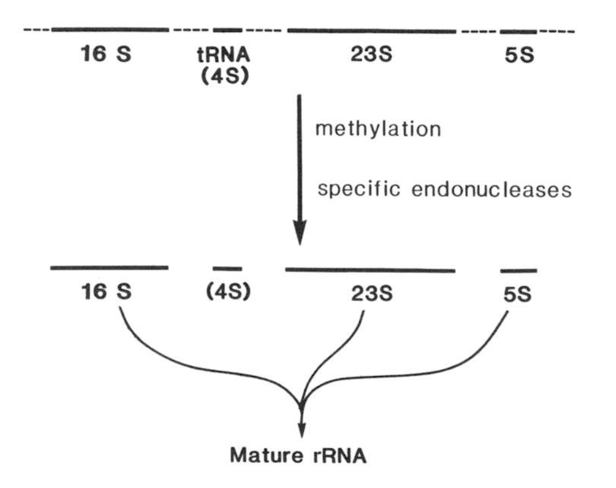

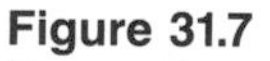

Figure 31.7
Processing of the ribosomal RNA transcript in prokaryotes.

notable exceptions, including those coding for the histone proteins) have a chain of 40 to 200 adenine nucleotides attached to the 3′-end (Figure 31.5). This ***poly(A) tail*** is not transcribed from the DNA, but rather is added after transcription by the nuclear enzyme *poly(A) polymerase*. These tails may help stabilize the mRNA and facilitate their exit from the nucleus. After the mRNA enters the cytoplasm, the poly(A) tail is gradually shortened.

3. ***Removal of introns:*** Maturation of eukaryotic mRNA may involve the removal of RNA sequences (***introns,*** or ***intervening sequences***) from the primary transcript that do not code for protein.
   a. Some eukaryotic primary transcripts contain no introns. Others contain a few introns, whereas some, such as the primary transcripts for the α-chains of collagen, contain more than 50 intervening sequences that must be removed before the mature mRNA is ready for translation. As far as is known, there is no analogous process of excision and splicing of RNA segments in prokaryotes.
   b. ***Small nuclear RNAs (snRNAs)*** facilitate the splicing of some exon segments by forming base pairs with each end of the intron (Figure 31.6). This binding brings the sequences of the neighboring exons into the correct alignment for enzymatic splicing, resulting in the excision of the intron.
   c. After removal of all the introns, the mature mRNA molecules leave the nucleus by passing into the cytoplasm through pores in the nuclear membrane.

B. Ribosomal RNA

1. Ribosomal RNAs of both prokaryotic and eukaryotic cells are synthesized from long precursor molecules called ***preribosomal RNAs***.
2. The 23S, 16S, and 5S ribosomal RNAs of prokaryotes are produced from a single 30S rRNA precursor molecule (Figure 31.7). This precursor is methylated at specific sites, then cleaved to yield intermediate-sized pieces of RNA. These are further "trimmed" to produce the required ribosomal RNA species.
3. Eukaryotic rRNA is produced by a similar series of methylation steps and enzymatic cleavages.

C. Transfer RNA:

1. Transfer RNAs are also made from longer precursor molecules which must be trimmed. Other post-transcriptional modifications include addition of a CCA sequence on the 3′-terminal end and modification of bases at specific positions to produce "unusual bases" (see p. 334).

Study Questions

Choose the ONE BEST answer:

31.1 One class of RNA characteristically contains methylated purines and pyrimidines. This RNA is

A. tRNA.
B. mRNA.
C. rRNA.
D. 16S RNA.
E. RNA with a 3′-poly(A) tail.

31.2 Which of the following statements about messenger RNA is INCORRECT?

A. The sugar moiety of mRNA is D-ribose.
B. The polynucleotide chain of mRNA is longer than that of DNA.
C. mRNA exists as single-stranded molecules.
D. mRNA has a 7-methylguanosine "cap" at its 5′-end.
E. mRNA has a 3′-poly(A) sequence.

31.3 During RNA synthesis, the DNA template sequence 5′-TpApGpCp-3′ would be transcribed to produce which of the following RNA sequences?

A. 5′-ApTpCpGp-3′
B. 5′-GpCpTpAp-5′
C. 5′-CpGpTpAp-3′
D. 5′-ApUpCpGp-3′
E. 5′-GpCpUpAp-3′

31.4 Which of the following statements about RNA polymerase activity is CORRECT?

A. Transcription of DNA by RNA polymerase is a semiconservative process because only one of the two strands of the DNA double-helix is copied into RNA.
B. Transcription of DNA by RNA polymerase requires the participation of a swivelase (topoisomerase I).
C. Helix-unwinding is an important catalytic activity of one of the subunits of RNA polymerase.
D. RNA polymerase cannot proofread its own products.
E. RNA polymerase catalyzes the removal of introns from the primary transcript.

Protein Synthesis

32

I. OVERVIEW

Genetic information, stored in the chromosomes and transmitted to daughter cells through DNA replication, is expressed through its transcription to RNA and subsequent translation into a polypeptide chain. This flow of information from DNA to RNA to protein is termed the "Central Dogma" and is descriptive of all organisms (with the exception of some viruses that have RNA as the repository of their genetic information). The process of translation requires a genetic code, through which the information contained in the nucleic acid sequence is expressed to produce a specific sequence of amino acids. Any alteration in the nucleic acid sequence may result in an improper amino acid being inserted into the polypeptide chain, potentially causing a disease or even death to the organism.

II. THE GENETIC CODE

A. Codons

1. The genetic code is a dictionary that gives the correspondence between a sequence of bases and a sequence of amino acids. The individual words in the code are each composed of three nucleotide bases. These genetic words are called codons.
2. The codons are found on the messenger RNA. The sequence of a codon is always read from its 5′-end to its 3′-end.
3. There are four nucleotide bases—adenine, guanine, cytosine and uracil—that can be used to produce a three-base codon. There are therefore 64 different ***combinations*** of bases, taken three at a time, as shown in Table 32.1 on page 378.

This table (or dictionary) can be used to translate any codon sequence and thus to determine which amino acids are coded for by the mRNA sequence. For example, the codon 5′-CAU-3′ codes for histidine, whereas 5′-AUG-3′ codes for methionine.

4. Three of the codons, UAG, UGA, and UAA, do not code for amino acids, but rather are ***termination codons***. When one of these codons appears in an mRNA sequence, it signals that synthesis of the peptide chain coded for by that mRNA has been completed.

TABLE 32.1 The Genetic Code

5′-OH Terminal Base	Middle Base U	C	A	G	3′-OH Terminal Base
U	Phe	Ser	Tyr	Cys	U
	Phe	Ser	Tyr	Cys	C
	Leu	Ser	Term	Term	A
	Leu	Ser	Term	Trp	G
C	Leu	Pro	His	Arg	U
	Leu	Pro	His	Arg	C
	Leu	Pro	Gln	Arg	A
	Leu	Pro	Gln	Arg	G
A	Ile	Thr	Asn	Ser	U
	Ile	Thr	Asn	Ser	C
	Ile	Thr	Lys	Arg	A
	Met	Thr	Lys	Arg	G
G	Val	Ala	Asp	Gly	U
	Val	Ala	Asp	Gly	C
	Val	Ala	Glu	Gly	A
	Val	Ala	Glu	Gly	G

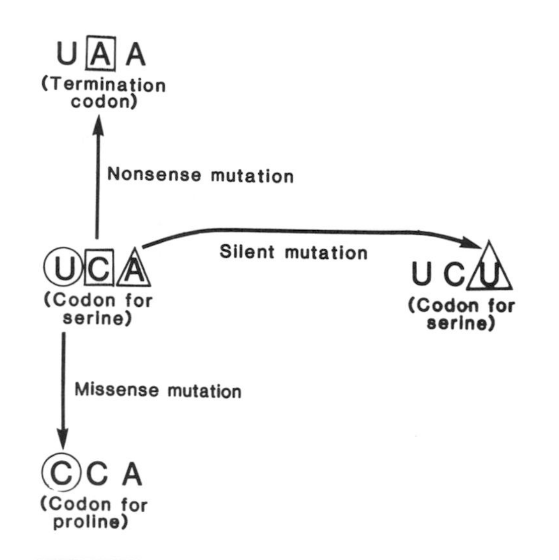

Figure 32.1
Possible effects of changing a single nucleotide base in the coding region of an mRNA chain.

5. Changing a single nucleotide base on the mRNA chain can lead to any one of three possible results (Figure 32.1):
   a. The codon containing the changed base may still code for the ***same amino acid***. For example, if the serine codon UCA is given a different third base (say, UC***U***), it will still code for serine. Therefore, this is a ***silent mutation***.
   b. The codon containing the changed base may code for a ***different amino acid***. For example, if the serine codon UCA is given a different first base (say, ***C***CA), the codon will code for a different amino acid, in this case, proline. This substitution of an amino acid is called a ***missense mutation***.
   c. The codon containing the changed base may become a ***termination codon***. For example, if the serine codon UCA is given a different second base (say, U***A***A), the new codon will cause the termination of translation at that point. The creation of a termination codon at an inappropriate place is called a ***nonsense mutation***.

B. Characteristics of the genetic code

1. The genetic code is ***specific:*** A specific codon always codes for a single amino acid.
2. The genetic code is usually stated to be ***universal*** (with a few minor exceptions); that is, the specificity of the genetic code has been conserved from very early stages of evolution, with only slight differences in the manner the code is translated.
3. The genetic code is ***redundant*** (sometimes called ***degenerate***). Although each triplet corresponds to a single amino acid, a given

amino acid may have more than one triplet coding for it. For example, arginine is specified by six different codons (Table 32.1).

4. The genetic code is ***nonoverlapping*** and ***commaless:*** The code is read from a fixed starting point as a continuous sequence of bases, taken three at a time. For example, ABCDEFGHIJKL... is read as ABC/DEF/GHI/JKL... without any "punctuation" between the codons. Note that if one or two nucleotides are either deleted from or added to the interior of a message sequence, the ***reading frame*** will be altered, and the resulting amino acid sequence may become radically different from this point onward (Figure 32.2).

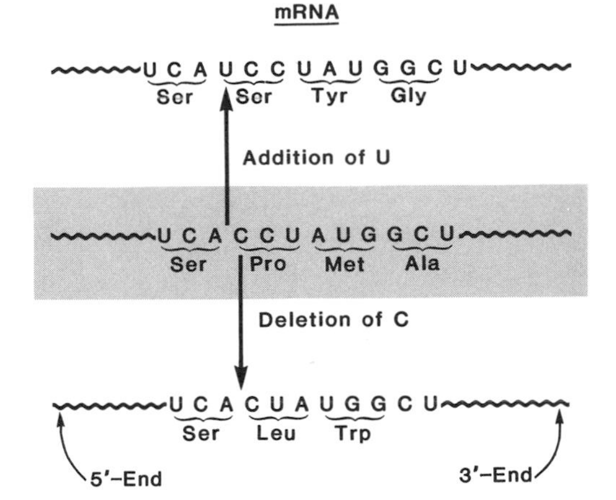

Figure 32.2
Frameshift mutations can cause an alteration in the reading frame of mRNA.

III. COMPONENTS REQUIRED FOR A TRANSLATIONAL SYSTEM

A. Amino acids

1. All the amino acids that will eventually appear in the finished protein must be present at the time of protein synthesis.

B. tRNA

1. At least one type of transfer RNA per amino acid is required.
2. In humans there are at least 31 species of tRNA in the cytoplasm and 22 in the mitochondria. Because there are only 20 species of amino acids commonly carried by tRNA, some amino acids have more than one specific tRNA molecule. This is particularly true of those amino acids that are coded for by several codons.
3. Each tRNA molecule contains a three-base nucleotide sequence—the ***anticodon***—that recognizes a specific codon on the mRNA. This codon specifies the insertion into the growing peptide chain of the amino acid carried by that tRNA (see Figure 28.16).
4. Each tRNA molecule has an attachment site for a ***specific*** amino acid at its ***3′-end***. When a tRNA has a covalently attached amino acid it is said to be ***charged;*** when tRNA is not bound to an amino acid it is defined as ***uncharged***. The amino acid that is attached to the tRNA molecule is said to be ***activated***.
5. Because of their ability to both carry a specific amino acid and to recognize the codon for that amino acid, tRNAs are known as ***adaptor molecules***.

C. Messenger RNA

1. The specific mRNA required as a template for the synthesis of the desired particular protein must be present.

D. Aminoacyl-tRNA synthetases

1. Each member of this family of enzymes recognizes both a specific amino acid and the tRNA that corresponds to that amino acid (Figure 32.3). The extreme specificity of the *synthetase* in recognizing these two structures is responsible for the high fidelity of translation of the genetic message.
2. At least one member of this family of enzymes is required for the ***activation*** of each type of amino acid.

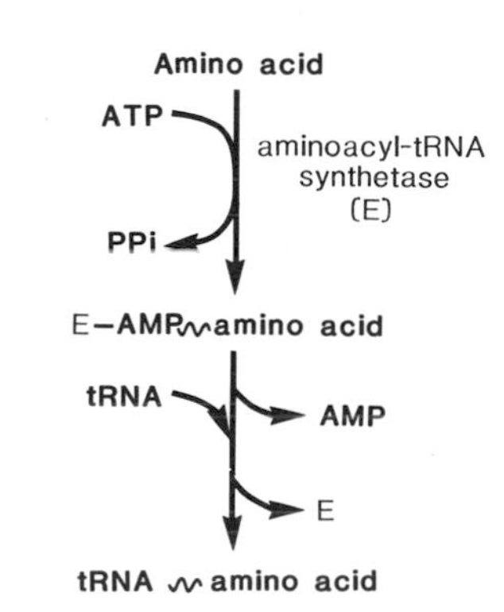

Figure 32.3
Attachment of a specific amino acid to its corresponding tRNA by *aminoacyl-tRNA synthetase*.

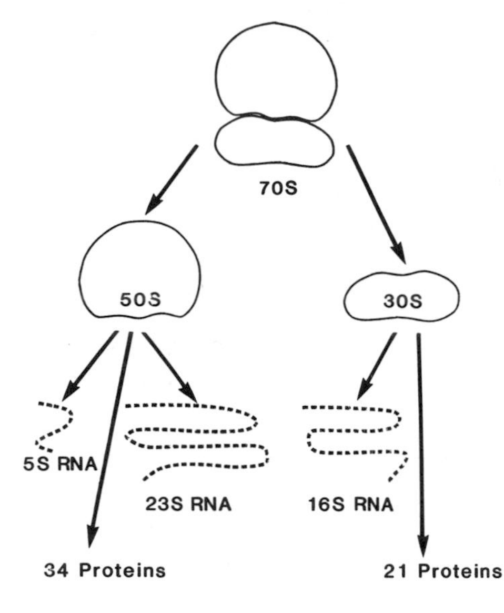

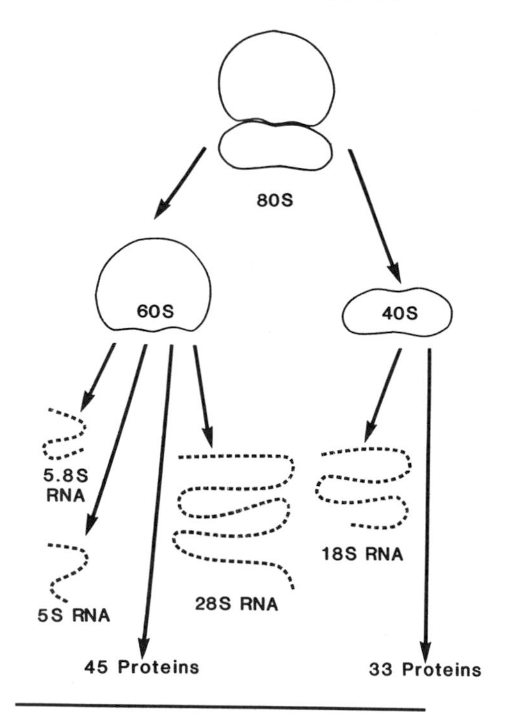

Figure 32.4
Ribosomal composition.

3. Each *aminoacyl-tRNA synthetase* catalyzes a two-step reaction that results in the covalent attachment of an amino acid to the 3′-end of its corresponding tRNA. The overall reaction requires ATP, which is cleaved to AMP and PP_i (Figure 32.3).

E. Functionally competent ribosomes

1. Ribosomes are large complexes of protein and rRNA (Figure 32.4). They consist of two subunits—one "large" and one "small", whose relative sizes are generally given in terms of their sedimentation coefficients, or S (**S**vedberg) values. (Note: Because the S values are determined both by ***shape*** and molecular weight, their numerical values are not strictly additive. For example, the prokaryotic 50S and 30S ribosomal subunits together form a ribosome with an S value of 70.) Prokaryotic and eukaryotic ribosomes are similar in structure, and both serve the same function in the cell, namely, as the "factories" responsible for the synthesis of proteins.
2. The ribosome has two ***binding sites*** for tRNA molecules, the A and the P sites, each of which extends over both subunits. Together, they cover two neighboring codons.
   a. During translation, the ***A site*** on the ribosome binds an incoming aminoacyl-tRNA as directed by the codon currently occupying this site. This codon specifies the next amino acid to be added to the growing peptide chain.
   b. The ***P site*** codon is occupied by peptidyl-tRNA. This tRNA carries the chain of amino acids that has already been synthesized (see Figure 32.7 for an illustration of the role of the A and P sites in translation).
3. In eukaryotic cells, the ribosomes are found either "free" in the cytoplasm or in close association with the endoplasmic reticulum (ER). The ER-associated ribosomes are responsible for synthesizing both the proteins that are to be exported from the cell and the proteins that become integrated into a cellular membrane.
4. The ribosomal RNAs have extensive regions of secondary structure arising from the base pairing of complementary sequences of nucleotides in different portions of the molecule. The formation of intramolecular double-stranded regions is similar to that found in tRNA (see Figure 28.16)..
5. Ribosomal proteins are present in considerably greater numbers in eukaryotic cells than in prokaryotic cells (see Figure 32.4). These additional proteins play numerous roles, including facilitating interaction of the ribosomes with receptors on the ER (these ribosomal proteins are called ***ribophorin I and II***) and in regulating the translational process.

F. Protein factors

1. Initiation, elongation, and termination (or release) factors are required for peptide synthesis (see Figure 32.7).
2. Some of these proteins perform a catalytic function, whereas others appear to stabilize the synthetic machinery.

G. ATP and GTP are required as sources of energy

1. Cleavage of a total of four high-energy bonds is required for the addition of one amino acid to the growing polypeptide chain: two

from ATP in the *aminoacyl-tRNA synthetase* reaction (one in removing PP_i and one in the subsequent hydrolysis of the PP_i to inorganic phosphate by *pyrophosphatase*) and two from GTPs—one for binding the aminoacyl-tRNA to the A site, and one for the translocation step (see Figure 32.7).

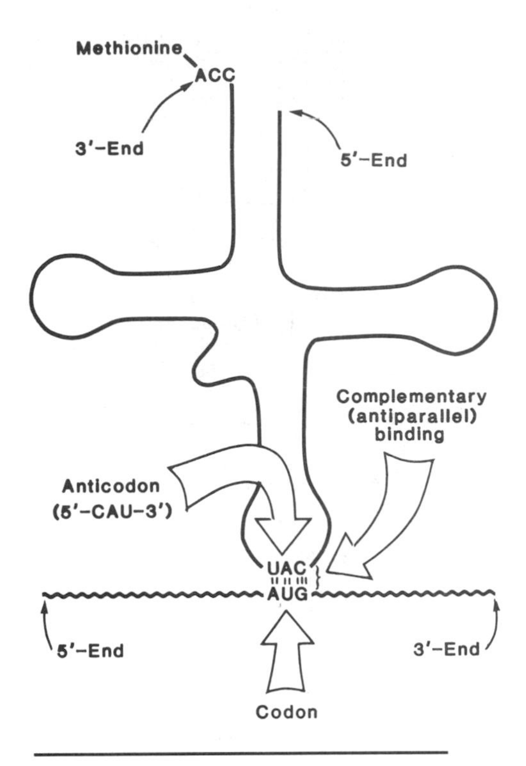

Figure 32.5
Complementary, antiparallel binding of the anticodon for methionyl-tRNA (CAU) to the mRNA codon for methionine (AUG).

IV. CODON RECOGNITION BY tRNA

A. Role of the anti-codon sequence

1. Recognition of a particular codon on an mRNA sequence is accomplished by the anticodon sequence of the tRNA (Figure 32.5).
2. The binding of the tRNA anticodon to the mRNA codon follows the rules of ***complementary, antiparallel*** binding, that is, the mRNA codon is "read" 5′→3′ by an anticodon pairing in the "flipped" (3′→5′) orientation (Figure 32.5). (Note: When writing the sequences of ***both*** codons and anticodons, the nucleotide sequence must ALWAYS be listed in the 5′→3′ order.)

B. Nontraditional base pairing

1. Some tRNAs recognize more than one codon for a given amino acid.
2. The base at the ***5′-end of the anticodon*** (the "first" base of the anticodon) is not as spatially defined as the other two bases. Movement of that first base allows nontraditional base-pairing with the ***3′-base of the codon*** (the "last" base of the codon). This movement is called ***wobble*** and allows a single tRNA to recognize several codons. Examples of these flexible pairings are shown in Figure 32.6. The result of this wobbling is that there need not be 61 tRNA species in order to read the 61 codons coding for amino acids.

V. STEPS IN PROTEIN SYNTHESIS

The pathway of protein synthesis is called ***translation*** because the "language" of the nucleotide sequence on the mRNA is translated into the language of an amino acid sequence. The mRNA is translated from its 5′-end to its 3′-end, producing a protein synthesized from its amino-terminal end to its carboxy-terminal end. Prokaryotic mRNAs may have several ***coding regions,*** each of which has its own initiation sequence and produces a separate species of polypeptide, whereas eukaryotic mRNAs each code only for one polypeptide chain. The process of translation is divided into three separate steps: initiation, elongation, and termination. The polypeptide chains produced by this pathway may be further modified by ***post-translational modification***.

A. Steps in protein synthesis

The steps in protein synthesis in the prokaryotic bacterium *E. coli* are summarized in detail in Figure 32.7. The points numbered in brackets below refer to those individual steps. Eukaryotic protein synthesis resembles that of prokaryotic protein synthesis in most details. Individual differences are mentioned in the text.

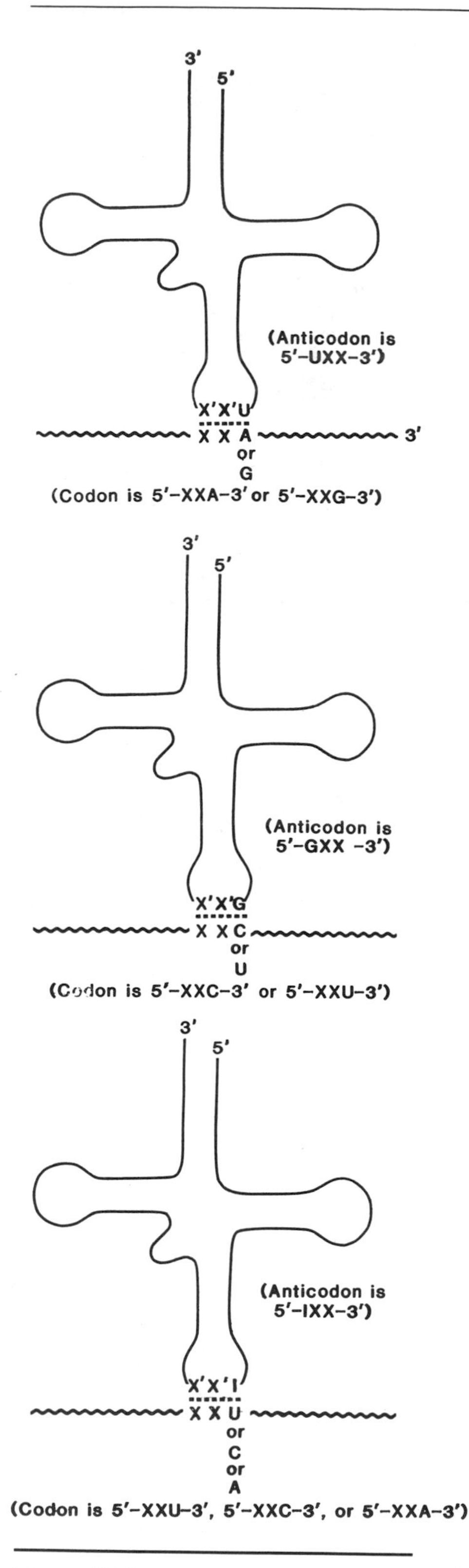

Figure 32.6
Wobble: Nontraditional base pairing between the 5′-nucleotide of the anticodon with the 3′-nucleotide of the codon.

[1] ***Initiation*** of protein synthesis involves the assembly of the components of the translational system before peptide bond formation. These components include the two ribosomal subunits, the mRNA to be translated, the aminoacyl-tRNA specified for by the first codon in the message, GTP (which provides energy for the process), and ***initiation factors*** that facilitate the assembly of this ***initiation complex***.

a. In prokaryotes, three initiation factors are known (IF-1, IF-2, and IF-3), whereas in eukaryotes there appear to be at least eight (designated eIF to show eukaryotic origin).

b. There are two mechanisms by which the ribosome recognizes the nucleotide sequence that initiates translation:

1) First, in *E. coli,* a sequence of nucleotide bases (5′-AGGAGG-3′) known as the ***Shine–Dalgarno sequence*** is located four to seven bases before the AUG codon on the mRNA molecule. The 16S ribosomal RNA component of the 30S ribosomal subunit has a nucleotide sequence that is complementary to all or part of the Shine–Dalgarno sequence, and therefore the mRNA 5′-end, and the 16S ribosomal RNA molecule can form complementary base pairs, thus facilitating the binding and positioning of the mRNA on the 30S ribosomal subunit (see Figure 32.8).

2) Second, the codon AUG at the beginning of the message is recognized by a special ***initiator tRNA***. In bacteria, this tRNA carries an ***N-formylated methionine***. The formyl group is added to the methionine after that amino acid is attached to the initiator tRNA by the enzyme *transformylase,* which uses N^{10}-formyl tetrahydrofolate as the carbon donor. In eukaryotes, the initiator tRNA carries a methionine that is ***not*** formylated. In both prokaryotic and eukaryotic cells, this N-terminal methionine may be removed before the functional protein has been completed.

[2] ***Elongation*** of the polypeptide chain involves the addition of amino acids to the carboxyl end of the growing polypeptide chain. During elongation, the ribosome moves from the 5′-end to the 3′-end of the mRNA that is being translated.

a. Elongation is facilitated by ***elongation factors*** (EF-Tu and EF-Ts) and requires GTP. (Note: Eukaryotic elongation factors are designated eEF.)

b. The formation of the peptide bonds is catalyzed by a 50S ribosomal subunit protein, *peptidyl transferase* (see Figure 32.9 for the reaction details).

c. After the peptide bond has been formed, the ribosome advances three nucleotides toward the 3′-end of the mRNA. This process is known as ***translocation***. It causes the release of the uncharged tRNA and the movement of the peptidyl-tRNA into the P site (see Figure 32.7).

[3] ***Termination*** occurs when one of the three termination codons moves into the A site. These codons are recognized by ***release factors***: RF-1, which recognizes the termination codons UAA and UAG; RF-2, which recognizes UGA and UAA; and RF-3, which stimulates the activity of RF-1 and RF-1). These factors cause the newly synthesized protein to be released from the ribosomal

complex and, at the same time, cause the dissociation of the ribosome from the mRNA (see Figure 32.7).

Inhibitors of the process of protein synthesis are illustrated in Figure 32.7.

B. Polysomes

1. Translation begins at the 5′-end of the mRNA, with the ribosome proceeding along the RNA molecule. Because of the length of the nucleotide sequence of most mRNAs, more than one ribosome at a time can generally translate the message (Figure 32.10). Such a complex of one mRNA and a number of ribosomes is called a ***polysome***.

VI. POST-TRANSLATIONAL MODIFICATION OF POLYPEPTIDE CHAIN

Many polypeptide chains are covalently modified, either while they are still attached to the ribosome or after their synthesis has been completed. Because the modifications usually occur after translation is complete, they are called post-translational modifications. There are several different types of post-translational modifications, a few of which are listed below:

A. Trimming

1. Many proteins destined for secretion from the cell are initially made as large, precursor molecules that are not functionally active. Portions of the protein chain can be removed by specialized ***endoproteases,*** resulting in the release of an active molecule.
2. The cellular site of the cleavage reaction depends on the protein to be modified. For example, some precursor proteins are cleaved in the Golgi apparatus, others in developing secretory vesicles, and still others after secretion.
3. Zymogens are inactive precursors of secreted enzymes (including the digestive proteases). The enzymes become activated through cleavage once they have reached their proper sites of action; for example, the pancreatic zymogen, trypsinogen, becomes active in the small intestine. The synthesis of potentially harmful enzymes in an inactive form protects the cell from being digested by its own products.

B. Phosphorylation

1. Phosphorylation occurs on hydroxyl groups of specific amino acid residues in a protein. This phosphorylation is catalyzed by a family of *protein kinases* and may be reversed by the action of cellular *protein phosphatases*. The result of the phosphorylation may either increase or decrease the functional activity of the protein. A good example of these phosphorylation reactions has been previously discussed (see p. 74 for the synthesis and degradation of glycogen).

C. Glycosylation

1. Many of the proteins that are destined to become either part of a cellular membrane or secreted from the cells receive carbo-

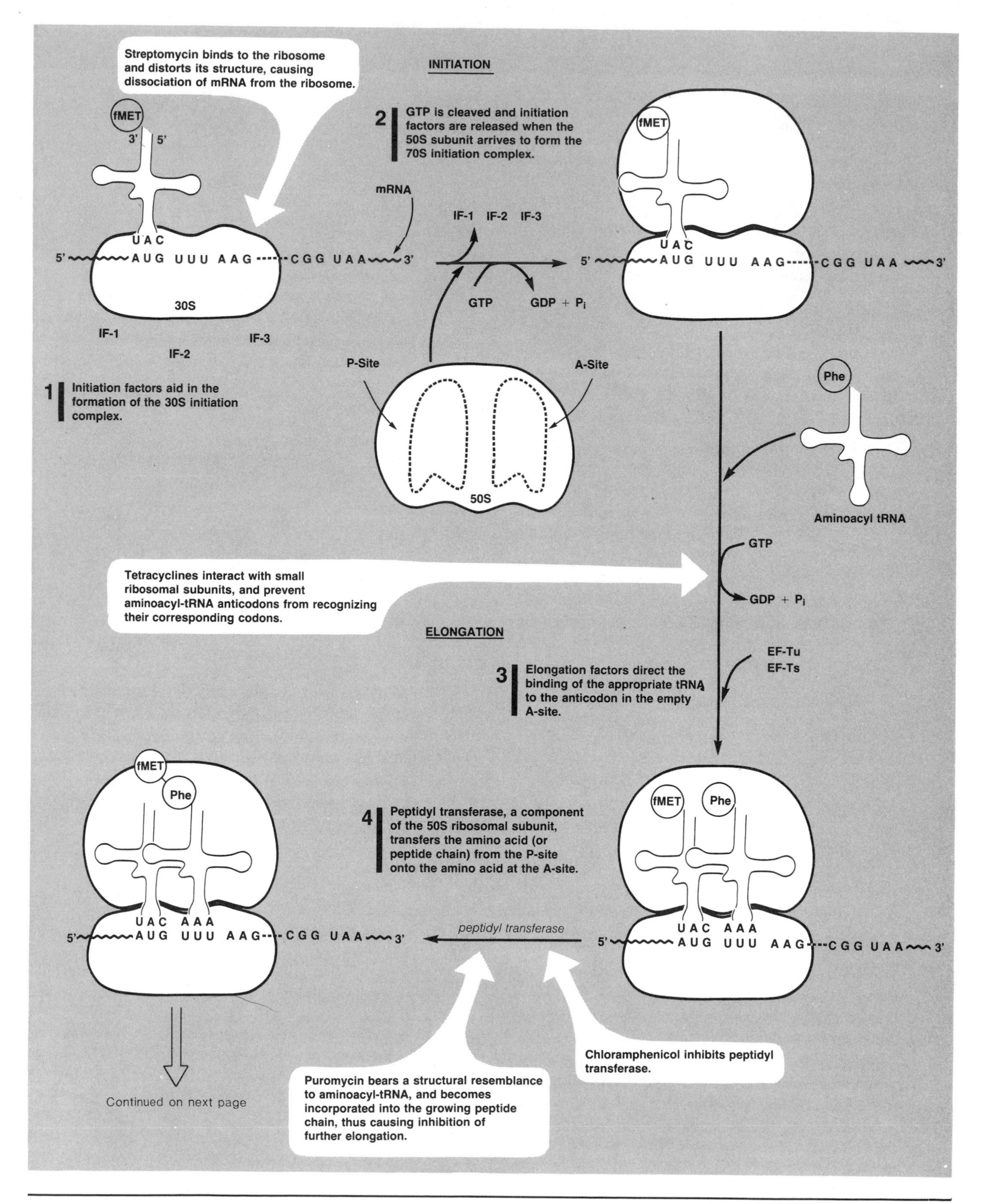

Continued on next page

Figure 32.7
Steps in protein synthesis (translation).

Continued from previous page

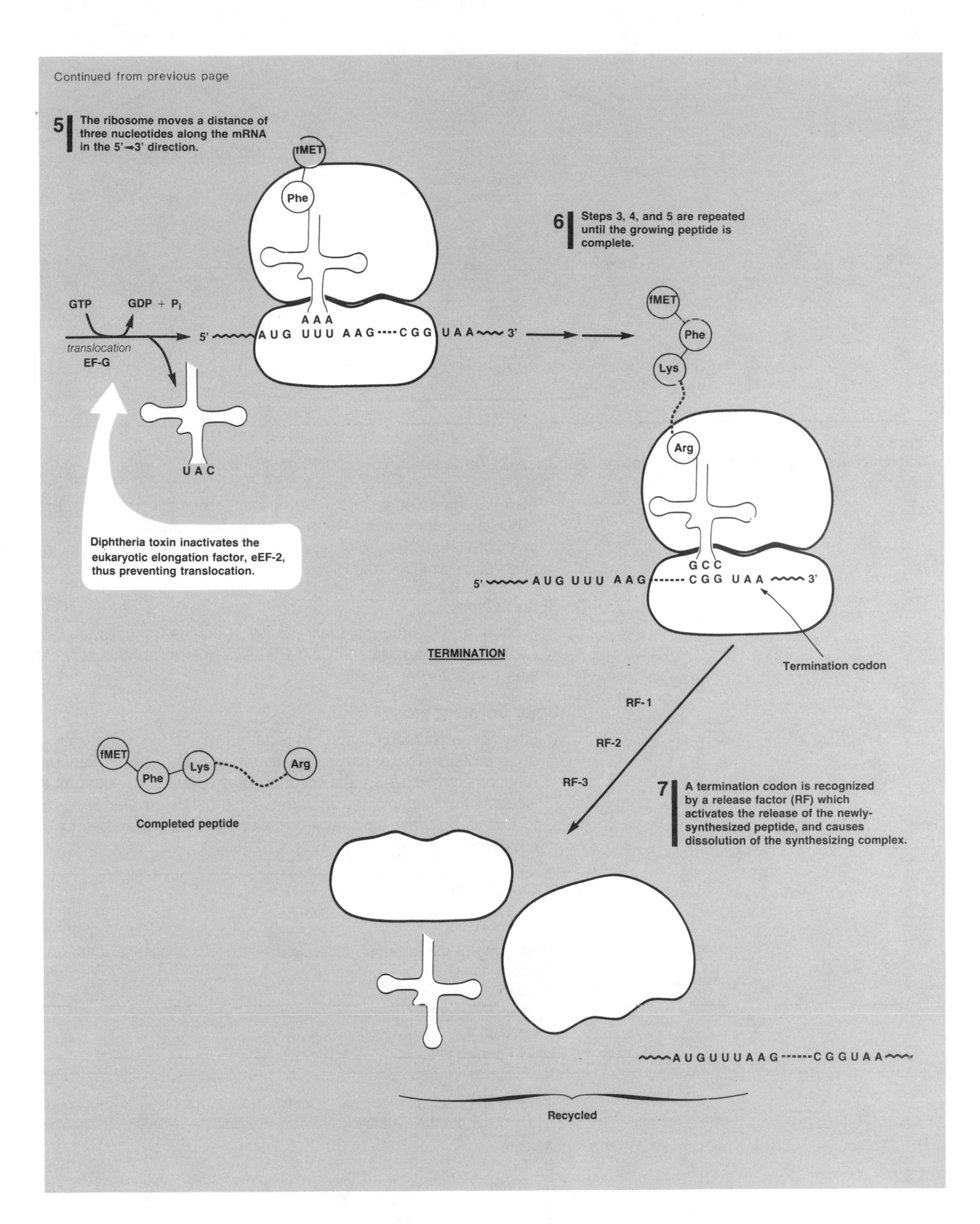

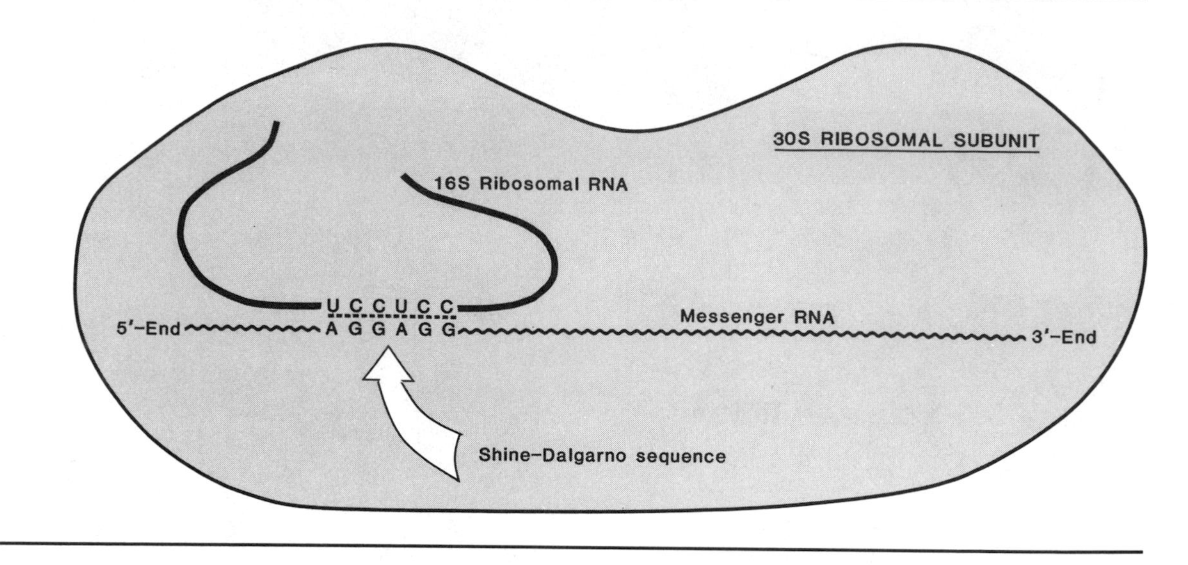

Figure 32.8
Complementary binding between prokaryotic mRNA Shine–Dalgarno sequence, and 16S ribosomal RNA.

hydrate chains attached to serine or threonine hydroxyl groups (O-linked) or asparagine (N-linked). This addition of sugars occurs in the ER and the Golgi apparatus. The process of producing such glycoproteins was discussed on p. 92.

D. Hydroxylation

1. Proline and lysine residues of the α-chains of collagen are extensively hydroxylated in the ER. A discussion of this process was presented on p. 32.

E. Other covalent modifications

1. Other covalent modification are required for the functional activity of a protein. There are many examples of proteins that are functionally inactive in the absence of a specific, covalent modification. For example, the vitamin biotin must be covalently bound to the carboxylase enzymes in order for these enzymes to be catalytically active (see p. 127).

Study Questions

Choose the ONE best answer:

32.1 Which one of the following molecules is NOT a component of the 30S initiation complex?.

A. GTP
B. Initiation factor 2 (IF-2)
C. mRNA
D. N-Formylmethionyl-tRNA
E. ATP

32.2 What is the maximum number of different amino acids in a polypeptide chain coded by the synthetic polyribonucleotide $(UCAG)_5$?

A. One
B. Two
C. Three
D. Four
E. Five

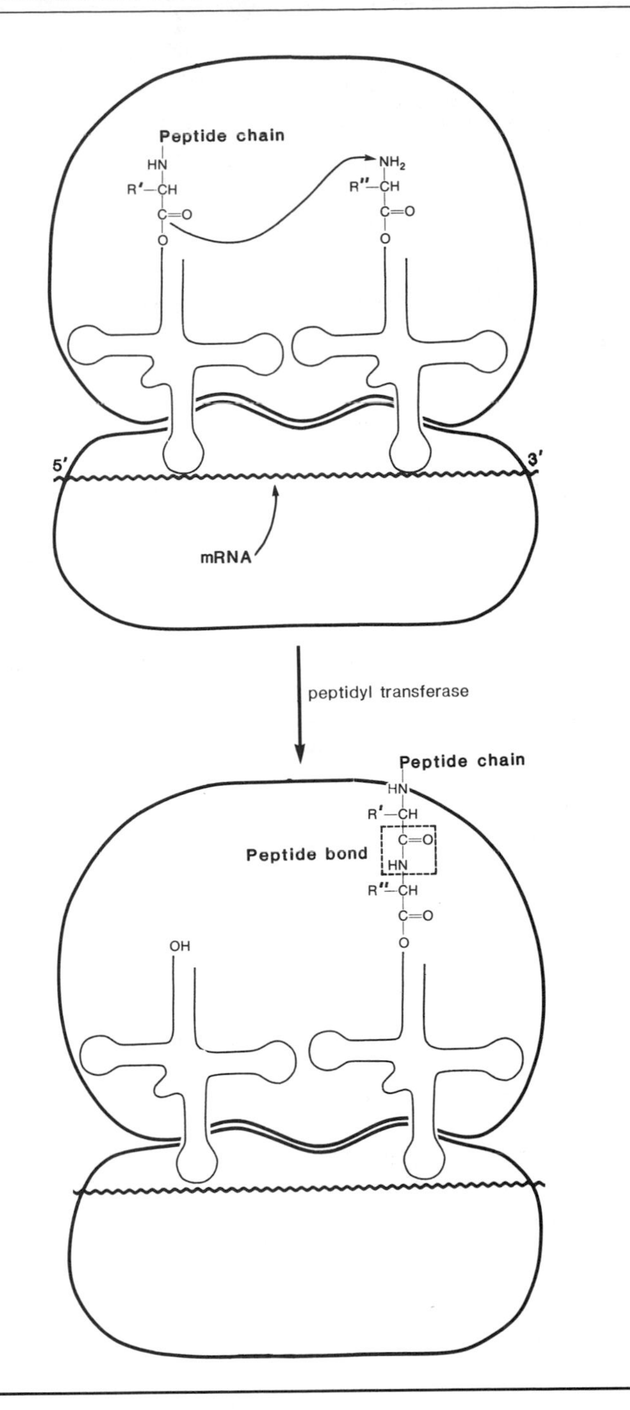

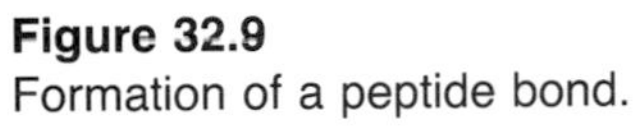

Figure 32.9
Formation of a peptide bond.

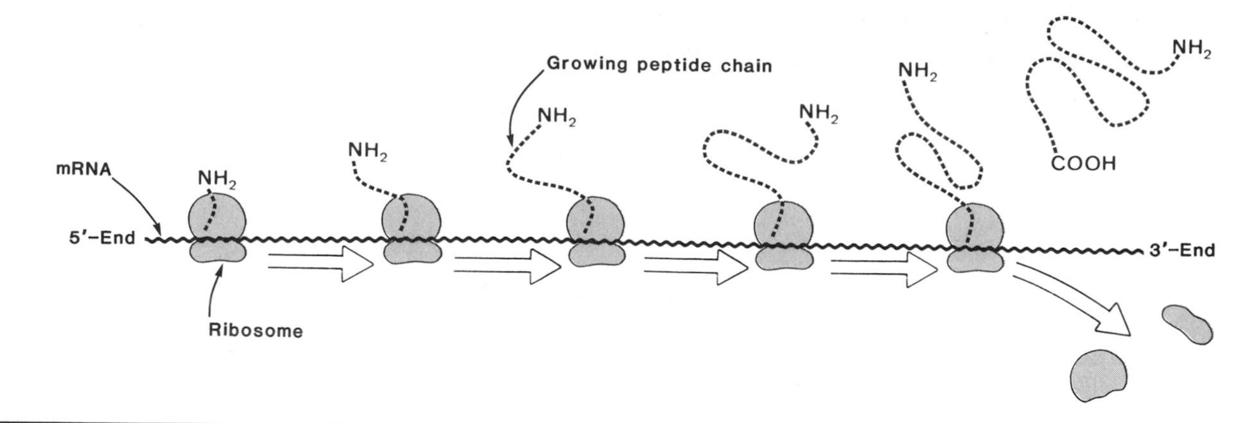

Figure 32.10
A polyribosome.

32.3 The genetic code ...

A. ... is degenerate in that many triplets code for more than one amino acid.
B. ... is read in the direction of 3′ to 5′.
C. ... triplet, CCA, is found at the beginning of nearly all mRNA coding sequences.
D. ... involves a number of minor bases that are associated with chain initiation and transcription.
E. ... is generally referred to as universal because it is nearly the same in all organisms.

32.4 In protein biosynthesis ...

A. ... each amino acid recognizes its own codon by a direct interaction with the mRNA template.
B. ... fidelity of translation is assured by the presence of traces of DNA on the ribosome.
C. ... each amino acid is first attached to an anticodon specific for the amino acid.
D. ... a given codon and its anticodon must have identical base sequences in order for there to be proper base-pairing.
E. ... each amino acid is added in its proper place to a growing peptide chain through the "adaptor" function of tRNA.

Answers to Study Questions

Study questions from the text are reprinted here along with explanations of the correct answers (indicated by a ✔).

Chapter 1: STRUCTURE OF AMINO ACIDS

Answer A if 1, 2, and 3 are correct
B if 1 and 3 are correct
C if 2 and 4 are correct
D if only 4 is correct
E if all are correct

1.1. Correct answer = B

Which of the following amino acids has(have) a charged side chain at physiologic pH?

✔1. Contains a hydroxyl group {***Yes: Serine is classified as an uncharged, polar amino acid because of the hydroxyl group in its side chain.***}

2. Can form disulfide bonds {***No: Only cysteine residues can form disulfide bonds.***}

✔3. Can participate in hydrogen bonds {***Yes: The hydroxyl group in the side chain can function as a hydrogen donor (—OH) in a hydrogen bond.***}

4. Is charged at physiologic pH {***No: The hydroxyl group in the side chain is not ionized at physiologic pH.***}

1.2. Correct answer = A

Which of the following amino acids has(have) a charged side chain at physiologic pH?

✔1. Aspartic acid {***Yes: Aspartic acid contains a carboxyl group (—COO^-) in its side chain that is ionized at physiologic pH.***}

✔2. Lysine {***Yes: Lysine contains an amino group (—NH_3^+) in its side chain that is ionized at physiologic pH.***}

✔3. Glutamic acid {***Yes: Glutamic acids contains a carboxyl group (—COO^-) in its side chain that is ionized at physiologic pH.***}

4. Asparagine {***No: Asparagine contains an amide group (—$CONH_2$) in its side chain that is uncharged at physiologic pH.***}

1.3. Correct answer = C

Glutamine

1. contains three titratable groups. {***No: Glutamine contains two titratable groups, α-carboxyl and α-amino groups.***}

✔2. contains an amide group. {***Yes***}

3. is classified as an acidic amino acid. {***No: Glutamine is classified as an uncharged, polar amino acid.***}

✔4. contains a side chain that can form hydrogen bonds in proteins. {***Yes***}

1.4. Correct answer = A

Which of the following statements about free amino acids is(are) true?

✔1. Glycine contains two dissociable hydrogens. {***Yes: Hydrogen ions can dissociate from the α-carboxyl group (—COOH) and from the protonated α-amino group (—NH_3^+).***}

✔2. Tyrosine is a site of attachment of phosphate groups in proteins. {***Yes***}

✔3. Cysteine is a sulfur-containing amino acid. {***Yes: cysteine contains a sulfhydryl group (—SH).***}

4. Glutamine is classified as a basic amino acid. {***No: Glutamine is a neutral amino acid that contains an amide group in the side chain***}

Choose the ONE best answer:

1.5. Correct answer = D

Lysine (pK_1 = 2.2, pK_2 = 9.0, pK_3 = 10.5)

A. contains an amide group. {***No: Lysine contains an ε-amino group.***}

B. has a charge of +1 when the carboxyl group is protonated. {***No: Lysine has a charge of +2 in acidic solutions (pH < 2) where the carboxyl group is uncharged (—COOH) but the α- and ε-amino groups are both positively charged (—NH_3^+).***}

C. has a pI of 5.6. {***No: The pH of lysine is the average of pK_2 and pK_3, ½ (9.0 + 10.5) = 9.75.***}

✔D. will migrate toward the cathode (negative electrode) during electrophoresis at pH 7.0. {***Yes: At pH = 7.0 the carboxyl group will be negatively charged (—COO^-) and the α- and ε-amino groups will both be positively charged (—NH_3^+), giving a net positive charge.***}

E. has a nonpolar side chain. {***No: Lysine is a basic amino acid.***}

1.6. Correct answer = D

Histidine has a side chain that has a $pK_2 = 6.0$. Which one of the following amino acids also has a side chain that titrates within about 1.5 pH units of neutrality?

A. Lysine {***No: The pK nearest neutrality for lysine is $pK_2 = 9.0$ (α-amino group).***}

B. Arginine {***No: The pK nearest neutrality for arginine is $pK_2 = 9.0$ (α-amino group).***}

C. Threonine {***No: The pK nearest neutrality for threonine is $pK_2 = 9.8$ (α-amino group).***}

✔ D. Cysteine {***Yes: The pK nearest neutrality for cysteine is $pK_2 = 8.3$ (sulfhydryl group).***}

E. Hydroxyproline {***No: The pK nearest neutrality for proline is $pK_2 = 9.8$ (imino group).***}

1.7. Correct answer = C

The letters A, B, C, D, and E designate regions on the titration curve of glycine ($pK_1 = 2.3$, $pK_2 = 9.6$) shown on page 9. Which one of the following descriptions is correct?

A. A is a region of maximal buffering. {***No: A is a region of minimal buffering.***}

B. B is a region of minimal buffering. {***No: B is a region of maximal buffering.***}

✔ C. C is at the isoelectric point (pI). {***Yes***}

D. The concentration of $+NH_3—CH_2—COOH$ is maximal in region D. {***No: At D, $+NH_3—CH_2—COO^-$ and $NH_2—CH_2—COO^-$ are the predominant species present.***}

E. The concentration of $+NH_3—CH_2—COO^-$ is maximal in region E. {***No: At E, $NH_2—CH_2—COO^-$ is the predominant species present.***}

Answer A if 1, 2, and 3 are correct
B if 1 and 3 are correct
C if 2 and 4 are correct
D if only 4 is correct
E if all are correct

1.8. Correct answer = A

The peptide bond

✔ 1. is a special type of amide linkage. {***Yes: The peptide bond is an amide linkage between an α-carboxyl group and an α-amino group (or imino group in the case of proline).***}

✔ 2. has a partial double bond character. {***Yes***}

✔ 3. is not ionized at physiologic pH. {***Yes***}

4. is cleaved by agents that denature proteins, such as organic solvents and high concentrations of urea. {***No: Acid hydrolysis at elevated temperatures is required to cleave completely the peptide bonds between amino acids.***}

1.9. Correct answer = B

The peptide alanylglycylserine

✔ 1. contains alanine with a free α-amino group. {***Yes: Alanine is the N-terminal residue and has a free α-amino group.***}

2. contains three peptide bonds. {***No: Alanylglycylserine is a tripeptide that contains two peptide bonds.***}

✔ 3. is optically active. {***Yes: The alanyl and serine residues contain asymmetric centers.***}

4. is a dipeptide. {***No: Alanylglycylserine is a tripeptide.***}

Chapter 2: STRUCTURE OF PROTEINS

Answer A if 1, 2, and 3 are correct
B if 1 and 3 are correct
C if 2 and 4 are correct
D if only 4 is correct
E if all are correct

2.1 Correct answer = B

Which of the following reagents would be useful in determining the N-terminal amino acid of a polypeptide?

✔ 1. Fluorodinitrobenzene {***Yes: This reagent is used in the Sanger method of N-terminal analysis.***}

2. Carboxypeptidase {***No: This enzyme is used to determine the C-terminal amino acid.***}

✔ 3. Phenylisothiocyanate {***Yes: This reagent is used in the Edman degradation for N-terminal analysis.***}

4. Cyanogen bromide {***No: This reagent is used to cleave at internal methionine residues in a polypeptide chain.***}

2.2. Correct answer = B

Which of the following correctly describes the expected products obtained when the polypeptide arg-gly-phe-leu-met-lys is treated as indicated below?.

✔ 1. Treatment with cyanogen bromide yields two fragments. {***Yes: Cyanogen bromide would cleave at the methionine residue to give two products, arg-gly-phe-leu-homoserine lactone and lys.***}

2. Treatment with trypsin gives three fragments. {***No: Trypsin would cleave between the arginine and glycine residues to yield two products.***}

✔ 3. Treatment with 6N HCl at 100° gives six products. {***Yes: Complete acid hydrolysis cleaves all the peptide bonds, liberating six free amino acids.***}

4. Treatment with hydrazine yields two fragments. {***No: Hydrazine will yield five amino acid hydrazones and lysine.***}

Choose the ONE best answer:

2.3. Correct answer = A

You are presented with the following information about a peptide composed of five amino acids:

(a) Amino acid analysis gives equimolar amounts of Ala, Glu, Gly, Lys, and Met;

(b) Digestion of the original peptide with trypsin gives rise to a free amino acid.

(c) Digestion of the original peptide with cyanogen bromide generates two fragments, one of which moves toward the anode and the other toward the cathode when electrophoresed at ph 7.

Which one of the following best describes the structure of the peptide?

✓ A. Lys-Gly-Met-Glu-Ala {***Yes:** **Treatment (b) would yield a free amino acid: lys and the polypeptide gly-met-gly-ala. Treatment (c) would produce lys-gly-homoserine, which at pH 7 has a net positive charge (due to protonated side chain of lysine) and would move toward the cathode on electrophoresis. The second product of treatment (c) would be glu-ala,which has a net negative charge at ph 7 (due to —COO⁻ in the side chain of glutamate) and would move toward the anode on electrophoresis.***}

B. Gly-Lys-Met-Glu-Ala {***No: Treatment (b) would not produce a free amino acid but would yield two peptides, gly-lys and met-glu-ala. Treatment (c) would produce gly-lys-homoserine (positively charged) and glu-ala (negatively charged).***}

C. Lys-Glu-Met-Ala-Gly {***No: Treatment (b) would yield a free amino acid: lys and the polypeptide glu-met-ala-gly. However, treatment (c) would produce lys-glu-homoserine and ala-gly, neither of which carries a net charge at pH 7.***}

D. Gly-Glu-Met-Ala-Lys {***No: Treatment (b) does not give a free amino acid. The original peptide has no susceptible bond to the action of trypsin. Treatment (c) would produce gly-glu-homoserine (negatively charged) and ala-lys (positively charged).***}

E. Glu-Gly-Met-Ala-Lys {***No: Treatment (b) would not give a free amino acid. The original peptide has no bond susceptible to the action of trypsin. Treatment (c) results in the formation of glu-gly-homoserine (negatively charged) and ala-lys (positively charged).***}

2.4 Correct answer = C

Which one of the following best describes the products obtained when the tripeptide alanylglycylleucine is treated with phenylisothiocyanate followed by mild acid hydrolysis?

✓ A. PTH-alanine, glycylleucine {***Yes: Phenylisothiocyanate forms a phenythiohydantoin (PTH) derivative with the amino terminal residue. Mild acid hydrolysis releases the PTH-derivative without cleaving the remaining polypeptide.***}

B. PTH-leucine, alanylglycine {***No***}

C. PTH-alanine, glycine, leucine {***No***}

D. PTH-alanylglycylleucine {***No***}

E. Alanine, glycine, leucine {***No***}

2.5 Correct answer = E

A mutation is most likely to alter the three-dimensional conformation of a protein if

A. it produces a substitution of a hydrophobic amino acid for a hydrophilic amino acid. {***No: This substitution may or may not produce a change in the structure since hydrophilic amino acids are usually located on the outside of a protein molecule.***}

B. valine is substituted for leucine. {***No: Substitution of one hydrophobic for another hydrophobic residue would be predicted to have little effect on the structure of the protein.***}

C. it changes the amino acid at the amino-terminus. {***No: This substitution may or may not produce a change in the protein structure.***}

D. it changes the amino acid at the carboxy-terminus. {***No: This substitution may or may not produce a change in the protein structure.***}

✓ E. it places proline in the middle of an α-helix. {***Yes: Proline disrupts the α-helix.***}

2.6 Correct answer = E

Which one of the following types of bonds or interactions is least important in determining the three-dimensional folding of most proteins?

A. Hydrogen bonds {***No: These bonds are important in stabilizing protein structure, particularly the α-helix and β-sheet.***}

B. Electrostatic bonds {***No: These bonds stabilize protein structure.***}

C. Hydrophobic interactions {***No: These bonds stabilize protein structure.***}

D. Disulfide bonds. {***No: These bonds stabilize protein structure.***}

✓ E. Ester bonds. {***Yes: Ester bonds are not important in stabilizing protein structure.***}

2.7. Correct answer = A

Which one of the following amino acids is most likely to be found in the interior of a typical globular protein?

{***Nonpolar amino acids are usually found in the interior of a globular protein, whereas polar and charged amino acids are most frequently found on the exterior of a globular protein.***}

✓ A. Leucine {***Yes***}

B. Glutamate {***No***}

C. Threonine {***No***}

D. Lysine {***No***}

E. Arginine {***No***}

2.8. Correct answer = E

Which one of the following statements about protein structure is correct?

A. The α-helix is stabilized primarily by ionic interactions between the side chains of amino acids. {***No: The α-helix is stable mainly because of hydrogen bonds and hydrophobic interactions.***}

B. The formation of a disulfide bond in a protein requires that the two participating cysteine residues be adjacent to each other in the primary sequence of the protein. {***No: The two cysteine residues that react to form the disulfide bond may be a great distance apart in the primary structure but are brought into proximity by the three-dimensional folding of the polypeptide chain.***}

C. The stability of quaternary structure in proteins is mainly due to covalent bonds among the subunits. {***No: Quaternary structure is stabilized by noncovalent interactions between subunits.***}

D. The denaturation of proteins always leads to irreversible loss of secondary and tertiary structure. {***No: Denaturation may either be reversible or irreversible.***}

✓ E. The information for the correct folding of a protein is contained in the specific sequence of amino acids along the polypeptide chain. {***Yes: Specific interactions among the side chains of the amino acid residues guide the folding of a polypeptide chain.***}

Chapter 3: SPECIALIZED PROTEINS

Answer A if 1, 2, and 3 are correct
B if 1 and 3 are correct
C if 2 and 4 are correct
D if only 4 is correct
E if all are correct

3.1. Correct answer = A

Which of the following statements about the binding of oxygen by hemoglobin is(are) correct?

✓1. The oxygen affinity of any one heme group depends on the quaternary structure of the molecule. {***Yes: As oxygen binds to the hemoglobin tetramer, the subunits change structure, causing an increase in oxygen affinity***}

✓2. Carbon dioxide lowers the oxygen affinity of hemoglobin by binding to the amino terminal groups of the polypeptide chains. {***Yes***}

✓3. The Bohr effect results in a greater affinity for oxygen at higher pHs. {***Yes***}

4. The hemoglobin tetramer binds four molecules of 2,3-DPG. {***No: One molecule of 2,3-DPG binds in the center of the hemoglobin tetramer.***}

3.2. Correct answer = D

Which of the following statements about hemoglobin is(are) correct?

1. The heme groups of hemoglobin are surrounded only by nonpolar side chains of the protein globin. {***No: The heme-binding cavity of globin includes some polar amino acids such as the proximal and distal histidines that interact with iron of the heme groups.***}

2. There are no proline residues in hemoglobin because their presence would disrupt the large number of α-helices present in the molecule. {***No: The proline in hemoglobin is found in the nonhelical regions of the molecule.***}

3. Oxyhemoglobin and deoxyhemoglobin have the same affinity for protons (H^+). {***No: Deoxyhemoglobin has a higher affinity for protons.***}

✓4. The polypeptide conformation of hemoglobin allows it to form a stable complex with oxygen without any oxidation of the iron in the heme. {***Yes: The heme binding pocket of globin provides a largely hydrophobic environment in which the ferrous (Fe^{+2}) is stable.***}

3.3. Correct answer = A

Which of the following statements is(are) correct about 2,3-diphosphoglycerate:

✓1. It is formed from an intermediate of the glycolytic pathway. {***Yes: 2,3-DPG is formed from 1,3-diphosphoglycerate by the action of a mutase.***}

✓2. By binding to hemoglobin, it stabilizes the deoxy form of hemoglobin and makes it more difficult for oxygen to bind. {***Yes***}

✓3. It is believed to form ionic bonds with positively charged amino acid R-groups in the center of the hemoglobin molecule. {***Yes***}

4. It markedly affects the sigmoidal shape of the oxygen saturation curve for hemoglobin. {***No***}

3.4. Correct answer = C

Which of the following heme proteins would be expected to show a lower (weaker) affinity for oxygen, compared to hemoglobin A at pH 7.4. (Assume that the concentration of 2,3-DPG is 5 mM, which is similar to that which occurs in the red blood cell).

1. Hemoglobin F {***No: HbF has a higher affinity for oxygen than does HbA, primarily because HbF has lower affinity for 2,3-DPG than does HbA.***}

✓2. Methemoglobin A {***Yes: Methemoglobin contains Fe^{+3} and does not bind oxygen.***}

3. Myoglobin {***No: Myoglobin has a higher affinity for oxygen than hemoglobin.***}

✓4. Hemoglobin A at ph 7.2 {***Yes: Lowering the pH decreases the affinity for oxygen.***}

3.5. Correct answer = D

You are presented with a patient who has mild anemia and whose hemoglobin has the same electrophoretic mobility (at pH 9.3) as sickle cell hemoglobin (HbS). However, the patient's cells do not sickle on deoxygenation. Which of the following genetic changes can explain the electrophoretic mobility?

1. A mutation that deletes a serine residue from the β-chain. {***No: Loss of a serine residue would not change the net charge of the molecule.***}

2. A substitution mutation that replaces a lysine residue in the β-chain with a phenylalanine. {***No: Lys → Phe results in a loss of positive charge, making the overall charge of the molecule more negative. This increases the electrophoretic mobility toward the anode (+).***}

3. A deletion mutation that deletes an arginine residue from the β-chain. {***No: Loss of an arginine residue results in a loss of positive charge, making the overall charge of the molecule more negative. This results in an increase in the electrophoretic mobility toward the anode (+).***}

✓4. A substitution mutation that replaces an alanine residue in the β-chain with an arginine. {***Yes: Ala → arg results in a gain of positive charge, making the overall charge of the molecule less negative. This produces a decrease in electrophoretic mobility toward the anode (+).***}

3.6 Correct answer = D

Hemoglobin A and hemoglobin S are the same with respect to which of the following?

1. Amino acid sequence of β-chain. {***No: HbS contains a valine (instead of glutamate) residue at position six of the β-chain.***}

2. Electrophoretic mobility at pH 8.6. {***No: HbS moves more slowly toward the anode (+).***}

3. Solubility in the deoxygenated form {***No: HbS is less soluble in the deoxy form.***}

✓4. Structure of the heme group {***Yes: The heme groups in HbA and HbS are identical.***}

3.7. Correct answer = E

Which of the following statements about the major collagen type from skin or bone is(are) correct?

✓ 1. One third of the amino acid composition of collagen is glycine. {***Yes: Glycine is located at every third position in the amino acid sequence. This small amino acid fits into the restricted space where three chains of the helix come together.***}

✓ 2. Ascorbate is required for the synthesis of triple-helical collagen. {***Yes: Ascorbate is required for the hydroxylation of proline and lysine residues of pro-α-chains. These hydroxylated amino acids are required for formation of the triple-helix of the finished collagen molecule.***}

✓ 3. Collagen molecules are trimers composed of three monomers each containing approximately 1000 amino acids. {***Yes***}

✓ 4. Collagen fibrils contain covalent cross-links. {***Yes***}

3.8. Complete the numbered statements below with the correct lettered terms.

A if item is associated with (A) only

B if item is associated with (B) only

C if item is associated with both (A) and (B)

D if item is associated with neither (A) nor (B)

(A) Mature collagen fibril

(B) Procollagen

1. contain(s) the amino acid glycine. {***Correct answer = C***}
2. contain(s) C- and N-terminal extensions (propeptides). {***Correct answer = B***}
3. contain(s) covalent cross links. {***Correct answer = C***}
4. is(are) globular proteins. {***Correct answer = D***}
5. is(are) intracellular proteins. {***Correct answer = B***}

Chapter 4: ENZYMES

Choose the ONE best answer:

4.1. Correct answer = A

A competitive inhibitor of an enzyme

✓ A. increases K_m without affecting V_m. {***Yes: In the presence of a competitive inhibitor an enzyme appears to have a lower affinity for the substrate, but as the substrate level is increased the observed velocity approaches V_m.***}

B. decreases K_m without affecting V_m. {***No***}

C. increases V_m without affecting K_m. {***No***}

D. decreases V_m without affecting K_m. {***No***}

E. decreases both V_m and K_m. {***No***}

4.2. Correct answer = D

The Michaelis constant, K_m, is

A. numerically equal to $\frac{1}{2} V_m$. {***No: K_m always has the dimension of concentration and is equal to the substrate concentration which produces a velocity that is $\frac{1}{2} V_m$.***}

B. dependent on the enzyme concentration. {***No: K_m is a characteristic of the enzyme under a given set of reaction conditions (pH, temperature, and so forth) and does not depend on the concentration of enzyme.***}

C. independent of pH. {***No: K_m can vary with pH as titratable groups in the enzyme or substrate either accept or release protons.***}

✓ D. numerically equal to the substrate concentration that gives half-maximal velocity.{***Yes***}

E. increased in the presence of a noncompetitive inhibitor. {***No: A noncompetitive inhibitor decreases the V_m but does not alter the K_m.***}

4.3. Correct answer = D

The rate of an enzyme-catalyzed reaction was measured using several substrate concentrations that were much lower than K_m. The dependence of reaction velocity on substrate concentration can best be described as

A. independent of enzyme concentration. {***No: Reaction velocity is proportional to enzyme concentration at all concentrations of substrate.***}

B. a constant fraction of V_m. {***No***}

C. equal to K_m. {***No***}

✓ D. proportional to the substrate concentration. {***Yes: The amount of the ES complex and hence the reaction velocity is proportional to the concentration of substrate.***}

E. zero order with respect to substrate. {***No: Zero order means that the reaction velocity is independent of substrate concentration. This is observed only when the substrate concentration is much greater than K_m.***}

4.4. Correct answer = D

Which one of the following statements is NOT characteristic of allosteric enzymes?

A. They frequently catalyze a committed step early in a metabolic pathway. {***Yes: Most metabolic pathways are regulated by changes in the activity of an early committed step in that pathway.***}

B. They are often composed of subunits. {***Yes: Allosteric effects are often mediated by alterations in the subunit interactions.***}

C. They frequently show cooperativity for substrate binding. {***Yes: Allosteric enzymes are often homotropic.***}

✓ D. They follow Michaelis-Menten kinetics. {***No: Allosteric enzymes usually show a complex relation between velocity and substrate concentration.***}

E. The binding of a positive allosteric effector results in an increase in enzymic activity. {***Yes***}

4.5. Correct answer = B

The presence of a noncompetitive inhibitor

A. leads to both an increase in the V_m of a reaction and an increase in the K_m. {***No: V_m is decreased, but K_m remains unchanged.***}

✔B. leads to a decrease in the observed V_m. {***Yes***}

C. leads to a decrease in K_m and V_m. {***No***}

D. leads to an increase in K_m without affecting V_m. {***No***}

E. increases the steady-state concentration of ES. {***No***}

4.6. Correct answer = C

The velocity, v_o, for an enzyme-catalyzed reaction was measured at several substrate concentrations:

[substrate] (moles per liter)	v_o (in millimoles product/min/mg protein)
0.25×10^{-4}	1.0
0.5×10^{-4}	1.7
1×10^{-4}	2.5
2×10^{-4}	5.0
5×10^{-4}	5.0

The K_m is approximately

A. 0.25×10^{-4} M. {***No***}

B. 0.5×10^{-4} M. {***No***}

✔C. 1×10^{-4} M. {***Yes: This concentration of substrate gives a velocity that is one half of V_m.***}

D. 2×10^{-4} M. {***No***}

E. 5×10^{-4} M. {***No***}

Chapter 5: CARBOHYDRATE METABOLISM

Choose the ONE best answer:

5.1. Correct answer = B

Which one of the following statements is INCORRECT regarding the predominant form of α-D-glucose?

A. It is a hemiacetal. {***Yes: 99% of aldose sugars with five or more carbons are found in a hemiacetal ring form rather than in an open chain form.***}

✔B. It contains five asymmetric carbon atoms. {***No: Glucose contains four asymmetric carbon atoms: carbon numbers 2, 3, 4, and 5.***}

C. It is a C-4 epimer of galactose. {***Yes: Glucose and galactose differ in structure only in the position of their hydrogen and hydroxyl groups at carbon #4.***}

D. It will rotate a plane of polarized light. {***Yes: Glucose is optically active because it has asymmetric carbon atoms, and therefore a solution of glucose will rotate a plane of polarized light.***}

E. In combination with fructose it forms sucrose, which is a nonreducing sugar. {***Yes: Carbon #1 of α-D-glucose forms a glycosidic bond with carbon #2 of fructose to form sucrose. Because the anomeric carbons of both sugars are involved in the glycosidic bond, sucrose is a nonreducing sugar.***}

5.2. Correct answer = E

Which one of the following oxidation-reduction reactions is ***not*** undergone by glucose?.

A. Oxidation of the aldehyde group (—CHO) at carbon #1 to a carboxyl group (—COOH) produces gluconic acid. {***Yes: Aldoses that have been oxidized at carbon #1 change their names from a word ending in -ose to one ending in -onic.***}

B. Oxidation of the hydroxymethyl group (—CH_2OH) at carbon #6 to a carboxyl (—COOH) group produces glucuronic acid. {***Yes: Aldoses that have been oxidized at carbon #6 change their names from a word ending in -ose to one ending in -uronic.***}

C. Reduction of the aldehyde group at carbon #1 produces sorbitol. {***Yes: Sorbitol is also called glucitol.***}

D. Reduction of the hydroxyl group at carbon #3 produces 3-deoxyglucose. {***Yes: Reduction of a hydroxyl group resulting in the replacement of the hydroxyl group with a hydrogen and the production of a molecule of water produces a deoxysugar.***}

✔E. Reduction of the hydroxyl group at carbon #2 produces fructose. {***No: Reduction of the hydroxyl group at carbon #2 produces 2-deoxyglucose, NOT fructose.***}

5.3. Correct answer = B

The structure shown on page 50 is

A. α-D-glucopyranose.{***No: α-D-Glucopyranose has the —OH group at carbon #1 below the plane of the ring rather than above.***}

✔B. β-D-glucopyranose.{***Yes***}

C. α-D-glucofuranose.{***No: The sugar shown has a β-structure, and has a six-membered (pyranose) ring rather than a five-membered (furanose) ring.***}

D. β-L-glucopyranose. {***No: The sugar shown is a D-sugar. β-L-Glucopyranose is its mirror image.***}

E. α-D-fructofuranose.{***No: α-D-Fructofuranose has a five-membered ring with carbon #1 (—CH_2OH) as well as with carbon #2, shown above the plane of the ring.***}

Answer	A if 1, 2, and 3 are correct	D if only 4 is correct
	B if 1 and 3 are correct	E if all are correct
	C if 2 and 4 are correct	

5.4. Correct answer = C

The disaccharide illustrated on page 50

1. contains a β(1 → 4) glycosidic bond. {***No: Although carbon #1 of the glucose molecule on the left is attached by a***

glycosidic bond to carbon #4 of the glucose molecule on the right, the bond is an α-bond.}

✓ 2. is a reducing sugar. {***Yes: The glucose residue on the right has a hydroxyl group at carbon #1 to which nothing else is attached. Therefore, the disaccharide is a reducing sugar.***}

3. contains a furanose ring. {***No: Furanose rings have five members, whereas pyranose rings have six. Therefore, both of the two component sugars of the disaccharide are pyranoses.***}

✓ 4. may undergo mutarotation. {***Yes: Any reducing sugar can undergo mutarotation.***}

5.5. Correct answer = C

D-Galactose and D-glucose are

1. enantiomers of each other. {***No: Enantiomers are mirror-images of each other.***}

✓ 2. isomers of each other. {***Yes: Galactose and glucose are isomers of each other because they have the same molecular formula.***}

3. anomers of each other. {***No: Anomers differ from each other by the position of the hydroxyl group at the anomeric carbon. For glucose and galactose, this carbon is #1.***}

✓ 4. epimers of each other. {***Yes: Epimers differ from each other only in the position of the hydroxyl and hydrogen groups at one carbon atom (other than the anomeric carbon). Glucose and galactose are C-4 epimers of each other.***}

5.6. Correct answer = C

Which of the following sugars is(are) ketose sugar(s)?

1. Galactose {***No: Galactose is an aldose sugar because it contains an aldehyde group at carbon #1.***}

✓ 2. Fructose {***Yes: Fructose is a ketose sugar because it contains a keto group at carbon #2.***}

3. Glucose {***No: Glucose is an aldose sugar.***}

✓ 4. Ribulose {***Yes: Ribulose is a ketose sugar, as are all monosaccharides whose names end in -"ulose."***}

5.7. Correct answer = B

Which of the following conditions result in the passage of undigested carbohydrate into the bowel?

✓ 1. Deficiency of intestinal lactase {***Yes: If intestinal lactase is deficient, lactose will not be digested in the small intestine and will pass into the bowel.***}

2. Deficiency of salivary α-amylase {***No: If salivary α-amylase is deficient, dietary starch will not be degraded in the mouth but will be sufficiently degraded in the small intestine by pancreatic α-amylase.***}

✓ 3. Malnutrition {***Yes: Malnutrition may result in a loss of digestive enzymes in the intestine.***}

4. Deficiency of intestinal glycogen phosphorylase {***No: Glycogen phosphorylase degrades glycogen in liver and muscle cells but is not a digestive enzyme in the gastrointestinal tract.***}

5.8. Correct answer = A

Which of the following compounds can be produced from dietary starch by salivary α-amylase?

✓ 1. Maltose {***Yes: Maltose, a disaccharide containing two glucose molecules in an α(1 → 4) linkage, is produced from dietary starch by salivary α-amylase.***}

✓ 2. Starch dextrins {***Yes: Starch dextrins, which are partial digestion products of dietary starch, are produced by salivary α-amylase.***}

✓ 3. Isomaltose {***Yes: Isomaltose, a disaccharide containing glucose in an α(1 → 6) linkage, is produced from dietary starch by salivary α-amylase.***}

4. Fructose {***No: Fructose is produced from dietary sucrose in the small intestine by sucrase.***}

5.9. Correct answer = B

Which of the following statements about human disaccharidases is(are) correct?

✓ 1. The disaccharidases are produced and secreted by the intestinal mucosal cells. {***Yes.***}

2. A specific intestinal disaccharidase cleaves β(1 → 4) glycosidic bonds. (***No: Human digestive enzymes cannot cleave β(1 → 4) glycosidic bonds.***}

✓ 3. The monosaccharides produced by the disaccharidases pass into the portal circulation. {***Yes.***}

4. Deficiency of a specific disaccharidase has little effect on an individual's ability to digest dietary carbohydrates. {***No: Deficiency of a specific disaccharidase results in a disaccharide passing into the large intestine undigested. Bacteria in the large intestine ferment the disaccharides, resulting in bloating, dehydration, and diarrhea.***}

Chapter 6: METABOLISM OF MONOSACCHARIDES AND DISACCHARIDES

Choose the ONE best answer:

6.1. Correct answer = B

In liver, the initial step in the utilization of fructose is its phosphorylation to fructose 1-phosphate. This is followed by

A. phosphorylation to fructose 1,6-bisphosphate. {***No: Fructose 1-phosphate cannot be phosphorylated to fructose 1,6-bisphosphate in humans.***}

✓ B. cleavage of fructose 1-phosphate to form glyceraldehyde and dihydroxyacetone phosphate. {***Yes: Fructose***

1-phosphate is cleaved by aldolase B to form glyceraldehyde and dihydroxyacetone phosphate.}

C. conversion to fructose 6-phosphate by action of a phosphofructomutase. {***No: Phosphoglucose isomerase converts glucose 6-phosphate to fructose 6-phosphate.***}

D. isomerization to glucose 1-phosphate. {***No: Isomerization of fructose 1-phosphate to glucose 1-phosphate does not occur in humans.***}

E. hydrolysis to fructose followed by isomerization to glucose. {***No: Fructose 1-phosphate is not hydrolyzed to fructose in humans.***}

6.2. Correct answer = A

An individual with fructose intolerance

✓A. cannot use fructose effectively in glycolysis because of a deficiency in liver fructose 1-phosphate aldolase. {***Yes: In fructose intolerance, aldolase B (fructose 1-phosphate aldolase) is deficient, and therefore, although fructose can be phosphorylated by fructokinase, the resulting fructose 1-phosphate cannot be further metabolized.***}

B. cannot produce glucose from fructose 6-phosphate. {***No: The production of glucose from fructose 6-phosphate (in gluconeogenesis) is not affected by aldolase B deficiency.***}

C. cannot convert fructose to fructose 1-phosphate. {***No: Fructokinase is not affected in an individual with fructose intolerance.***}

D. cannot convert fructose 6-phosphate into fructose 1,6-bisphosphate. {***No: Phosphofructokinase is not affected in an individual with fructose intolerance.***}

E. cannot produce lactic acid from fructose 6-phosphate. {***No: The enzymes of glycolysis that convert fructose 6-phosphate to lactic acid are not deficient in an individual with fructose intolerance.***}

6.3 Correct answer = B

Fructosuria is the result of

A. a deficiency of phosphofructokinase. {***No: Phosphofructokinase converts fructose 6-phosphate to fructose 1,6-bisphosphate.***}

✓B. a deficiency of liver fructokinase. {***Yes: Fructokinase, which converts fructose to fructose 1-phosphate, is deficient in individuals with fructosuria.***}

C. elevated levels of liver aldolase B. {***No: Aldolase B is deficient in fructose intolerance (fructose poisoning.***}

D. a deficiency of liver hexokinase. {***No: Hexokinase phosphorylates glucose to glucose 6-phosphate.***}

E. elevated levels of liver fructose 1,6-bisphosphatase. {***No: Fructose 1,6-bisphosphatase converts fructose 1,6-bisphosphate to fructose 6-phosphate during gluconeogenesis.***}

6.4. Correct answer = B

A galactosemic female can produce lactose because

A. free (nonphosphorylated) galactose is the acceptor of glucose transferred by lactose synthase in the synthesis of lactose. {***No: UDP-Galactose, not free galactose, is the source of the galactose portion of lactose.***}

✓B. she is able to produce galactose from a glucose metabolite by epimerization. {***Yes: UDP-Hexose 4-epimerase converts UDP-glucose to UDP-galactose, thus providing the appropriate form of galactose for lactose synthesis.***}

C. hexokinase can efficiently phosphorylate dietary galactose to galactose 1-phosphate. {***No: Galactose is not converted to galactose 1-phosphate by hexokinase.***}

D. the enzyme deficient in galactosemia is activated by a hormone produced in the mammary gland. {***No: A mammary gland hormone does not play a role in activating the enzyme deficient in galactosemia—galactose 1-phosphate uridyl transferase.***}

E. she is able to produce galactose from fructose by isomerization. {***No: Isomerization of fructose to galactose does not occur in the human body.***}

6.5. Correct answer = D

Which one of the following compounds is NOT involved as an intermediate in the metabolic conversion of dietary galactose into blood glucose?

A. UDP-glucose {***Is involved: Dietary galactose is converted to UDP-galactose in a two-step pathway described below in choice "B." UDP-galactose is converted to UDP-glucose by UDP-hexose 4-epimerase. UDP-glucose serves as a substrate for the synthesis of glycogen, which is subsequently degraded, releasing free glucose.***}

B. UDP-galactose {***Is involved: Dietary galactose is first phosphorylated to galactose 1-phosphate and then converted to UDP-galactose. This compound is metabolized as described above in choice "A" to produce glucose.***}

C. Glucose 6-phosphate {***Is involved: Dietary galactose is converted to glucose units found in glycogen as described in the choices above. Degradation of glycogen releases glucose 1-phosphate, which is converted to glucose 6-phosphate by phosphofructomutase. The phosphate group is removed by glucose 6-phosphatase, releasing free glucose.***}

✓D. Galactose 6-phosphate {***Is not involved: Galactose 6-phosphate does not enter the pathways of intermediary metabolism that produce glucose.***}

E. Glycogen {***Is involved: As described in the choices above.***}

6.6. Correct answer = D

Which of the following statements is true for a mature woman with galactosemia?

A. She can use both hexoses arising from dietary lactose as energy sources. {***No: She can use the glucose, but not the galactose, produced by the hydrolysis of lactate.***}

B. She cannot produce lactose in her mammary glands. {***No: She can produce the necessary UDP-galactose building block of lactose from UDP-glucose by using the enzyme UDP-hexose 4-epimerase.***}

C. She will show a marked decrease in ability to synthesize galactosyl-containing carbohydrates when on a galactose-free diet. {***No: The UDP-galactose needed to produce galactosyl-containing carbohydrates can be supplied as described in choice "B" above.***}

✔D. When consuming a diet that contains galactose, she will accumulate both galactose 1-phosphate and galactitol in various tissues. {***Yes: Because she is missing galactose 1-phosphate uridyltransferase, she will be unable to convert galactose 1-phosphate to UDP-galactose. Therefore, galactose 1-phosphate will accumulate, causing galactose also to accumulate (since the major pathway for galactose metabolism requires its conversion to galactose 1-phosphate). Thus side-pathways, such as the conversion of galactose to galactitol, will occur.***}

E. She will not be able to convert glucose into UDP-galactose. {***No: She will be able to convert glucose into UDP-galactose as described in choice "B" above.***}

6.7. Correct answer = C

A hereditary childhood disease, galactosemia, is characterized by a

A. high level of liver UDP-galactose. {***No: The enzyme producing UDP-galactose from galactose 1-phosphate is missing. Therefore, the body produces only as much as it requires through the UDP-hexose 4-epimerase reaction.***}

B. lack of glucose 1-phosphate. {***No: Glucose 1-phosphate is synthesized from glucose 6-phosphate by phosphoglucomutase.***}

✔C. very low galactose 1-phosphate uridyltransferase activity in liver. {***Yes: This is the enzyme deficient in the major form of galactosemia.***}

D. lack of galactokinase. {***No: This enzyme phosphorylates dietary galactose, producing galactose 1-phosphate.***}

E. lack of UDP-hexose 4-epimerase. {***No: This enzyme interconverts UDP-glucose and UDP-galactose, and is used both to provide an alternative source of UDP-galactose and to allow excess dietary galactose (in an individual without galactosemia) to enter the pathways of intermediary metabolism.***}

6.8. Correct answer = E

N-Acetylneuraminic acid arises biologically from the condensation of which one of the following pairs of compounds?

A. Erythrose and N-acetylxylosamine {***No***}

B. Erythrose and N-acetylribosamine {***No***}

C. Pyruvate and N-acetylglucosamine {***No***}

D. Glyceraldehyde 3-phosphate and N-acetylglucosamine {***No***}

✔E. Phosphoenolpyruvate and N-acetylmannosamine {***Yes***}

6.9. Correct answer = C

Which one of the following statements about an individual with hereditary pentosuria is INCORRECT?

A. Dietary xylitol can be metabolized by the liver. {***Correct statement: The step in which hereditary pentosuria is blocked occurs before the entry of xylitol into the glucuronic acid pathway. Therefore, the liver can metabolize dietary xylitol.***}

B. Most dietary glucuronic acid will be converted to pentoses, which will be found in the urine. {***Correct statement: Glucuronic acid will be converted to L-xylulose by the reactions of the uronic acid pathway. In hereditary pentosuria, L-xylulose cannot be further metabolized, and therefore large amounts of this pentose may appear in the urine, for example, after glucuronic acid ingestion.***}

✔C. The patient will be unable to synthesize inositol and will require it in the diet. {***Incorrect statement: The glucuronic acid pathway does not synthesize inositol, although dietary inositol does serve as a precursor for the synthesis of glucuronic acid. Therefore, a defect in that pathway (such as that causing hereditary pentosuria) will not affect inositol synthesis.***}

D. The patient's ability to synthesize glucuronylated bilirubin will not be impaired. {***Correct statement: A sufficient supply of UDP-glucuronic acid needed for the glucuronylation of bilirubin can be provided by the oxidation of UDP-glucose.***}

E. A normal supply of ribose required for the biosynthesis of nucleic acids will be provided via the hexose monophosphate pathway. {***Correct statement: Under normal conditions, the intermediates of the glycolytic pathway are the major source of carbons for synthesis of ribose 5-phosphate.***}

6.10. Correct answer = A

Biosynthesis of glucuronic acid requires the

✔A. oxidation of UDP-glucose. {***Yes: UDP-glucose is oxidized at carbon #6 (—CH_2OH) to produce UDP-glucuronic acid (—COOH).***}

B. oxidation of glucose 6-phosphate. {***No***}

C. oxidation of 6-phosphogluconate. {***No***}

D. oxidation of glucose. {***No***}

E. reduction of sorbitol. {***No***}

6.11. Correct answer = B

A major contributing factor to cataract formation in diabetes may be the accumulation of sorbitol in the lens. For that to occur, glucose has to interact with

A. glucose oxidase. {***No: Glucose oxidase converts glucose, in the presence of molecular oxygen, to gluconolactone plus H_2O_2 (peroxide).***}

✔B. NADPH-dependent aldose reductase. {***Yes: This enzyme reduces glucose, forming sorbitol (glucitol).***}

C. glucokinase. {***No: Glucokinase phosphorylates glucose to glucose 6-phosphate.***}

D. hexokinase and glucose 6-phosphate dehydrogenase. {***No: These two sequential reactions provide an entrance for glucose into the hexose monophosphate pathway.***}

E. hexokinase and phosphoglucoisomerase. {***No: These two sequential reactions result in the production of glucose 1-phosphate—a precursor of UDP-glucose.***}

6.12. Correct answer = B

In lactose biosynthesis, an immediate precursor for lactose is

A. UDP-glucose. {***No: Glucose is a precursor of lactose.***}

✔B. UDP-galactose. {***Yes***}

C. galactose 1-phosphate. {***No: Galactose 1-phosphate is the immediate precursor of UDP-galactose.***}

D. glucose 1-phosphate. {***No: Glucose 1-phosphate is the immediate precursor of UDP-glucose.***}

E. galactose. {***No: Galactose is the immediate precursor of galactose 1-phosphate.***}

6.13 Correct answer = E

No lactose is metabolized after its intravenous injection into a rat; however ingestion of lactose leads to rapid metabolism of galactose. The difference in these results is due to

A. the absence of lactase in the serum. {***Yes: Lactase is an intestinal enzyme. Therefore, lactose is not degraded in the serum and cannot be utilized by the cells.***}

B. the absence of hepatic galactokinase. {***No: If hepatic galactokinase is absent, the galactose segment of the lactose will not be metabolized. However, the glucose segment of the lactose will be metabolized, and therefore 50% of the component monosaccharides of lactose will contribute to the overall body's metabolism.***}

C. the presence of maltase in the serum. {***No: Maltase, which degrades the disaccharide maltose, is an intestinal enzyme.***}

D. the presence of lactase in the intestine. {***Yes: Ingested lactose will be degraded by the intestinal enzyme lactase.***}

✔ E. a combination of A and D above. {***Correct answer: Ingested lactose is degraded; injected lactose is not.***}

6.14 Correct answer = E

Which one of the following statements is NOT correct about lactose?

A. It can undergo mutarotation. {***Correct: Carbon #1 of the glucose moiety of lactose is not attached to another compound. Therefore, it is a reducing sugar and can undergo mutarotation.***}

B. It is a reducing sugar. {***Correct: See choice "A."***}

C. It is hydrolyzed by β-galactosidase to glucose and galactose. {***Correct: β-Galactosidase (lactase) is an intestinal enzyme that digests lactose, hydrolytically producing galactose and glucose.***}

D. It is synthesized in the mammary gland by galactosyl transferase. {***Correct: Lactose is synthesized in the lactating mammary gland from UDP-galactose and glucose.***}

✔ E. It can be converted into sucrose by epimerization of its galactose residue, so that the two disaccharides are freely interchangeable. {***Incorrect: Sucrose is synthesized from glucose and fructose; lactose and sucrose are not interconvertable.***}

Questions 6.15–6.17:

For each of the disaccharides listed below, choose the monosaccharides of which it is composed:

A. Fructose only

B. Glucose only

C. Glucose and fructose

D. Glucose and galactose

E. Fructose and galactose

6.15. Sucrose {***Correct answer = C***}

6.16. Lactose {***Correct answer = D***}

6.17. Maltose {***Correct answer = B***}

Chapter 7: GLYCOGEN METABOLISM

Choose the ONE best answer:

7.1. Correct answer = E

An abnormal, poorly branched glycogen was isolated from the liver of a patient with type IV glycogen storage disease. The deficiency is most probably in

A. phosphorylase kinase. {***No: Phosphorylase kinase activates glycogen phosphorylase by transferring a phosphate group from ATP to the enzyme. A deficiency of phosphorylase kinase would therefore result in an overall decrease in glycogen degradation.***}

B. glycogen phosphorylase a. {***No: Glycogen phosphorylase a is the active form of glycogen phosphorylase. A deficiency in this enzyme would result in an overall decrease in glycogen degradation.***}

C. protein kinase. {***No: Protein kinase activates the cascade of enzymes that results in the activation of glycogen degradation. A deficiency in protein kinase activity would prevent the activation of the entire glycogen degradation pathway.***}

D. amylo-α-(1,6)-glucosidase. {***No: This enzyme removes single glucosyl residues attached to the glycogen chain through an α-1 → 6 glycosidic bond. A deficiency in this enzyme would result in a decreased ability of the cell to degrade glycogen branches.***}

✔ E. amylo-α-(1,4),(1,6)-transglycosylase. {***Yes: This enzyme transfers a chain of 5 to 8 glucosyl residues from the nonreducing end of the glycogen chain to another location on the chain, attaching the 5 to 8 glucosyl residue chain by an α-1 → 6 glycosidic linkage. If there is a deficiency of this enzymatic activity, fewer than normal branches are made.***}

7.2. Correct answer = B

Epinephrine and glucagon have the following effects on glycogen metabolism in the liver:

A. The net synthesis of glycogen is increased. {***No: The net synthesis of glycogen is decreased.***}

✔ B. Glycogen phosphorylase is activated, whereas glycogen synthetase is inactivated. {***Yes: A cascade of enzymes are activated that result in the degradation of glycogen and a decrease in glycogen synthesis.***}

C. Both glycogen phosphorylase and glycogen synthase are activated but at markedly different rates. {***No: Glycogen phosphorylase is activated, whereas glycogen synthase activity is decreased.***}

D. Glycogen phosphorylase is inactivated, whereas glycogen synthase is activated. {***No: See choice "C."***}

E. Cyclic AMP-dependent protein kinase is activated, while phosphorylase kinase is inactivated. {***No: Activation of protein kinase results in the activation of phosphorylase kinase.***}

7.3. Correct answer = D

In the muscle, a sudden elevation of the Ca^{++} concentration will cause

A. activation of cyclic AMP-dependent protein kinase. {***No: This enzyme is activated only by cAMP.***}

B. dissociation of cyclic AMP-dependent protein kinase into catalytic and regulatory subunits. {***No: Dissociation of protein kinase into its catalytic and regulatory subunits occurs in the absence of cAMP.***}

C. inactivation of phosphorylase kinase owing to the action of a protein phosphatase. {***No: Phosphorylation kinase is activated by*** Ca^{++}.}

✓D. conversion of glycogen phosphorylase b to phosphorylase a. {***Yes: An elevated*** Ca^{++} ***concentration results in the activation of phosphorylase kinase. Phosphorylase kinase converts glycogen phosphorylase b to its active form, phosphorylase a.***}

E. conversion of cyclic AMP to AMP by phosphodiesterase. {***No: Elevated*** Ca^{++} ***does not stimulate the activity of phosphodiesterase.***}

7.4. Correct answer = B

Muscle glycogen cannot contribute directly to blood glucose levels because

A. muscle glycogen cannot be converted to glucose 6-phosphate. {***No: When muscle glycogen is degraded, glucose 1-phosphate is produced, which is then converted to glucose 6-phosphate by phosphoglucomutase.***}

✓B. muscle lacks glucose 6-phosphate phosphatase. {***Yes: This enzyme, which converts glucose 6-phosphate to glucose, is present in the liver but not in the muscle. Therefore, because glucose 6-phosphate cannot cross cell membranes, the major product of muscle glycogen degradation is not able to contribute to blood glucose levels.***}

C. muscle contains no glucokinase. {***No: In the liver, glucokinase converts glucose to glucose 6-phosphate, thus trapping glucose in its phosphorylated form inside the cell. Muscle contains no glucokinase.***}

D. muscle contains no glycogen phosphorylase. {***No: Both liver and muscle contain glycogen phosphorylase, a necessary enzyme for glycogen degradation.***}

E. muscle lacks phosphoglucoisomerase. {***No: Phosphoglucoisomerase is necessary for the interconversion of glucose 6-phosphate and fructose 6-phosphate in the glycolytic pathway.***}

7.5. Correct answer = A

In the liver, a significant increase in the activities of protein phosphatase(s) that act on the enzymes responsible for glycogen synthesis and degradation will most probably lead to

✓A. increased rate of glycogen synthesis and decreased rate of degradation. {***Yes: Protein phosphatases result in the inactivation of glycogen phosphorylase and activation of glycogen synthase.***}

B. decreased rate of glycogen synthesis and increased rate of degradation. {***No: See answer to choice "A."***}

C. increased rate of glycogen synthesis and increased rate of degradation. {***No: See answer to choice "A."***}

D. decreased rate of glycogen synthesis and decreased rate of degradation. {***No: See answer to choice "A".***}

E. no net change in the rates of either synthesis or degradation of glycogen. {***No: See answer to choice "A."***}

7.6. Correct answer = A

How does 3′,5′-cyclic AMP increase the rate of glycogenolysis?

✓A. It promotes the formation of a phosphorylated form of glycogen phosphorylase. {***Yes: Cyclic AMP activates the cascade of reactions that results in increased glycogen phosphorylase activity.***}

B. It serves as a cofactor for glycogen phosphorylase. {***No: It serves as an activator of protein kinase.***}

C. It serves as a precursor of 5′-AMP, which is a cofactor for glycogen phosphorylase. {***No: Cyclic AMP is converted to 5′-AMP by the enzyme phosphodiesterase. 5′-AMP is not a cofactor for glycogen phosphorylase.***}

D. It furnishes phosphate for the phosphorolysis of glycogen. {***No: It is necessary for only small amounts of cyclic AMP to be synthesized for the activation of the glycogen degradative pathway.***}

E. It serves as a potential source of ATP. {***No: Cyclic AMP must first be converted to AMP, which can then, at the expense of an additional ATP, be converted to ADP. The ADP can be phosphorylated by substrate level or oxidative phosphorylation to ATP. Energy is thus required for the reconversion of AMP to ATP.***}

7.7. Correct answer = D

Which of the following conditions would exist in a mutant tissue culture line derived from ***liver*** that is unable to synthesize 3′,5′-cyclic AMP?.

A. An abnormally low cellular content of glycogen {***No: A liver cell unable to synthesize 3′,5′-cyclic AMP would have a decreased ability to degrade glycogen.***}

B. A high phosphorylase a/phosphorylase b ratio {***No: The synthesis of 3′,5′-cyclic AMP in the liver is required for the conversion of phosphorylase b to phosphorylase a.***}

C. An increased level of protein kinase activity after incubating the cells with glucagon {***No: Incubation of these mutant liver cells with glucagon would not increase 3′,5′-cyclic AMP (as it would in normal cells). Therefore, protein kinase activity would not be stimulated.***}

✓D. Little effect of glucose 6-phosphate on the activity of glycogen synthase {***Yes: In the absence of 3′,5′-cyclic AMP, glycogen synthase will be in the I (active) form. Glucose***

6-phosphate affects the activity of the normally inactive (D) form of glycogen synthase.}

E. Increased phosphodiesterase activity {***No: Phosphodiesterase converts 3′,5′-cyclic AMP to AMP.***}

7.8. Correct answer = E

The laboratory report on a patient with glycogen storage disease was as follows: fasting blood glucose, 45 mg/dl; blood glucose after epinephrine infusion, 41 mg/dl; blood glucose after oral fructose administration, 95 mg/dl; blood lactate in the resting condition, 18 mg/dl; blood lactate after exercise, 39 mg/dl. Glycogen from both liver and muscle was structurally normal. The laboratory results suggest an absence of

A. liver and muscle α-1,6 glucosidase. {***No: If this enzyme were absent, the structure of both liver and muscle glycogen would be abnormal.***}

B. liver glycogen synthase. {***No: An absence of glycogen synthase would result in a lack of glycogen in the liver.***}

C. muscle phosphorylase. {***No: If this enzyme were absent, exercise would not result in an increase of blood lactate, since the muscle glycogen could not be degraded to produce glucose 6-phosphate, the precursor for anaerobic glycolysis.***}

D. liver fructokinase. {***No: If this enzyme were absent, oral fructose would not contribute to blood glucose levels.***}

✓E. liver glucose 6-phosphatase. {***Yes: In this patient, epinephrine infusion does not result in an increase in blood glucose levels, yet liver glycogen is structurally normal. Therefore, the glycogen is degraded to glucose-phosphate units but cannot be dephosphorylated, releasing free glucose to the blood.***}

Chapter 8: GLYCOSAMINOGLYCANS

Choose the ONE best answer:

8.1. Correct answer = C

Mucopolysaccharidoses are inherited storage diseases. They are caused by

A. an increased rate of synthesis of proteoglycans. {***No: In mucopolysaccharidoses, synthesis of proteoglycans is unaffected.***}

B. the synthesis of polysaccharides with an altered structure. {***No: Synthesis is unaffected.***}

✓C. defects in the degradation of proteoglycans. {***Yes: Mucopolysaccharidoses are caused by a deficiency of one of the lysosomal, hydrolytic enzymes responsible for the degradation of glycosaminoglycans.***}

D. the synthesis of abnormally small amounts of protein cores. {***No: Synthesis of the protein cores to which the carbohydrate chains are attached in the glycosaminoglycan structure is not affected in mucopolysaccharidoses.***}

E. an insufficient amount of proteolytic enzymes. {***No: Lysosomal degradation of the core protein of glycosaminoglycans is not affected in mucopolysaccharidoses.***}

8.2. Correct answer = E

Mucopolysaccharidoses are a family of diseases characterized by each of the following EXCEPT

A. elevated urinary excretion of oligosaccharides containing glucuronic acid. {***Yes: Polysaccharides are not excreted.***}

B. elevated urinary excretion of oligosaccharides containing hexosamine. {***Yes: Polysaccharides are not excreted.***}

C. tissue accumulation of glycosaminoglycans. {***Yes: Because there is a deficiency in the enzymes required for the degradation of glycosaminoglycans, these compounds accumulate in the tissues.***}

D. deficiency in lysosomal enzymes. {***Yes: Mucopolysaccharidoses are caused by a deficiency in lysosomal enzymes.***}

✓E. elevated urinary excretion of hyaluronic acid. {***No: Polysaccharides such as hyaluronic acid are not excreted.***}

Questions 8.3–8.6 refer to the structure shown on page 89.

8.3. Correct answer = D

The polymeric substance shown above belongs to a group of compounds known as

A. amylose. {***No: Amylose is an unbranched polysaccharide composed of glucose that is found in plants.***}

B. amylopectin. {***No: Amylopectin is a branched polysaccharide composed of glucose that is found in plants.***}

C. glycogen. {***No: Glycogen is highly branched polysaccharide composed of glucose that is found in mammalian muscle and liver.***}

✓D. proteoglycan. {***Yes: The structure shown is the repeating disaccharide unit of hyaluronic acid.***}

E. keratin. {***No: Keratin is a structural protein.***}

8.4. Correct answer = B

The substance shown on page 89 is

A. lactose. {***No: Lactose is a disaccharide composed of galactose and glucose.***}

✓B. hyaluronic acid. {***Yes: Hyaluronic acid is a glycosaminoglycan composed of alternating residues of glucuronic acid and N-acetylglucosamine.***}

C. heparin. {***No: Heparin is a glycosaminoglycan composed of sulfated glucuronic acid and glucosamine.***}

D. N-acetylneuraminic acid. {***No: N-Acetylneuraminic acid (NANA) is a monosaccharide component of glycoproteins.***}

E. sucrose. {***No: Sucrose is a disaccharide composed of glucose and fructose.***}

8.5. Correct answer = E

The component monosaccharides shown above are

A. gluconic acid and N-acetyl glucosamine. {***No: Gluconic acid has a —COOH group at carbon #1.***}

B. N-acetyl glucosamine and N-acetylneuraminic acid. {***No: N-Acetylneuraminic acid is a nine-carbon monosaccharide with a carboxyl group.***}

C. glucuronic acid and N-acetylneuraminic acid. {***No: See choice "B."***}

D. gluconic acid and N-acetylneuraminic acid. {***No: See choices "A" and "B."***}

✓E. glucuronic acid and N-acetylglucosamine. {***Yes***}

8.6. Correct answer = B

This compound is of particular functional importance in

A. blood clotting. {***No: The glycosaminoglycan heparin is of particular functional importance in blood clotting.***}

✓B. synovial fluid. {***Yes: Hyaluronic acid is an important component of synovial fluid, the vitreous humor of the eye, and the umbilical cord.***}

C. liver cells. {***No.***}

D. mast cells. {***No: The glycosaminoglycan heparin is found in mast cells.***}

E. skin. {***No: The glycosaminoglycans dermatan sulfate and heparin are found in significant amounts in skin.***}

8.7. Correct answer = C

The predominant proteoglycan in cartilage is

A. keratin sulfate. {***No: Keratin sulfate is found in cartilage proteoglycan (in smaller amounts than chondroitin sulfate), cornea, and bone.***}

B. dermatan sulfate. {***No: Dermatan sulfate is found predominantly in skin, blood vessels, and heart valves.***}

✓C. chondroitin sulfate. {***Yes: Chondroitin sulfate, the most abundant glycosaminoglycan in the body, is found in cartilage, bone, and heart valves.***}

D. heparan sulfate. {***No: Heparan sulfate is found in basement membrane and as a component of cell surface.***}

E. heparin. {***No: Heparin is an intracellular component of mast cells.***}

Answer	A if 1, 2, and 3 are correct	D if only 4 is correct
	B if 1 and 3 are correct	E if all are correct
	C if 2 and 4 are correct	

8.8. Correct answer = E

Which of the following statements about proteoglycans is(are) CORRECT?

✓1. In proteoglycans, a carbohydrate chain is linked to a protein through a unique linkage region that contains xylosyl and galactosyl residues. {***Yes.***}

✓2. Proteoglycans are generally composed of a disaccharide repeating unit containing an acidic and an amino sugar. {***Yes.***}

✓3. The iduronic acid of dermatan sulfate is synthesized by an epimerase that acts on a glucuronic acid residue in the polysaccharide. {***Yes.***}

✓4. Sulfation of the proteoglycan occurs after monosaccharides have already been incorporated into the carbohydrate chain. {***Yes.***}

Chapter 9: GLYCOPROTEINS

Choose the ONE best answer:

9.1. Correct answer = B

The presence of the following compound in the urine of a patient suggests a deficiency in which one of the enzymes listed below?

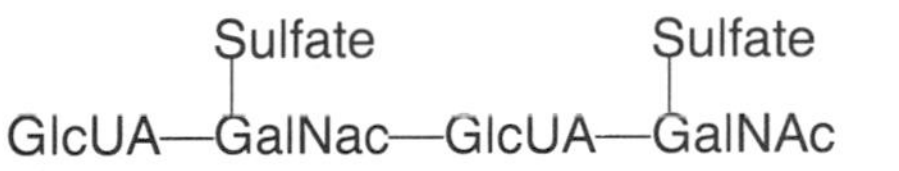

A. Galactosidase {***No: Degradation of glycoproteins follows the rule "last on, first off." Therefore, since sulfation occurs among the last steps in the synthesis of a glycoprotein, a sulfatase is the enzyme required for the next step in the degradation of the above compound.***}

✓B. Sulfatase {***Yes.***}

C. Glucuronidase {***No: Although after the sulfatase, a glucuronidase is the next enzyme required***}

D. Mannosidase {***No: There is no mannose in the above structure.***}

E. Glucosidase {***No: There is no glucose in the above structure.***}

9.2. Correct answer = D

Which one of the following is NOT a common feature of the carbohydrate structure in N-linked and O-linked glycoproteins?

A. They may contain N-acetylneuraminic acid. {***Yes.***}

B. They may contain glucose. {***Yes.***}

C. Their degradation *in vivo* involves action of lysosomal enzymes. {***Yes.***}

✓D. Their synthesis involves participation of a lipid carrier. {***No: Only synthesis of the N-linked glycoproteins requires the lipid carrier dolichol.***}

E. They are synthesized in the endoplasmic reticulum and the Golgi apparatus. {***Yes.***}

9.3. Correct answer = A

The synthesis of the carbohydrate portion of glycoproteins

✓A. is catalyzed by specific enzymes, each of which synthesizes a specific glycosidic bond in a determined sequence. {***Yes: Glycoproteins are synthesized by the sequential addition of monosaccharides at the nonreducing ends of the growing carbohydrate chains.***}

B. is a process catalyzed by the action of specific glycosidic hydrolases present in most cells. {***No: Hydrolases degrade glycoproteins.***}

C. is usually initiated by the addition of N-acetylneuraminic acid. {***No: N-Acetylneuraminic acid (and fucose) are added at the ends of chains.***}

D. is initiated at a glutamine or methionine residue on the protein. {***No: The carbohydrate chains of glycoproteins are attached at serine or threonine residues ("O-linked") or at asparagine residues ("N-linked").***}

E. produces an oligosaccharide with a reducing end belonging to the last monosaccharide added. {***No: The last monosaccharide added has a nonreducing end.***}

Chapter 10: BIOENERGETICS AND OXIDATIVE PHOSPHORYLATION

Choose the ONE best answer:

10.1. Correct answer = B

The free energy change, ΔG,

A. is directly proportional to the standard free energy change, ΔG°. {***No: The free energy change is proportional to the sum of the standard free energy change plus RTln([P]/[S]), where R is the gas constant, T is the absolute temperature, [P] is the product of the concentrations of all products of the reaction, and [S] is the product of the concentrations of all substrates of the reaction.***}

✓B. is equal to zero at equilibrium. {***Yes.***}

C. can be calculated only when the reactants and products are present at 1 M concentrations. {***No: The free energy change can be calculated at any concentrations of substrates and products except 0. When all substrates and products are at 1 M concentrations (which is defined as being under standard conditions), the free energy change is equal to the standard free energy change.***}

D. will indicate the rate and direction of the reaction, if you also know the standard free energy change and the concentrations of products and reactants. {***No: The free energy change of a reaction does not indicate the rate at which the reaction will go.***}

E. is equal to $-RT \ln K_{eq}$. {***No: This is the equation for the standard free energy change.***}

10.2. Correct answer = C

Under standard conditions (i.e., where all substrates and products are present at 1 M concentrations),

A. the free energy change, ΔG, is equal to 0. {***No: Under standard conditions, the free energy change, ΔG, is equal to the standard free energy change, ΔG°.***}

B. the standard free energy change, ΔG°, is equal to 0. {***No: Because it is a constant, the standard free energy change is not influenced by concentrations of substrates and products.***}

✓C. the free energy change, ΔG, is equal to the standard free energy change, ΔG°. {***Yes.***}

D. K_{eq} is equal to 1. {***No: Because the K_{eq} is a constant, it is not influenced by the concentrations of substrate and product.***}

E. K_{eq} is equal to 0. {***No: K_{eq} cannot be equal to 0 since it represents the ratio between the concentrations of products and substrates at equilibrium.***}

10.3. Correct answer = A

Consider the following reaction:

Fructose 6-P + P_i → fructose 1,6-bisphosphate + H_2O

This reaction has an equilibrium constant (K_{eq}) of 0.001 at pH 7, where T = 25°C = 298°K, R = 1.98 cal/mole degree. (The ln of a number is equal to 2.303 log of the number.)

The standard free energy change, ΔG°, for this reaction is equal to approximately

✓A. +4.0 kcal/mole. {***Yes: $\Delta G° = -(1.98)(298)(2.3 \log 10^{-3})$.***}

B. −4.0 kcal/mole.

C. +2.0 kcal/mole.

D. −2.0 kcal/mole.

E. none of the above.

10.4. Correct answer = D

The complete oxidation of 1 mole of glucose results in the release of about 700,000 calories of free energy. If this process is coupled to ATP biosynthesis from ADP + P_i with approximately 40% efficiency, the number of moles of ATP that could be produced would be approximately

A. 2.

B. 7.

C. 20.

✓D. 40. {***Yes: If 40% of 700,000 cal of free energy are coupled to ATP synthesis (i.e., a total of 280,000 cal) and approximately 7000 cal are required to convert a molecule of ADP to ATP, then 280,000/7000 = 40 ATP can be produced from the complete oxidation of 1 mole of glucose.***}

E. 100

10.5. Correct answer = C

Under physiologic conditions, each of the following contains a high-energy phosphate group EXCEPT

A. ATP. {***Contains two high-energy phosphate groups***}

B. ADP. {***Contains one high-energy phosphate group***}

✓C. AMP. {***Correct choice: Contains no high-energy phosphate groups***}

D. phosphoenolpyruvate. {***Contains one high-energy phosphate group and is found in the glycolytic pathway***}

E. phosphocreatine. {***Contains one high-energy phosphate group and is found in the muscle, where it serves as a source of energy during muscle contraction***}

Answer A if 1, 2, and 3 are correct
B if 1 and 3 are correct
C if 2 and 4 are correct
D if only 4 is correct
E if all are correct

10.6. Correct answer = D

Given the following sequence of reactions where the components A through D are present at steady-state concentrations and where X is present in an inexhaustible reservoir,

X →A ↔ B ↔ C ↔ D → products

Which of the following statements about that pathway is(are) correct?

1. If the observed concentration ratio of [B]/[A] equals the equilibrium constant for the reaction A↔B, the overall pathway would be at equilibrium and no products would be made. {**No: Even if one reaction in the pathway is at or near equilibrium, the other reactions may be far from equilibrium, and products could be made.**}
2. None of the individual reactions could be rate-limiting unless its ΔG° was equal to zero. {**No: Any reaction in the pathway may be rate-limiting regardless of the value of its ΔG°.**}
3. The reactant A could not be converted to D unless the sum of all of the ΔG° values for the individual reactions of A to D is negative. {**No: As long as the overall value of ΔG (the free energy change) for the pathway is negative, A can be converted to D. Individual reactions may or may not have a positive ΔG° value.**}
4. ✔ The ΔG° for the conversion of A to D is equal to the sum of the ΔG° values for each individual reaction. {**Yes: Standard free energy changes (ΔG°) for sequential steps in a reaction pathway are additive.**}

Choose the ONE best answer:

10.7. Correct answer = B

An uncoupler of oxidative phosphorylation such as dinitrophenol

A. inhibits respiration and ATP synthesis. {**No: Uncouplers inhibit ATP synthesis while allowing respiration (i.e., operation of the electron transport chain) to continue.**}

✔ B. allows electron transport to proceed without ATP synthesis. {**Yes: See answer to choice A above.**}

C. inhibits respiration without impairment of ATP synthesis. {**No: The opposite is true.**}

D. specifically inhibits cytochrome b. {**No: Uncouplers are not site-specific inhibitors.**}

E. acts as a competitive inhibitor of NAD^+-requiring reactions in the mitochondrion. {**No: Uncouplers are not competitive inhibitors.**}

10.8. Correct answer = A

In an intact mitochondrial suspension, rotenone or amytal inhibits the one-step oxidation of malate to oxaloacetate but not that of succinate to fumarate. The reason why these two agents have this discriminatory effect is because they

✔ A. restrict the flow of electrons between NADH and coenzyme Q. {**Yes: By preventing the oxidation of NADH to NAD^+, insufficient NAD^+ will be available to participate as a cosubstrate in the oxidation of malate to oxaloacetate, and the reaction will be unable to proceed. In the oxidation of succinate to fumarate, $FADH_2$ is produced, which donates its electrons to the electron transport chain at a point after the rotenone or amytal block. Therefore, $FADH_2$-producing reactions are unaffected by these inhibitors.**}

B. prevent mitochondria from accumulating calcium. {**No**}

C. inhibit the ATP synthesizing complex. {**No: An example of an inhibitor of the ATP synthesizing complex is oligomycin.**}

D. compete with ATP in substrate level phosphorylation reactions. {**No**}

E. make the inner mitochondrial membrane permeable to protons. {**No: Uncouplers such as dinitrophenol cause such permeability.**}

10.9. Correct answer = E

Which one of the statements listed below about the enzymic complex that carries out the synthesis of ATP during oxidative phosphorylation is INCORRECT?

A. It is located on the matrix side of the inner mitochondrial membrane. {**Correct**}

B. It is inhibited by oligomycin. {**Correct: Oligomycin inhibits the dissolution of the proton gradient across the inner mitochondrial membrane. As a result, electron transport as well as ATP synthesis is inhibited by oligomycin.**}

C. It contains a proton channel. {**Correct: The proton gradient is dissolved by passage of electrons through this channel from the cytoplasmic to the matrix side of the inner mitochondrial membrane.**}

D. It can exhibit ATPase activity. {**Correct: In a test tube, it can hydrolyze ATP to ADP + P_i (the reverse of its function in the mitochondria, where it is responsible for synthesizing ATP.)**}

✔ E. It can bind molecular oxygen. {**Incorrect.**}

For questions 10.10–10.14:

Answer	
A if 1, 2, and 3 are correct	D if only 4 is correct
B if 1 and 3 are correct	E if all are correct
C if 2 and 4 are correct	

10.10. Correct answer = A

Which of the following statements correctly completes the sentence "NADH dehydrogenase. . ."

✔ 1. . . . contains FMN and iron/sulfur centers. {**Correct**}

✔ 2. . . . has a standard reduction potential (E_o) less positive than that of cytochrome c. {**Correct**}

✔ 3. . . . is oxidized by coenzyme Q. {**Correct**}

4. . . . is inhibited directly by oligomycin. {**Incorrect: Oligomycin is an inhibitor of the ATP synthesizing complex.**}

10.11. Correct answer = A

According to the Mitchell chemiosmotic hypothesis for oxidative phosphorylation, which of the following statements is(are) CORRECT?

✓1. The cytoplasmic side of the inner mitochondrial membrane becomes positively charged with respect to the matrix as respiration occurs in normal functioning mitochondria. {*Yes: As protons are pumped from the inside to the outside of the inner mitochondrial membrane, the outside (cytoplasmic side) becomes positively charged with respect to the matrix side.*}

✓2. ATP formation in mitochondria is accompanied by movement of protons from the cytoplasmic to the matrix side of the inner mitochondrial membrane. {*Yes: Movement of the protons back into the mitochondrion provides energy for the synthesis of ATP.*}

✓3. The electron transport chain consists of loops of alternating hydrogen and electron carriers. {*Yes: These loops span the inner mitochondrial membrane.*}

4. The inner mitochondrial membrane must be permeable to protons in order to build up a proton gradient. {*No: If the inner mitochondrial membrane is made permeable to protons, for example by dinitrophenol, a proton gradient cannot be established.*}

10.12. Correct answer = C

Which of the following statements about mitochondria is(are) CORRECT?

1. Calcium ions can diffuse freely across the inner mitochondrial membrane. {*No: Calcium ions must be transported across the inner mitochondrial membrane.*}

✓2. The outer mitochondrial membrane is permeable to most small molecules, whereas the inner membrane is impermeable to most. {*Yes.*}

3. The matrix is a protein-rich gel that contains the enzymes involved in oxidation/reduction reactions. {*No: The TCA cycle enzymes are present in the mitochondria, but glycolysis exists in the cytosol.*}

✓4. The inner mitochondrial membrane is folded into cristae so as to increase its surface area. {*Yes.*}

10.13. Correct answer = E

From the known effects of 2,4-dinitrophenol on the process of oxidative phosphorylation, one may infer that its administration might cause which of the following physiologic manifestations?

✓1. Muscle weakness or general fatigue due to a deficiency in ATP synthesis. {*Yes: 2,4-Dinitrophenol serves as an uncoupler of ATP synthesis and electron transport.*}

✓2. Weight loss owing to an increased catabolism of carbohydrate, lipid, and protein reserves to generate ATP by way of substrate level phosphorylation. {*Yes: A decrease in the ability to synthesize ATP by oxidative phosphorylation would necessitate elevated ATP production through substrate level phosphorylation.*}

✓3. Fever, since the energy from respiration would be converted to heat instead of being used for the formation of ATP. {*Yes: Since electron transport (but not ATP synthesis) can continue in the presence of an uncoupler, all energy produced by electron transport chain would be released as heat.*}

✓4. Increased need for oxygen by the body, and therefore an increased rate of breathing. {*Yes: When electron transport is uncoupled from ATP synthesis its rate increases, and therefore has an increased need for molecular oxygen.*}

10.14. Correct answer = D

Given the following reaction:

Succinate + FAD ↔ Fumarate + $FADH_2$

where the standard reduction potential, E_o, for succinate/fumarate is −0.03 v and the E_o for $FADH_2$/FAD is −0.06 v, which of the following statements is(are) CORRECT?

1. There would be a net production of fumarate under standard conditions. {*No: Under standard conditions (i.e., where all substrates and products are present at 1 M concentrations), the reaction would run in the direction of succinate production.*}

2. Under standard conditions, the overall ΔG would be less than $\Delta G°$. {*No: Under standard conditions, ΔG is equal to $\Delta G°$.*}

3. Since the reduction potential for $FADH_2$/FAD is lower than that of succinate/fumarate, $FADH_2$ could not be used as a reducing agent in the mitochondria. {*No: $FADH_2$ is an important reducing agent in the mitochondria because it can reduce Coenzyme Q, an important member of the electron transport chain.*}

✓4. The $\Delta G°$ for the conversion of succinate to fumarate would be $(+0.03)(n)(\mathcal{F})$, where n is the number of electrons transferred to FAD and $\mathcal{F}$ is the Faraday constant. {*Yes*}

Chapter 11: GLYCOLYSIS

Answer A if 1, 2, and 3 are correct
B if 1 and 3 are correct
C if 2 and 4 are correct
D if only 4 is correct
E if all are correct

11.1. Correct answer = C

Glucokinase

1. is widely distributed and occurs in most mammalian tissues. {*No: Glucokinase occurs primarily in the liver.*}

✓2. has a high K_m for glucose and, hence is important in the phosphorylation of glucose primarily after ingestion of a carbohydrate-rich meal. {*Yes*}

3. is inhibited by glucose 6-phosphate. {*No*}

✓4. is specific for the phosphorylation of glucose. {*Yes*}

11.2. Correct answer = B

The reaction catalyzed by phosphofructokinase

✓1. is inhibited by high concentrations of ATP and citrate. {*Yes*}

2. uses fructose 1-phosphate as substrate. {*No: Fructose 6-phosphate is the substrate for phosphofructokinase.*}

✓3. is an important control point in the glycolytic pathway. {***Yes: Phosphofructokinase is the pace-setting enzyme of glycolysis.***}

4. is near equilibrium in most tissues. {***No: Phosphofructokinase catalyzes a reaction that is rate-limiting with substrate and product far from equilibrium.***}

11.3. Correct answer = A

Compared to the resting state, vigorously contracting muscle shows

✓1. increased lactate formation. {***Yes: Anaerobic glycolysis increases during vigorous muscular contraction.***}

✓2. increased oxidation of pyruvate to CO_2 and water. {***Yes: Contracting muscle will derive as much energy as possible from aerobic metabolism. When oxygen is limited, additional energy is provided by anaerobic glycolysis.***}

✓3. an increased NADH/NAD^+ ratio. {***Yes: The production of NADH by the glyceraldehyde dehydrogenase reaction is only partially counterbalanced by NADH oxidation by the mitochondria and lactate dehydrogenase (pyruvate → lactate). Thus, the steady-state ratio of NADH/NAD^+ increases.***}

4. increased conversion of pyruvate to acetaldehyde. {***No: The reaction occurs only in certain bacteria and yeasts.***}

11.4. Correct answer = D

Under anoxic (low oxygen concentration) conditions, glycolysis in muscle becomes more rapid because of an increase in the intracellular concentration of

1. NAD^+. {***No: The concentration of NAD^+ decreases as it is converted to NADH (see question 11.3).***}

2. ATP. {***No: The [ATP] decreases slightly as the energy stores of the muscle are depleted.***}

3. glycogen. {***No: Glycogen stores are depleted during anoxia.***}

✓4. AMP. {***Yes: The concentration of AMP (and that of ADP) increases as the energy stores of muscle are depleted***}

11.5. Correct answer = A

The rate of glycolysis is controlled in part by inhibition of

✓1. hexokinase by glucose 6-phosphate. {***Yes: Glucose 6-phosphate inhibits hexokinase, one of the rate-limiting enzymes of glycolysis.***}

✓2. phosphofructokinase by citrate. {***Yes: The concentrations of citrate increase when the TCA cycle is inhibited and signal an "energy-rich" state.***}

✓3. phosphofructokinase by ATP. {***Yes: High concentrations of ATP signals an "energy-rich" state.***}

4. glucokinase by ATP. {***No***}

Choose the ONE best answer

11.6. Correct answer = C

The conversion of glucose 6-phosphate to lactate in the glycolytic pathway is accompanied by a net gain of

A. 1 mole of ATP. {***No***}

B. 2 moles of ATP. {***No***}

✓C. 3 moles of ATP. {***Yes***}

D. 1 mole of NADH. {***No***}

E. none of the above. {***No***}

11.7. Correct answer = B

During strenuous exercise, the NADH formed in the glyceraldehyde 3-phosphate dehydrogenase reaction in skeletal muscle must be reoxidized to NAD^+ if glycolysis is to continue. The most important reaction involved in the reoxidation of NADH is

A. oxaloacetate → malate. {***No***}

✓B. pyruvate → lactate. {***Yes***}

C. dihydroxyacetone phosphate → glycerol phosphate. {***No***}

D. isocitrate → α-ketoglutarate. {***No***}

E. glucose 6-phosphate → fructose 6-phosphate. {***No***}

11.8. Correct answer = C

In pyruvate kinase (PK) deficiency, hemolysis of red cells occurs primarily because of increased intracellular levels of

A. lactate. {***No: Lactate and pyruvate formation would be expected to decrease in pyruvate kinase deficiency.***}

B. pyruvate. {***No***}

✓C. the ratio of ADP to ATP. {***Yes: A deficiency in PK causes a decrease in the rate of ATP production. This leads to a small increase in the ADP/ATP ratio, which in turn results in alterations in the cell membrane and ultimately in lysis.***}

D. 2,3-diphosphoglycerate. {***No: While 2,3-diphosphoglycerate (and other intermediates "upstream" from the enzyme deficiency) might be expected to increase in PK deficiency, these altered concentrations appear not to play a major role in hemolysis.***}

E. fructose 1,6-bisphosphate. {***No: See above***}

Chapter 12: GLUCONEOGENESIS

Choose the ONE best answer:

12.1. Correct answer = C

The synthesis of glucose from pyruvate by gluconeogenesis

A. occurs exclusively in the cytoplasm. {***No: The carboxylation of pyruvate occurs in the mitochondria.***}

B. is inhibited by elevated levels of glucagon. {***No: Glucagon stimulates both gluconeogenesis and ketogenesis.***}

✓C. requires the participation of biotin. {***Yes: Biotin is the cofactor of pyruvate carboxylase.***}

D. involves lactate as an intermediate. {***No: Lactate is a "dead-end" intermediate whose only metabolic fate is oxidation back to pyruvate.***}

E. requires the oxidation/reduction of FAD. {***No: All the reactions of gluconeogenesis are*** NAD^+***-linked.***}

12.2. Correct answer = D

Which one of the following is NOT a characteristic of gluconeogenesis?

A. It requires energy in the form of ATP or GTP. {***Yes: The formation of phosphoenolpyruvate and 1,3-diphosphoglycerate requires ATP.***}

B. It is important in maintaining blood glucose during the normal overnight fast. {***Yes: Hepatic glycogen stores are not sufficient to maintain blood sugar level during the latter part of an overnight fast.***}

C. It uses carbon skeletons provided by degradation of amino acids. {***Yes: Gluconeogenesis also uses lactate and glycerol as a precursor for glucose.***}

✔D. It consists of the reactions of glycolysis functioning in the reverse direction. {***No: Three reactions of glycolysis are irreversible and are by-passed by reactions unique to gluconeogenesis.***}

E. It involves the enzyme fructose 1,6-bisphosphatase. {***Yes***}

12.3. Correct answer = C

Which one of the following reactions is unique to gluconeogenesis?

A. Lactate→pyruvate {***No***}

B. Phosphoenolpyruvate (PEP)→pyruvate {***No***}

✔C. Oxaloacetate→phosphoenolpyruvate {***Yes***}

D. Glucose 6-phosphate→fructose 6-phosphate {***No***}

E. 1,3-Diphosphoglycerate→3-phosphoglycerate {***No***}

12.4. Correct answer = E

Which of the following compounds CANNOT give rise to the net synthesis of glucose?

A. Lactate {***gluconeogenic***}

B. Glycerol {***gluconeogenic***}

C. α-Ketoglutarate {***gluconeogenic***}

D. Oxaloacetate {***gluconeogenic***}

✔E. Acetyl-CoA {***not gluconeogenic***}

Chapter 13: CITRIC ACID CYCLE

Answer A if 1, 2, and 3 are correct
B if 1 and 3 are correct
C if 2 and 4 are correct
D if only 4 is correct
E if all are correct

13.1. Correct answer = A

The conversion of pyruvate to acetyl-CoA and CO_2

✔1. is essentially irreversible. {***Yes***}

✔2. involves the participation of lipoic acid. {***Yes: Lipoic acid is an intermediate acceptor of the acetyl group formed in the reaction.***}

✔3. is inhibited when pyruvate dehydrogenase is phosphorylated by a protein kinase in the presence of ATP. {***Yes***}

4. involves the participation of biotin. {***No: Thiamine pyrophosphate is the cofactor of pyruvate dehydrogenase.***}

13.2. Correct answer = D

Which of the following enzymic activities would you expect to be decreased in thiamine deficiency:

1. Pyruvate carboxylase {***No: This enzyme contains biotin as a cofactor.***}

2. Isocitrate dehydrogenase {***No: This enzyme does not require an organic cofactor.***}

3. Fumarase {***No: This enzyme does not require an organic cofactor.***}

✔4. α-Ketoglutarate dehydrogenase {***Yes: Thiamine pyrophosphate is a cofactor for this enzyme.***}

13.3. Correct answer = B

Which of the following statements about the citric acid cycle is(are) correct:

✔1. The cycle produces 3 moles of NADH and 1 mole of $FADH_2$ per mole of acetyl CoA oxidized to CO_2 and H_2O. {***Yes: Four pairs of electrons are transferred during the oxidation of acetyl CoA.***}

2. The cycle is inhibited by malate. {***No: The cycle is inhibited by malonate (*** $^-OOC—CH_2—COO^-$***), not malate.***}

✔3. The conversion of isocitrate to α-ketoglutarate is the key regulatory step in the citric acid cycle. {***Yes***}

4. The oxidation of acetate leads to a net consumption (loss) of oxaloacetate. {***No: Each turn of the cycle both consumes and produces one molecule of oxaloacetate. There is thus no net change in the concentration of this intermediate.***}

Choose the ONE BEST answer:

13.4. Correct answer = D

The conversion of 1 mole of isocitrate to 1 mole of succinate by the citric acid cycle results in the formation of how many moles of high-energy phosphate?

A. 3 {***No***}

B. 5 {***No***}

C. 6 {***No***}

✔D. 7 {***Yes: The conversion of isocitrate to succinate yields 2 NADH (each worth 3ATP via oxidative phosphorylation) and 1 GTP in the conversion of succinyl CoA to succinate.***}

E. 8 {***No***}

13.5. Correct answer = E

Entry of acetyl CoA into the citric acid cycle is decreased when

A. the ratio of ATP/ADP is low. {***No: The citric acid cycle is stimulated when [ATP] is low and [ADP] is high.***}

B. NADH is rapidly oxidized through the respiratory chain. {***No: The rapid oxidation of NADH provides*** NAD^+ ***that is essential for the oxidations of the cycle.***}

C. the ratio of $NAD^+/NADH$ is high. {***No: NAD^+ is required for the oxidation of the cycle.***}

D. the concentration of AMP is high. {***No: Elevated levels of AMP (along with ADP) is an "energy-poor" signal that stimulates the cycle.***}

✓E. The GTP/GDP ratio is high. {***Yes: Low levels of GDP would decrease the rate of the succinate thiokinase reaction, leading to an overall inhibition of the cycle.***}

Chapter 14: HEXOSE MONOPHOSPHATE SHUNT

Choose the ONE best answer:

14.1. Correct answer = C

Which one of the following is NOT characteristic of the hexose monophosphate pathway?

A. It produces CO_2. {***Yes: Glucose 6-phosphate is converted to hexose and CO_2 in the HMP pathway.***}

B. It uses $NADP^+$ as a cofactor. {***Yes: The HMP pathway contains 2 $NADP^+$-linked dehydrogenases.***}

✓C. It requires ATP for phosphorylation. {***No: The HMP pathway does not directly consume or produce ATP.***}

D. It produces ribose 5-phosphate. {***Yes***}

E. It involves the breakage and formation of C—C bonds. {***Yes***}

14.2. Correct answer = C

Which one of the following reactions does NOT consume NADPH?

A. Reduction of oxidized glutathione (G—S—S—G) {***Yes: NADPH is used by glutathione reductase.***}

B. Synthesis of steroids {***Yes: NADPH is used in the hydroxylation of the steriod ring.***}

✓C. Conversion of glucose 6-phosphate to 6-phosphogluconolactone {***No: NADPH is produced, not consumed.***}

D. Microsomal hydroxylation with the cytochrome P_{450} oxygenase system {***Yes***}

E. Fatty acid synthesis {***Yes***}

14.3. Correct answer = E

Glutathione functions in red blood cells largely to

A. produce NADPH. {***No***}

B. reduce methemoglobin to hemoglobin. {***No***}

C. produce NADH. {***No***}

D. reduce pyruvate to lactate. {***No***}

✓E. reduce oxidizing agents such as H_2O_2. {***Yes***}

14.4. Correct answer = B

Which one of the following metabolites is NOT directly produced in the hexose monophosphate pathway?

A. Fructose 6-phosphate {***Yes***}

✓B. Dihydroxyacetone phosphate {***No***}

C. CO_2 {***Yes***}

C. Erythrose 4-phosphate {***Yes***}

D. Gluconolactone 6-phosphate {***Yes***}

Chapter 15: METABOLISM OF DIETARY LIPIDS

Choose the ONE best answer:

15.1. Correct answer = A

Which one of the following statements about the absorption of lipids from the intestine is correct?

✓A. Dietary triacylglycerol is partially hydrolyzed and absorbed as free fatty acids and monoacylglycerol. {***Yes: Pancreatic lipase hydrolyzes dietary triacylglycerol primarily to 2-monoacylglycerol plus two fatty acids. These products of hydrolysis can all be absorbed by the intestinal mucosal cells.***}

B. Dietary triacylglycerol must be completely hydrolyzed to free fatty acids and glycerol before absorption. {***No: See answer to choice A above.***}

C. Release of fatty acids from triacylglycerol in the intestine is inhibited by bile salts. {***No: Bile salts are necessary for the proper solubilization and hydrolysis of dietary triacylglycerol in the small intestine.***}

D. Fatty acids that contain ten carbons or fewer are absorbed and enter the circulation primarily by way of the lymphatic system. {***No: Short-chain fatty acids (ten carbons or fewer) enter the portal circulation after absorption in the small intestine.***}

E. Formation of chylomicrons does not require protein synthesis in the intestinal mucosa. {***No: The synthesis of apoproteins by the intestinal mucosal cells is required for assembly and secretion of chylomicrons.***}

15.2. Correct answer = E

The form in which dietary lipids are packaged and exported from the intestinal mucosal cells is as

A. free fatty acids. {***No: Free fatty acids are esterified primarily to glycerol, forming triacylglycerol, which is exported from the intestine in chylomicrons.***}

B. mixed micelles. {***No: Mixed micelles are found in the small intestine and are composed primarily of dietary lipids and bile salts.***}

C. free triacylglycerol. {***No: Triacylglycerol is secreted by the intestinal mucosal cells as a component of chylomicrons.***}

D. 2-monoacylglycerol. {***No: 2-Monoacylglycerol is the primary degradative product of pancreatic lipase in the small intestine. It is absorbed by the intestinal mucosal cells and reesterified to fatty acids forming triacylglycerol.***}

✓E. chylomicrons. {***Yes: Chylomicrons contains a lipid core that has dietary lipid and lipid synthesized in the intestinal mucosal cells.***}

15.3. Correct answer = C

Which one of the following enzymes is NOT involved in the degradation of total dietary lipid during digestion?

A. Gastric lipase {***Incorrect choice: Gastric lipase in the stomach hydrolyzes triacylglycerol containing short-chain fatty acids. This enzyme may be of importance only in the degradation of dietary lipids in infants.***}

B. Pancreatic lipase {***Incorrect choice: Pancreatic lipase, synthesized by the pancreas and present in pancreatic juice hydrolyzes dietary triacylglycerol in the small intestine.***}

✓C. Lipoprotein lipase {***Correct choice: Lipoprotein lipase degrades triacylglycerol contained in chylomicrons and very low-density lipoproteins circulating through the peripheral tissues.***}

D. Phospholipase A_2 {***Incorrect choice: Phospholipase A_2 is also synthesized by the pancreas and hydrolyzes dietary phospholipids in the small intestine.***}

E. Cholesterol esterase {***Incorrect choice: Cholesterol esterase is also a pancreatic enzyme, and hydrolyzes cholesterol esters found in dietary lipid in the small intestine.***}

Chapter 16: FATTY ACID AND TRIACYLGLYCEROL METABOLISM

Choose the ONE best answer

16.1. Correct answer = E

Palmitic acid

A. is one of the most abundant monounsaturated fatty acids. {***No: Palmitic acid is a fully saturated fatty acid.***}

B. contains a double bond at carbon # 9. {***No: Palmitic acid has no carbon–carbon double bonds.***}

C. is a short-chain fatty acid. {***No: Fatty acids with ten carbons or fewer) are considered "short-chain"; palmitic acid contains 16 carbons.***}

D. contains more double bonds than arachidonic acid. {***No: Palmitic acid contains no carbon–carbon double bonds.***}

✓E. has a negative charge at ph 7.4. {***Yes: Palmitic acid contains a carboxyl group (—COOH) that is ionized (to —COO⁻) at physiologic pH.***}

16.2. Correct answer = B

Which one of the following fatty acids is not synthesized in humans?

A. Oleic acid

✓B. Linoleic acid {***Correct choice: Linoleic and linolenic acids are not synthesized by humans and therefore must be obtained through the diet. They are called "essential" fatty acids.***}

C. Palmitic acid

D. Stearic acid

E. Propionic acid

16.3 Correct choice = B

Which one of the following statements about fatty acids is INCORRECT?

A. Almost all fatty acids found in mammalian tissues are of the straight chain variety, but branched chain fatty acids do exist in nature. {***Correct.***}

✓B. More than 90% of the fatty acids found in plasma are "free," that is, are not esterified to another compound. {***Incorrect: Fatty acids in the plasma are generally esterified to glycerol (forming triacylglycerol), cholesterol (forming cholesteryl esters), or phospholipids.***}

C. Addition of double bonds to a fatty acid chain lowers its melting temperature. {***Correct.***}

D. Linoleic acid cannot be synthesized by humans and thus must be supplied by the diet. {***Correct: Linoleic and linolenic acids cannot be synthesized by humans, and therefore are called "essential fatty acids."***}

E. In general, the longer the chain length of a saturated fatty acid, the higher is its melting temperature. {***Correct.***}

16.4. Correct answer = D

Which one of the following compounds is obtained on complete hydrogenation (i.e., saturation) of linoleic acid?

A. Palmitic acid {***No: Palmitate is a fully saturated, 16-carbon fatty acid.***}

B. Oleic acid {***No: Oleic acid is an 18-carbon fatty acid with one double bond.***}

C. Myristic acid {***No: Myristic acid is a 14-carbon, fully saturated fatty acid.***}

✓D. Stearic acid {***Yes: Linoleic acid is an 18-carbon fatty acid with three double bonds. When it is fully saturated, it becomes stearic acid.***}

E. Fumaric acid {***No: Fumaric acid is a four-carbon compound that is a component of the tricarboxylic acid cycle.***}

16.5. Correct answer = E

If radioactively labeled carbon dioxide ($^{14}CO_2$) is used to make malonyl CoA from acetyl CoA, and if the labeled malonyl CoA is then used in fatty acid biosynthesis, which positions in the fatty acid would be labeled?

A. Only the carbonyl carbon (carbon #1)

B. All odd-numbered carbons

C. All even-numbered carbons

D. Only the methyl terminal carbon

✓E. None of the carbons {***Correct: The CO_2 used to make malonyl CoA from acetyl CoA (by acetyl CoA carboxylase) is subsequently removed during fatty acid synthesis. Therefore none of the labeled carbons remain in the completed fatty acid.***}

16.6. Correct answer = C

The formation of fatty acids from malonyl CoA

A. is stimulated by citrate. {***No: Citrate is a positive modulator for acetyl CoA carboxylase that synthesizes malonyl CoA from***

acetyl CoA. It does not stimulate the formation of fatty acids from malonyl CoA.}

B. directly requires biotin as a cofactor. {***No: Biotin is a cofactor for acetyl CoA carboxylase, not for fatty acid synthase, the enzyme complex that synthesizes fatty acids from malonyl CoA.***}

✓C. uses NADPH as a reductant. {***Yes: Two molecules of NADPH are required for each —C=O group reduced to —CH_2.***}

D. requires FAD as an oxidant. {***No: FAD is a cofactor in the degradation of fatty acids but not in their synthesis.***}

E. requires ATP {***No: ATP is required for the synthesis of malonyl CoA by acetyl CoA carboxylase but not for the formation of fatty acids from malonyl CoA.***}

Answer A if 1, 2, and 3 are correct
B if 1 and 3 are correct
C if 2 and 4 are correct
D if only 4 is correct
E if all are correct

16.7. Correct answer = A

Characteristics of acetyl CoA carboxylase include which of the following

✓1. Biotin is an essential cofactor. {***Yes***}

✓2. Citrate catalyzes the polymerization of the enzyme into its active form. {***Yes***}

✓3. It synthesizes malonyl CoA from acetyl CoA. {***Yes***}

4. It is found in the tricarboxylic acid cycle. {***No***}

16.8. Correct answer = B

Substances that play a direct role in the synthesis of palmitate by the fatty acid synthase complex include

✓1. covalently bound phosphopantetheine. {***Yes***}

2. covalently bound lipoic acid. {***No***}

✓3. malonyl CoA. {***Yes***}

4. thiamine pyrophosphate. {***No***}

16.9. Correct answer = E

When glucose is converted to triacylglycerol in adipose tissue,

✓1. citrate serves to transport acetyl units across the mitochondrial membrane. {***Yes: Citrate is formed by citrate synthetase in the mitochondria from acetyl CoA and oxaloacetate. It is transported through the mitochondrial membrane to the cytoplasm where it is cleaved by citrate lyase, producing cytoplasmic acetyl CoA and oxaloacetate.***}

✓2. some reducing equivalents required for this synthesis are provided by the reactions in glycolysis. {***Yes: In adipose, glycerol phosphate can be produced only by reducing dihydroxyacetone phosphate. The NADH reducing units required by the enzyme glycerol dehydrogenase that catalyzes the reduction can be produced during glycolysis.***}

✓3. CO_2 is a participant. {***Yes: CO_2 is required for the synthesis of malonyl CoA, an intermediate in the synthesis of triacylglycerol.***}

✓4. free glycerol is not an intermediate. {***Yes: Adipocytes lack glycerol kinase and therefore cannot utilize nonphosphorylated glycerol to make triacylglycerol.***}

Choose the ONE best answer

16.10. Correct answer = C

The lipolysis of triacylglycerol in adipose tissue leads to the formation of

A. glycerol 3-phosphate, which leaves the adipose cell and is metabolized by the liver. {***No: Lipolysis of triacylglycerol produces free fatty acids and nonphosphorylated glycerol.***}

B. glycerol, which is converted to glycerol 3-phosphate in the fat cell. {***No: Adipocytes are lacking in glycerol kinase and therefore cannot phosphorylate glycerol.***}

✓C. glycerol, which is converted to glucose in the liver. {***Yes: Hepatocytes do contain glycerol kinase, which can phosphorylate glycerol to glycerol 3-phosphate. Glycerol 3-phosphate can be oxidized to dihydroxyacetone phosphate (DHAP) by glycerol dehydrogenase, which may enter the gluconeogenic pathway.***}

D. glycerol, which is oxidized by muscle. {***No: Muscle also lacks glycerol kinase and therefore cannot utilize nonphosphorylated glycerol.***}

E. glycerol 3-phosphate, which is converted to glucose in the fat cell. {***No: See answer to choice B above.***}

16.11. Correct answer = D

Which of the following best describes the number of ATPs produced by the oxidation of palmitic acid to CO_2 and H_2O?

A. 40 ATP

B. 70 ATP

C. 100 ATP

✓D. 130 ATP {***Yes: Palmitic acid is a 16-carbon, fully saturated fatty acid. When it is degraded, it is first converted by seven cleavage steps to eight acetyl CoA units. Each cleavage step results in the production of one NADH and one $FADH_2$. These can be oxidized by the electron transport chain: Each NADH oxidized produces sufficient energy to produce three ATP; each $FADH_2$ oxidized produces sufficient energy to produce two ATP. Therefore from NADH, 7 x 3 = 21 ATP, and from $FADH_2$, 7 x 2 = 14 ATP. Each of the eight acetyl CoA molecules can enter the tricarboxylic acid cycle, resulting in the production of three NADHs, one $FADH_2$, and one GTP per acetyl CoA. These are equivalent to 3 x 3 = 9 ATP, plus 1 x 2 = 2 ATP, plus GTP (which is energeticaly the "same" as ATP) = 12. ATP is produced for each of the eight acetyl CoAs entering the TCA cycle (i.e., 8 x 12 = 96 ATP). Therefore, the total number of ATP obtained from the oxidation of a molecule of palmitate is 21 + 14 + 96 = 131 ATP.***}

E. 160 ATP

Answer A if 1, 2, and 3 are correct
B if 1 and 3 are correct
C if 2 and 4 are correct
D if only 4 is correct
E if all are correct

16.12. Correct answer = A

Among the differences between fatty acid synthesis and fatty acid oxidation are the fact(s) that

✓1. synthesis uses NADPH and oxidation uses NAD^+ as a cofactor. {***Yes***}

✓2. synthesis is accelerated and oxidation depressed in the presence of insulin. {***Yes***}

✓3. malonyl CoA is an intermediate in synthesis but not oxidation. {***Yes***}

4. synthesis occurs in the mitochondria whereas oxidation occurs in the cytoplasm. {***No: Synthesis occurs in the cytoplasm, whereas oxidation occurs in the mitochondria.***}

16.13. Correct answer = A

Propionyl CoA

✓1. arises from the oxidation of a fatty acid with an odd number of carbon atoms. {***Yes: Fatty acids with an odd number of carbons are degraded by the same pathway as those with an even number of carbons until the final three carbons attached to a molecule of coenzyme A are reached. This remaining structure is propionyl CoA.***}

✓2. enters the tricarboxylic acid cycle after being converted to succinyl CoA. {***Yes: Propionyl CoA is first carboxylated to methylmalonyl CoA. This structure is then converted to succinyl CoA by a mutase.***}

✓3. metabolism is affected in patients with vitamin B_{12} deficiency. {***Yes: Vitamin B_{12} is required as a cofactor for the mutase reaction that converts methylmalonyl CoA to succinyl CoA.***}

4. is a direct precursor of acetyl CoA. {***No.***}

16.14. Correct answer = C

In humans, carnitine

1. stimulates the activity of acetyl CoA carboxylase. {***No: Citrate stimulates the activity of acetyl CoA carboxylase.***}

✓2. is important for fatty acid oxidation. {***Yes: Carnitine provides a shuttle that transports fatty acids from the cytoplasmic side to the mitochondrial side of the inner mitochondrial membrane.***}

3. inhibits the formation of triacylglycerol. {***No***}

✓4. cannot serve its function in the presence of malonyl CoA. {***Yes: Malonyl CoA inhibits the activity of the carnitine shuttle.***}

Choose the ONE best answer:

16.15. Correct answer = B

Which one of the following statements about prostaglandins is INCORRECT?

A. Prostaglandins have a very short half-life. {***Yes***}

✓B. Prostaglandins are synthesized only in the liver and the adrenal cortex. {***No: Prostaglandins are synthesized by a broad variety of tissues.***}

C. Prostaglandins generally act locally on or near the tissue that produced them. {***Yes***}

D. The common precursor of the prostaglandins is arachidonic acid. {***Yes***}

E. Prostaglandin synthesis can be inhibited by a number of unrelated compounds, including cortisol and aspirin. {***Yes***}

16.16. Correct answer = B

Which of the following has as one of its major effects the ability to inhibit platelet aggregation?

A. Leukotriene A_4 {***No***}

✓B. Prostacyclin {***Yes***}

C. Thromboxane A_2 {***No***}

D. Prostaglandin H_2 {***No***}

E. Arachidonic acid {***No***}

16.17. Correct answer = C

In the major pathway by which liver produces ketone bodies, the immediate precursor of acetoacetate is

A. acetoacetyl CoA. {***No: Acetoacetyl CoA must first be converted to 3-hydroxy-3-methylglutaryl CoA, which is the immediate precursor of acetoacetate in the liver.***}

B. β-hydroxybutyrate. {***No: β-Hydroxybutyrate is the reduced form of acetoacetate.***}

✓C. 3-hydroxy-3-methylglutaryl CoA. {***Yes***}

D. two molecules of acetyl CoA. {***No***}

E. malonyl CoA. {***No: Malonyl CoA is a precursor of fatty acids but not of ketone bodies.***}

16.18. Correct answer = E

Which one of the following statements about use of ketone bodies as a fuel by the body is INCORRECT?

A. They are soluble in aqueous solution and therefore do not require carriers in the blood. {***Yes***}

B. They are made in response to elevated levels of fatty acids in the liver, where the amount of acetyl CoA exceeds the oxidative capacity of the liver. {***Yes: For example, during times of fasting or starvation when the triacylglycerol stores of the adipose are being degraded, with large amounts of fatty acids coming to the liver***}

C. Acetone is not used by the body as a fuel. {***Yes: It is a spontaneous breakdown product of acetoacetate that cannot be metabolized by the body. It is volatile and can be blown out in the breath.***}

D. Unlike fatty acids, they can be oxidized by the brain. {***Yes: Fatty acids are unable to cross the blood-brain barrier, but ketone bodies can.***}

✓E. When plasma ketone body levels are elevated, the liver efficiently oxidizes them for energy. {***No: The liver cannot utilize ketone bodies because it lacks the enzyme necessary to convert acetoacetate into its acetoacetyl CoA form.***}

Chapter 17: PHOSPHOLIPID METABOLISM

Choose the ONE best answer:

17.1. Correct answer = D

The neurologic disturbances seen in Niemann-Pick disease are associated with the accumulation in central nervous tissue of which one of the following:

A. Prostaglandins

B. Gangliosides

C. Cerebrosides

✓ D. Sphingomyelin {***Correct: Individuals with Niemann-Pick disease lack the lysosomal hydrolytic enzyme sphingomyelinase. This enzyme catalyzes the degradation of sphingomyelin to ceramide + phosphocholine. In its absence, sphingomyelin will accumulate in vacuoles of the cells, especially in cells of the nervous tissue where large amounts of sphingomyelin are found.***}

E. Phosphatidylserine

Answer A if 1, 2, and 3 are correct
B if 1 and 3 are correct
C if 2 and 4 are correct
D if only 4 is correct
E if all are correct

17.2 Correct answer = B

Phospholipid(s) that contain glycerol is(are)

✓ 1. lecithin. {***Correct: Lecithin (or phosphatidylcholine) contains glycerol phosphate, two fatty acids, and choline.***}

2. sphingomyelin. {***Incorrect: Sphingomyelin is composed of sphingosine, a fatty acid, and phosphorylcholine. It contains no glycerol.***}

✓ 3. cardiolipin. {***Correct: Cardiolipin (diphosphatidylglycerol) is composed of two phosphatidyl glycerol molecules attached to each other by a glycerol bridge between the two phosphate groups.***}

4. cerebroside. {***Incorrect: A cerebroside is composed of a ceramide attached to one or more monosaccharides such as glucose or galactose.***}

17.3. Correct answer = A

Which of the following statements about phosphatidylcholine (PC) metabolism in humans is(are) correct?

✓ 1. PC can give rise to lysophosphatidylcholine by the action of phospholipase A. {***Yes: Phospholipase A can remove one fatty acid from PC, producing a lysophosphatidylcholine.***}

✓ 2. PC can be synthesized from phosphatidylethanolamine (PE) by transmethylation. {***Yes: Three methyl groups are added to PE to produce PC. The source of the methyl groups is S-adenosylmethionine.***}

✓ 3. Cytidine triphosphate (CTP) is required for PC synthesis from 1,2-diacylglycerol. {***Yes: 1,2-Diacylglycerol is activated by being converted to its CDP derivative, after which it can participate in PC synthesis.***}

4. PC is derived exclusively from dietary choline. {***No: See choice 2 above.***}

17.4. Correct answer = E

Hydrolysis of a mixture of phosphoglycerides will yield which of the following compounds?

✓ 1. Choline {***Yes: From phosphatidylcholine.***}

✓ 2. Glycerol {***Yes: From any of the phosphoglycerides.***}

✓ 3. Phosphate {***Yes: From any of the phosphoglycerides.***}

✓ 4. Serine {***Yes: From phosphatidylserine.***}

Chapter 18: GLYCOLIPID METABOLISM

Answer A if 1, 2, and 3 are correct
B if 1 and 3 are correct
C if 2 and 4 are correct
D if only 4 is correct
E if all are correct

18.1. Correct answer = E

Sphingolipidoses are a group of diseases caused by related enzyme deficiencies. Which of the following statements about sphingolipidoses is(are) correct?

✓ 1. A specific catabolic enzyme is missing in each disorder. {***Yes: These catabolic enzymes are specific, lysosomal hydrolases.***}

✓ 2. Specific sphingolipidosis can be diagnosed by analyzing tissue samples for the presence of enzyme activity and for accumulation of a particular lipid. {***Yes: If a specific enzyme is deficient, the normal substrate for that enzyme will accumulate.***}

✓ 3. Usually only a single species of sphingolipid accumulates in the affected organs in each disease. {***Yes***}

✓ 4. The rate of biosynthesis of the accumulating lipid is normal. {***Yes: These diseases are characterized by deficiencies in degradative, not synthetic, lysosomal enzymes.***}

18.2. Correct answer = C

Which of the following compounds is(are) direct precursor(s) for the synthesis of the sphingosine found in glycolipids?

1. Asparagine {***No***}

✓ 2. Serine {***Yes***}

3. Malonyl CoA {***No***}

✓ 4. Palmitoyl CoA {***Yes***}

Choose the ONE best answer:

18.3. Correct answer = E

Which one of the following compounds would be found in a total hydrolysate of a typical mammalian tissue glycolipid?

A. Serine {***No: Serine is not found in glycolipid.***}

B. Choline {***No: Choline is found in phospholipids, not glycolipids.***}

C. Lecithin {***No: Lecithin (phosphatidylcholine) is a phospholipid.***}

D. Glucosylceramide {***No: Glucosylceramide can be further hydrolyzed to glucose, sphingosine, and a fatty acid.***}

✓ E. Fatty acid {***Yes.***}

18.4. Correct answer = A

To be defined as a ganglioside, a lipid substance isolated from nerve tissue must contain in its structure

✓ A. N-acetylneuraminic acid (NANA), hexoses, sphingosine, long chain fatty acid. {***Yes.***}

B. NANA, a hexose, a fatty acid, sphingosine, phosphorylcholine. {***No: Phosphorylcholine is not a component of a ganglioside.***}

C. NANA, sphingosine, ethanolamine. {***No: Ethanolamine is not a component of a ganglioside.***}

D. an N-acyl fatty acid derivative of sphingosine, hexose. {***No: NANA is also present.***}

E. NANA, hexoses, fatty acid, glycerol. {***No: Glycerol is not a component of a ganglioside.***}

Chapter 19: CHOLESTEROL AND STEROID METABOLISM

Choose the ONE best answer:

19.1. Correct answer = D

The immediate precursor of mevalonic acid is

A. mevalonyl CoA.

B. mevalonyl pyrophosphate.

C. acetoacetyl CoA.

✔ D. 3-hydroxy-3-methylglutaryl CoA. {***Correct***}

E. isopentenyl pyrophosphate.

19.2. Correct answer = D

Which one of the following statements about sterols found in nature is INCORRECT?

A. Cholesterol is the most abundant sterol found in animal tissue. {***Correct***}

B. All the carbon atoms of cholesterol are derived from acetyl CoA. {***Correct***}

C. β-Sitosterol is the most abundant plant sterol. {***Correct***}

✔ D. Dietary β-sitosterol and cholesterol are absorbed to about the same extent in the intestine of normal humans. {***Incorrect: Normal humans absorb almost no β-sitosterol.***}

E. The cholesterol ring structure cannot be broken down enzymatically by humans into smaller molecules for excretion. {***Correct: Cholesterol must be excreted either as unmodified cholesterol or as its modified form—bile salts or acids.***}

19.3. Correct answer = C

Which one of the following compounds is a precursor in the biosynthesis of cholesterol?

A. Cholestanol {***No: Cholestanol is produced from cholesterol by intestinal bacteria.***}

B. Progesterone {***No: Cholesterol is a precursor of progesterone.***}

✔ C. Lanosterol {***Yes***}

D. Cholic acid {***No: Cholic acid, produced from cholesterol, is a bile acid.***}

E. Pregnenolone {***No: Cholesterol is a precursor of pregnenolone.***}

19.4. Correct choice = D

Which one of the following compounds is NOT a precursor for the biosynthesis of cholesterol?

A. Mevalonic acid

B. Squalene

C. Isopentenyl pyrophosphate

✔ D. Aldosterone {***Correct choice: Aldosterone is a steroid hormone of which cholesterol is a precursor.***}

E. Farnesyl pyrophosphate

19.5. Correct choice = B

Animals fed a high cholesterol diet exhibit decreased cholesterol synthesis by liver because of the inhibition of which one of the following enzymes?

A. 3-Hydroxy-3-methyl glutaryl CoA (HMG CoA) synthetase

✔ B. HMG CoA reductase {***Correct choice: HMG CoA reductase is the major regulatory enzyme of cholesterol synthesis.***}

C. Mevalonate kinase

D. HMG CoA lyase

E. Squalene synthetase

19.6. Correct choice = A

Which one of the following is NOT a bile acid?

✔ A. Glycocholate {***Correct choice: Glycocholate is a bile salt.***}

B. Deoxycholate

C. Lithocholate

D. Cholate

E. Chenodeoxycholate

19.7. Correct choice = D

Which of the following functions is NOT performed by high density lipoproteins (HDL)?

A. HDL contains apoprotein apoA-I, which activates phosphatidylcholine:cholesterol acyl transferase. {***Is performed: PCAT transfers a fatty acid from phosphatidylcholine to cholesterol, producing a cholesterol ester and leaving a lysophosphatidylcholine.***}

B. HDL contains apoA-III, which transfers cholesterol esters from the HDL to other circulating lipoproteins in exchange for triacylglycerol. {***Is performed: Because of their hydrophobicity, the cholesterol esters remain "trapped" in the other serum lipoproteins until they are endocytosed by cells and degraded.***}

C. HDL carries cholesterol from the peripheral tissues to the liver. {***Is performed: HDL collects excess free cholesterol from the surface of cells. HDL are then endocytosed and degraded by hepatocytes.***}

✔ D. HDL is an important source of cholesterol esters for the extrahepatic tissues. {***Is NOT performed.***}

E. HDL donates apoprotein E to chylomicra. This apoprotein, together with apoprotein B, is recognized by the chylomicron receptor on hepatocytes. {***Is performed.***}

19.8. Correct answer = C

Which one of the following statements about serum lipoproteins is CORRECT?

A. Chylomicrons are synthesized primarily in adipose tissue and transport triacylglycerol to the liver. {***Incorrect: Chylomicrons are synthesized in intestinal mucosal cells and transport triacylglycerol to the peripheral tissues.***}

B. HDL are produced from LDL particles (LDL) in the circulation by the action of lipoprotein lipase. {***Incorrect: HDL are produced de novo by the liver.***}

C. VLDL are the precursors of LDL in the circulation. {***Correct: After triacylglycerol is removed from the VLDL by lipoprotein lipase in the peripheral tissues, the VLDL become LDL.***}

D. HDL competes with LDL for binding to receptors on the surface of cells in extrahepatic tissues. {***Incorrect: HDL and LDL each have their own specific cell surface receptors.***}

E. Cholesterol ester transfer protein in HDL is important for the efficient uptake of cellular cholesteryl esters by HDL in extrahepatic tissues. {***Incorrect: Cholesterol ester transfer protein exchanges cholesteryl esters from HDL for triacylglycerol from other circulating lipoproteins.***}

19.9. Correct choice = D

Which one of the following statements about familial hypercholesterolemia is INCORRECT?

A. This is a group of disorders characterized by elevations of total serum and especially LDL cholesterol. {***Yes***}

B. The disease is manifested clinically by xanthomas and accelerated atherosclerosis. {***Yes***}

C. Heterozygotes for this disease may have plasma cholesterol levels that are approximately twice normal. {***Yes***}

✔ D. The primary metabolic defect is a lack of binding of LDL to cell surface receptors caused by a lack of LDL apoprotein B. {***No: The lack of binding of LDL is due to a defect in the cell surface receptors for LDL.***}

E. Homozygotes for this disease are able to metabolize chylomicrons normally. {***Yes***}

19.10. Correct choice = B

Which one of the following changes would you expect in a patient with decreased activity of lipoprotein lipase?

A. Elevation of serum chylomicrons only. {***No: Serum VLDL will also be elevated.***}

✔ B. Elevation of both serum chylomicrons and VLDL. {***Yes: Lipoprotein lipase is required for the degradation of triacylglycerol in circulating chylomicrons and VLDLs. If much of the triacylglycerol is not removed from these particles, they cannot be further metabolized efficiently.***}

C. Elevation of serum HDL only. {***No: HDL carry relatively little triacylglycerol.***}

D. Elevation of serum LDL only. {***No: LDL carry relatively little triacylglycerol.***}

E. Elevation of both serum HDL and LDL. {***No.***}

19.11. Correct choice = C

The lipoprotein particles that have the highest percent concentration of cholesterol are

A. the chylomicrons.

B. the VLDL.

✔ C. the LDL. {***Yes***}

D. the HDL.

E. serum albumin-associated lipid.

19.12. Correct choice = A

The lipoprotein particles that have the highest percent concentration of triacylglycerol are

✔ A. the chylomicrons.{***Yes***}

B. the VLDL.

C. the LDL.

D. the HDL.

E. serum albumin-associated lipid.

19.13. Correct choice = A

A patient has a genetic defect that results in a deficiency of lipoprotein lipase. After eating a meal containing a large amount of fat, one would expect to see a plasma elevation of

✔ A. the chylomicrons. {***Yes: Chylomicrons are produced by the intestinal mucosal cells from dietary lipid. They contain primarily triacylglycerol, which is normally degraded by lipoprotein lipase. If this enzyme is deficient, chylomicrons would accumulate in the plasma after a lipid-rich meal.***}

B. the VLDL.

C. the LDL.

D. the HDL.

E. serum albumin-associated lipid.

19.14. Correct choice = A

Which one of the following steroids is synthesized from cholesterol WITHOUT being hydroxylated by 17 α-hydroxylase?

✔ A. Corticosterone {***Yes***}

B. Cortisol

C. Testosterone

D. Estradiol

E. Androstenedione

19.15. Correct choice = E

Which one of the following steroids is synthesized from cholesterol WITHOUT being hydroxylated by 21-hydroxylase?

A. Corticosterone

B. Cortisol

C. Aldosterone

D. 11-Deoxycorticosterone

✔ E. 17 α-Hydroxyprogesterone {***Yes***}

Chapter 20: DISPOSAL OF NITROGEN

Answer A if 1, 2, and 3 are correct
B if 1 and 3 are correct
C if 2 and 4 are correct
D if only 4 is correct
E if all are correct

20.1. Correct answer = A

In humans, amino acids can be used

✓1. as building blocks for the biosynthesis of proteins and other nitrogen-containing molecules. {***Yes***}

✓2. for the synthesis of tissue proteins. {***Yes***}

✓3. as sources of energy. {***Yes: After removal of the amino group, the carbon skeletons of the amino acids can enter glycolysis or the citric acid cycle***}

4. as carriers for other small molecules in body fluids. {***No: Proteins, rather than free amino acids, serve as transport molecules***}

20.2. Correct answer = D

Chymotrypsin acts

1. in the stomach on peptide bonds formed by the amino acid glycine. {***No: Chymotrypsin acts in the intestine on peptide bonds formed by any of several amino acids, particularly the aromatic amino acids, tryptophan, tyrosine, or phenylalanine.***}

2. in the intestinal mucosa on carboxy-terminal amino acids in proteins and peptides. {***No: Chymotrypsin is an endopeptidase that cleaves internal peptide bonds.***}

3. in the intestine on peptide bonds formed by the amino acids arginine or aspartate. {***No: Chymotrypsin does not favor cleavage next to arginine or aspartate (see 1 above).***}

✓4. in the intestine on peptide bonds formed by amino acids with aromatic side chains. {***Yes***}

20.3. Correct answer = E

Which of the following statements about glutamine is(are) correct?:

✓1. Glutamine is responsible for the transport and excretion of ammonium ions in a nontoxic form. {***Yes***}

✓2. The high level of activity of glutamine synthetase in the liver effectively traps ammonium ions as glutamine. {***Yes***}

✓3. ATP is required for the reaction leading to the synthesis of glutamine from glutamate and ammonia. {***Yes***}

✓4. The kidneys can hydrolyze glutamine to glutamate and ammonia. {***Yes***}

20.4. Correct answer = A

Given the following reactions, numbered I to IV,

I.

$$^{-}OOC-CH(NH_3^{+})-CH_2-CH_2-COO^{-} + NAD^{+} \rightarrow$$
$$^{-}OOC-C(=O)-CH_2-CH_2-COO^{-} + NADH + NH_3$$

II.

$$^{-}OOC-CH(NH_3^{+})-CH_2-COO^{-} + {}^{-}OOC-C(=O)-CH_2-CH_2-COO^{-} \rightleftharpoons$$
$$^{-}OOC-C(=O)-CH_2-COO^{-} + {}^{-}OOC-CH(NH_3^{+})-CH_2-CH_2-COO^{-}$$

III.

$$^{-}OOC-CH(NH_3^{+})-CH_2-CH_2-COO^{-} + NH_3 \rightarrow$$
$$^{-}OOC-CH(NH_3^{+})-CH_2-CH_2-CONH_2$$

IV.

$$NH_3 + CO_2 + 2ATP \rightarrow NH_2-C(=O)-O-P(=O)(OH)-OH + 2ADP + P_i$$

Which of the following statements about these amino acids is(are) correct?

✓1. Reaction IV is activated by N-acetyl glutamate. {**Yes: *Reaction IV is catalyzed by carbamyl phosphate synthetase, which is allosterically activated by N-acetyl glutamate***}

✓2. Reaction II is catalyzed by aspartate aminotransferase. {***Yes***}

✓3. Reaction III requires ATP. {***Yes: Reaction III is catalyzed by glutamine synthetase, which requires ATP in the synthesis of glutamine***}

4. Reaction I is catalyzed by glutaminase. {***No: Reaction I is catalyzed by glutamate dehydrogenase***}

20.5. Correct answer = B

Which of the following statements about the urea cycle is(are) correct?

✓1. The two nitrogen atoms that are incorporated into urea enter the cycle as ammonia and aspartate. {***Yes***}

2. Urea is produced directly by the hydrolysis of ornithine. {***No: Urea is formed by the cleavage of arginine.***}

✓3. ATP is required for the reaction in which argininosuccinate is formed. {***Yes***}

4. The urea cycle occurs primarily in the kidney. {***No: Urea is formed primarily in the liver.***}

Choose the ONE best answer:

20.6. Correct answer = D

In humans, the major route of nitrogen metabolism from amino acids to urea is catalyzed by which of the following enzymatic activities?

A. Amino acid oxidases and decarboxylases {***No: These enzymes are important for the metabolism of certain amino acids but are not major participants in nitrogen metabolism.***}

B. Amino acid decarboxylases and amino acid oxidases {***No***}

C. Transaminases and glutaminase {***No***}

✓D. Glutamate dehydrogenase and transaminases {***Yes: The combined action of these two enzymes leads to the removal of the amino group from most of the amino acids.***}

E. Glutaminase and amino oxidase {***No***}

20.7. Correct answer = D

Which of the following statements about the synthesis of carbamoyl phosphate by carbamoyl phosphate synthetase I is NOT true?

A. The enzyme catalyzes the rate-limiting reaction in the urea cycle. {***Yes***}

B. The reaction occurs in the mitochondria. {***Yes***}

C. The reaction requires two high-energy phosphates for each carbamoyl phosphate molecule synthesized. {***Yes***}

✓D. The enzyme requires biotin. {***No***}

E. The reaction is irreversible. {***Yes***}

Chapter 21: METABOLISM OF AMINO ACIDS

Answer A if 1, 2, and 3 are correct
B if 1 and 3 are correct
C if 2 and 4 are correct
D if only 4 is correct
E if all are correct

21.1. Correct answer = E

In the degradation of amino acids,

✓1. arginine, proline, histidine, and glutamine all lead to the production of α-ketoglutarate by glutamate. {***Yes***}

✓2. valine, isoleucine, and methionine all lead to the production of succinyl CoA by way of propionyl CoA and methylmalonyl CoA. {***Yes***}

✓3. phenylalanine leads to the production of fumarate and acetoacetyl CoA via tyrosine and homogentisic acid. {***Yes***}

✓4. asparagine and aspartic acid lead to the production of oxaloacetate. {***Yes***}

21.2. Correct answer = B

The structures of four amino acids are listed below:

I. $^{-}OOC-CH(NH_3^+)-CH_2-COO^-$

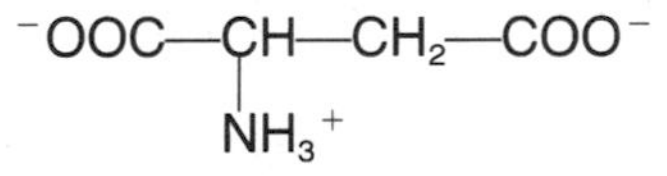

II. $^{-}OOC-CH(NH_3^+)-CH_2-CH_2-S-CH_3$

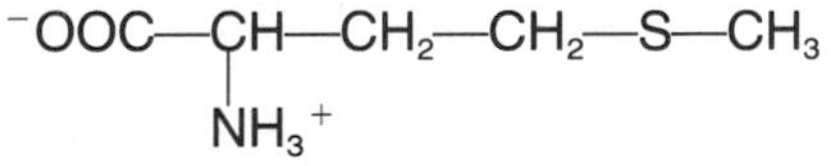

III. $^{-}OOC-CH(NH_3^+)-CH_2-CH_2-COO^-$

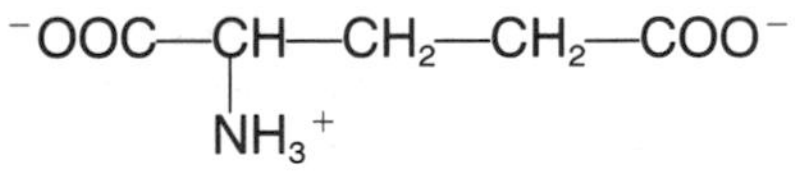

IV. $^{-}OOC-CH(NH_3^+)-CH_2-CH(CH_3^+)-CH_3$

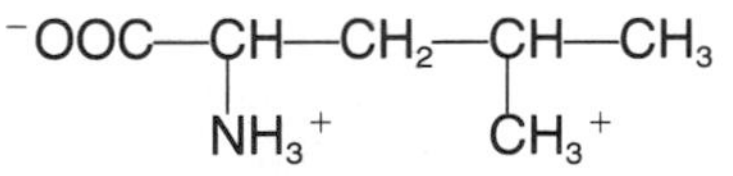

Which of the following statements about these amino acids (is/are) correct?

✓1. Amino acids I and II are glucogenic. {***Yes: I is aspartate and II is methionine, both glucogenic amino acids.***}

2. Amino acids II, III, and IV are essential amino acids. {***No: II is methionine (essential), III is glutamate (nonessential), and IV is leucine (essential).***}

✓3. Amino acid IV is ketogenic. {***Yes: IV is leucine, which is ketogenic.***}

4. Amino Acid III is degraded to pyruvate after transamination. {***No: III is glutamate, which is degraded to α-ketoglutarate.***}

21.3. Correct answer = D

Which of the following are synthesized from essential amino acids?

1. Alanine {***No***}
2. Cysteine {***No***}
3. Proline {***No***}
✓4. Tyrosine {***Yes: Tyrosine is formed from phenylalanine.***}

21.4. Correct answer = B

From which of the following amino acids can the α-amino group be removed by a dehydration reaction?

✓1. Serine {***Yes***}
2. Phenylalanine {***No***}
✓3. Threonine {***Yes***}
4. Arginine {***No***}

Choose the ONE best answer:

21.5. Correct answer = D

In humans, essential amino acids (with two exceptions) may be replaced in the diet by which one of the following?

A. Reducing caloric requirements {***No: The need for essential amino acids is independent of activity levels.***}
B. Increasing tricarboxylic acid cycle activity {***No: TCA cycle provides energy and does not influence requirement for essential amino acids.***}
C. Adding an excess of all other essential amino acids {***No: All the essential amino acids must be present simultaneously for protein synthesis to occur.***}
✓D. Adding the keto acids corresponding to the essential amino acids {***Yes: The ketoacids can be transaminated to the correspond amino acid.***}
E. None of the above. {***No***}

21.6. Correct answer = D

A normal adult is placed on a diet deficient only in phenylalanine. Which of the following statements is CORRECT?

A. Synthesis of proteins by the liver continues normally. {***No: Phenylalanine is an essential amino acid, and all essential amino acids must be present for protein synthesis to occur.***}
B. Tyrosine in the diet will be used to compensate for the missing phenylalanine. {***No: Tyrosine cannot be converted to phenylalanine.***}
C. Phenylalanine will be formed from alanine and benzoic acid, and therefore no metabolic changes will be observed. {***No: Phenylalanine is an essential and therefore cannot be synthesized in the body.***}
✓D. Tyrosine becomes an essential amino acid because it is synthesized from phenylalanine by hydroxylation. {***Yes***}
E. An increased dietary intake of both vitamin B_{12} and biotin will be required to remain in nitrogen balance. {***No***}

21.7. The correct answer = B

Which one of the following statements about amino acid metabolism in a growing child is INCORRECT?

A. The basic (positively charged) amino acids are all essential, whereas the acidic (negatively charged) amino acids are nonessential. {***Yes: Lysine, arginine, and histidine (positively charged) are all essential in growing children, whereas glutamate and aspartate (negatively charged) are nonessential.***}
✓B. The basic amino acids and acidic amino acids are all glycogenic and not ketogenic. {***No: Arginine and histidine are glycogenic, but the other basic amino acid, lysine, is both glycogenic and ketogenic; the acidic amino acids glutamate and aspartate are both glycogenic.***}
C. The aromatic amino acids are ketogenic and glycogenic. {***Yes: Phenylalanine, tyrosine, and tryptophan are ketogenic and glycogenic.***}
D. Proline is degraded to glutamic acid by way of glutamic acid semialdehyde, and glutamic acid is converted to α-ketoglutarate by transamination. {***Yes***}
E. The dietary requirement for the essential amino acid methionine is lowered if cysteine is included in the diet. {***Yes***}

Chapter 22: CONVERSION OF AMINO ACIDS TO SPECIALIZED PRODUCTS

Answer A if 1, 2, and 3 are correct
B if 1 and 3 are correct
C if 2 and 4 are correct
D if only 4 is correct
E if all are correct

22.1. Correct answer = E

Which of the following is(are) heme proteins?

✓1. Catalase {***Yes***}
✓2. Hemoglobin {***Yes***}
✓3. Cytochrome oxidase {***Yes***}
✓4. Myoglobin {***Yes***}

22.2. Correct answer = A

δ-Aminolevulinic acid synthetase activity

✓1. is frequently increased in individuals treated with drugs, such as the barbiturate phenobarbital. {***Yes: Drug metabolism leads to an increase in the synthesis of the cytochrome P_{450} system. This depletes intracellular heme levels and de-***

represses (increases) the synthesis of δ-aminolevulinic acid synthetase.}

✔ 2. catalyzes a rate-limiting reaction in porphyrin biosynthesis. {***Yes***}

✔ 3. requires the cofactor pyridoxal phosphate. {***Yes***}

4. is strongly inhibited by heavy metal ions such as lead. {***No: Another enzyme in the pathway (δ-aminolevulinic acid dehydrase) is extremely sensitive to heavy metals.***}

22.3. Correct answer = A

The catabolism of heme

✔ 1. occurs in the cells of the reticuloendothelial system. {***Yes***}

✔ 2. involves the oxidative cleavage of the porphyrin ring. {***Yes***}

✔ 3. results in the liberation of carbon monoxide. {***Yes***}

4. results in the formation of protoporphrinogen. {***No***}

22.4. Correct answer = B

In intermittent acute porphyria,

✔ 1. the severity of the symptoms can be diminished by intravenous injection of hemin. {***Yes: Hemin represses (decreases) the synthesis of δ-aminolevulinic acid synthetase.***}

2. the disease is associated with a decreased activity of ALA synthetase. {***No: Decreased intracellular levels of heme results in an increase in ALA synthetase.***}

✔ 3. skin photosensitivity does not occur. {***Yes***}

4. protoporphyrin accumulates in the liver and in the blood. {***No: The enzyme deficiency occurs before the formation of protoporphyrin, and, hence, it does not accumulate.***}

Choose the ONE best answer

22.5. Correct answer = A

The normal brown-red color of feces results from the presence of

✔ A. stercobilinogen. {***Yes: Stercobilinogen is oxidized to stercobilin, a red-orange pigment***}

B. urobilin. {***No: Urobilin gives urine its characteristic yellow color.***}

C. bilirubin diglucuronide. {***No***}

D. coproporphyrin III. {***No***}

E. biliverdin. {***No***}

22.6. Correct answer = D

Which one of the following is a direct precursor for the carbon atoms of the heme portion of hemoglobin?

A. Alanine {***No***}

B. ALA {***No***}

C. Aspartate {***No***}

✔ D. Succinyl CoA {***Yes***}

E. Carbon monoxide {***No***}

Chapter 23: METABOLIC EFFECTS OF INSULIN AND GLUCAGON

Choose the ONE best answer:

23.1. Correct answer = D

In which of the following tissues is glucose transport into the cell enhanced by insulin?

A. Brain {***No***}

B. Lens {***No***}

C. Red blood cell {***No***}

✔ D. Adipose tissue {***Yes: This tissue very sensitive to insulin***}

E. Nerve {***No***}

23.2. Correct answer = D

Insulin does all of the following EXCEPT

A. enhance glucose transport into muscle. {***Yes***}

B. enhance glycogen formation by liver. {***Yes***}

C. decrease lipolysis in adipose tissue. {***Yes***}

✔ D. enhance gluconeogenesis in liver. {***No: Insulin decreases the rate of hepatic gluconeogenesis.***}

E. enhance amino acid transport into muscle. {***Yes***}

23.3. Correct answer = D

Which one of the following statements about glucagon is INCORRECT?

A. High levels of blood glucose decrease the release of glucagon from the α-cells of the pancreas. {***Yes***}

B. Glucagon levels increase after ingestion of a protein-rich meal. {***Yes***}

C. Glucagon increases the intracellular levels of cAMP in liver cells, causing an increase in glycogen breakdown. {***Yes***}

✔ D. Glucagon and insulin are produced by the β-cells of the islets of Langerhans in the pancreas. {***No: Glucagon is produced by the α-cells, whereas insulin is produced by the β-cells of the islets of Langerhans.***}

E. Glucagon stimulates the formation of ketone bodies by the liver. {***Yes***}

23.4. Correct answer = D

Insulin causes the deposition of triacylglycerols in adipose tissue because it

A. inhibits glycolysis in adipose tissue. {***No***}

B. increases the concentration of blood glucose. {***No***}

C. stimulates gluconeogenesis, providing glucose that can serve as a precursor for triacylglycerol synthesis. {***No***}

✔ D. inhibits the activation of the hormone-sensitive lipase in adipose tissue. {***Yes***}

E. stimulates the uptake of glycerol by adipose tissue. {***No***}

Chapter 24: THE ABSORPTIVE STATE

Answer A if 1, 2, and 3 are correct
B if 1 and 3 are correct
C if 2 and 4 are correct
D if only 4 is correct
E if all are correct

24.1. Correct answer = A

Which of the following is(are) elevated in plasma during the absorptive period (compared to the postabsorptive state)?

✓1. Insulin {***Yes:** During the absorptive period the concentration of blood glucose and amino acids rise, prompting a release of insulin from the pancreas.*}

✓2. VLDL {***Yes:** Dietary triacylglycerols are repackaged in the intestine and secreted into the blood as chylomicra. These are taken up by the liver and repackaged and exported as VLDL.*}

✓3. Chylomicra {***Yes:** See 2 above.*}

4. Free fatty acids {***No:** During the absorptive period, fatty acids in the plasma exist primarily as triacylglycerol components of lipoproteins.*}

24.2. Correct answer = D

Which of the following fuel molecules is(are) used by the brain in the absorptive period?

1. β-Hydroxybutyrate {***No:** During the absorptive period, β-hydroxybutyrate and acetoacetate (ketone bodies) are not present in the blood at sufficiently high concentrations to function as a fuel for the brain.*}

2. Free fatty acids {***No:** Fatty acids do not cross the blood–brain barrier.*}

3. Amino acids {***No:** With a few exceptions, amino acids do not readily cross the blood–brain barrier.*}

✓4. Glucose {***Yes:** Glucose is present at relatively high concentration in blood and freely crosses the blood–brain barrier.*}

24.3. Correct answer = B

Ingestion of a meal consisting exclusively of protein would result in which of the following?

✓1. An increased release of insulin {***Yes:** The β-cells of the pancreas respond to elevated levels of circulating amino acids (derived from the dietary protein) by releasing insulin.*}

2. Hypoglycemia {***No:** Ingestion of protein causes a release of both insulin and glucagon, the latter stimulating gluconeogenesis and averting hypoglycemia (see 1 above and 3 below).*}

✓3. An increased release of glucagon {***Yes:** The α-cells of the pancreas respond to elevated level of circulating amino acid by releasing glucagon.*}

4. Ketoacidosis caused by the metabolism of ketogenic amino acids {***No:** Although ketoacidosis is, in principle, possible, the metabolism of the glycogenic amino acids tends to prevent ketoacidosis.*}

24.4. Correct answer = E

In the absorptive period (as compared to the postabsorptive state), the adipose tissue shows

✓1. increased transport of glucose into the adipocyte. {***Yes***}

✓2. increased production of NADPH. {***Yes***}

✓3. increased rate of glycolysis. {***Yes***}

✓4. decreased activity of hormone-sensitive lipase. {***Yes***}

Chapter 25: STARVATION AND DIABETES

Choose the ONE best answer:

25.1. Correct answer = B

Increased formation of ketone bodies during starvation is due to

A. mobilization of high-density lipoproteins. {***No***}

✓B. formation of acetyl CoA in amounts that exceed the oxidative capacity of the liver. {***Yes:** Adipose tissues release massive quantities of fatty acids, which overwhelm the oxidative capacity of the liver.*}

C. decreased levels of free fatty acids in serum. {***No***}

D. inhibition of β-oxidation of fatty acids in the liver. {***No***}

E. a decreased mobilization of triacylglycerols from adipose tissue. {***No***}

25.2. Correct answer = D

Which one of the following is the most important source of blood glucose during the last hours of a 48-hour fast?

A. Muscle glycogen {***No***}

B. Fatty acids {***No***}

C. Liver glycogen {***No:** Liver glycogen is largely depleted after 2 days of starvation.*}

✓D. Amino acids {***Yes:** During starvation, amino acids are metabolized to the corresponding ketoacids which serve as substrates for gluconeogenesis.*}

E. Acetyl CoA {***No***}

25.3. Correct answer = E

Starvation results in all of the following EXCEPT

A. decreased levels of VLDL. {***Yes***}

B. stimulation of adipose tissue hormone-sensitive lipase. {***Yes***}

C. increased levels of ketone bodies in the blood. {***Yes***}

D. increased fatty acid oxidation. {***Yes***}

✓E. increased synthesis of fatty acids in adipose tissue. {***No***}

25.4. The correct answer = C.

Which one of the following series best describes the chronological sequence of events that occurs during the first week of starvation?

A. Glycogenolysis, gluconeogenesis, ketogenesis, hypoglycemia. {**_No: Hypoglycemia does not occur._**}

B. Gluconeogenesis, glycogenolysis, fatty acid mobilization, ketogenesis. {**_No: Gluconeogenesis does not precede glycolysis._**}

✓ C. Glycogenolysis, gluconeogenesis, fatty acid mobilization, ketogenesis. {**_Yes: Fatty acid mobilization and ketogenesis occur together._**}

D. Gluconeogenesis, glycogenolysis, ketogenesis, fatty acid mobilization. {**_No: Gluconeogenesis does not precede glycolysis._**}

E. Glycogenolysis, fat mobilization, gluconeogenesis, hypoglycemia. {**_No: Hypoglycemia does not occur._**}

25.5. Correct answer = B

Relative or absolute lack of insulin in humans would result in which one of the following reactions in the liver:

A. Increased glycogen synthesis. {**_No_**}

✓ B. Increased gluconeogenesis from lactate. {**_Yes_**}

C. Decreased glycogenolysis. {**_No_**}

D. Decreased formation of acetoacetate. {**_No_**}

E. Increased action of hormone-sensitive lipase. {**_No_**}

25.6. Correct answer = A

Which one of the following is always found in patients with diabetes mellitus?

✓ A. An inability to metabolize glucose appropriately {**_Yes_**}

B. Extremely low levels of insulin synthesis and secretion {**_No_**}

C. Synthesis of an insulin with an abnormal amino acid sequence {**_No_**}

D. A simple pattern of genetic inheritance {**_No_**}

E. Microangiopathy {**_No_**}

25.7. Correct answer = C

An individual with obesity-associated diabetes (type II)

A. usually shows a normal glucose tolerance test. {**_No_**}

B. usually has a lower plasma level of insulin than a normal individual. {**_No: Insulin levels are often elevated but in some patients are lower than normal._**}

✓ C. usually develops a normal glucose tolerance test if his weight returns to normal. {**_Yes_**}

D. usually benefits from receiving insulin about 6 hours after a meal. {**_No_**}

E. usually has lower plasma levels of glucagon than a normal individual. {**_No_**}

25.8. The correct answer is A

Relative or absolute lack of insulin in humans would result in which one of the following reactions in the skeletal muscle:

✓ A. Increased use of muscle proteins for production of amino acids {**_Yes: Mobilization of amino acids favors hepatic gluconeogenesis._**}

B. Increased glycogen synthesis {**_No_**}

C. Increased uptake of glucose from the blood {**_No_**}

D. Increased gluconeogenesis from amino acids {**_No: Gluconeogenesis occurs in liver, not muscle._**}

E. Increased rate of glucose 6-phosphate oxidation in the pentose phosphate pathway {**_No_**}

Chapter 26: NUTRITION

Answer A if 1, 2, and 3 are correct
B if 1 and 3 are correct
C if 2 and 4 are correct
D if only 4 is correct
E if all are correct

26.1. Correct answer = A

Kwashiorkor

✓ 1. is characterized by growth retardation, anemia, hypoproteinemia, edema, and fatty infiltration of the liver. {**_Yes_**}

✓ 2. symptoms respond therapeutically to a high protein diet containing meat and milk products. {**_Yes_**}

✓ 3. affects populations largely dependent on cereals and grains or other products of low biological value. {**_Yes_**}

4. is a disease observed primarily in highly developed industrial areas. {**_No_**}

26.2. Correct answer = D

You are to design a new formula diet "Ultima Plus!," taking into account established nutritional guidelines. Which of the following statements about the composition of "Ultima Plus!" is INCORRECT?

1. The quantity of protein should be 0.8 g/kg/day or about 50 to 75 g/day. {**_Yes_**}

2. About 30% of calories should come from fat. {**_Yes_**}

3. About 100 g/day of carbohydrate should be included to avoid ketosis. {**_Yes_**}

✓ 4. To maintain the weight of a normally active 70-kg individual, the formula should contain 1200 to 1500 calories per day. {**_No: The RDA for calories is approximately 2900 for a 70-kg individual._**}

26.3. Correct answer = C

Given the information that a 70-kg man is consuming a daily average of 275 g of carbohydrate, 75 g of protein, and 65 g of lipid, one can draw the following conclusions:

1. Total energy intake per day is about 3000 kcal. {**_No: Total energy intake is (275 g carbohydrate × 4 kcal/_**

g) + (75 g protein × 4 kcal/g) + (65 g lipid × 9 kcal/g) = 1100 + 300 + 585 = 1985 total kcal/day.}

✔2. About 30% of the calories are derived from lipid. {***Yes: 585/1985 = 30%.***}

3. The diet does not contain a sufficient amount of dietary fiber. {***No: The amount of fiber cannot be deduced from the data presented.***}

✔4. The proportions of carbohydrate, protein, and lipid in the diet conform to the recommendations of the Senate Select Committee on Nutrition. {***Yes***}

Chapter 27: VITAMINS

Choose the ONE best answer:

27.1. Correct answer = E

The coenzyme required in oxidative decarboxylation is

A. biotin. {***No***}

B. vitamin B_{12}. {***No***}

C. pyridoxal phosphate. {***No***}

D. ascorbic acid. {***No***}

✔E. thiamine pyrophosphate. {***Yes***}

27.2. Correct answer = C

Which one of the following compounds is synthesized from glutamic acid, p-aminobenzoic acid, and a pteridine nucleus?

A. Vitamin B_{12} {***No***}

B. Cyanocobalamin {***No***}

✔C. Folic acid {***Yes***}

D. Biotin {***No***}

E. Coenzyme A {***No***}

27.3. Correct answer = E

Which one of the following statements about vitamin B_{12} is INCORRECT?

A. It can be converted to cofactor forms containing a 5′-deoxyadenosine or methyl group attached to cobalt. {***Yes***}

B. It can serve as a source of a cofactor required for the conversion of methylmalonyl CoA to succinyl CoA. {***Yes***}

C. It requires a specific glycoprotein for its absorption. {***Yes***}

D. It may be present in inadequate quantities in a strictly vegetarian diet. {***Yes***}

✔E. It contains a heme group. {***No: Vitamin B_{12} contains a corrin ring, not the protoporphyrin ring of heme.***}

27.4. Correct answer = C

Which one of the following statements about ascorbic acid is INCORRECT?

A. It is readily oxidized, particularly in the presence of divalent metal ions. {***Yes***}

B. It is a cofactor required for the hydroxylation of proline and lysine. {***Yes***}

✔C. Its requirement varies with the caloric intake. {***No***}

D. It is metabolized in part to oxalate, which can form an insoluble salt with calcium. {***Yes***}

E. It facilitates the absorption of dietary iron. {***Yes***}

Answer A if 1, 2, and 3 are correct
B if 1 and 3 are correct
C if 2 and 4 are correct
D if only 4 is correct
E if all are correct

27.5. Correct answer = D

The nutritional requirement for niacin in humans is

1. increased when the diet includes large amounts of raw egg white. {***No***}

2. decreased when the diet is supplemented with commercial "liquid protein" consisting largely of hydrolyzed collagen (which does not contain tryptophan). {***No***}

3. independent of the composition of the diet. {***No***}

✔4. decreased when the diet contains large amounts of animal protein. {***Yes: Animal proteins are a good source of tryptophan, which can be metabolized, in part, to niacin.***}

27.6. Correct answer = D

A deficiency of biotin in a higher animal is likely to be accompanied by

1. defective oxidation of fatty acids to acetyl CoA. {***No***}

2. decreased formation of lactate in skeletal muscular contraction. {***No***}

3. decreased oxidation of succinate by mitochondria isolated from the liver of such animals. {***No***}

✔4. defective synthesis of fatty acids. {***Yes: Biotin is a cofactor for acetyl CoA carboxylase, an enzyme essential to fatty acid synthesis.***}

27.7. Correct answer = C

Which of the following reactions involve the participation of thiamine?

1. Lactate → pyruvate {***No***}

✔2. α-Ketoglutarate → succinyl CoA {***Yes***}

3. Acetyl CoA → malonyl CoA {***No***}

✔4. Ribose 5-phosphate → sedoheptulose 7-phosphate {***Yes***}

27.8. Correct answer = A

Which of the following statements about niacin is(are) true?

✔1. Niacin forms part of the structure of $NADP^+$. {***Yes***}

✔2. Niacin is derived from the degradation of tryptophan. {*Yes*}

✔3. Niacin is involved as a cofactor in oxidation-reduction reactions. {*Yes*}

4. Niacin is a constituent of FAD. {*No*}

27.9. Correct answer = A

Vitamin B_{12}

✔1. participates in the conversion of homocysteine to methionine. {*Yes*}

✔2. contains cobalt. {*Yes*}

✔3. when injected into patients with pernicious anemia overcomes the lack of intrinsic factor. {*Yes*}

4. can be obtained in the diet from peas and carrots. {*No*}

27.10. Correct answer = A

Vitamin A (or one of its derivatives)

✔1. can be enzymically formed from dietary β-carotene. {*Yes*}

✔2. is transported from the intestine to the liver in chylomicrons. {*Yes*}

✔3. is the light-absorbing portion of rhodopsin. {*Yes*}

4. is phosphorylated and dephosphorylated during the visual cycle. {*No*}

27.11. Correct answer = D

Prolonged deficiency of vitamin D will result in

1. increased secretion of calcitonin. {*No*}
2. increased urinary excretion of calcium. {*No*}
3. increased density of bone. {*No*}

✔4. increased secretion of parathyroid hormone. {*Yes*}

27.12. Correct answer = A

Vitamin D

✔1. increases absorption of calcium from the intestine. {*Yes*}

✔2. is not required in the diet of individuals exposed to sunlight. {*Yes*}

✔3. is not really a vitamin because the active form, 1,25-dihydroxycholecalciferol, is synthesized in humans. {*Yes*}

4. opposes the effect of parathyroid hormone. {*No*}

27.13. Correct answer = C

Vitamin K

1. plays an essential role in preventing thrombosis. {*No*}

✔2. decreases the coagulation time in newborn infants with hemorrhagic disease. {*Yes*}

3. is present in high concentration in cow's or breast milk. {*No*}

✔4. is synthesized by intestinal bacteria. {*Yes*}

27.14. Correct answer = B

α-Tocopherol

✔1. functions primarily as an antioxidant. {*Yes*}

2. deficiency is commonly found in adults. {*No*}

✔3. requirements increase with the amount of polyunsaturated fatty acids in the diet. {*Yes*}

4. is found in high concentrations in whole grains and cereals. {*No*}

Chapter 28: STRUCTURE OF NUCLEIC ACIDS

Choose the ONE best answer:

28.1. Correct answer = E

Which one of the following statements about the structure of double-helical DNA is INCORRECT?

A. Within the double-helix there are ten base pairs per turn of the helix. {***Yes: The B form is a right-handed helix with ten residues per 360° turn of the helix.***}

B. The forces that stabilize the DNA double-helix are hydrogen bonds between complementary bases and stacking interactions between bases. {***Yes: A forms two hydrogen bonds with T, whereas G forms two hydrogen bonds with C. The "flat plates" of the nucleotide bases form π-bonds, stabilizing the DNA double-helix.***}

C. Separation of the two strands of the double-helix requires untwisting of the helix. {***Yes: In order to separate the two strands of the double-helix so that they can be replicated, the helix must untwist.***}

D. The double-helix contains antiparallel chains that form a major and a minor groove on the surface of the helix. {***Yes: The B form of DNA has characteristic grooves on its surface.***}

✔E. The molar amount of adenine plus thymine equals the molar amount of guanine plus cytosine. {***No: In double-stranded DNA, the molar amount of adenine equals that of thymine, and the molar amount of guanine equals that of thymine. Therefore, A + G = T + C, and A + G/T + C = 1.***}

28.2. Correct answer = D

Complete acid hydrolysis of nucleic acids yields all of the following except

A. phosphoric acid. {***Yes: Phosphoric acid is the terminal group of nucleotides.***}

B. purines. {***Yes: Adenine and guanine.***}

C. pentoses. {***Yes: Ribose (RNA) or deoxyribose (DNA).***}

✔D. adenosine. {***No: Adenosine is a nucleoside and is composed of adenine plus ribose (or deoxyribose). These components would be separated by acid hydrolysis.***}

E. cytosine. {***Yes: DNA contains the pyrimidines cytosine and thymine, whereas RNA contains cytosine and uracil.***}

28.3. Correct answer: B

Which one of the following choices best completes the following sentence?

Transfer RNA...

A. ...contains the information necessary for the synthesis of a specific protein. {***No: Messenger RNA contains this information. Transfer RNA is the adaptor molecule that carries a specific amino acid and also recognizes the codon on the mRNA that codes for that specific amino acid.***}

✓B. ...must exist in at least 20 different forms, one for each amino acid. {***Yes: Since each amino acid is coded for by at least one unique codon, there must exist at least one species of transfer RNA molecule per species of amino acid.***}

C. ...is the largest of the RNA species. {***No: Transfer RNAs are among the smallest RNAs in the cell.***}

D. ...has little or no secondary structure. {***No: Transfer RNAs have extensive secondary structure due to intramolecular base pairing between stretches of complementary sequences within the RNA chain. This gives the transfer RNA its characteristic "cloverleaf" (actually upside-down "L") shape.***}

E. ...exists in the cytoplasm associated with histones. {***No: Histones are found associated with DNA in the nucleus of eukaryotic cells.***}

28.4. Correct answer: A

Which one of the following choices best completes the following sentence?

Histones...

✓A. ...are basic proteins rich in lysine or arginine, or both. {***Yes: These basic amino acids give histones their positive charge at physiologic pH.***}

B. ...are bound covalently to DNA. {***No: Histones interact with the negatively charged DNA through electrostatic interactions.***}

C. ...have relatively high molecular weights (200,000 daltons or higher). {***No: Histones are relatively small proteins.***}

D. ...are identical to protamines. {***No: Protamines are a separate class of small, positively charged proteins that bind to DNA.***}

E. ...are found in high concentrations in ribosomes. {***No: Histones are found in the nucleus, whereas ribosomes are found in the cytoplasm.***}

28.5. Correct answer: E

Which one of the following statements about most eukaryotic messenger RNA is INCORRECT?

A. The pentose found in mRNA is D-ribose. {***Yes: Ribose is found in RNA, whereas deoxyribose is found in DNA.***}

B. mRNA exists as a single-stranded molecule. {***Yes: With the exception of some double-stranded RNA-containing viruses, RNA is a single-stranded molecule.***}

C. mRNA has a long sequence of adenine nucleotides on its 3′-end. {***Yes: This 3′-"poly(A) tail" is characteristic of most mRNA molecules. A notable exception are the mRNAs that code for histones.***}

D. mRNA has a molecule of 7-methylguanosine at its 5′-end. {***Yes: This 7-methylguanosine is called a "cap" and is attached to the 5′-end through an unusual triphosphate linkage.***}

✓E. The mRNA chain is longer than that of DNA. {***No: mRNA is a complementary copy of a small portion of a strand of DNA.***}

Chapter 29: NUCLEOTIDE METABOLISM

Choose the ONE BEST answer:

29.1. Correct choice is E

The formation of uric acid from purines is catalyzed by

A. adenylate deaminase. {***No: Adenylate deaminase converts only adenosine to inosine.***}

B. uricase. {***No: Uricase oxidizes uric acid to allantoin in animals.***}

C. allantoinase. {***No: Allantoinase hydrolyzes allantoin.***}

D. urease. {***No: Urease cleaves urea to CO_2 and NH_3.***}

✓E. xanthine oxidase. {***Yes: Xanthine oxidase converts both hypoxanthine to xanthine, and xanthine to uric acid, thus acting on the degradation products of all purines.***}

29.2. Correct choice is C

The committed step in pyrimidine biosynthesis

A. provides a classic example of positive feedback control. {***No: Negative feedback control.***}

B. results in the formation of dihydroorotic acid. {***No: See choice C below.***}

✓C. is the formation of N-carbamoylaspartic acid. {***Yes: Aspartate transcarbamoylase, which synthesizes carbamoyl aspartate from carbamoyl phosphate and aspartic acid, catalyzes the committed step in pyrimidine biosynthesis.***}

D. is catalyzed by orotate decarboxylase. {***No: See choice C above.***}

E. requires ATP. {***No.***}

29.3. Correct choice is A

The four nitrogen atoms of the purine ring are derived from

✓A. aspartate, glutamine, and glycine. {***Yes***}

B. glutamine, ammonia, and aspartate.

C. glycine and aspartate.

D. ammonia, glycine, and glutamate.

E. urea and ammonia.

29.4. Correct choice = A

The absence of which enzyme involved in the "salvage pathways" of nucleotide metabolism results in the genetic disease Lesch–Nyhan syndrome?

✓A. Hypoxanthine-guanine phosphoribosyl transferase {***Yes: This enzyme catalyzes the transfer of a ribose-phosphate unit from phosphoribosylpyrophosphate to the purine bases hypoxanthine and guanine.***}

B. Aspartate transcarbamoylase {**No: This enzyme catalyzes the committed step in de novo pyrimidine biosynthesis.**}

C. Thymidylate kinase {**No: This enzyme converts dTMP to dTDP.**}

D. Adenylate deaminase {**No: This enzyme removes an ammonia group from adenosine or AMP.**}

E. Xanthine oxidase {**No: This enzyme catalyzes the oxidation of purine bases to uric acid.**}

29.5. Correct choice = A

6-Mercaptopurine, which has been used to treat acute leukemia, is converted to the nucleotide 6-mercaptopurine-9-ribose-5′-phosphate in the body. This nucleotide interferes with the conversion of inosine 5′-phosphate (IMP) to adenosine 5′-phosphate (AMP). Which one of the following compounds is the immediate source of the amino group that is introduced into IMP during this conversion?

✔A. Aspartate {**Yes**}

B. NH_4^+

C. S-Adenosylmethionine

D. Glutamine

E. Asparagine

Answer A if 1, 2, and 3 are correct
B if 1 and 3 are correct
C if 2 and 4 are correct
D if only 4 is correct
E if all are correct

29.6. Correct choice = B

In the formation of purine and pyrimidine nucleotides,

✔1. both pathways require ATP. {**Yes**}

2. all intermediates of the pyrimidine nucleotides are derivatives of ribose 5′-phosphate. {**No: Ribose 5′-phosphate is added to the pyrimidine base after the ring structure has been completed.**}

✔3. all intermediates of the purine nucleotides are derivatives of ribose 5′-phosphate. {**Yes: The purine ring grows attached to ribose 5′-phosphate.**}

4. 5-phosphoribosyl-1-pyrophosphate is not involved in the synthesis of pyrimidine nucleotides. {**No: PRPP is the source of the ribose 5′-phosphate found in both purine and pyrimidine rings.**}

29.7. Correct choice = A

Uric acid is a breakdown product of

✔1. AMP. {**Yes: Uric acid is the end product of purine catabolism in humans.**}

✔2. IMP. {**Yes: See choice 1 above.**}

✔3. GMP. {**Yes: See choice 1 above.**}

4. CMP. {**No: The base in CMP is a pyrimidine.**}

29.8. Correct choice = A

Which of the following statements about purine and pyrimidine biosynthesis is(are) CORRECT?

✔1. The formation of 5-phosphoribosyl-1-amine is an important regulatory step in purine biosynthesis. {**Yes: This step, catalyzed by glutamine phosphoribosyl pyrophosphate amidotransferase, is the major committed step in purine biosynthesis.**}

✔2. The *de novo* synthesis of purines requires the participation of tetrahydrofolate-derivatives. {**Yes: Tetrahydrofolate derivatives contribute two carbons to the growing purine ring.**}

✔3. 5-Phosphoribosyl-1-pyrophosphate (PRPP) is used for the synthesis of uridine 5′-phosphate (UMP) from orotate. {**Yes: PRPP provides the ribose 5′-phosphate component of both purines and pyrimidines.**}

4. Thymidine 5′-phosphate is formed in a reaction involving the direct participation of PRPP and thymidine. {**No: Thymidine 5′-phosphate (dTMP) is synthesized from dUMP by thymidylate synthase.**}

Chapter 30: DNA SYNTHESIS

Choose the ONE best answer:

30.1. Correct answer = D

Which one of the choices below BEST completes the statement: The fact that DNA polymerase I from E. coli has a 5′→3′ exonuclease activity. . . .

A. . . . implies that the enzyme has multiple subunits. {**No: This is not implied.**}

B. . . . implies that DNA polymerase I can use both RNA and DNA as primers. {**No: This is not implied.**}

C. . . . makes the enzyme able to detect thymine-dimers in double-stranded DNA. {**No: Thymine-dimers are detected by specific endonucleases present in the cell for that purpose.**}

✔D. . . . enables the enzyme to play an important role in DNA replication. {**Yes: The 5′ → 3′ exonuclease activity of DNA polymerase I is used to excise RNA primers.**}

E. . . . makes the enzyme able to correct errors during elongation of a primer. {**No: Errors are corrected by the polymerase's 3′ → 5′ exonuclease ("proofreading") activity.**}

30.2. Correct choice = A

During DNA replication, the sequence 5′-TpApGpAp-3′ would produce which of the following complementary structures:

✔A. 5′-TpCpTpAp-3′ {**Yes: The newly synthesized DNA strand binds to its template in an antiparallel, complementary orientation. Nucleotide sequences, however, must always be written in the 5′ to 3′ order.**}

A. 5′-TpCpTpAp-3′

B. 5′-ApTpCpTp-3′

C. 5′-UpCpUpAp-3′

D. 5′-GpCpGpAp-3′

E. 3′-TpCpTpAp-3′

Answer A if 1, 2, and 3 are correct
B if 1 and 3 are correct
C if 2 and 4 are correct
D if only 4 is correct
E if all are correct

30.3. Correct choice = B

Which of the following statements about DNA polymerases is(are) CORRECT?

✓1. DNA polymerases require primers. {***Yes: DNA polymerases cannot copy single strands of DNA; rather, they require that at least a short stretch of the template be double stranded, with a free 3'-hydroxyl group on the shorter "primer" strand.***}

2. DNA polymerases can add nucleotides at both the 3'- and the 5'-ends of the growing polynucleotide chain. {***No: DNA polymerases can only add nucleotides to the 3'-end of the growing chain.***}

✓3. In addition to their polymerizing activity, DNA polymerases have a 3'→5'-exonuclease activity. {***Yes: The 3' → 5'-exonuclease activity is responsible for "proofreading" the newly synthesized chain.***}

4. DNA polymerases can synthesize DNA only in the presence of an RNA template. {***No: Only RNA-dependent DNA polymerase (reverse transcriptases synthesized by some viruses) can synthesize DNA in the presence of an RNA template.***}

30.4. Correct choice = D

Which of the following statements about DNA ligase is(are) CORRECT?

1. DNA ligase is an important enzyme in replication of DNA because it seals the gaps between RNA primers and the growing DNA strands. {***No: The gaps between RNA primers and the growing DNA strands are not sealed. DNA ligase can seal single-stranded nicks between DNA strands.***}

2. DNA ligase requires free 3'- and 5'-hydroxyl ends plus ATP. The terminal phosphate group of ATP is used to form the phosphodiester bond between the two DNA strands that are joined. {***No: DNA ligase does not require ATP to seal single-stranded nicks.***}

3. DNA ligase fills in gaps in double-helical DNA. {***No: DNA ligase cannot add nucleotides to fill gaps in double-helical DNA.***}

✓4. DNA ligase participates in the process of excision-repair of damaged DNA. {***Yes: DNA ligase seals the single-stranded nick remaining after the defective base(s) in damaged DNA have been excised and replaced.***}

Chapter 31: RNA SYNTHESIS

Choose the ONE best answer:

31.1. Correct answer = A

One class of RNA characteristically contains methylated purines and pyrimidines. This RNA is

✓A. tRNA. {***Yes: tRNA is characterized by containing a number of unusual bases, including methylated purines and pyrimidines.***}

B. mRNA.

C. rRNA.

D. 16S RNA.

E. RNA with a 3'-poly(A) tail.

31.2. Correct answer = B

Which of the following statements about messenger RNA is INCORRECT?

A. The sugar moiety of mRNA is D-ribose. {***Yes: RNA contains D-ribose, DNA contains D-2'-deoxyribose.***}

✓B. The polynucleotide chain of mRNA is longer than that of DNA. {***No: DNA contains the genetic information coding for all the mRNA species.***}

C. mRNA exists as single-stranded molecules. {***Yes***}

D. mRNA has a 7'-methylguanosine "cap" at its 5'-end. {***Yes***}

E. mRNA has a 3'-poly(A) sequence. {***Yes***}

31.3. Correct choice = E

During RNA synthesis, the DNA template sequence 5'-TpApGpCp-3' would be transcribed to produce which of the following RNA sequences?

A. 5'-ApTpCpGp-3'

B. 5'-GpCpTpAp-5'

C. 5'-CpGpTpAp-3'

D. 5'-ApUpCpGp-3'

✓E. 5'-GpCpUpAp-3' {***Correct: The RNA sequence is transcribed antiparallel to the DNA sequence ("3'-ApUpCpGp-5' "). However, all nucleotide sequences must be reported in the 5' → 3' direction. Also, the RNA transcript contains uridine (U) instead of thymidine (T).***}

31.4. Correct choice = D

Which one of the following statements about RNA polymerase activity is CORRECT?

A. Transcription of DNA by RNA polymerase is a semi-conservative process because only one of the two strands of the DNA double-helix is copied into RNA. {***No: Transcription is a conservative process. However, both DNA strands can serve as templates for RNA synthesis, although within a given region of the double-helix generally only one strand will be transcribed.***}

B. Transcription of DNA by RNA polymerase requires the participation of a swivelase (topoisomerase I). {***No: RNA polymerase does not require the action of topoisomerases for transcription.***}

C. Helix-unwinding is an important catalytic activity of one of the subunits of RNA polymerase. {***No***}

✓D. RNA polymerase cannot proofread its own products. {***Yes: Unlike DNA polymerase, RNA polymerase has no proofreading ability.***}

E. RNA polymerase catalyzes the removal of introns from the primary transcript. {***No***}

Chapter 32: PROTEIN SYNTHESIS

Choose the ONE best answer:

32.1. Correct choice = E

Which one of the following molecules is NOT a component of the 30S initiation complex?

A. GTP

B. Initiation factor 2 (IF-2)

C. mRNA

D. N-Formylmethionyl-tRNA

✓E. ATP {***Yes: ATP participates in protein synthesis only in the initial aminoacyl:tRNA synthetase reaction. The rest of the energy required for protein synthesis is provided by GTP.***}

32.2. Correct choice = D

What is the maximum number of different amino acids in a polypeptide chain coded by the synthetic polyribonucleotide (UCAG)5?

A. One

B. Two

C. Three

✓D. Four {***Yes: Write out the sequence: UCAGUCAGUCAGUCAGUCAG. If you count the nucleotides three at a time, you find the codons: UCA, GUC, AGU, CAG, and then you begin to repeat . . . UCA, GUC, and so forth. Therefore, the sequence can code for four amino acids.***}

E. Five

32.3. Correct choice = E

The genetic code. . . .

A. . . . is degenerate in that many triplets code for more than one amino acid. {***No: Each codon codes for only one amino acid.***}

B. . . . is read in the direction of 3′ to 5′. {***No: The genetic code sequence on the mRNA is read in the 5′ → 3′ direction.***}

C. . . . triplet, CCA, is found at the beginning of nearly all mRNA coding sequences. {***No: AUG, coding for methionine (which is formylated in E. coli), is found at the beginning of many mRNA coding sequences.***}

D. . . . involves a number of minor bases that are associated with chain initiation and transcription. {***No: The genetic code utilizes only adenine, guanine, uracil, and cytosine.***}

✓E. . . . is generally referred to as universal because it is nearly the same in all organisms. {***Yes: The genetic code appears to be universal with some minor exceptions.***}

32.4. Correct choice = E

In protein biosynthesis. . . .

A. . . . each amino acid recognizes its own codon by a direct interaction with the mRNA template. {***No: A tRNA molecule is required as an "adaptor molecule" to allow recognition of a codon for a specific amino acid carried by that tRNA.***}

B. . . . fidelity of translation is assured by the presence of traces of DNA on the ribosome. {***No: There are no "traces" of DNA on the ribosome.***}

C. . . . each amino acid is first attached to an anticodon specific for the amino acid. {***No: An amino acid is attached to the 3′-CCA sequence on a tRNA able to recognize an mRNA codon specific for that amino acid.***}

D. . . . a given codon and its anticodon must have identical base sequences in order for there to be proper base-pairing. {***No: The codon and anticodon must have complementary three-base sequences for there to be proper base-pairing.***}

✓E. . . . each amino acid is added in its proper place to a growing peptide chain through the "adaptor" function of tRNA. {***Yes***}

Figure Sources

2.1 Geoffrey Zubay, Biochemistry, Addison-Wesley (1983)
2.7 Geoffrey Zubay, Biochemistry, Addison-Wesley (1983)
2.8 Geoffrey Zubay, Biochemistry, Addison-Wesley (1983)
2.11 Geoffrey Zubay, Biochemistry, Addison-Wesley (1983)
3.2 Lubert Stryer, Biochemistry, 2nd Ed., W. H. Freeman and Company (1981)
3.3 Geoffrey Zubay, Biochemistry, Addison-Wesley (1983)
3.9 Robert M. Windslow and W. French Anderson, in The Metabolic Basis of Inherited Diseases, 4th Ed., J. B. Stansbury, J. Wyngaarden, D. Fredrickson, McGraw Hill (1978)
3.14 Darwin Prockop, Genetic defects of collagen, Hospital Practice (1986)
10.8 Geoffrey Zubay, Biochemistry, Addison-Wesley (1983)
10.12 Geoffrey Zubay, Biochemistry, Addison-Wesley (1983)
16.20 Laurence Demers, The effects of prostaglandins, Diagnostic Medicine (1984)
19.15 M. S. Brown and J. L. Goldstein, How LDL receptors influence cholesterol and atherosclerosis, Scientific American (1984)
23.2 Lubert Stryer, Biochemistry, 2nd Ed., W. H. Freeman and Company (1981)
23.4 R. H. Unger, Glucagon physiology and pathophysiology, New England Journal of Medicine 285:445 (1971)
25.2 Neil Ruderman, T. T. Aoki, and George Cahil, Jr., Gluconeogenesis: Its Regulation in Mammalian Species, John Wiley & Sons, (1976)
26.7 E. Newbrun, Sugar and dental caries: A review of human studies, Science 217:419 (1982)
28.12 Geoffrey Zubay, Biochemistry, Addison-Wesley (1983)
28.14 Geoffrey Zubay, Biochemistry, Addison-Wesley (1983)
28.15 Lehninger, Principles of Biochemistry, Worth Publisher, Inc. (1982)
30.4 Benjamin Lewin, Genes, John Wiley & Sons (1982)
30.5 Benjamin Lewin, Genes, John Wiley & Sons (1982)
30.10 Benjamin Lewin, Genes, John Wiley & Sons (1982)
30.12 Benjamin Lewin, Genes, John Wiley & Sons (1982)

Index

The numbers in **boldface** indicate pages on which the structure of a substance is given. Page numbers in *italics* indicate the location of summary diagrams.